Handbuch der experimentellen Pharmakologie

Handbook of Experimental Pharmacology

Handbuch der experimentellen Pharmakologie

Handbook of Experimental Pharmacology

Heffter-Heubner New Series

Vol. XVI/5

Springer-Verlag Berlin Heidelberg New York 1976

Experimental Production of Diseases

Part 5

LIVER

With Contributions by

J. Harenberg · R. Lesch · I. R. Mackay · H. J. Zimmermann

Edited by

Oskar Eichler

With 60 Figures

Springer-Verlag Berlin Heidelberg New York 1976

Professor Dr. OSKAR EICHLER, Gutleuthofweg 18, D 6900 Heidelberg-Schlierbach

ISBN-13: 978-3-642-45485-1 e-ISBN-13: 978-3-642-45483-7
DOI: 10.1007/978-3-642-45483-7

Library of Congress Cataloging in Publication Data. Main entry under title: Experimental production of diseases. (Handbook of experimental pharmacology: New series; v. 16/). Includes bibliographies and index. CONTENTS: pt. 3. Heart and circulation. – pt. 5. Liver. 1. Pathology, Experimental. I. Betz, Eberhard, 1926– II. Schmier, Johannes, 1922– III. Eichler, Oskar, 1898– IV. Series: Handbuch der experimentellen Pharmakologie: New series; v. 16/3, [etc.] [DNLM: 1. Cardiovascular diseases. 2. Pharmacology. QV34 H236 v. 16 pt. 3]. QP905.H3 vol. 16, pt. 3 615'.1'08s [616.07'07'24] 75-28458

Softcover reprint of the hardcover 1st edition 1976

Table of Contents

Experimental Hepatotoxicity. H.J. ZIMMERMAN. With 13 Figures

Radiation-Induced Injury of the Liver. R. Lesch. With 32 Figures

List of Contributors

J. HARENBERG, Dr. med., Medizinische Universitätsklinik, Bergheimer Straße 58, D-6900 Heidelberg

R. LESCH, Professor Dr., Ludwig-Aschoff-Haus, Pathologisches Institut der Universität Freiburg, Abteilung für Experimentelle Pathologie und Hepato-Gastroenterologie, Albertstraße 19, D-7800 Freiburg

I.R. MACKAY, M.D., F.R.C.P., F.R.A.C.P., F.R.C.P.A., Head of the Clinical Research Unit, The Walter and Eliza Hall Institute of Medical Research, Post Office, Royal Melbourne Hospital, Victoria 3050, Australia

H.J. ZIMMERMAN, M.D., Veterans Administration Hospital, 50 Irving Street, N.W., Washington, DC 20422, USA

Experimental Hepatotoxicity*

HYMAN J. ZIMMERMAN

With 13 Figures

The literature of experimental hepatotoxicity has become so enormous as to overwhelm the effort to summarize the current state of knowledge. Excellent reviews [126, 498, 472, 348, 342, 418, 325, 430, 190, 269, 240, 286, 517, 490, 432] that have been published during the past several decades have assisted the present effort considerably. This review includes a survey of the broad aspects of hepatotoxicity, categorization of types of hepatic injury and discussion of presumed mechanisms followed by a description of the details of the injury produced by a few specific agents. Reference made to hepatocarcinogenicity is restricted to its relationship to hepatotoxicity. The last section contains an analysis of the character of injury according to the source and chemical nature of the individual agents.

A. Introductory Considerations

Chemical hepatic injury includes a number of diverse phenomena. A huge number and variety of compounds have been identified as hepatotoxins of clinical or experimental relevance. Some are found in nature as mycotoxins or other toxic botanical products or as minerals [498, 472, 190, 269, 240, 286, 490, 638]. Others are products of the chemical or pharmaceutical industry, and several (nitrosamines [18], ethionine [140]) may conceivably be produced within the individual animal. They may be as simple as inorganic elements and compounds or as complex as heterocyclic, steroid and peptide [472, 638].

The spectrum of susceptibility to individual agents may extend from substances that injure the livers of almost all individuals in a variety of species to those that produce hepatic damage in uniquely susceptible humans [638]. The hepatic damage may involve mainly the hepatic parenchymal cells, cells of the excretory tree or both [638]. In the case of some hepatotoxic agents, vascular structures are the primary locus of injury [498]. Acute hepatic injury may be translated into chronic liver disease, expressed as cirrhosis or even as carcinoma [472].

A *hepatotoxin* might be defined as any chemical agent that can produce injury to the liver. The term, however, is usually employed to describe agents that are *predictably* toxic to the liver and not those (drugs) that produce hepatic injury unpredictably only in uniquely susceptible humans [472, 269].

* Supported in part by Veterans Administration Research Fund.

Studies of experimental hepatotoxicity necessarily focus on, or begin with, reference to the phenomena of human disease. Accordingly, a glance at the scope of human hepatotoxicity is relevant to the present discussion.

Some natural toxins, like the peptides of *Amanita phalloides* [610, 612], the pyrrolidizine alkaloids [498, 286, 352] and the toxin of the cycad nut [498] are encountered as environmental hazards that are ingested in ignorance of their toxicity or taken as folk medicine [498, 286, 352]. Others, e.g. mycotoxins, are encountered because of climatic conditions in some parts of the world that favor their presence as unsuspected contaminants of food [286].

Hepatotoxic agents that have been employed in industrial operations have proved to be, or are potentially, important sources of liver disease in humans [393, 394]. Most prominent have been the chlorinated hydrocarbons widely used as solvents [394]; although a large number of agents in this category are known. Recently the development of angiosarcoma of the liver, cirrhosis, and of noncirrhotic portal hypertension in workers exposed to vinyl chloride has focused the attention of clinical and experimental hepatotoxicologists on the toxicity of this compound [568].

Hepatotoxins encountered in domestic settings include not only the botanical and mycotoxins cited above, but also various chemical agents to which exposure occurs by inhalation or ingestion, as the result of carelessness or during suicidal attempts, or because of accidental contamination of food by toxic chemicals [280, 497]. Contamination of flour by the hepatotoxic chemical 4′,4-diaminodiphenylmethane recently led to a curious epidemic of jaundice in Epping, England [280]; and contamination of wheat with hexachlorabenzene (employed as a fungistatic) led to a severe outbreak of hepatic porphyria in Turkey several decades ago [497]. A unique form of hepatotoxicity has become a matter of at least theoretical concern in recent years. The demonstration that certain preserved fish may contain nitrosamines [483, 309], and that nitrosamines may be formed by intestinal bacteria in experimental animals which ingest food preserved with nitrites [18], has led to the concern with this possible mode of human exposure to the hepatotoxicity and hepatocarcinogenicity of dimethylnitrosamine [631]. (See Section on Dialkylnitrosamines.)

B. Historical Aspects

Hepatotoxicity has been the subject of experimental study for over 100 years. In 1866, NOTHNAGEL [389] first produced hepatic injury in dogs by the administration of chloroform, 18 years after the first deaths in patients anesthetized with that agent [81], and over two decades before a report (1889) [565] that showed "delayed" chloroform poisoning to include severe, acute liver disease. Studies by ROSENBAUM in 1882 [469] on the effects of inorganic phosphorous and arsenic on hepatic glycogen, and by ZIEGLER and OBOLONSKY in 1888 [637] on experimental arsenic poisoning, mark the only other contributions to experimental hepatotoxicity prior to the present century; although hepatic injury had been recognized in a fatal case of phosphorous poisoning as early as 1860 [198].

By the turn of the century, experimental hepatotoxicity began to be employed as a tool to study problems encountered in human or veterinary medicine. Between

1900 and 1910 systematic studies, conducted in Canada [406] and Australia [170], confirmed the etiologic role of plants of the Senecio and Heliotropum family in liver disease of grazing cattle and sheep [352]. At about the same time a series of thoughtful studies [581, 396, 547, 218, 604, 605, 606, 395] on the toxicity of $CHCl_3$ for experimental animals and on the role of dietary [395] and other modifying factors [218, 604, 605, 606] were undertaken. Some of these [218, 604, 605, 606, 395] reports are now among the classics of experimental hepatotoxicity. Interest in the experimental toxicity of the related compound, CCl_4 came only during the third decade of this century when the use of the agent as a vermifuge led to unexpected liver disease and death in humans [527, 360]. During the intervening half-century, CCl_4 has been subjected to an enormous number of studies [126, 472, 348, 430, 190, 269, 240, 432] as a model for the study of hepatic disease and as an experimental cause of necrosis.

By the end of the first quarter of the 20th century, a number of hepatotoxic agents had become clearly identified as the result of experience with disease in humans and domestic animals and of experimental observations [126, 638]. Experimental hepatotoxicity was at first descriptive in its thrust, defining the forms of injury that some chemical agents induce, demonstrating differential susceptibility of various species and attempting to define age, sex and dietary factors that modify susceptibility. The descriptive phase continued until the mid-forties. The fifth and sixth decades of this century, comprised an era of pathophysiologic approach to experimental toxicity. During the mid-fifties studies began to be directed at the subcellular and molecular basis for chemical hepatic unjury [430]. The unravelling of the enzyme mechanisms for the metabolism of foreign compounds and of the phenomenon of enhancement ("induction") of this mechanism during this period has clarified the mechanisms of hepatotoxicity [430, 432, 347, 146]. In turn experimental hepatotoxic states have been of value in the study of the enzymatic machinery of the endoplasmic reticulum [146].

Most attention by clinicans to chemical hepatic injury during the past 50 years has focused on the type induced by medicinal agents. From the midpoint of the 19th century until the fourth decade of this century, the recognized hepatotoxins included chloroform, carbon tetrachloride, inorganic phosphorous and arsenical compounds encountered accidentally or occupationally [126, 638] and some botanical hepatotoxins of interest to animal husbandry [352]. Iatrogenic hepatic injury was restricted to instances of hepatic necrosis after chloroform anesthesia or after ingestion of CCl_4 employed as a vermifuge, or of hepatic necrosis or cirrhosis induced by inorganic arsenicals [638]. Such agents were, accordingly, removed from clinical use. In 1923, the first report [633] of an instance of hepatic injury induced by a drug (cinchophen) apparently innocuous for most exposed individuals, appeared. By the mid-thirties several hundred cases had been reported [398]; and the development of hepatic disease as the result of unique susceptibility to a drug was recognized [638]. During the intervening half-century many others drugs have been incriminated in the production of liver damage [418, 269, 639]. Relatively few of these have been found to be toxic for experimental animals and the mechanism of injury has been the subject of inference, speculation and hypothesis [638]. Nevertheless, some drugs that are not ordinarily considered hepatotoxic for experimental animals can be shown to produce injury in experimental settings [638, 368].

C. Relevance of Experimental Hepatotoxicity

The huge volume of literature on experimental hepatotoxicity includes many facets relevant to clinical medicine. The studies conducted have been useful in the understanding of the character and mechanism of production of hepatotoxic states in humans (e.g. acute hepatic injury induced by carbon tetrachloride, inorganic phosphorous or Amanita phalloides). Studies of experimental hepatotoxicity also provide increased understanding of chronic disease that might be due to hepatotoxins (e.g. cirrhosis [195, 399] or carcinoma of the liver [410, 226]). Experimental hepatotoxic states also have provided useful models for the study of the genesis of tissue injury in general [74] and the histogenesis, biochemical features and manifestations of spontaneous hepatic disease (e.g. viral hepatitis) [252] in particular. Hepatic necrosis induced by chemical agents has been a useful model for the study of biochemical pathology of the death of cells [348, 74, 328]. Experimental hepatic injury is a fundamental tool for the development of diagnostic methods; and it has become traditional for tests of liver function and serum enzyme tests to be evaluated in animals with experimental hepatic injury before assessing their usefulness in clinical settings [587, 52].

Experimental hepatic injury has been extensively employed to study hepatic physiology and pathophysiology [428] applying the oft-cited [551, 141] principle enunciated by CLAUDE BERNARD [40] that poisons are useful tools for the study of physiological processes. The unravelling of the role of the hepatocyte in the synthesis of proteins [472] and plasma coagulation factors [49], in protein [143], carbohydrate [472, 592] and lipid [145, 539] metabolism; in storage of vitamins [243]; in the metabolism of hormones [537]; in electrolyte and water balance [363]; in bile formation [242, 523], and in the transport and metabolism of drugs [414, 24], has been greatly enhanced by the study of staged hepatic injury utilizing known hepatoxins. The relationship of hepatic physiology to homeostatic mechanisms also has been clarified by the employment of experimental hepatotoxic models. For example, the ability to produce experimental hypertension has been shown to be blunted by producing experimental CCl_4 poisoning [314], and pressor responses to be modified by ethionine administration [588]. Employment of a number of hepatotoxins has helped unravel the role of DNA and RNA in cell economy [142]; and studies with CCl_4 and galactosamine [570] have helped clarify the role of the liver in the immune response to antigens absorbed from the gastrointestinal tract.

Studies of the role of the organelles in cell life and death also have employed models of experimental toxicity. Lesions of smooth or rough endoplasmic reticulum [472, 531, 555], changes in chromatin, nucleus and nucleolus [142, 544], lysozomes [256, 25] and mitochondria [472] induced by various toxic agents, have assisted in identification of the role of these organelles in hepatic pathology. Studies of the mechanism by which hepatic steatosis is induced by hepatotoxins has helped to clarify the pathogenesis of fatty metamorphosis of other etiology [430] and the role of Golgi apparatus in the assembly of the lipid–protein complex for the movement of lipid from the liver [539, 514].

Considerable light has been shed on hepatic histopathology by experimental hepatotoxicity studies. Almost all of the lesions that can be seen in the liver

Table 1. Morphologic types of toxic hepatic injury

Type of injury	Example
Acute	
A. Cytotoxic	
1. Necrosis[a]	
a) Zonal—1. Central	CCl_4, Acetominophen, Thioacetamide
2. Mid	Ngaione
3. Peripheral	Allyl formate, Albitocin
b) Massive	Tetrachlorethane
c) Diffuse	Galactosamine
d) Focal	(also see Table 7)
2. Steatosis	
a) Microvesicular	Ethionine, Tetracycline, Phosphorous
b) Macrovesicular	Ethanol (also see Table 8)
3. Necrosis plus steatosis	CCl_4, DMN
B. Cholestatic	
1. Without overt bile duct injury	Icterogenin Anabolic steroids C-17 alkylated
2. With overt bile duct injury	ANIT (also see Table 10)
C. Vascular (hepatic veins and branches)	Pyrrolidizine alkaloids
Chronic	
A. Cirrhosis	
1. Macronodular	CCl_4
2. Micronodular	CCl_4; AFB, TAA
3. Congestive ("cardiac" type)	Pyrrolidizine alkaloids
4. Biliary	ANIT, AFB_1 (monkey)
B. Neoplasm	
1. Carcinoma	
a) Hepatocellular	AFB, TAA, CCl_4, PAs
b) Cholangiocellular	Rare TAA
2. Adenoma	Acetamide
3. Sarcoma	DMN (mice)
4. Angiosarcoma	Vinyl chloride Inorganic arsenic

[a] Degenerative changes including acidophilic bodies, hyalinization, ballooning, precede necrosis.

as the result of spontaneous disease can be induced by hepatotoxic agents (Table 1). Necrosis, zonal, massive or diffuse [472, 418, 269, 517, 639]; steatosis [472, 418, 269, 517, 639]; hepatic venule lesions [498]; cirrhosis of several morphologic types [195, 70]; hepatocellular and cholangiocellular carcinoma [410, 226] and angiosarcoma [568]; cholestasis with and without evidence of hepatocyte injury or bile duct lesions [472, 342, 418, 190, 269, 517]; all can be induced by various hepatotoxic agents. Specific lesions such as sinusoidal ("free") acidophilic bodies [418, 269, 639], nucleolar and nuclear abnormalities [226, 142] and megalocytes [498] can be produced by various toxic insults to the liver. The ability to produce examples of types of hepatic injury permits experimental hepatotoxic states to be elegant tools for the study or teaching of hepatic histopathology.

The ability of the liver to regenerate after resection or injury has long a puzzling, interesting and important phenomenon. While most studies have focused on the regenerative response to surgical resection of a portion of the liver, some probing questions regarding regeneration have employed toxic injury [70, 420, 475, 298]. For example, the adequacy and briskness of regenerative activity were found to be inversely related to age in response to hepatic injury induced by CCl_4 [420].

Studies regarding the pathogenesis of cirrhosis have employed hepatotoxicity as the model [70, 419, 420, 475, 298, 339, 340, 211, 213, 466]. The observation that fibrosis after hepatic injury may be "passive" i.e. collapse after necrosis, or "active" i.e. involving synthesis and breakdown of collagen is derived from studies with CCl_4 [475, 298, 339, 340, 211, 213, 466]. Potential reversibility of cirrhosis and the use of pharmacologic agents to prevent or reverse fibrosis also have been explored in chronic CCl_4 toxic states [211, 466].

D. Vulnerability of the Liver to Toxic Injury

The great susceptibility of the liver to damage by chemical agents appears to be a consequence of its primary role in the metabolism of foreign substances [126, 430]. The concentration of foreign chemicals in the liver [615], the metabolic conversions that occur in the hepatocyte [325, 432, 368, 169] and perhaps the position of the liver as a portal to the tissues for ingested agents [28], all may be presumed [638] to contribute to the vulnerability of the liver to chemical injury.

I. Concentration of Agents in Liver

Foreign compounds are concentrated in the liver, perhaps related to unique binding proteins of the hepatocytes [615, 345] and to attachment to sites wherein metabolic conversions occur [345]. Nevertheless, the observation that some potent hepatotoxins (e.g. CCl_4) [394] can reach even higher concentration in organs that sustain relatively little injury [28], indicates that uniquely high concentration of foreign substances in the liver is not necessarily the decisive factor in the unique vulnerability of the liver to toxic injury.

II. Liver as Portal to Tissues

The position of the liver as a portal to the tissues may contribute to the toxicity of ingested agents [638, 615, 28]. Furthermore, a relatively sustained or repeated exposure of the liver to toxic agents may be the result of, or enhanced by, the enterohepatic circulation of some toxins [615]. Nevertheless, most agents that are toxic by the oral route or by intraportal administration are also hepatotoxic by a parenteral route. For agents (e.g. cycasin), which are inocuous until converted by intestinal or bacterial enzymes to a toxic product [28] or for dialkylnitrosamines that might be synthesized by intestinal bacteria [631], the portal site of the liver is particularly relevant to hepatic vulnerability to injury.

III. Metabolism of Foreign Compounds

Perhaps the most important factor in the special hepatic vulnerability to toxins is the role of the liver in the metabolism of foreign compounds [325, 432, 368, 169, 402]. The strategic location which permits a defense role against ingested toxins is presumed to explain the evolution of the hepatic enzyme systems involved in the metabolism of foreign compounds [402]. PARKE and WILLIAMS [402] have emphasized that the enzymes which metabolize foreign compounds are strategically located at sites of entry or exit of substances from the body and have suggested that those in the liver may have developed as a defense mechanism against the naturally occurring toxic agents taken in the diet. Often referred to as the "detoxifying" function of the liver, the main effect of the metabolism of foreign compounds is the biotransformation of the lipid-soluble foreign compounds to more polar metabolites which can be excreted in the bile or urine [402]. The process includes two phases [402]. The first ("Phase I") introduces an atom of oxygen into the foreign compounds, which leads to hydroxylation, dealkylation, oxidative deamination or oxidation. The second ("Phase II") consists of conjugation of the initial compound or of a metabolic product with glucuronate, sulfate, glycine or other groups [402]. Phase II is usually a detoxifying process permitting excretion of potentially harmful substances. Phase I, performed by mixed function oxidases of the ER, however, may increase or decrease the toxicity of a foreign compound [432, 368, 169, 402]. Native molecules which are far less toxic than their metabolites include CCl_4 [240, 432, 345), dimethylnitrosamine [402, 349], carcinogenic azo dyes [366, 367], allyl compounds [441] and other substances listed in Table 2. The hepatotoxicity of these compounds is enhanced by conditions that increase their metabolism and decreased by manipulations that inhibit conversion to metabolic products. Conversely, the product(s) of metabolism of a compound may be less hepatotoxic than the native molecule, as may be deduced when the toxicity is decreased by enhancement of drug metabolism [355, 240]. In some instances the relationship between the metabolism of a foreign compound and its hepatotoxicity may be more complicated [240]. One metabolite may be more toxic than the original compound; yet another metabolite, subsequent to the first or derived by another pathway, may be less toxic [240]. In such instances, unravelling of the relationships may be difficult (see Sections on Aflatoxins and Pyrrolidizine Alkaloids).

Table 2. Relation of metabolism to toxicity for a few agents[a]

Metabolite of agent proximate toxin[b]	Agent proximate toxin
CCl_4 *et al.* haloalkanes	Phosphorous
Carcinogenic azo dyes	Ethionine
Allyl compounds	GALN
Phalloidin	α-Amanitin
Brombenzene	
Acetominophen	
Ngaione	
ANIT	
TAA[b]	
PAs[b]	
AF[b]	
DMN[b]	

[a] This information is available and reasonably clear for only a few agents.

[b] Relationship of metabolism to toxicity is not as clear for these as for the other members of group (see text).

IV. Enzyme Induction

Relevant to the understanding of some of the phenomena of hepatotoxicity [240, 432, 347, 639, 368, 169, 28, 345, 402, 349, 557, 366, 367, 441, 355] is the modification of the ability of the liver to metabolize foreign chemicals, that results from exposure to a variety of compounds [99]. Administration of phenobarbital, and a wide variety of other chemical agents enhances the ability of the liver to metabolize a large number of compounds [99]. The enhancement is accompanied by an increase in the amount of smooth endoplasmic reticulum (SER) and in its content of drug-metabolizing enzymatic machinery. This phenomenon is referred to as "induction" of the relevant enzyme system [99]. The ability to enhance the metabolism of foreign compounds by the administration of "inducing drugs" [99] and to inhibit the enzymatic machinery by compounds [402, 83] such as piperonyl butoxide or SKF 525a or by protein deprivation, has provided a powerful tool for the study of mechanisms of toxicity of a number of compounds [83].

Hepatotoxins which are less toxic than their metabolites have their toxic effect enhanced by pretreatment of the animal with an enzyme-inducing drug, and decreased by pretreatment which inhibits drug-metabolizing enzymes [240]. Substances that are more toxic than their metabolites would have their toxic effects inhibited by enzyme induction and enhanced by treatment that depresses drug-metabolizing activity [240].

Animals of a species well supplied with the enzyme system responsible for the metabolism of CCl_4 (and other foreign agents) are susceptible to the adverse effects of this hepatotoxin [432, 345]. In the liver of the newborn rat which is resistant to CCl_4 toxicity [432, 70, 345] there is practically none of this metabolizing system [432, 345]. The adult animal on a standard diet, which has a liver well supplied with the hydroxylating system and its marker, cytochrome P-450 [432, 345], is susceptible [432, 70, 345]. This susceptibility can be enhanced by exposure to phenobarbital or DDT which "induce" the metabolizing system [432, 345]. The susceptibility can be decreased by the feeding of a low protein diet which decreases hydroxylating enzyme mechanisms [345, 347]. Inhibition of this system by specific agents [83] leads to a reduced ability to metabolize foreign compounds and to a decrease in toxicity of CCl_4. These observations indicate the metabolite to be the mediator of toxicity [432]. Conversely, where an enhancement of the metabolizing ability decreases the toxicity of a hepatotoxin, it may be inferred that the native compound (or some other metabolite) is more toxic than the metabolite, the production of which is enhanced.

Conversion of compounds to toxic metabolites also can occur by enzyme activity other than the P-450 system. Thioacetamide is toxic to the adult but not the neonatal rat liver and, appears to exert its toxic effect by activation to a necrogenic compound, perhaps the "S-oxide", yet the toxicity of thioacetamide is not enhanced by pretreatment with phenobarbital or inhibited by SK 525a. These and other studies have led CASTRO *et al.* to conclude that activation of thioacetamide to its toxic metabolite does not involve the P-450 dependent mixed function oxidase [83].

These and other factors which affect the metabolism of foreign compounds are discussed elsewhere in this volume. The relative ability to perform the task can be evaluated *in vivo* by measuring the physiological effect of a drug (e.g. hexobarbital sleeping time) or *in vitro* by measuring drug-metabolizing activity or amount of cytochrome P-450 of liver slices, homogenates or microsomes [221]. It is also reflected in the amount of SER seen under the electron microscope; [292] although in some instances dissociation between increase in the amount of SER and the drug-metabolizing ability of the liver is noted [221]. Genetic factors [291] (species, strains) [64, 614, 334]; age and sex [334]; and other endocrine factors [191]; diet [334]; stress [334]; diurnal variation [86]; and, as cited above, the exposure to a variety of chemical agents, modify the ability of metabolize foreign compounds.

V. Factors That Modify Susceptibility

1. Species

For many hepatotoxins differences in susceptibility of various species have not been systematically explored. For others, CCl_4, [432, 70], aflatoxins [175], pyrrolidizine alkaloids [352, 60] dialkylnitrosamines [80] galactosamine [113] and ethionine [140], there is a considerable amount of information (Table 3). Rats

Table 3. Susceptibility and resistance of various species to several hepatotoxins[a]

	CCl_4	DMN	Ethionine	PAs[b]	AF[b]	Amanitin	Orotic Acid	GALN[b]
Rats	S	S	S	S	VS	R	S	S
Mice	S	S	S	S	R	S	R	R
GP	S	S	S	R	VS	S	R	S
Rabbits	S	S	S	S	S	S	R	S
Hamsters	S	S	S	S	S	S	R	S
Dogs	S	S	S	S	S	S	R	?
Cats	S	S	S	S	S	S	?	?
Chickens	R	S	S	S	R	S	R	?
Fish	R	S	?	?	VS	R	?	S
Cattle	S	S	?	S	S	?	?	?
Pigs	S	S	?	S	S*	?	?	?
Goats	S	S	?	S	?	S	?	?
Sheep	S	S	?	R	R	S	?	?
Monkeys	S		S	S	S	?	R	S
Humans	S	S	S	S	S(?)	S	R	?

[a] Supporting references given in the sections devoted to the respective agents.
[b] See Appendix for Meaning of Abbreviations.
S = Sensitive; R = Resistant; ? = no or insufficient data available.

for example, are susceptible to a variety of toxic agents, particularly evident in the extensive studies with carbon tetrachloride, thiocetamide, and ethionine [472, 348, 240, 432, 140]. Mammals in general are all somewhat susceptible to CCl_4. Chickens, ducks, frogs, pigeons and terrapins, however, are resistant [70]. There are important differences between different species in the susceptibility to aflatoxins [175].

Several theoretical or demonstrated factors (Table 6) that may determine the differential susceptibility of different species to the adverse effect of hepatotoxins have been suggested by MCLEAN [345]. The affinity of toxic chemicals for sites on cells of the target organ required to express the toxic effects or to undergo an activation step might be important. Differences between species and between individuals of the same species, in the amino acid sequence of the binding protein would allow a toxin to attack only species or individuals that carry the proper binding site. MCLEAN [345] has suggested that organ specificity of toxic injury might be, in part, linked to the organ specificity of proteins which develop during differentiation. Accordingly, toxins that selectively affect the liver might be expected to be selectively bound by hepatospecific proteins [345] of which ligandin [186] is a possible example. Needless to say, the variability of response to hepatotoxins is importantly related to the metabolism of foreign compounds by the liver. For hepatotoxins that express their adverse effect by means of a metabolite of the native molecule (Table 2), the degree to which the compound can be metabolized to the toxic product by a species would determine the vulnerability of members of that species to the toxicity of the substance. Thus, the resistance of chickens to hepatotoxic effects of CCl_4 is attributed to their inability to metabolize this compound [432]. Unfortunately, there is still no systematic body of knowledge on the relationship between metabolizing ability and the susceptibility of various species to hepatotoxins.

2. Age

The effect of age on the susceptibility to hepatotoxic agents appears to depend, in part at least, on the relevance of metabolism of the respective agent to its toxicity. The neonatal rat is far less susceptible to CCl_4 toxicity than is the adult animal [432]. This difference appears to reflect the fact that CCl_4 is less hepatotoxic than its metabolic product, and it disappears as the P-450 metabolizing system for foreign compounds matures [432]. However, aflatoxin B_1 [68] and Senecio alkaloids [472] are examples of hepatotoxins to which the neonatal rat is more susceptible than the adult. Yet, evidence suggests that these compounds also must be metabolized to exert their toxic effects [352, 403].

The resistance to galactosamine (GALN) toxicity of the newborn rat appears to reflect a higher rate of uridylate biosynthesis and so the ability to cope with the uridylate trapping presumed to account for the toxic effects of GALN [113]. Comprehension of these phenomena and of differences in susceptibility of the newborn to other hepatotoxins awaits systematic studies of the development of pathways of drug metabolism in relation to vulnerability to hepatic injury.

Analysis of the effect of age on susceptibility of animals that have reached maturity is also difficult [437, 357, 446, 478]. Weanling rats have been reported to be more [437] and less [357] susceptible than adults to CCl_4-induced cirrhosis; several studies suggest, that "old" animals are somewhat more susceptible than younger, but mature, ones to development of injury [357, 446, 478]. Regenerative response of aging rats to CCl_4-induced hepatic injury also is less vigorous than that of younger ones [420, 357, 446, 478].

3. Sex and Other Endocrine Factors

Differences between male and females in susceptibility to a number of toxic agents have been described [472, 348, 190]. Males in some [472] but not all [348] studies have appeared to be more susceptible to the hepatotoxic effects of CCl_4. Indeed, the described [472] greater susceptibility of males to CCl_4, pyrrolidizine alkaloids, thioacetamide and tannic acid, and of females to trichlorethylene and ethanol seems to be, at most, modestly quantitative, and to a varying degree unconvincing [348]. To ethionine [140], however, and apparently to Amanita phalloides [573] toxicity, females are more susceptible.

The information bearing on other endocrine factors in hepatotoxicity has been well review [472, 194]. It is, fragmentary [348] however, and does not permit useful generalization. Thyroid hormone appears to enhance hepatotoxicity of CCl_4 and other agents [472, 636] and to convert the necrosis induced by CCl_4 from a centrizonal to a midzonal lesion [472]. Hypothyroidion seems to protect somewhat against various hepatotoxic insults [472]. Pituitary, hypothalamic, adrenal and gonadal effects apparently include the role of fat accumulation induced by some hormonal perturbations [472], altered hepatic blood flow and/or body temperature [296] induced by neuroendocrine manipulations, "protective" effects of glucocorticoids activity [303], and other complex and insufficiently delineated factors.

4. Nutritional State

The effect of dietary status on susceptibility to toxic hepatic injury has been the subject of confusion and remains somewhat controversial [347]. For many years it had been widely accepted that malnutrition in general and protein deficiency in particular, enhance the adverse effects of all hepatotoxic agents [347]. McLean and his associates [347, 349, 557], however, have drawn attention to the inhibitory effects of protein deprivation on the hepatotoxic effects of some agents (CCl_4, DMN), enhancement of the hepatotoxic effects of other agents (AFB_1) [240], and lack of significant effect or a qualitative alteration of the effects of others. Among the factors that have led to confusion has been the failure to separate the direct effects of protein-deprivation on drug-metabolizing systems (i.e. inhibition) from the indirect effect, i.e., the nutritional fatty metamorphosis which can enhance the toxic effects of lipid-soluble substances by increasing hepatic storage of them [472, 347].

The important, indirect effect of low dietary protein on drug metabolizing systems consists of decrease in the amount of cytochrome P-450 and in the activity of the hydroxylating system of the SER [347]. Accordingly, agents that are less toxic than their metabolic products would have their hepatotoxicity decreased by a low protein diet (i.e. CCl_4). Confusingly, the acute toxicity of AFB_1 for rats also is decreased, but the chronic hepatic toxicity and the hepatocarcinogenicity are enhanced by a protein-deficient diet [464]. The earlier presumption [240] that AFB_1 is a more potent acute hepatotoxin than its metabolite awaits clarification. An explanation of the lack of the effect of diet and enzyme induction on the toxicity of retrorsine (pyrrolidizine alkaloid) has been offered [240]; namely, a combination of lesser and greater hepatotoxic products. Judah *et al.* [240] have proposed that the initial metabolite might be more, and a secondary or other one, less, hepatotoxic than the native molecule. Such a possibility seems supported by the demonstration of CHESNEY and ALLEN [87] that resistance of the guinea pig to a pyrrolidizine alkaloid relates to its conversion of the agent to a non-toxic metabolite.

Qualitative changes in toxic effects of a foreign agent may result from the metabolic effects of diet. For example, there is a reduction in the hepatotoxicity and hepatocarcinogenicity of DMN induced by a diet deficient in proteins [349]. Accompanying this decrease in hepatic injury, however, is an increased incidence of renal carcinoma presumably reflecting a longer period of circulation of intact toxin [347]. This illustrates the role of the drug-metabolizing function of the liver in protecting extrahepatic tissue from the effects of foreign chemicals at the expense of hepatic injury induced by the metabolite; and, in turn, the possible adverse effect on a peripheral organ of inhibition of conversion of the foreign compound to a metabolite.

The fatty liver that results from protein- and choline-deficient diets can contribute to hepatotoxicity or confuse the analysis of dietary modification of vulnerability to liver—damaging effects of chemical agents [472]. The hypothetical role of increased liver fat in permitting greater affinity for a more prolonged storage of lipid-soluble toxins has long been invoked [502] to explain the enhancement of susceptibility to CCl_4 by ethanol and alcoholism. Evidence is strong, however, that the enhancement of CCl_4 toxicity by ethanol and other alcohols includes other mechanisms [308, 267, 102, 572, 599] (see Section on CCl_4 poisoning).

Fasting must be distinguished from prolonged, specifically (i.e. protein) deficient diets [347]. Fasting enhances the toxicity of CCl_4 and $CHCl_3$. It also leads to glycogen depletion. This observation, coupled with the moderately protective effect of a high carbohydrate diet against $CHCl_3$ poisoning [395, 347], suggests that glycogen depletion has an adverse influence on hepatotoxicity [347]. The mechanism, however, is unknown.

E. Types of Experimental Models

I. Whole Animals

The studies performed during the past 100 years have employed a variety of species. Most popular have been rats because of their size and relatively low cost. Furthermore, comparison of results obtained in widely separated laboratories is facilitated by the general employment of a relatively uniform experimental model. Other, less widely employed species include mice, hamsters, guinea pigs, rabbits and dogs. Relatively few studies have involved cats, cattle, swine, horses, sheep and several species of birds. During recent years, primates have come into use, for the obvious reason of the reater presumed relevance to disease of humans. Several species of fowl have been employed in the study of mycotoxins; in theses studies the day-old duckling has been particularly useful.

The employment of various animal models has permitted exploration of the effect of species, on susceptibility as in the early studies of CAMERON and KARUNARATNE [70] and the recent ones of Recknagel and his associates [430, 432] of

CCl_4 poisoning. The greatest amount of information bearing on other modifiers of susceptibility to hepatotoxins such as age, sex, stage of development, diet and exposure to other toxic substances applies to the rat [472].

Utilization of the whole animal has involved various parameters of hepatic injury. These have included lethality, histologic study by light and electron microscopy, chemical study of changes in the liver and physiologic and biochemical tests that measure the functional status or that reflect the type or intensity of hepatic injury.

1. Parameters of Injury

Death of the animal has served as a measure of hepatotoxic potency, applicable mainly to known hepatotoxins. Employment of the LD_{50} or an equivalent measure of lethal potency has permitted comparison of various hepaotoxic agents. It is, however, a gross parameter, subject to the pitfall that adverse effects other than hepatic injury may contribute to death, and so obscure the effort to define the hepatotoxic potency [126]

2. Histology

Light Microscopy (LM). Studies with LM have been the traditional means for the demonstration of toxic hqatic injury and for categorization of the type of injury. It also has provided the yardstick against which other abnormalities are measured. The ultimate significance of biochemical abnormalities, inferred to reflect hepatic injury, has had to be judged by the supporting evidence of demonstrable steatosis or necrosis provided by LM. Efforts to quantitate the degree of injury are better served by chemical measurement of liver or blood and efforts to define mechanisms have involved electron microscopic and biochemical studies. The demonstration of characteristic hepatic lesions by LM, however, continues to be an important end-point in the study of toxicity of unknown agents or of the modifying effects of physiologic manipulations or drugs on the hepatic injury induced by known hepatotoxins. The first steps in the unravelling of aflatoxin toxicity [175, 529], the demonstrations of the effects of enzyme induction and inhibition on CCl_4 toxicity [161, 343], and the basic observations of galactosamine hepatotoxicity [252, 113] are examples of the continued dependence of experimental hepatotoxicity on traditional histology with LM.

Electron Microscopy (EM). Ultrastructural studies have provided an extremely important tool for experimental hepatotoxicology [472, 190, 240, 490, 146, 226, 539, 142, 514]. They provide a much earlier demonstration of hepatocyte injury, permit the recognition of damage too subtle to be appreciated by LM [472, 531, 181] and provide clues to the mechanisms of injury [142]. Hepatocyte abnormalities are apparent by EM in minutes and by LM in hours after CCl_4 administration [472]. The demonstration that changes in the RER are at least as early as any demonstrable functional deficit after CCl_4 administration [432] and that characteristic changes occur in the Golgi apparatus [539, 420] and in the nucleoli [226, 142, 555, 514] have shed light on the mechanisms of toxicity of various agents. While EM does not permit useful quantitation of injury, it has been a very helpful tool for the evaluation of factors and manipulations that modify hepatotoxic effects.

3. Chemical Changes in Hepatic Tissue

Analysis of changes in the chevcal composition of the liver has served to quantitate hepatic injury and has shed useful light on mechanisms of injury. Measurement of the amount of fat in the liver serves to quantitate the intensity of adverse effect of agents that produce hepatic steatosis [181], to compare the toxicity of different agents [121] and to evaluate potentiating and protective manipulations [84]. For agents that produce fatty metamorphosis with little or no necrosis (ethionine, phosphorous, tetracycline) and which are insensitively reflected by serum enzyme measurement [640], microscopic demonstration of fat or chemical measurement of amount of fat remain reliable and useful techniques for demonstration of injury.

Chemical demonstration of diene producpon [432] and of qualitative changes in fatty acids [432], polysomes [142], and nucleic acids [142] of the hepatocytes has provided important information on possible mechanisms of injury. Diene formation has been cited as evidence by proponents of the view that lipid peroxidation is the mechanisms for hepatic injury induced by CCl_4 and other agent432]. More difficult to measure is malonic dialdehyde content of liver, also a measure of lipid peroxidation [432]. The decrease in proportion of unsaturated, and increase in proportion of saturated fatty acids, and the production of abnormal fatty acids, in CCl_4 toxicity are considered keys to understanding the mechanism of injury [432]. The disaggregation of polysomes, demonstrable by physical biochemical techniques, is considered [141, 143] an important factor in the pathogenesis of chemical hepatic injury. The changes induced in purine and pyrimidine components of DNA and RNA by the alkylating nitrosamines are presumed to be relevant to the hepatocarcinogenicity and hepatotoxicity of these agents [348, 325, 142].

Demonstration of covalent binding, to glutathione and to tissue proteins, of metabolic products of hepatotoxic agents appears to be relevant to the production of hepatic injury [368, 169]. This phenomenon has been shown to play an important role in the hepatotoxicity of brombenzene [169, 56], acetaminophen [368] and several other agents [368]. It has been interpreted [368, 169] as representing a protective role of the glutathione against chemical injury with the inference that tissue injury occurs when the binding capacity of the available glutathione is exceeded.

Changes in enzyme and coenzyme content of the liver have been of interest, but the information relevant to hepatotoxic phenomena is somewhat controversial and confusing. The hepatic content of a large number of enzymes has been reported to be decreased after a dose of CCl_4 [208, 534, 329]. Of the tissue enzymes, however, only the tryptotophane pyrrolase [329] has received serious consideration as a useful quantitative measure of hepatic injury and glucose-6-phosphatase as a measure of microsomal injury [432].

Measurement of cytochrome P-450 has served to identify the site of injury of some toxins [432] and as a quantitative measure of the degree of injury [32, 450]. While quantitation of cytochrome P-450 levels and study of changes in this molecule have become one of the widely employed measures of hepatotoxicity [450], the precise correlation between this measure and hepatic injury remains to be proved. Assay of levels of cytochrome B_5 has been employed infrequently, and for the purpose of demonstrating qualitative differences between the effects of various forms of hepatic injury [79].

4. Physiological and Biochemical Measure of Hepatic Function and Injury

The ability of the liver to metabolize drugs [138], excrete foreign ions [299], synthesize urea [306], cholesterol and its esters [371], and plasma proteins including clotting factors [554], and to maintain normal blood sugar levels [404], provides time-honored reflections of hepatic injury in experimental animals [182]. Demonstration of abnormality of various of these functional responsibilities has served to document the hepatic injury inkced by foreign agents. Most of these measures, however, have been too insensitive, non-specific or cumbersome to be useful in measuring the degree of injury, comparing the relative toxicity of different agents, or assessing the potentiating or protective effect of various treatments on the toxicity of an agent.

Drug Metabolism. Measurement of the role of the liver in drug metabolism has been applied by a number of workers to the study of hepatic injury [138, 182]. The effects of toxic agents on the hexobarbital sleeping time or on zoxazolamine-induced paralysis or lethality have become standard tests of hepatic injury and show a reasonable correlation with other quantitative measures of hepatic function [182]. Specifically, hepatic injury leads to an enhanced effect of the respective drug, a phenomenon which, when appropriately standardized, permits some assessment of degree of hepatic injury [182].

Amino Acid Levels. Measurement of blood and urine levels of amino acids serves as a reflection of parenchymal injury [105] but has provided more of a qualitative confirmation of damage to hepatocytes than a ueful quantitative measure of degree of injury [165]. The aminoacidemia and aminoaciduria, evidence of severe injury, appear to reflect necrosis of cells with consequent release into the blood as well as deficient utilization of amino acids owing to impairment of the protein-synthesizing ability of the liver.

Excretion of Dyes. Measurement of the ability of the liver to excrete foreign dyes has served for a half-century as a measure of hepatic injury [166]. For many years sulfobromophthalein (BSP) [166], and more recently indocyanine green (ICG) [167] have been useful measures of hepatic damage. Until recent years, however, the ability of the liver to excrete foreign dyes was employed much more extensively to demonstrate hepatic disease in humans than experimental hepatic damage in animals. Recent studies have led to the development of techniques applicable to the measurementof dye clearance in experimental animals, even small ones; and have demonstrated differences between various experimental species that must be taken into account in using dye excretion as a parameter of experimental hepatotoxicity [411]. Plaa [411] has demonstrated that the optimal dose for measuring BSP clearance differs with different species and has suggested doses for the dog, rat and rabbit, of 15, 50 and 75 mg/kg, respectively. Other aspects of employment of BSP excretory ability as a measure of experimental hepatotoxicity have been analyzed by Plaa [411].

Impaired excretion of BSP has been shown to reflect sensitively several forms of parenchymal injury. Available technique permits measurement of uptake from the blood, or storage in the hepatocyte, of conjugation and of excretion into bile as affected by the administration of hepatotoxins [411, 169]. The degree of impairment of BSP excretion has been found to compare favorably with the degree of impaired drug metabolism, with enzymologic measures of hepatic injury, and with histologic evidence of hepatic damage as an index of damage [411, 268]. Nevertheless, relatively limited use has been make of BSP excretion as a test for the assessment of hepatotoxicity in experimental animals.

Indocyanine green has found even less application in experimental hepatotoxicology [48]. Since it can be excreted by the liver without conjugation, while BSP must be conjugated for adequate excretion, employment of both dyes in parallel experiments can serve to distinguish impaired conjugation from impaired uptake or secretion into the bile [589].

Bilirubin Levels. The elevation of bilirubin levels of the serum that accompanies sufficiently severe parenchymal injury provides an insensitive measure of chemical hepatic injury [411]. Bilirubin clearance studies, in which the ability to clear from the blood an administered bilirubin load is measured, have found special and limited usefulness in the study of agents that lead to cholestatic phenomena [202].

Blood Levels of Substances of Hepatic Origin. Release into the blood of substances normally found in the lver provides a useful group of biochemical measures of hepatic injury. Increased blood levels of free and transferrin-bound iron [442], of vitamin B_{12} [243, 540] and of a group of proteins released by the damaged liver ("liver antigens") [137, 128] have been demonstrated after acute toxic doses of CCl_4. While these are interesting manifestations of liver injury, none has found useful application in experimental hepatotoxicology. Of the proteins released by the damaged liver, the most useful as tools in the study of hepatotoxicity are the enzymes.

Serum Enzymology has become the standard approach to the measurement of hepatic injury during the past 20 years [640, 411, 206, 372, 115, 207, 109, 496, 634, 284, 440, 644, 101, 238, 104, 344, 157, 123, 108, 16, 647, 167, 510, 641, 100, 85, 77, 171, 78, 103, 643, 152, 51, 380, 122]. Studies during the 1930's and 1940's demonstrated abnormal serum levels of alkaline phosphatase and pseudocholinesterase in liver damage [206]. It was not until the recognition in 1955 that transaminase (aminotransferase) levels of the serum are sensitive measures of hepatic injury [372, 115], however, that the use of serum enzyme assay as a tool for studies in experimental hepatotoxicity came into its own.

Measurement of enzyme levels of the serum or plasma has permitted detection of hepatic toxicity with far less labor than that involved in histologic analysis [640, 207, 634]. It has provided a tool for detection of early damage, and for demonstration of hepatic injury without sacrifice of animals [640, 115, 207, 109, 496]. It also has permitted serial measurements, especially in larger animals [207, 109, 496]. Serum enzymology, as a parameter of injury, has been applied to the study of possible hepatotoxicity of unknown agents [207, 109, 496], to comparison of relative toxicity of different agents [284], to demonstration of the onset of injury [440, 644] and to study of he potentiation or inhibition of the toxic phenomena by physiologic manipulations or administration of various agents [207, 109, 496].

There are limitations to the use of serum enzyme levels for the study of hepatotoxicity [181, 182, 207, 109, 496]. The inference [101] of hepatotoxic effects deduced from studies of levels of serum enzymes should be corroborated by at least some histologic studies [207, 109]. The levels may increase in the serum as a result of leakage from cells with altered permeability of membranes rather than frank necrosis [647]. Some of the enzymes considered to reflect hepatic injury also may derive from organs other than the liver [647]. Furthermore, some forms of hepatic injury (e.g. that induced by ethionine and phosphorous) [16, 647] are accompanied by little or no elevation of serum enzyme levels [640].

The general aspects of the application of serum enzymology to the study of experimental hepatotoxicity have been considered by a number of authors [640, 411, 207, 109, 496, 634, 284, 440, 644]. Selection of the enzyme(s) to be measured in testing for hepatic injury requires analysis of specificity for and sensitivity to liver damage [207, 109, 496]. The large number of enzymes identified in the serum or plasma of animals may be categorized into four groups with regard to sensitivity as measures of hepatic disease [640, 647] (Table 4). One group contains enzymes elevated levels of which appear to reflect cholestasis more sensitivity than parenchymal injury. In a second group are enzymes that are more sensitive to parenchymal injury than to decreased biliary flow. The third group includes enzymes that reflect the hepatic injury relatively little or not at all; but serum levels of which are elevated in disease of other tissues. In the fourth group are enzymes the value which is depressed in hepatic injury. It is the enzymes in the first and second groups that have been most useful for the study of hepatic disease in general; and those of the second group that have been most useful in the study of toxic hepatic injury.

The employment of serum enzymology to test for the hepatotocity of an unknown agent requires that the enzyme test be hepatospecific [207, 109, 496]. Some of the enzymes, elevated serum levels of which reflect parenchymal hepatic injury, are non-specific, however, and can also reflect injury of a number of tissues.

Table 4. Groups of serum enzymes according to their levels in experimental hepatic injury

Group		Enzymes	Obstructive jaundice and intrahepatic cholestasis	Acute necrosis	Chronic Injury	Injury of other organs
I		AL PH, 5′N, LAP, GTP	Markedly increased	Increased	Increased	±
II	A	GOT, MDH, LDH, ALD	Increased	Markedly increased	Increased	Increased
	B	GPT, ICDH, GDH	Increased	Markedly increased	Increased	Increased
	C	OCT, SDH, LDH_5, guanase, F-P-ALD, arginase	Increased	Markedly increased	Increased	±
III		CPK	Normal	Normal	Normal	Increased
IV		CHE	Normal	Decreased	Decreased	±

AL PH = alkaline phosphatase; 5′N = 5′nucleotidase; LAP = leucine aminopeptidase; GTP = glutamyl transpeptidase; LDH_5 = isoenzyme of lactate dehydrogenase; CPK = creatine phosphokinase; CHE = cholinesterase; ± = insignificant or minimal change. See Appendix for Explanation of Other Abbreviations.

Table 5. Relative degree of increase of several serum enzymes in toxic hepatic injury

Toxin	Lesion		Degree increase Serum enzyme[a] levels			
	Zonal necrosis	Steatosis	GOT	GPT	ICDH MDH	GDH
CCl_4	+	+	4+	3+	4+	2+
Thioacetamide	+	−	4+	3+	4+	2+
Tetracycline	−	+	2+	1+	2+	−
Ethioline	−	+	+	−	1	−

[a] See Appendix for Necessary Abbreviations.

For example, GOT*, LD*, MD*, ICD* and aldolase (fructose diphosphate aldolase) are found in sufficiently high concentrations in liver, muscle, myocardium, kidney and other tissues to reflect injury of the respective organs by increased serum levels [647]. Others, however, are found mainly (GPT*) or almost exclusively (OCT*, SDH*, LDH_5*, F-I-P*-aldolase, arginase, guanase) in the liver and, when elevated in the serum, are reliable reflections of hepatic injury [640, 647].

Despite the greater hepatospecificity of several other serum enzymes, the most widely employed and generally accepted measures of hepatic injury are the transaminase levels. The ease of measurement of the transaminases, the extensive experience with the use of them and their high degree of sensitivity to acute hepatic injury accounts for the general dependence on these measures of toxic liver damage [647]. Many investigators have employed only the GOT levels as the guide to the time course or intensity of injury. Others have employed both GOT and GPT; and a number of investigators have employed only the GPT value as the measure of hepatic injury. The relative usefulness of the two transaminases, however, relates to the nature of the injury (Table 5) and to the species under study. In the rat, the GPT is almost as sensitive a measure as the GOT for hepatic fcrosis Hepatic steatosis, not accompanied by necrosis (e.g. ethionine- [16], phosphorous- [167] or tetracycline-induced [510] hepatic steatosis), leads to much higher values for GOT than of GPT [510] or low values of both enzymes [640, 167]. The GPT in those instances is an insensitive measure of hepatic injury in the rat. Furthermore, while both GOT and GPT are present in large amounts in the liver of the rat and other small animals, other species show differing concentrations [641]. For example, the horse has very low values for GPT in the liver, and hepatic necrosis leads to rather slight elevations, although the GOT values are useful measures in this species [100]. Accordingly, the literature on the relative distribution of the enzymes under study in various species should be consulted before the selection of a parameter of injury for a particular species.

Assay of serum transaminase levels is useful for monitoring the severity and course of hepatic injury induced by *known* hepatotoxins, but serum enzymes which are more hepatospecific may be more useful in the study of agents with unknown potential for hepatic injury. Elevated values for OCT [85], SD [17], guanase [171], arginase [78] and LD_5 [103] would provide support for the inference that elevated

* See Appendix for Meaning of Abbreviations.

Table 6. Serum enzyme levels of which are increased in CCl_4 poisoning

GOT (Total and mitochondrial isoenzyme)
GPT
OCT
ICDH (TPN-linked)
MDH
ALD
F-1-P ALD
PHI
GR
LDH
GDH
Xanthine oxidase
Quinine oxidase
Amylase
Tributyrinase
Alkaline phosphatase
5-Nucleotidase
Leucine aminopeptidase
Urocanase
Histidase
Phosphomonoesterase I and II

Enzymes below line only slightly elevated.

values for GOT and GPT reflect injury to the liver rather than to another organ (heart, skeletal muscle, kidney [640]). Of this group of enzymes OCT [100] and SD [85] have seemed particularly useful. To insure that involvement of an organ (e.g. muscle), other than the liver, is not contributing to hypertransaminasemia, enzymes that do not rise in hepatic disease (e.g. CPK) have been studied [647, 643].

A number of investigators have attempted to employ serum enzymology as a reflection of organelle injury [640, 440, 644, 101, 238, 108]. Demonstration of elevated serum levels of glutamate dehydrogenase, an enzyme found almost exclusively in the mitochondira, has been generally accepted as a biochemical reflection of mitochondrial injury [440, 644, 108]. Indeed, demonstrations of delayed elevation of this enzyme in the serum of animals exposed to CCl_4 has been interpreted as support for the view that mitochondrial injury occurs later than that of other organelle [440, 644]. While this inference appears to be correct, the rate of entry of an enzyme into the serum after hepatic injury may be modified by factors other than intracellular organelle location. Values for GPT after CCl_4 administration to the rat increase as belatedly as do those of glutamate dehydrogenase [644], yet the GPT of the rat hepatocyte is found mainly in the cytosol [51]. Perhaps, the slower release of this enzyme relates to the binding of it to an intracellular component not necessarily an identified organelle. Measurement of the mitochondrial isozyme of GOT also has been employed as a measure of mitochondrial injury [152].

The type of injury induced by a chemical agent determines the main aspects of the enzymologic response. The acute hepatic necrosis induced by carbon tetrachloride leads to a sharp and prompt rise of a number of cytoplasmic enzymes followed by an increase in mitochondrial enzymes (glutamate dehydrogenase, mitochondrial isoenzyme of GOT) [644, 152] (The paradoxically delayed elevation of GPT levels has received comment). The rate and degree of increase in levels of the enzymes show a relationship to the dose of CCl_4; and in this type of necrogenic damage, the levels of transaminases and of a number of other enzymes listed in Table 6, are a useful measure of the severity of injury and of its development [440]. As suggested above, they *may* provide a clue to the organelle injured. On the other hand, acute toxic steatosis leads to much lesser elevation of serum transaminase levels and apparently leads to no abnormality of glutamate dehydrogenase levels [640, 510]. Values appear to be even lower for ethionine-induced hepatic steatosis [193] (Table 5).

Utilization of serum enzyme measurement has been of little help in determining injury of organelles other than mitochrondria [108]. Serum levels of several enzymes ordinarily found in lysozomes (acid phosphatase, B-glucuronidase) have been studied as a possible reflection of lysozomal injury, an effort that has not proved to be helpful [108]. Similarly, efforts to demonstrate leakage into the serum of enzymes from endoplasmic reticulum (ER) have led to conflicting results [108]. Increased values of glucose 6-phosphatase have been considered by some [380] to reflect ER injury, but other workers have been unable to confirm the reliability of this measure [108]. Curtis *et al.* [108] have demonstrated that elevated values of the monoesterase of the liver are a measure of ER injury.

Many workers have considered serum enzyme measures to be more sensitive, although perhaps less reliable, measures of toxicity than electron microscopic studies of histologic changes [122]. Grice [181], however, has reported the sensitivity of EM changes to early CCl_4 toxicity to be greater than that of elevated levels of serum enzymes.

Early in the application of serum enzyme measurement to hepatotoxicity, it was confidently expected and reported by some investigators [634, 104] that, as serum enzyme levels increased in response to injury, tissues levels would decrease [222]. This has, however, not been consistantly true [104, 122, 222]. Failure to find decreased amounts in hepatic tissue of an enzyme (e.g. GOT or GPT), which is found in strikingly increased amounts in the serum as a response to hepatic injury, is a puzzling phenomenon which has been postulated [222] to reflect increased synthesis, keeping pace with leakage. There is little concrete evidence bearing on this matter, and it remains an interesting and obscure aspect of the problem of toxicologic enzymology. Further understanding of this aspect, of the kinetics of the disappearance of enzymes from the circulation and of the mechanism for their disposal would be useful for optimal application of serum enzymology to hepatotoxicity studies.

II. *In Vitro* Models

A number of models have been employed for study of hepatotoxicity *in vitro*. These include the perfused liver [53, 111], liver homogenates and slices [472, 432, 141, 142, 260, 533, 460, 237], suspensions of hepatocytes freshly isolated from the liver [110, 642, 127, 41] or grown in tissue or organ culture [106, 200, 228, 646, 648, 649, 276, 433, 90], or isolated organelles from hepatocytes [472, 432, 141, 532, 521, 114, 548].

1. Liver Perfusion

Development of the technique of perfusion of the liver *in vitro* for the study of hepatic physiology has permitted study of the effects of a number of toxic agents [53, 333, 234, 210, 452, 34, 54, 479, 111]. Most experiments utilizing the *in vitro* perfused liver have selected the rat liver, although the liver of other species also has served [210]. Studies of the effect of toxic agents on synthetic or other metabolic activity, bile flow, dye extraction or excretion and lipid secretion by the isolated liver into efferent venous flow or into bile all have served to elucidate mechanisms of injury. The problem has been approached by pretreating the intact animal with the agent under study prior to sacrifice and removal of the liver for perfusion [54] or by adding the agent under study to the perfusate [53, 333, 234, 210, 452, 34]. The nature of the hepatic injury also has been studied by observing the effect of hepatotoxic agents on leakage of intracellular enzymes. into the perfusate [479].

2. Tissue Homogenates and Slices

Homogenates of liver tissue have generally served to test the adverse effects of toxic agents on functions of the liver that can be measured less directly *in vivo*. Metabolism of drugs [260] and incorporation of labelled amino acid as a measure of protein synthesis [533] are examples. Slices of liver tissue have served not only this purpose, but also have been used to measure the inhibition of lipid secretion [460] by the toxin-damaged liver and have been used to demonstrate an adverse effect on the plasma membrane of the hepatocyte (e.g. potassium or enzyx leakage into the medium) [237].

3. Hepatocyte Suspensions

The use of suspensions of hepatocytes [110, 642, 127, 41], rather than homogenates or slices for studies of hepatotoxicity is a relatively recent development. During the past few years, mzhbs have been developed for the isolation of suspensions of hepatocytes that have retained sufficiently intact metabolic function to mimic that of the normal liver [41]. Relatively few studies relevant to hepatotoxicity have employed this model, t more may be expected. Cells, of human embryo [106], of normal animal liver [200], or of animal hepatocellular carcinoma [228], grown in tissue culture also have been xployed to study the effects of known hepatotoxins and drugs on the liver. While cells grown in tissue culture undergo sufficient dedifferentiation to lose important characteristics of hepatocytes, they have served to study the adverse effects of tetracycline [648], aflatoxins [649], chlorinated hydrocarbons [646], and galactosamine [276].

4. Organelles

Organelles, isolated from hepatocytes of normal animals or from animal pretreated with hepatotoxic agents have served to pose some important questions [433, 90, 532, 521, 114, 548, 288]. The adverse effects of such hepatotoxic agents as CCl_4 [432], ethionine [142], phosphorous [532], mycotoxins [175] and other agents on the protein-synthetic function of the liver, have been studied by measuring the ability of ribosomes isolated from animals pretretreated with the respective agent to incorporate labelled amino acid [472, 190,40, 432, 141]. Also the integrity of lysozomes [521, the functional status and integrity of mitochondria [472] and the chemical changes in ccleus and nucleoli [142], isolated from the livers of animals pretreated with hepatotoxic agents have been the subject of considerable study by hepatotoxicologists. The adverse effects of adding hepatotoxic agents *in vitro* to isolated ribosomes [432], mitochondria [432], lysozomes [114], nuclei [548] and plasma membranes [288] also have provided useful information.

5. Nuclear Components

Study of the effects of known hepatotoxins on DNA, RNA, nuclei and synthesizing enzymes has provided key information of mechanisms of injury [142]. This facet has been approached by examining the various compounds isolated from the liver after pretreatment of the experimental animw with toxic agents or by isolating the respective compounds from normal animals and examining the effect of the particular toxic agent *in vitro* on the nucleic acid or enzymes [142].

F. Types of Toxic Hepatic Injury

An understanding of the mechanisms of heqtic injury is facilitated by an analysis of the forms of injury produced by various chemical agents. Indeed, combining the available information of the type of injury with information on mechanisms permits a useful classification of toxic agents [638].

I. Changes Observed by Light Microscopy

Chemical or biologic substances can produce mainly damage to hepatocytes or mainly interference with bile flow [342, 418, 269, 638, 639]. The former is often referred to as the *cytotoxic* type and the latter as the *cholestatic* type of hepatic injury (Table 1). The injury may be acute or chronic.

1. Acute Hepatic Injury

The cytotoxic form of damage includes necrosis, steatosis or both *Necrosis* induced by most predictable hepatotxins is usually zonal; it may involve the central, mid or peripheral portion of the lobule. Carbon tetrachloride [472], chloroform [472], iodoform [506], brombenzene [472], thiocetamide [472], the dialkylnitrosamines [472], pyrrolidizine alkaloids [352], tannic acid [472], toxins of Amanita phalloides [610] and a number of other agents usually produce centrizonal necrosis (Table 7). Occasionally the lesion of carbon tetrachloride is modified by other circumstances. (It may be midzonal in the hyperthyroid animal [472].) Some agents e.g. the chlorinated diphenyls and naphthalenes and tetrachlorethane produce massive rather than zonal injury [269]. A few agents (Table 10) produce, selectively, peripheral (periportal) necrosis [472] Aflatoxins produce central necrosis in some species (rat), peripheral in others (e.g. guinea pig) and midzonal in others (e.g. rabbit) [175]. A pattern of diffuse or multiple small areas of necrosis is characteristic of idiosyncrasy-dependent hepatic injury in humans [639] but not in general of that produced by predictable hepatotoxins. However, the recently recognized intrinsic hepatotoxin, galactosamine [252] and, in some species, the aflatoxins produce diffuse rather than zonal necrosis.

Hepatic steatosis is produced by a large umber of agents [472]. Most extensively studied is ethionine [140]. It produces in the rat a characteristic form of small-droplet fat (microvesicular steatosis) which is initially or mainly periportal in location. Tetracycline, in large doses, produces hepatic steatosis of similar appearance which is initially centrizonal in location [639]. The fatty liver induced by elemental phosphorous is at first periportal [472]. Recent studies have demonstrated the ability of ethanol to lead to steatosis [308]. Other agents that can produce a fatty liver are listed in Table 8.

Table 7. Agents[a] that produce hepatic necrosis[b], with or without steatosis

Necrosis only	Necrosis and steatosis
Acetominophen (CZ)	Aflatoxins (CZ, PZ)
Allyl compounds (PZ)	Amanitin (CZ)
Albitocin (PZ)	Arsenic compounds (inorganic) (CZ, M)
Aniline (M)	Brombenzene (CZ)
Alloxan (PZ)	CCl_4 (CZ)
ANIT (CZ, MZ, PZ)	Chloroform (CZ)
Beryllium (MZ)	Chloroprene (CZ)
Chlorinated benzenes (M)	Chlorinated diphenyls (M)
Dioxane (M)	Chlorinated naphthalene (M)
Diphtheria toxin (CZ)	2-Chloropropane (CZ)
Divinyl ether (CZ)	Dichloropropane (CZ)
Ferrous sultate (PZ)	DDT
Manganese compunds (PZ)	Dimethylnitrosamine[a]
Methylene chloride (M)	Dinitrobenzone (CZ, M)
Ngaione (MZ)	Dinitrophenol (M)
Paraquat (CZ, MZ)	Dinitrotoluene (CZ, M)
Phalloidin (CZ)	Galactosamine (D)
P. vulgaris endotoxin (PZ)	Iodoform (CZ)
Rubratoxin (CZ)	Islandicum (CZ)
Selenium (M)	Luteoskyrin (CZ)
Sporidesmin (PZ)	Ethylene dibromide (CZ)
Thioacetamide (CZ)	Ethylene dichloride (CZ)
Urethane (CZ)	Methylchloroform (CZ)
	Naphthalene (CZ)
	Pyrrolidizine alkaloids (CZ)
	Synthalin (PZ)
	Tannic acid (CZ)
	Tetrachloroethane (M)
	TNT (CZ or M)

[a] Partial list. See Rouillier [472] for other agents.
[b] CZ = centrizonal necrosis. PZ = peripheral necrosis. MZ = midzonal necrosis. M = massive necrosis. D = diffuse necrosis.

Table 8. Agents that produce steatosis[a]

Acetamide	Ethyl chloride
Antimony	Flectol H
L-Asparaginase	Hydrazine
Azacytidine	Hypoglycin
Azaserine	Methyl bromide
Azauridine	Methyl chlorobromide
BAL	Methyl chloride
Barium salts	Methyl dichloride
Bleomycin	Orotic acid
Bojtes	Phosphorous[c]
Carbon disulfide	Puromycin
Cerium salts[b]	Rare earths[b]
Chromates	Satrole
Dichloroethylene	Tetracycline
Dimethylhydrazine	Thallium compounds
Ethanol	Uranium compounds
Ethionine	Warfarin
Ethylbromide	

[a] Partial list of agents that produce fatty liver in rats. Fg other agents ROUILLIER [472] should be consulted.
[b] Only rare earths of low atomic number (57–61) produce fatty liver.
[c] Phosphorous causes mainly fatty liver; may be some peripheral necrosis as well.

Some agents produce both steatosis and necrosis (Tables 7, 8). Examples are carbon tetrachloride, chloroform, tetrachlorethane [269] extracts of Amanita phalloides [610, 612], tannic acid [472] and in some species, several aflatoxins [175].

Cytotoxicity also is manifested by changes in individual hepatocytes. Decrease in cytoplasmic basophilia followed by progressively intense acidophilic staining and eventuating in acidophilic degeneration and "ballooning" of cells also reflects hepatocyte injury induced by some toxins [472, 531, 70]. For example, an early lesion of acute CCl_4 poisoning is midzonal and centrizonal ballooning [70].

Cholestatic injury may consist of bile casts in the canalicular spaces with little or no injury to the ducts or ductules [639] or may consist of bile duct and ductule injury or destruction [584]. Icterogenin and several anabolic and estrogenic steroids lead mainly to interference with bile flow [639], while α-naphthylisothiocyanate (ANIT) produces in most species a selective cholangiodestructive and cholangioproliferative lesion [584]. Either form of cholestatic injury may be accompanied by some degree of parenchymal injury. Furthermore, agents that produce mainly hepatic injury e.g. ethionine [140], aflatoxin [175] also lead to some degree of ductal injury. Nevertheless, hepatotoxic agents can be categorized generally as mainly cytotoxic or mainly cholestatic [638, 639].

Inflammatory response to toxic injury is of variable prominence, depending on the form of injury. Acute necrosis of CCl_4 poisoning is usually accompanied by aggregates of leucocytes, both polymorphonuclear and mononuclear, in the area of early necrosis [472]. Aflatoxicosis in chickens, but not in other species, is accompanied by striking lymphocyte infiltration and even by the formation of aggregates that resemble lymph follicles [175].

Injury of hepatic vasculature, RE system and supporting structure which has been less extensively studied than that of the parenchymal cells has been well summarized by ROULLIER [472]. Collapse of reticulum, fibroblast stimulation, collagen formation and collagenolytic activity that have been shown in the liver of rats with experimental cirrhosis [339, 340, 211, 213, 466, 212, 259], have commanded considerable interest.

2. Chronic Hepatic Injury

Chronic changes include fibrosis, cirrhosis [195] and neoplasia [410, 226]. The degree and type of fibrosis produced by hepatotoxins varies with the agent, its mode of administration, the species and other circumstances. CCl_4-induced massive necrosis, if not lethal, may be followed by micronodular cirrhosis [125] or by restitution of normal architecture [7 . Small dosegiven repeatedly, at intervals too short to permit recovery from each dose, can lead to diffuse, micronodular cirrhosu [70]. Pyrrolidizine alkaloids, which lead to central necrosis and, usually, occlusion of hepatic venules, can lead to a "congestive" type of cirrhosis resembling cardiac cirrhosis ("venoocclusive disease") [352]. Aflatoxins, in many species can lead to a macronodular or micronodular cirrhosis and, in monkeys, to a "biliary"type of cirrhosis [175]. ANIT can lead to a form of biliary cirrhosis [584].

3. Carcinogenesis

The enormous literature [410, 226, 142] devoted to chemical hepatocarcinogenicity is beyond summarizing in this review. Many hepatotoxins are also hepatocarcinogenic [410, 226]. Indeed, most hepatocarcinogens are also hepatotoxins. The two, however, are not necessarily synonymous. Some hepatotoxins can lead to hepatic carcinoma without producing overt acute hepatic injury or cirrhosis, a phenomenon observed with low doses of aflatoxin B_1 [175]. Some aflatoxins, on the other hand, are acutely hepatotoxic, but not carcinogenic [175]. Nevertheless, the possibility that related abnormalities induced in the hepatocyte may be responsible for both phenomena remains.

Alkylation, arylation and addition of heterocyclic radicals to macromolecules of the cell, especially nucleic acids, appears to trigger the neoplastic process [142]. Apparently the reactivity of the carcinogens in altering control molecules in the hepatocyte also leads to metabolic changes in the cell that provoke degeneration and necrosis. Most attention has focused on the organelles of the cytoplasm [531, 544]; although recent studies have concentrated on ultrastructural changes in the nucleus [555, 410, 226].

Changes in Endoplasmic Reticulum. A wide variety of agents, some of which are discussed below, lead to disorganization of the RER. Indeed, the disorganization, distortion, dispersal, redistribution and fragmentation of the RER are the most consistent and striking ultrastructural abnormalities of early CCl_4 poisoning. The earliest manifestation of injury to the RER is dilation of the rough-surfaced cisternae and loss of attached ribosomes. These appear to have been dissociated from the membranous surface; since decrease in numbers of attached ribosomes is accompanied by an increase in free ribosomes scattered through the cytoplasm. Detachment of ribosomes may be reversible when induced by some agents (orotic acid) but not by others (CCl_4, tannic acid) [472, 531, 544].

Carbon tetrachloride, phosphorous, allyl formate and other toxins also produce a dose-related, more drastic abnormality of the RER which includes disruption of cisterna and fragmentation and dissolution of the membranes [472]. The striking disruption, fragmentation and dissolution of the RER appears almost immediately after CCl_4 administration and appears to be responsible for distorted function of the hepatocyte and the metabolic effect of the injury [432]. Indeed, this relationship between organelle injury and metabolic effect permits distinction of two main types of predictable hepatotoxins. Agents that lead to almost instant destruction of this critical component of the metabolic machinery of the hepatocyte, we have classified as *direct* hepatotoxins; whereas agents that may produce similar changes but do so apparenly as the result of specific interferences with a cellular metabolic pathway we have labeled *indirect* hepatotoxins. (See Section on Classification.)

The SER also is vulnerable to hepatotoxic agents. As the site of the drug-metabolizing enzyme system, it is extremely important in the modification of a number of the hepatotoxins to their toxic metabolic products [472, 531, 544]. Accordingly, it also may be the initial site of the injury [432]. Almost immediately after the administration of CCl_4 there is a decrease of NADP and a diminution of the drug-detoxifying enzyme activity of the SER. A decline of cytochrome P-450 content occurs more slowly (after two hours). Thereafter, the vesicles of the SER become dilated. These changes in the SER are less dramatically evident than the dilation of the cisternae of the RER [472, 531, 544].

Small doses of hepatotoxins and a large variety of nontoxic or oligotoxic chemical agents produce increased amounts of SER. The hypertrophy of the endoplasmic reticulum and the metabolic significance of this change is discussed elsewhere in this chapter and in other chapters with reference to the phenomenon of enzyme "induction". While this is usually an adaptive and potentially useful one, HUTTERER and his associates [221] have described a phase of this phenomenon that is counterproductive. They have demonstrated an ultimate, *decreased*, metabolic activity of SER even though it is increased in amount as the result of exposure to some agents. Initially these produce hypertrophy of the SER with increased activity of its enzymes; but, subsequently, these dissociate with *decreased* drug-detoxifying activity in association with *increased* amounts of SER. This has been referred to as "hyperplastic-hypoactive endoplasmic reticulum" and an early ultrastructural manifestation of toxicity [221].

A curious, additional, ultrastructural change induced by a number of chemical agents is the development of *lamellar* formations [531, 555, 544]. These consist of multiple layers of concentric membranes, surrounding a core of one or more amorphous, lipid bodies apparently derived from mitochondria, microbodies, lysosomes or glycogen residues. The concentric lamellar membranes may be tightly packed ("myelin figures") or loosely arranged ("fingerprint" formations). While the significance of the lamellar formations is unclear, "fingerprint" formation appears to reflect hepatocyte injury (ANIT*, ethionine), and the myelin figures apparently represent a physiologic response to metabolism of large doses of nontoxic drugs (phenobarbital) [531]. Chronic CCl_4 administration, however, leads to both forms of response, presumably representing both the injurious and the inducing effects of small doses of the agent.

The changes observed by LM can be related to those observed by EM. The loss of basophilia, cloudy swelling and hydropic degeneration observed sequentially in CCl_4 poisoning appear to reflect changes in the RER. Loss of basophilia mirrors loss of RNA, cloudy swelling corresponds to moderate dilation of RER cisternae, while hydropic degeneration appears to reflect more severe dilation of the cisternae and imbition of water. Increase in the amount of SER can be correlated with increased cytoplasmic acidophilia of hepatocytes in H and E stained sections. When hyperplastic SER membranes are densely compacted, sinusoidal acidophilic ("hyaline") bodies are seen. On the other hand when proliferated SER membranes are aggregated relatively loosely, as in the case of ANIT-induced hepatic injury, such acidophilic bodies are not seen. Concentric lamellar formations are reflected in light microscopy as round or ovoid cytoplasmic inclusions [544].

Nuclear Changes. The most prominent changes in the nucleus are those produced by hepatotoxic agents that are also potent hepatocarcinogens. The nuclei increase in size and there may be striking anisonucleosis. The most prominent changes in the nucleus involve the nucleolus, but there also are changes in the nucleoplasm. These include the production of increased amounts of "interchromatin" and of "satellite" granules in the nucleoplasm as is seen with toxic effects of aflatoxins, dimethylnitrosamine, pyrrolidizine alkaloids, tannic acid and thiocetamide; and of curious nuclear inclusions induced by tannic acid [226, 555].

Nucleolar changes produced by some agents appear to be important and striking. These seem to be related to the mechanism of injury and the type of interference with RNA synthesis. The most dramatic change, referred to as *segregation*, consists of two types, macrosegregation and microsegregation [555].

Macrosegregation refers to the presence of distinct, relatively large zones, each composed of pure granules or fibrils. The granular component of the nucleolus appears to be reduced, and the nucleolus has a compact appearance. The presence of one or more of the condensed fibrillar zones at the periphery of the nucleolus leads to an appearance referred to as "nuclear capping". Aflatoxin B_1, a pyrrolidizine alkaloid (lasiocarpine), and 3′MeDAB have been reported to produce this change [555].

Microsegregation describes compact condensations of the fibrillar component of the nucleolus which normally is arranged in multiple small aggregates throughout a granular environment. The condensation, or segregation of the fibrillar component from the granular environment, is less clear cut than that of macrosegregation. There are differences in the degree of microsegregation produced by various hepatotoxic substances. It is characteristically induced by dimethylnitrosamine and thioacetamide. The microsegregation induced by thioacetamide may resemble compact knots ("whorls") within the granular background [555].

Some hepatotoxic agents, e.g. ethionine and α-amanitin induce a pattern of nucleolar fragmentation as well as or instead of microsegregation. This pattern has been attributed [226, 142] to inhibition of RNA synthesis by mechanisms other than those of the segregation-producing toxins.

Still another type of nuclear change is produced by CCl_4, which also does not produce nucleolar segregation. As necrosis develops, shortly after the onset of the CCl_4-injury, nuclear pyknosis and fragmentation is observed [392]. During recovery from CCl_4-injury, there is binucleation and striking anisonucleosis as in regeneration from other acute injury.

Significance of Ultrastructural Abnormalities. Changes in the ultrastructure of the cell can be related to pathogenesis of injury. Injury of the RER, the site of protein synthesis, can be held accountable for the impairment of protein synthesis induced by toxic agfts that damage this organelle [432]. Injury of the SER seems relatable to impairment of drug metabolism and of glycogen synthesis [531, 544]. Changes in the Golgi apparatus may be relatable to impairment of processing of lipids and apolipoprotein to form the lipoprotein needed to permit exit of lipids from the hepatocyte [539] to, and changes in the nucleolus and nucleus reflect the fundamental alterations in DNA and RNA that may be central to hepatotoxicity and hepatocarcinogenicity [226, 555]. Changes in the mitochondria are difficult to interpret because of the array of substances and circumstances that leads to similar abnormalities [472].

G. Classification of Hepatotoxins

Hepatotoxic agents, theoretically, might be classified according to mechanism of injury, types of liver damage, fundamental chemical nature or source of the agent. Understanding of mechanisms of hepatic injury, while still burdened with important gaps, has advanced sufficiently during the past few years to permit assignment of a number of agents to the categories of the classification proposed in this discussion (Table 9) [638, 639]. Inclusion of types of injury with mechanisms permits greater refinement of the categories.

Classification of hepatotoxic agents according to chemical structure would be desirable but is impossible [472]. The fundamental chemical nature of *some* liver-damaging agents (e.g. ethionine [140], DMN [490], azo dyes [410], chlorinated hydrocarbons [432]), clearly has a bearing on the mechanism and type of hepatic injury. Information on the relationship of chemical structure to mechanism of injury, for most compounds, however, is too limited and the chemical variety of toxic agents much too great to permit useful generalization. The following discussion presents a classification based on apparent mechanisms, and types of injury [638, 639]. The evidence in support of the presumed mechanisms is presented for examples in each category.

Clinical and experimental observations have led to general agreement that there are two main categories of agents that can produce hepatic injury (Table 9) [638]. One consists of agents that are *predictable* (*true*, *intrinsic*) hepatotoxins; the other contains agents that are not predictably hepatotoxic but produce hepatic injury in only a small proportion of exposed individuals, who are uniquely susceptible (host *idiosyncrasy*).

Intrinsic hepatotoxins are recognized by the high incidence of hepatic injury in exposed individuals, the production of a similar lesion in experimental animals, the consistent latent period between exposure to a particular agent and the development of hepatic injury, and the dose-dependence of the phenomenon [342, 418, 269, 638]. With agents that produce hepatic damage in only a small proportion of exposed individuals, the injury does not appear to be dose related, is not reproducible in experimental animals and appears after a variable latent period.

Table 9. Classification of hepatotoxic agents

Category of agent	Characteristics[a]					
	Inc.	Exp. repr.	Dose Dep.	Mechanism	Histol. lesion	Examples
Intrinsic toxicity						
Direct	High	Yes	Yes	Membrane injury destruction of structural basis cell metabolism	Necrosis (zonal) and/or steatosis	CCl_4 $CHCl_3$ Phosphorous
Indirect						
Cytotoxic	High	Yes	Yes	Interference with specific metabolic pathways leads to structural injury	Steatosis or necrosis	Ethionine mycotoxins (see Table 10)
Cholestatic	High	Yes	Yes	Interference with hepatic excretory pathways leads to cholestasis	Bile casts	Icterogenin C-17 alkylated anabolic and contraceptive steroids (see Table 10)
Host idiosyncracy						
Hypersensitivity	Low	No	No	Drug allergy	Necrosis or cholestasis	Sulfonamides Paramino-salycilate Halothane
Metabolic Abnormality	Low	No	No	Production of hepatotoxic metabolites?	Necrosis or cholestasis	Iproniazid, Isoniazid

[a] Inc. = Incidence; Exp. repr. = Experimental reproducibility; Dose Dep. = Dose Dependent; Histol. = Histologic.

These substances are recognized to depend on host idiosyncracy for their adverse effect.

This chapter deals mainly with intrinsic hepatotoxins which, by definition, are experimental toxins; while agents that depend on host idiosyncracy are not. Nevertheless, some agents that appear to produce injury only in uniquely susceptible humans have been found to have an adverse effect on experimental models [638, 639, 368].

I. Intrinsic Hepatotoxins

Hepatotoxic agents produce hepatic injury by a variety of mechanisms (472, 190, 638]. Search for common denominators, however, suggest that there are two types of intrinsic hepatotoxins [638, 226] that we have categorized as *direct* and *indirect* (Table 9). These categories are approximately equivalent to the "toxipathic" and "trophopathic" forms of hepatic injury, respectively, which were proposed by HIMSWORTH [209].

Direct hepatotoxins may be so called because they (or their metabolic products) produce *directly* injury to the hepatocyte and its organelles, especially the ER. CCl_4, the prototype produces peroxidation of the membrane lipids [432] or other

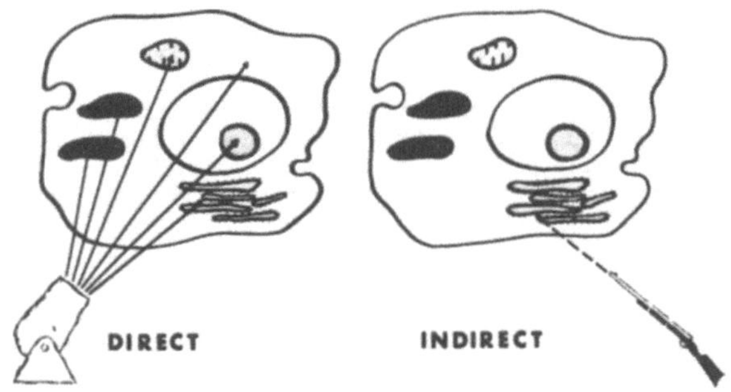

Fig. 1. Diagrammatic representation of presumed differences between mode of action of direct and indirect intrinsic hepatotoxins. Direct injures all elements of cell, while indirect are more precise and selective. (From ZIMMERMAN [638], with permission of Perspectives in Biology and Medicine and the University of Chicago Press)

chemical changes that lead to denaturation [449] of the membranes. These changes which begin almost immediately, after administration of the toxic are the first stages in the injury that culminates in the characteristic cytotoxic effect, i.e., hepatic necrosis, steatosis or both [432]. We would epitomize *direct hepatotoxicity as destruction of the structural basis of hepatocyte metabolism.*

Indirect hepatotoxins are more selective. They are antimetabolites and related compounds that produce hepatic injury by interference with a specific metabolic pathway or process [638] (Fig. 1). *The structural injury produced by indirect hepatotoxins appears to* be secondary to a metabolic lesion (hence *indirect*); while in that produced by *direct hepatotoxins* the metabolic derangement is secondary to the structural injury. The hepatic damage produced by indirect hepatotoxins may be mainly *cytotoxic* expressed as steatosis or necrosis, or may be mainly *cholestatic*, expressed as arrested bile flow with or without bile duct injury.

The distinction between "direct" and "indirect" hepatotoxins is somewhat arbitrary and there are substances that we have categorized at this time as indirect (e.g. brombenzene, DMN) that others might prefer to place in the same category as CCl_4. Nevertheless, the distinction between the mechanism for injury by CCl_4 as the prototype of the direct category and ethionine as the prototype of the indirect suggests this general categorization to be valid [638].

II. Hepatic Injury Owing to Host Idiosyncracy

A number of drugs produce hepatic injury, unpredictably, in a small proportion of recipients [126, 342, 418, 269, 517, 638, 639]. The hepatic injury appears to be an expression of unique, individual susceptibility instead of intrinsic toxicity of the offending agent [638]. At least two types of mechanisms seem to be involved [638, 639]. Some agents produce hepatic injury under circumstances and accompanied by clinical and other features that suggest the mechanism to be hypersensitivity (drug allergy) [638, 639]. Other drugs produce hepatic injury not accompanied by collateral features indicative of hypersensitivity [638, 639]. Accordingly they are inferred to depend on a metabolic aberration, in the susceptible patient, that permits conversion of the respective drug to hepatotoxic metabolites [638, 639, 368].

Recent studies in experimental animals by MITCHELL *et al.* [368] have provided evidence in support of the view [638, 639] that at least one form of host idiosyncracy-dependent hepatic injury can be the expression of conversion of the respective drug (e.g. isoniazid) to a hepatotoxic metabolite. Furthermore, we [638, 639] and others [127] have employed several *in vitro* experimental models (of Chang cells, rat hepatocytes, rabbit liver slices, perfused rat liver) to provide evidence in support of the hypothesis [638, 639] that even the drugs that produce hepatic injury in a setting suggestive of hypersensitivity are also intrinsically, albeit mildly, hepatotoxic.

H. Direct Hepatotoxins

Agents in this category (or their metabolites) have a directly injurious effect on membranes of the hepatocyte, prior to or not dependent on selective interference with a metabolic pathway [638]. In our view, an agent assigned to this category, should like CCl_4 [432] produce injury to the cell or its components at least as early or earlier than any alteration of DNA, or RNA, or before impaired synthesis of protein, depression of levels of ATP or glutathione or other metabolic aspect which when altered can lead to heaptic injury. The directly injurious effect on the hepatocytes involves a physiochemical alteration of membrane integrity, perhaps as the result of lipid peroxidation of the unsaturated fatty acids that are key parts of the structure [432] or by other chemical changes [449]. (Other characteristics of direct hepatotoxins emphasized by us in the past [638] such as the very brief interval between exposure to them and evidence of hepatic injury, the ability to produce zonal hepatic injury in many species and to injure a wide variety of living things are shared by some of the indirect hepatotoxins.) Substances that appear to be categorizable as direct hepatotoxins include CCl_4, tetrachlorethane, $BrCCl_3$, carbon tetraiodide, chloroform, iodoform, perhaps some other halogenated hydrocarbons and inorganic phosphorous. While the nature of phalloidin toxicity suggests that it might also be in this category [610, 612, 142], we have included it with the amatoxins in the discussion of indirect hepatotoxins.

Some agents that we have categorized as direct hepatotoxins depend on metabolic transformation to exert their toxic effect; while others appear not to require conversion to a metabolite to produce hepatic injury. Carbon tetrachloride is in the former group [432], and elemental phosphorous appears to be in the latter category [220]. Even more variety can be expected in the type of physiochemical alteration of cellular membranes that leads to hepatocyte injury [432]. The following description of the features of carbon tetrachloride and phosphorous hepatotoxicity will serve to illustrate some of these differences.

I. Carbon Tetrachloride

The prototype of direct hepatotoxins [638], and the best-studied [432] of hepatotoxic agents is CCl_4. During the half century since the first demonstration of its hepatotoxic effects on experimental animals [360], thousands of reports have been devoted to this agent. CCl_4-poisoning has been a widely-used model to study the phenomena of hepatic necrosis and to study the effects of induced hepatic injury on hepatic function. In the course of unravelling the mechanism by which it produces fatty liver, CCl_4 has served to elucidate the pathogenesis of fatty metamorphosis induced by other ethiologic factors [430]. While it can lead to damage to a number of tissues [394], it is particularly prone to produce hepatic and renal injury in man and in a variety of experimental animals [126, 472, 430].

This agent is a potent hepatotoxin. Single doses lead to centrizonal necrosis and steatosis after a very short latent period [472]. Within a few minutes there is injury to the ER which leads to functional defects of the hepatocyte and multiple biochemical manifestations of hepatic injury [432]. Steatosis develops because movement of fat from the cell is blocked by disruption of the mechanism for coupling triglycerides to the appropriate apoprotein to form the lipoprotein carrier molecule [430, 432]; perhaps in part by defective synthesis of the apolipoprotein and perhaps by a defect in transport of the lipoprotein across the plasma membrane [240]. The relevance of the proposed [69, 492], increased mobilization of tissue lipids to the pathogenesis of steatosis remains controversial [432, 539].

Necrosis, the pathogenesis of which is unclear [240, 432], may be the result of the abruptly developing, intracellular biochemical chaos and the consequent loss of bioenergetics needed to maintain cellular integrity [638]. Prolonged administration of CCl_4 can lead to *cirrhosis* [70], and in some species, to hepatic *carcinoma* [443, 444, 447]. Most of the acute and chronic hepatic injury appears to result from the action of a metabolite of the toxin [432].

1. Chemical Properties

CCl_4 is a simple, strongly non-polar molecule [394] which undergoes metabolism in the endoplasmic reticulum [432]. A chemical characteristic of relevance to the hepatotoxic potential of this compound emphasized by SLATER [520] and by RECKNAGEL and GLINDE [432], is the relatively low association energy for the C-Cl bond. The bond association energy is progressively higher in less toxic ($CHCl_3$) and lower in more toxic ($CBrCl_3$) chlorinated hydrocarbons [432].

2. Toxicity in Humans

Clinical hepatotoxicity results from inhalation or ingestion of the agent [269, 375, 232]. There is little experimental or clinical evidence to support the view [526] that poisoning by inhalation produces mainly renal injury and by ingestion leads mainly to hepatic injury. Most adults who have carbon tetrachloride poisoning are alcoholics [269, 375, 332, 526, 341], since alcoholism appears to enhance susceptibility to the hepatotoxin and leads to increased carelessness with the use of CCl_4. Accidental ingestion of the agent during the state of alcoholic intoxication or inhalation of it during careless domestic use, are the usual circumstances of injury.

The clinical *syndrome* consists of hepatic failure usually accompanied by renal failure [269, 394, 375, 341]. Prior to the appearance of the hepatic injury there are usually neurologic and gastrointestinal manifestations, and a varying degree of vascular collapse. Cardiac arrhythmias may occur shortly after exposure; and, late in the course, cardiac failure and often pulmonary edema are part of the syndrome [394].

The evidence of hepatic disease appears early, usually within 2 to 4 days of exposure. Hepatocellular jaundice may proceed to severe hepatic failure. Renal failure becomes manifest shortly after hepatic failure [375, 232, 526, 341].

Biochemical reflections of hepatic injury include elevated, often strikingly, serum values for the transaminases (GOT and GPT) and a variety of other enzymes (Table 6) [634, 647]. Alkaline phosphatase values are usually only slightly elevated. Prolonged "1-stage" prothrombin time presumably reflects depressed levels of plasma coagulation factors, intravascular coagulation, or both [546]. Fibrinogen levels are low in severe CCl_4 toxicity [579].

The chief *histopathologic* abnormalities include centrolobular hepatic necrosis and some hepatic steatosis [269, 375, 232, 526, 341]. Renal abnormalities include necrosis and fatty changes of tubular epithelium [526]. Evidence of injury to the lungs, by way of a pseudomomembrane and thickened alveolar walls may be seen [580].

3. Experimental Models

Most investigators have employed rats, mice, dogs and rabbits; guinea pigs, hamsters, cats, horses, cattle, pigs, monkeys and other species have been used in relatively few studies [472]. In recent years rats have been employed far more extensively than any other species.

Administration of the agent intragastrically, subcutaneously, intraperitoneally and by inhalation all lead to the characteristic lesion of centrizonal necrosis and steatosis [472]. The effect is dose related, with the minimal toxic dose in the adult rat approximately 0.02 ml/kg by these routes. The subcutaneous route appears, however, to lead to somewhat more irregular and less predictable results [338]. Intrasplenic and intraportal administration employed in a few studies lead to massive necrosis [71].

The effects of CCl_4 on a number of *in-vitro* models also have been studied in an effort to define the mechanisms of injury [432]. These have included liver slices and homogenates [67, 600, 530], cell suspensions [110, 646], and the *ex-vivo* perfused liver [53, 452, 111, 203]; even studies of the effects of the CCl_4 on isolated organelles *in-vitro* have been conducted [432, 533, 451, 431].

4. Factors in Susceptibility

Species. Rats, mice, rabbits, guinea pigs, hamsters, cats, dogs, sheep and cattle all are susceptible to the liver-damaging effects. Chickens and other birds and amphibians are very resistant. Some early studies suggested monkeys to be relatively resistant [70], not borne out by recent observations [89].

Sex and Age. Males have been reported to be somewhat more susceptible than females [472], but some studies show little difference or even greater susceptibility of females [348]. Newborn animals (rats) are resistant; susceptibility appears in the animals (e.g. 7-day old rats) at the time that the enzyme system for metabolism of foreign compounds appears in the hepatocytes [432]. Old rats appear to recover less rapidly and well from acute CCl_4-induced injury and to be somewhat more susceptible than younger, mature animals [357, 446, 478].

Diet. Early studies suggested that starvation in general and low carbohydrate and protein diets, in particular, increased susceptibility to CCl_4 toxicity [472]. McLEAN and his associates [347], who have contributed very importantly to an understanding of the problem, have demonstrated that protein deficiency not only does not enhance CCl_4 toxicity, but actually seems to protect against it. They have demonstrated that protein deficiency decreases the activity of the enzyme system which metabolizes CCl_4 and by a variety of observations confirmed the relevance of this change to inhibition of CCl_4 toxicity by protein deprivation [345, 347]. The adverse effects, reported in the past, of carbohydrate-depleted diet, appear to have been, at least in part, owing to the high fat content of the diet and the resultant fatty liver which perhaps increased localization of CCl_4 in the liver.

5. Experimental Injury

Carbon tetrachloride, even in a single dose, produces hepatic necrosis and steatosis in a variety of experimental animals and man, usually accompanied by lesions of other organs [472]. Necrosis when fully developed is centrizonal in all species when the agent is given by any route except direct injection into the portal system (see above). The necrosis may be midzonal rather than centrizonal in animals made thyrotoxic by administration of thyroid hormones before giving the CCl_4 [472]. Hydropic degeneration (balloon cells) in the midzonal area [70], and acidophilic degeneration and formation of free acidophilic bodies in the centrizonal area precede the centrolobular necrosis. These disappear when necrosis is maximal. To a varying degree neutrophilic and mononuclear leukocytes accumulate at the site of early single cell necrosis [472]. Fat accumulates first in the centrizonal area; as the lesion proceeds fat is seen in the cells peripheral to the necrosis.

Biochemical changes in the blood reflect the injury sensitively. Serum enzyme levels, are elevated within 3 hrs and reach a peak at 12 to 36 hrs, depending on the intracellular locus of the respective enzyme and the dose of CCl_4 [496, 440]. Levels of LD, aldolase, PHI, sorbitol dehydrogenase reach a peak at 12 hrs; those of GOT and MD peak by 24 hrs and those of glutamate dehydrogenase and GPT are highest at 36 hrs [440]. In general, this follows the pattern of elevation of levels of enzymes derived from the cytosol before the increased values of those leaked from mitochondria [440].

Recovery begins by 24 hrs with the appearance of mitotic figures. Removal of necrotic debris begins by 48 hrs and is usually complete by one week. By 14 days the liver is restored to normal [472, 70].

6. Evolution of Hepatic Injury

The interval between administration of the agent to experimental animals and the development of hepatic injury is very brief. By 12 hrs after the toxin is given there is early evidence in the central zone of necrosis, that consists of individually degenerated and necrotic cells and acidophilic bodies accompanied by hydropic degeneration (ballooning) of cells in the midzonal area. By 24 to 48 hrs the necrosis is maximal [472, 70, 295, 594, 214].

More subtle changes occur earlier. Within the first hour the central zone shows loss of hepatocyte basophilia, and pyrinophilia and ultrastructural evidence of increased cytoplasmic lipids in the central zone [472]. The fat can be seen as droplets by EM at 1 hr and by light microscopy at 3 hrs. By 5 to 6 hrs initial evidence of single cell necrosis appears. Lipid droplets can be seen at this time in surviving centrizonal cells and in midzonal cells which also show hydropic degeneration (balloon cells) [472].

Ultrastructural studies in many laboratories have revealed changes in the hepatocyte almost immediately after administration of the toxin [432]. By 15 min the endoplasmic reticulum shows evidence of injury. Vacuoles form in the cisternae; and the ribsomes disappear from the RER and are seen scattered through the cytoplasm. The SER, normally in parallel arrays closely oriented to the mitochondria, develops a chaotic, fragmented appearance. Ultimately the SER and degranulated RER coalesce into labyrinthine tubular aggregates [472, 531, 544]. These changes in the ER ("membrane denaturation") [449] are the ultrastructural equivalent of the loss of basophilia and pyrinophilia observed by light microscopy. Abnormalities and destruction of lysozomes become apparent by 5 to 6 hrs and mitochondrial abnormalities can be seen by 10 to 20 hrs. The mitochondrial changes consist of enlargement, disappearance of cristae and degranulation [472]. GOLGI apparatus changes consist of a loss of the normally present dense particles which is presumed to reflect depressed lipoprotein assembly [432].

Biochemical changes can be correlated with the histologic abnormalities. Within one hour ribosomal enzyme (glucose-6-phosphatase, NADPH reductase, aminopyrine demethylase, aniline demethylase, cytochrome P-450 activity is depressed, protein synthesis is inhibited, and there is polysome disaggregation (80s polysomes decrease). Impairment of protein synthesis can be demonstrated by decreased incorporation of leucine 1-C^{14} into hepatic lipoprotein and of glycine C^{14} into plasma albumin, fibrinogen and gamma globulin [432] within 1 hr. Chemical measurement demonstrates that lipid content is increased by over 30% at 1 hr and by 140% at 3 hrs [432]. Recently RECKNAGEL and GLINDE [432] have demonstrated striking qualitative as well as quantitative change in hepatic lipids to be induced promptly (within minutes) after CCl_4 administration. The earliest and main changes appear to involve the phospholipids of the ER. Within one hour there is a decrease in unsaturated fatty acids, accompanied by the presence of a variety of saturated, long-chain, branched fatty acids some of which are chlorinated or methylchlorinated. The remaining polyunsaturated fatty acids have undergone shifts in the hydrocarbons tails and there is cross-linking between fatty acids. Those changes which can be assumed to alter the physical properties of the ER and are the apparent biochemical counterparts of the ultrastructural changes observed, have been attributed to peroxidation of the membrane lipids [121].

Biochemical evidence of mitochondrial injury occurs relatively late. Although enzymologic evidence of injury to mitochondria has been demonstrated by a number of workers [240], it does not become demonstrable for a number of hours after damage to other organelles [432]. Very large doses of CCl_4, however, can lead by two hours to decrease in the P/O ratio and to a doubling of Ca^{++} ion content of mitochondria, but more significant biochemical evidence of mitochondrial injury usually does not occur until 10 to 20 hrs. At 10 to 15 hrs change in the mitochondrial membrane can be deduced from the observation that aged mitochondria rapidly lose pyridine nucleotides *in vitro*, and the tricarboxylic acid cycle is disorganized [517]. By 10 hrs there is abnormality of mitochondrial ATPase, loss of respiratory control by mitochondria and impaired mitochondrial oxidation of fatty acids [472]. The role of mitochondrial damage in the pathogenesis of the lesion of CCl_4 poisoning remains unclear, and continues to be the subject of study [317, 318]. Recent data suggest that it may be significant [317, 318].

7. Mechanism of Injury

Studies of the past quarter-century have clarified the mechanism of hepatic injury [430, 432]. An early concept [209] attributed the hepatic necrosis to the centrizonal ischemia, secondary to the decrease in blood flow through sinusoids partially obliterated by swollen parenchymal cells initially injured because of their location at the periphery of the lobule. While GLYNN and HIMSWORTH [173] provided evidence that sinusoidal flow was impaired at some stages of CCl_4 poisoning, there has been a wealth of subsequent data (SENEVIRATNE [508], STONER [550]) which indicates that the sinusoids remain fully patent and that blood flow to the central zone remains adequate until *after* centrizonal injury has occurred. Furthermore, the demonstration by BRAUER [53] that perfusion of the liver *in vitro* by $CHCl_3$ led to the centrizonal locus of injury even when blood flow was reversed by use of the hepatic vein as the afferent vessel, indicated the site of necrosis to be a characteristic of the toxin and not a consequence of the effect on hepatic blood flow.

The "catecholamine hypothesis" has attributed the hepatic effects of carbon tetrachloride to its stimulation of central autonomic centers and the resultant massive increase in the catecholamine levels of the blood [430, 526]. Proposed by BRODY and his associates [69, 57], it attributed the fatty changes in the liver to the excessive mobilization of free fatty acids from the fat depots induced by the lipolytic effects of the increased circulating catecholamines, and the centrobular necrosis to the catecholamine-induced decrease in hepatic blood flow. While these workers marshalled considerable evidence that seemed to support their view, the critical studies by LARSON and PLAA [296] demonstrated that intact autonomic responses *permitted* CCl_4 toxicity to be expressed, but that autonomic discharge could not be held accountable for the hepatotoxicity. The demonstration by BRAUER [53] of a toxic effect of $CHCl_3$ on the *ex-vivo* perfused rat liver, excluded an important role of altered blood flow and autonomic factors from the mechanism of toxicity. While the essence of the theory of BRODY *et al.* [57] appears not to describe the main pathogenesis of the hepatic injury, evidence that some mobilization of lipid from the depots contributes to the hepatic steatosis has been offered by SCHAFFRIR [492]. The available evidence [430, 432] suggests that the factors proposed by BRODY *et al.* are less important than the direct effect of the hepatotoxins on the liver.

Crucial to an understanding of the mechanism for CCl_4 – induced hepatic injury are the recent investigations [430, 432, 240] which indicate that the fatty metamorphosis and hepatic necrosis are independent toxic effects of carbon tetrachloride. Fat accumulation begins in experimental animals with one hour after the toxin is administered, at a time of peak concentration of the CCl_4 in the liver. Hepatic necrosis occurs later, at about 12 hrs, and reaches its maximum approximately 24 to 36 hrs after the hepatotoxin has been administered. Most critical in demonstrating the independence of steatosis and necrosis, is the observation that these two histologic sequela of carbon tetrachloride administration can be dissociated by pretreatment with a number of "surface-protective" agents which prevent the hepatic necrosis, but not the fatty metamorphosis, or by other agents that permit the necrosis by not the steatosis. The mechanism for the production of steatosis seems quite clear; that for the production of necrosis is subject to much more speculation.

The *fatty metamorphosis* appears to result from inability of the liver to rid itself of lipid transported to it in normal amounts as proposed by RECKNAGEL and GLINDE [430, 432] or in increased amounts as suggested by BRODY and his associates [69] and by SCHAFFRIR [492]. This defect in transport of fat out of the liver has been attributed by Recknagel [430, 432] to damage of the endoplasmic reticulum and to the resulting inability to convert the lipid to the molecular form necessary for secretion into the blood. Consistent with this hypothesis are the observations of ROBINSON and SEAKINS [460], REES and SHOTLANDER [439], SMUCKLER and his associates [96, 532, 533, 451] and others [432] who have demonstrated a defect in synthesis of the lipoprotein necessary for transport of fat from the liver.

The pathogenosis of the necrosis remains obscure [240]. It has been attributed to the alteration of the permeability of cell and mitochondrial membranes, that is induced by carbon tetrachloride. The altered cell membrane permeability leads to the loss of intracellular potassium and soluble protein, including cytoplasmic enzymes and coenzymes and to an intracellular accumulation of water and calcium with an adverse effect on the mitochondrial membrane which leads to a loss of mitochondrial enzymes and coenzymes [240]. The resulting disruption of the energy-yielding oxidative phosphorylation has been suggested [348, 236] to be possibly responsible for the development of hepatic necrosis. The prevention of hepatic necrosis by pretreatment with antihistaminic and other compounds has been attributed [348, 240] to the ability of these substances to inhibit changes in membrane permeability, induced by an effect of carbon tetrachloride (and its metabolites) on the lipids of the membranes.

Early view held that CCl_4 exerted its hepatotoxic effect as a powerful lipid solvent which injured the lipid-rich membranes of the hepatocyte [430, 235]. Evidence is now conclusive that it is a metabolite of this agent, rather than the native molecule which is mainly responsible foe the hepatic injury [432]. The very low doses of CCl_4 that can produce hepatic injury, and the striking predilection of the liver for injury, despite equally high concentration of the agent in blood, bone marrow and heart clearly indicate that the hepatotoxicity cannot be primarily a result of the lipid-solvent properties of this toxin [432].

The view that the toxic actions of CCl_4 are mediated through a metabolite is strongly supported by the available evidence [432]. Circumstances and manipulations that enhance its metabolism increases its hepatotoxicity and *vice versa* [432]. Members of species susceptible to CCl_4 toxicity are able to metaboolize the agent; those that are resistant cannot [432]. The newborn rat fails to metabolize CCl_4 and is resistant to its adverse effect; the resistance disappears as soon as metabolizing ability appears in the 1-week-old rat [432]. The hepatotoxicity of the agent is diminished by a protein-restricted diet and by the administration of dibenamine, cobaltous chloride and other agents that inhibit the drug-metabolizing activity of the ER. An extremely interesting manifestation of this phenomenon is the effect of very small doses of CCl_4 on the subsequent toxicity of the agent [432]. RECKNAGEL and his associates have demonstrated that the subtle injury induced by small doses of the toxin interfered with drug-metabolizing ability sufficiently to render a subsequent dose of CCl_4 virtually non-toxic [432]. Conversely, administration of phenobarbitol, DDT or other agents that enhance the drug-metabolizing activity of the rat ER, enhances strikingly the hepatotoxic effects of CCl_4. The centrolobular location of CCl_4-induced hepatic necrosis has been attributed [520] to the concentration in the central zone of the enzyme system for the metabolism of this and other foreign compounds.

The metabolism of CCl_4 has been studied by a number of workers [432]. It appears to consist of a series of reactions, the first being homolytic cleavage of the molecule to yield the free radicals $CCl_3^{\cdot}$ and $Cl^{\cdot}$. Subsequent metabolism would be expected to yield $CHCl_3$ and ultimately CO_2 as confirmed by studies after administration of $C^{14}Cl_4$ [432]. Small amounts of hexachlorethane, presumably the result of condensation of two molecules of trichloromethyl free radicals, are formed; and, when demonstrated, are a useful measure of the metabolism of CCl_4 [432].

There is a consensus in the literature that the metabolite responsible for hepatic injury is a free radical ($CCl_3^{\cdot}$), formed by homolytic cleavage of CCl_4. Originally proposed by BUTLER [67] and by WIRTSCHAFTER and CRONYN [623], this view has been supported by a large body of evidence recently summarized by RECKNAGEL and GLENDE [432]. They have coined the term "lethal cleavage" for this conversion of a non-toxic molecule to a toxic product. The mechanism by which the free radical produces damage remains controversial. RECKNAGEL and GLINDE [432] have proposed that the free radical produces peroxidation of the unsaturated lipids of the ER, which results in distortion and destruction of the membranes and produces new free radicals derived from the lipids of the membrane, a form of chain reaction. They attribute damage to other hepatocyte organelles to these secondary free radicals derived from the initial effect of the $CCl_3^{\cdot}$ on the lipids of the ER. In a closely reasoned argument RECKNAGEL and GLENDE [432] have marshalled the evidence in support of the role of peroxidation of lipids as the cause of hepatic injury and against the importance of alkylation or oxidation of thiol groups or direct attacks on proteins, nuclei acid polymers or nucleotides. While there is general agreement on the importance of the metabolism of CCl_4 in its hepatotoxicity and of the probable role of a free radical metabolite, there are others who believe peroxidation to be a relatively minor accompaniment of CCl_4 injury rather than a pathogenic mechanism of importance [432].

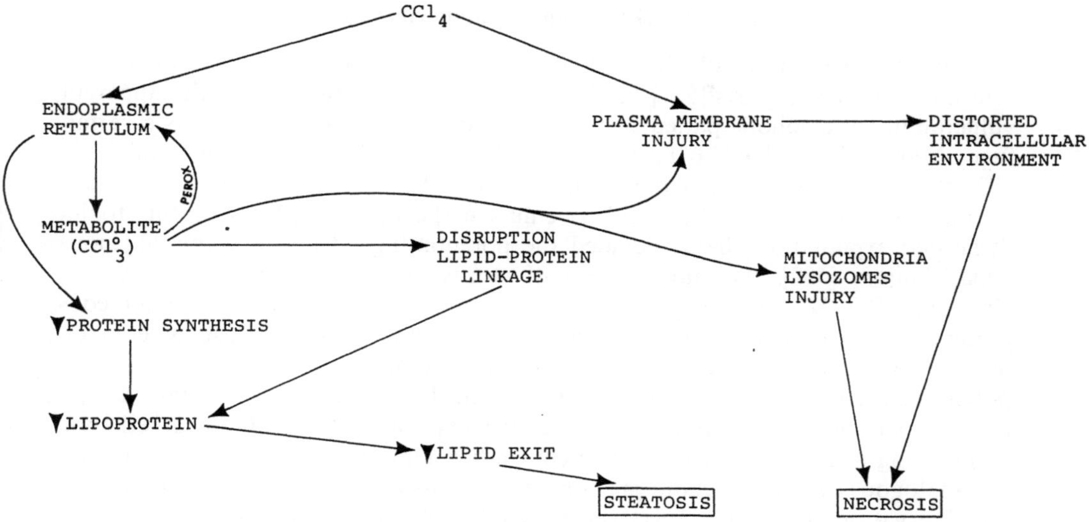

Fig. 2. Presumed mechanism for CCl_4-induced hepatic injury

Despite the general agreement that the hepatotoxicity depends mainly on conversion of CCl_4 to a toxic metabolite, there is evidence that native non-metabolized CCl_4 may contribute to the injury [638, 276, 645], particularly that of the plasma membrane [645, 302] of the hepatocyte. This is suggested by the almost immediate, adverse effects of CCl_4 on cells that are presumably unable to metabolize the agent [276] the demonstration of a deleterious effect of CCl_4 on isolated membranes [645] and mitochondria [433] *in vitro* and by the demonstration of some tissue injury by CCl_4 in chickens and ducks, species unable to metabolize the agent [432]. The 10-fold greater toxicity of CCl_4 for rats than for chickens [432], however, would indicate that the adverse effect of unmetabolized CCl_4 is a minor component of the toxicity of this agent.

Summary of the available evidence, according to the interpretation of this reviewer, would suggest the hypothetical scheme for the pathogenesis of CCl_4 toxicity formulated in Fig. 2.

Immediate injury to the plasma membrane by nonmetabolized CCl_4 leads to loss of intracellular enzymes and electrolytes and entry of ions from the extracellular environment (e.g. Ca^{++}). Almost simultaneously with this beginning distortion of this intracellular environment, there may be prompt metabolism of CCl_4 to the damaging metabolite (free radical) in the endoplasmic reticulum. This organelle, the site of the earliest and greatest concentration of the metabolite, suffers peroxidative disruption of membranes and dissociation of the lipoprotein transport system from the lipids which require transport. The result is steatosis. Subsequently, as the metabolite accumulates and leads to secondary free radicals, peroxidative injury of mitochondrial, lysosomal and plasma membranes occurs and, presumably, leads to necrosis.

8. Alcohol and Carbon Tetrachloride Toxicity

Ethanol potentiation of CCl_4 hepatotoxicity has been recognized for a half-century. The early reports [527] of CCl_4 poisoning drew attention to the apparent vulnerability of alcoholic patients to hepatotoxic effects of CCl_4, given as a vermifuge. Many clinical [269, 638, 394, 520, 341, 294, 165] and experimental [102, 572, 599, 165, 470, 598, 22] observations which have appeared since then have documented the ability of alcohol to enhance the adverse effects of this toxin. Suggested explanations have included the potentiating effects of alcohologenous hepatic injury [402], the enhancement of storage of CCl_4 in the fatty liver of alcoholics [502, 22], and the enhancement of absorption of CCl_4 by the simultaneous presence of ethanol in the gastrointestinal tract [269]. A single dose of ethanol, however, given to an experimental animal many hours before the CCl_4 also can potentiate the hepatotoxicity without pre-existent liver damage, in general, or steatosis in particular [102]. Even the attractive hypothesis [638, 308] that ethanol, by inducing microsomal metabolizing enzymes potentiates CCl_4 toxicity in a manner analogous to phenobarbital pre-treatment seems belied by the acute experimental observations [102]. The mechanism of ethanol potentiation remains obscure. Future hypotheses will need to explain the potentiating ability of a variety of other alcohols [102, 599] (Isopropanol, n-propanol, n-butyl, isobutyl, secondary butyl and tertiary butyl alcohol) and the demonstration that peak potentiation is achieved when the alcohol is given 18 hrs before the CCl_4 [102]. The selective potentiation by ethanol of only some manifestations of CCl_4 toxicity (elevated serum enzyme levels) but not of others (impairment of drug metabolism and accumulation of fat) reported by WEI *et al.* [599] while not in agreement with the studies of TRAEGER and PLAA [102] also may prove to be an important clue to the mechanism of ethanol potentiation. WEI *et al.* [599] have proposed that ethanol may provoke output of catecholamines, which have been shown [504] to potentiate CCl_4 toxicity.

9. Chronic Toxicity of Carbon Tetrachloride

a) Cirrhosis

Chronic injury can result from prolonged exposure to the agent. Repeated administration of sublethal doses can lead to cirrhosis in a variety of species (dogs, rats, rabbits, guinea pigs, mice, hamsters). In order to produce cirrhosis, the dose of CCl_4 must be small enough to permit survival, large enough to produce overt injury, and given at intervals that permit only partial recovery from each insult [70]. CAMERON and KARUNARATNE [70] found that does of 1 ml/kg administered to rats at intervals of 3 or 4 days led to cirrhosis by 5 weeks or before. Similar doses at intervals of 10 days and tiny doses (0.02 ml/kg) at intervals of 3 days failed to produce cirrhosis. Administration of the toxin by feeding, gastric intubation, subcutaneous or intraperitoneal injection or by inhalation all are successful in producing the cirrhosis, provided the principles cited above are observed. The rate of development of cirrhosis can be strikingly accelerated by administration of phenobarbital to enhance metabolism of the CCl_4 (instant cirrhosis) [351].

The morphological character of the cirrhosis as described by most investigators is micronodular and resembles that of Laennec's cirrhosis in humans. DOMINIS *et al.* [125], however, have described macronodular cirrhosis ("postnecrotic cirrhosis") in rats sacrificed at 8 to 12 weeks and "diffuse nonseptal cirrhosis" in animals sacrificed 5 to 7 weeks after repeated exposure to CCl_4 vapors.

The microscopic changes include architectural distortion with marked fibrosis, many small pseudolobules that have no identifiable relationship to the normal hepatic vasculature or excretory tree and distortion of the hepatic vasculature and microvasculature [70, 376, 233, 20, 21, 473, 475, 582, 596, 196, 31, 488, 445, 562, 543, 560, 197]. The destruction of the hepatic venous drainage system of lobular sinudoidal channels leads to a postsinusoidal block of hepatic blood flow, the development of venular communications between the portal and hepatic veins within the fibrous septa, and an irreversible portal hypertension [376, 233, 20, 21, 473, 475, 582, 596, 196, 31, 488, 445, 560, 562, 543]. Thrombosis of the central veins indicative of CCl_4-induced injury to the venous endothelium has been described by REUBER and GLOVER [445]. Indeed, the model of cirrhosis produced by CCl_4 reproduces most of the features of cirrhosis in humans; portal hypertension, an elaborate collateral venous development, ascites and abnormal hepatic function [376, 233, 20, 21, 473, 475, 582, 596, 196, 31, 488, 445, 560, 562, 543]. The model, accordingly, has been called on repeatedly for the study of cirrhotogenesis. The extensive studies have demonstrated that the hepatic injury provokes both hepatocyte proliferation and fibrogenesis [213]. The latter is an expression of an active metabolic role of connective tissue manifested by increased hepatic and plasma content of hydroxyproline-containing peptides and sulfated mucopolysaccharides [211, 213]. The studies, which have demonstrated that there is a balance between the fibrogenesis and fibrolysis, have provided a foundation for the efforts at therapy that include steps to inhibit fibrogenesis or enhance collagenolysis [466]. *Biochemical manifestations* of hepatic injury during the development of cirrhosis are prominent only at the times of acute injury from the intermittent doses [66]. Elevated serum enzyme levels like those of acute toxicity are seen at these times [66]. After administration of CCl_4 has been discontinued, however, enzyme levels are minimally abnormal. Low serum albumin levels, impaired dye clearance and depressed plasma coagulation factors are characteristic [217]. Fibrinogen levels may be low, apparently both because of decreased synthesis and increased catabolism [579].

b) *Carcinogenesis*

The carcinogen potency of CCl_4 is relatively low grade. Prolonged administration can lead to "hyperplastic nodules" and carcinogenesis in mice, rats, hamsters and rabbits. The *buffalo* strain of rats is described to be particularly susceptible [443]. Only rare instances of metastases from the CCl_4-induced hepatocellular carcinoma have been [443, 444, 447].

10. Other Halogenated Hydrocarbons

Several other halogenated hydrocarbons produce hepatic injury similar to that of CCl_4 poisoning presumably by similar distortion of the ultrastructure of the cell. Apparently haloalkanes with bond dissociation energies lower than that of CCl_4 are even more potent hepatotoxins than CCl_4 and are also lipoperoxidant; while those with higher bond dissociation energies ($CHCl_3$, trichlorethylene) are less potent toxins and apparently lead to less or no lipid peroxidation (432]. There is evidence that, for at least some members of the latter group (e.g. $CHCl_3$), enhanced metabolism of the compound enhances toxicity [240]. Some halogenated hydrocarbons produce only fatty metamorphosis, even more trivial hepatic injury or none [394].

II. Phosphorous

The white allomorph of elemental phosphorous also appears to produce its hepatic injury by a direct attack on cell constituents. The injury consists of hepatic steatosies and, when severe, necrosis [472, 297, 92, 7, 331, 42, 364, 293, 477, 118, 231, 153, 505, 163, 400]. It develops much less rapidly than that of CCl_4, however, and the role of lipid peroxidation is in dispute [167, 505, 163]. Phosphorous toxicity also appears to differ from that of CCl_4 in that it does not require conversion to a tissue damaging metabolite [220]; it produces drastic injury to many tissues [293, 477, 231, 602] and does not appear to be enhanced by phenobarbital pretreatment [220].

Phosphorous poisoning has been a known cause of hepatic injury for a century. Indeed, it was included in the earliest studies [637, 98] of experimental studies of hepatotoxicity.

1. Chemical Properties

Elemental phosphorous is a protoplasmic poison, but only the white (yellow) allomorph is toxic when ingested [477, 118]. The red allomorph is insoluble and unabsorbable; but the white form is soluble in fats and in bile, and forms a colloidal solution in water. It is absorbed rapidly from the gastro-intestinal tract [477, 168]. It also can be absorbed from the skin [477] and from subcutanous [3] and intraperitoneal sites [231].

2. Toxicity in Humans

Poisoning of humans has occurred after accidental or suicidal ingestion of rodenticides, insecticides, firecrackers or matches that contain phosphorous [293, 118, 153, 505]. Tiny amounts of phosphorous (15 to 60 mg) can produce toxic manifestations or even death [118]. Outlawing of the use of phosphorous in the manufacture of match tips and fireworks in industrial countries has decreased the incidence of poisoning; although cases continue to occur in some parts of the world [484].

The syndrome is highly fatal with mortality rates of 50% or more [293, 477, 118, 484]. Initial manifestations include vomiting, hematemesis and abdominal pain, peripheral vascular collapse, delirium and convulsions. After a period of symptomatic improvement, hepatic and renal failure appear, often accompanied by heart failure and neurologic involvement [602].

a) Histopathology

Histologic changes in the liver include fatty metamorphosis and other degenerative changes in hepatocytes and necrosis [331, 484]. The long-accepted view of the lesion has emphasized the periportal location of the main hepatic injury. Some recent reports have challenged this view [484] and autopsy studies usually show panlobular fatty metamorphosis [484]. Nevertheless, biopsy studies of patients [293, 153] and observations in experimental phosphorous poisoning [231] have indicated that fat accumulates first or mainly in the periportal hepatocytes. Fat droplets are small [331] yielding a pattern of microvesicular steatosis somewhat similar to that observed in ethionine or tetracycline toxicity. Necrosis when present also begins in the periportal zone [484], although scattered areas and foci of necrosis may be found throughout the lobule.

b) Blood Changes

There is only fragmentary information on *biochemical* abnormalities in the blood. In general they appear to resemble those produced by toxic steatosis of other causation (e.g. tetracycline). Jaundice, even in fatal human cases is modest [118]. Levels of the transaminases (both GOT and GPT) are increased only slightly in experimental injury [167]. This is in striking contrast to the markedly elevated values observed after CCl_4 administration [644, 647]. Depressed plasma coagulation factors are reflected in the prolonged one-stage prothrombin time [153]. Depressed urea formation has been cited [117], but levels of blood urea are not depressed in most instances [293, 118, 153], probably because of the usually concomitant renal injury. Plasma triglyceride levels are depressed in experimental animals given phosphorous [167]. Hypoglycemia is frequent in fatal cases [118]. Hyperphosphatemia, curiously, is a late development, occurring four to 5 days after the phosphorous has been taken [118].

3. Experimental Animals and Susceptibility

There have not been the extensive studies on species susceptibility to phosphorous poisoning that have marked the investigation of CCl_4 and other hepatotoxins. Dogs [596], rats [42, 231, 505, 163, 400, 168], guinea pigs [297] and rabbits [118] all are vulnerable. Even invertebrates such as the lobster are vulnerable and show severe damage to the hepatopancreas on exposure to white phosphorous [3]. There is no evidence of dependence of susceptibility on age or sex. Most studies have employed rats.

4. Acute Toxicity

In rats fat appears, by light microscopy, at 12 to 18 hrs and reaches a peak by 72 to 96 hrs, after a single intraperitoneal dose (0.5—1.0 mg/100 g). First seen in the periportal hepatocytes the steatosis progresses toward the central vein. Regression of the lesion in surviving animals is in the opposite direction, the centrolobular hepatocytes being the first to lose the fat.

Loss of basophilia by parenchymal cells, which is apparent by 12 hrs, also is first seen in cells at the periphery of the lobule. It involves the entire lobule by 36 hrs.

Ultrastructural studies [297, 400] show small amounts of fat at 12 hrs, but according to GANOTE and OTIS [400] no other significant abnormalities after single doses (0.75 to 0.9 mg/100 g). By 24 hrs there is a marked increase in RER [400]. With small doses there are no further changes. After larger doses there is progression of the lesion, with formation by 48 hrs of concentric lamellae surrounding mitochondria and nucleus. Smooth ER remains relatively unaffected unless injury is severe. In cells undergoing necrosis, SER increases strikingly while RER and ribosomes may virtually disappear; and in cells that have become necrotic all ER may have disappeared. GOLGI cisternae seem empty, but otherwise show little structural abnormality. GANOTE and OTIS [400] consider these ultrastructural abnormalities to be relatively characteristic of elemental phosphorous poisoning and to differ distinctly from those of several other hepatotoxins. JEZEQUEL has described ultrastructural evidence of organelle injury to occur somewhat earlier [118].

5. Chronic Toxicity

Administration of small daily oral doses (1 mg/Kg) to rabbits and guinea pigs for 4 to 6 months leads to cirrhosis [331]. According to MALLORY [331] injury of fibroblasts and of hepatocytes leads to the fibrotic response. The cirrhotic process begins in the periportal zone but thereafter involves all segments of the lobule and eventuates in a micronodular form of cirrhosis [331].

6. Mechanism of Injury

The mechanism for the hepatotoxicity of elemental phosphorous remains unclear. The accumulation of fat seems clearly to be the result of impaired exit of fat from the liver [400, 311, 574, 575, 119]. Impaired protein synthesis has been demonstrated [505] to occur as early as 2 hrs after a dose of phosphorous, and deficient production of apolipoprotein may be suspected to be responsible at least in part for the steatosis [505, 311, 575]. The basis for the necrosis remains obscure.

Efforts to unravel the significance, with regard to mechanism of injury, of the chronological events in phosphorous poisoning have led to conflicting interpretations. Impressive organelle (RER) injury and fat accumulation is seen only at 24 hrs [231, 163]; yet 70% of an oral dose accumulates in the liver by 2 hrs [168]. This has led GHOSHAL *et al.* [167] to propose that the delay reflects the time required for the conversion of phosphorus to a metabolite responsible for the hepatic injury. The demonstration by PANI *et al.* [400] that phenobarbital pretreatment does not enhance the toxic effects of phosphorous, however, seems to belie the view that a metabolite is responsible for the injury.

Evidence for [167, 119] and against lipoperoxidation [400] as the mechanism for organelle injury has been presented.

DI LUZIO [119] has interpreted the effectiveness of an antioxidant in preventing the development of fatty liver in phosphorous-intoxicated rats as evidence for the importance of lipoperoxidation in the production of the lesion. GHOSHAL *et al.* [167] demonstrated increased diene conjugation at 4 and 24 hrs after a dose of phosphorous. They found this evidence of lipoperoxidation to be largely evident in the microsomal fraction of the hepatocyte, and attributed the phenomenon to the preferential attachment of phosphorous to microsomes. PANI *et al.* [400], however, were unable to demonstrate lipid peroxidation in the phosphorous-poisoned rats but found that antioxidants which are also free radical scavengers (propyl gallate, glutathione) can protect against the adverse effect on the liver.

The available information, accordingly, suggests that phosphorous toxicity leads to hepatic steatosis by a somewhat delayed effect on fat transport from the liver by a mechanism that remains to be understood. Lipoperoxidation seems to play a minor role [167, 163]; but free radicals, conceivably generated by the effect of phosphorus on membrane lipids [297], may play a role in the injury to polysomes, RER and the consequent impairment of protein synthesis. We have chosen to categorize phosphorus with CCl_4 and several other chlorinated hydrocarbons, as direct hepatotoxins, since it has a directly disruptive effect on metabolic machinery, not recognizably dependent on a selective metabolic block.

I. Indirect Hepatotoxins

Agents that damage the liver by diversion or competitive inhibition of essential metabolites were dubbed by HIMSWORTH [209] "trophopathic" toxic agents. We have referred [638, 639] to these as *indirect* hepatotoxins and have included in this category antimetabolites and other compounds that by modifying key molecules in the cell (e.g. alkylation of purines and pyrimidines of nucleic acids by DMN) or by other selective metabolic blocks lead to metabolic aberration and hepatocyte injury. The selective interference with metabolism results in structural or functional damage of the liver. For a number of agents such selective metabolic injury to the liver has been identified (e.g. ethionine) and a reasonable formulation for the probable pathway by which the injurious effect is produced (Table 10). For others, the known antimetabolic effect in other biologic systems (e.g. tetracycline in bacteria) permits the inference that a similar effect in mammals can account for the liver damage [638, 639].

Two types of indirect hepatotoxins can be recognized (Table 10). One produces *cytotoxic* injury by interfering with metabolic pathways or processes essential for parenchymal cell integrity. The other produces *cholestasis,* interfering only or mainly with biliary secretion, but usually sparing the parenchyma [638, 639].

I. Cytotoxic Indirect Hepatotoxins

A large number of synthetic compounds, a number of agents of botanical origin and even some drugs employed in clinical medicine appear to warrant inclusion in this category [638, 639] (Table 10). Ethionine [140], puromycin [141, 469] dialkylnitrosamines [325], brombenzene [56], galactosamine [113] and thioacetamide [460] have been well studied and the information on the apparent mechanism of injury leads us to consider them useful prototypes of indirect hepatotoxicity.

Table 10. Types of indirect hepatotoxins

Type	Mechanism	Lesion	Agents
Cytotoxic	Selective interference with metabolic pathways (antimetabolites and related compounds)	Steatosis	L-Asparaginase Azacytidine Azaserine Azauridine Ethanol Ethionine Orotic acid Paromycin Tetracycline
		Necrosis	Brombenzene Phalloidin Thioacetamide Urethane
		Necrosis and steatosis	Aflatoxins cycasin DMN GALN Luteoskyrin PAS Tannic acid
Cholestatic	Selective interference with hepatic secretory mechanisms or injury of excretory pathway	Bile casts	Icterogenin, C-17 alkylated anabolic and estrogenic steroids
		Bile casts and bile duct injury[a]	ANIT
		Bile casts, bile[a] duct injury and periportal parenchymal injury	ANIT Sporidesmin
	Selective interference with sinusoid-hepatocyte transport or with bilirubin conjugation	No lesion-only unconjugated hyperbilirubinemia	Novobiocin Flavaspidic acid Rifampicin

[a] Character of injury varies with species.

Aflatoxin [68], ochratoxin [327], luteoskyrin [498], cycasin [498, 348] some toxins (amatoxins) of A. phalloides [612] and of Senecio and related species (pyrrolidizine alkaloids) [352, 60] tannic acid [435] and other agents of plant origin [498, 477, 348, 190, 269, 286, 638] produce hepatic injury by a selective interference with hepatocyte metabolism and hence, warrant categorization as indirect cytotoxic hepatotoxins (Table 10). Others of interest to clinicians are ethanol [308] and antibotics and antimetabolites which are employed as therapeutic agents, and can act as indirect hepatotoxins [639]. For example, tetracycline, L-asparaginase, urethane and 6-mercaptopurine are medicinal agents which can induce hepatic injury by mechanisms that probably are related to their selective interference with cell metabolism [639].

1. Types of Injury

Many of these agents produce steatosis (ethionine [140], ethanol [137], tetracycline [639], puromycin [460], asparaginase [639], aflatoxin [175]*. Some produce

* Under some conditions, and in some species, aflatoxins produce steatosis and under other conditions necrosis or both steatosis and necrosis. (See Section on Aflatoxins.)

mainly necrosis (bromobenzene [274], urethane [124], thioacetamide [65], 6-mercaptopurine [639], galactosamine [113]). Some indirect hepatotoxins produce both (amatoxins of A. phalloides [610, 612], tannic acid [472, 435], aflatoxins* [175] and dialkylnitrosamines [348]).

2. Mechanisms

The mechanism for the production of steatosis by hepatotoxins in all of the instances that have been studied [311], except that induced by a single intoxicating dose of ethanol [539, 227], involves inhibition of formation of the transport system for movement of lipid from the liver, or defective movement of the assembled lipoprotein across an altered plasma membrane. Many of the indirect cytotoxic hepatotoxins have the ability to interfere with protein synthesis by introducing a selective biochemical lesion into the cell, at the ribosomal level, by interference with DNA or RNA synthesis, or by some other form of injury to RNA or DNA [143] (Fig. 3). The steatosis has been attributed to deficient synthesis of the apoprotein moiety of the very low density lipoprotein (VLDL) by which lipids are transported from the liver [141] or interference with assembly of the VLDL [432]. The defect may be that of insufficient synthesis of the apoproteins *per se* [141] or of formation of an abnormal apoprotein, perhaps in its glycosylation [539]. Defective protein synthesis characterizes the adverse effect of a number of hepatotoxins [142]. However, there are agents that produce hepatic steatosis without inhibition of protein formation and agents that inhibit protein formation and yet produce little or no steatosis [539]. Orotic acid, for example, does not inhibit

Possible loci for mechanism of adverse effect of cytotoxic indirect hepatotoxins

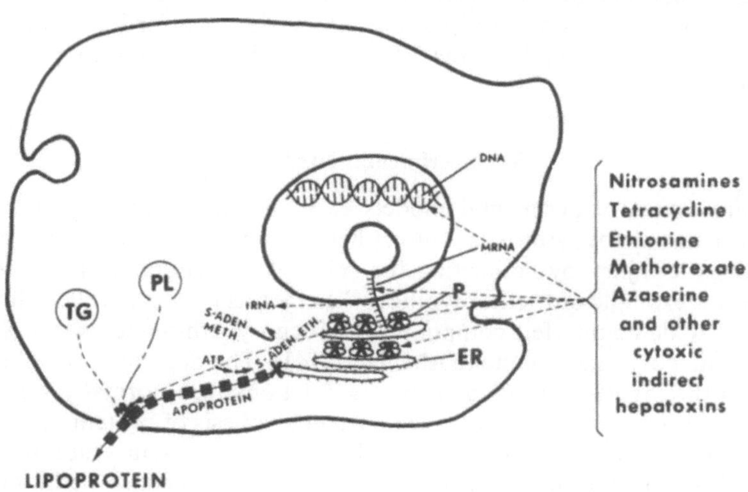

Fig. 3. Diagrammatic representation of loci and probable mechanism for production of hepatic injury (steatosis) induced by indirect, cytotoxic hepatotoxins. TG, triglycerides; PL, phospholipids; P, polysomes; ER, endoplasmic reticulum; S-ADEN-METH, *S*-adenosylmethionine; S-ADEN-ETH, *S*-adenosylethionine; ATP, mRNA, DNA, and tRNA have the usual meaning. (From ZIMMERMAN [639] with permission of editor and publisher)

protein formation, but can lead to fatty liver by interference with exit of lipid from the liver [539, 619]. STEIN *et al.* [539] have suggested that this may be the result of the demonstrated [421] impaired glycosylation of one of the apoprotein components of the VLDL. Defective assembly of the components of VLDL by which lipids are transported from the liver also may be responsible for the hepatic steatosis induced by some hepatotoxins [430, 432]. Altered properties of the membrane across which transport of VLDL occurs also might contribute to the hepatic steatosis induced by some agents [349]. MCLEAN and VERSCHUDDOREN [349] also have suggested that injury to the plasma membrane can lead to loss of potassium from the cell, which in turn can introduce a defect in lipoprotein transfer across the plasma membrane.

Evidence from several sources indicates that defective transport of lipid from the cell alone does not necessarily lead to fatty liver. There are agents (cycloheximide, actinomycin D) that inhibit protein synthesis to a marked degree without producing a significant degree of fatty metamorphosis [141]. FARBER [141] has suggested that, since these agents inhibit synthesis of triglycerides (TG) and synthesis of protein and yet do not lead to steatosis, TG synthesis must be intact in order to have depressed protein synthesis or assembly of lipoproteins lead to fatty liver. STEIN *et al.* [539] also have proposed that agents that produce steatosis do so by increased flow of free fatty acids from depots to the liver as well as by decreased exit of lipid from the liver.

Hepatic steatosis induced by these agents, accordingly, is the result of impaired exit of TG from the liver because of *defective synthesis* of the apoprotein moiety or *impaired assembly* of lipid with the apoprotein to form the VLDL by which lipid is transported from the liver, or alteration of cell membranes that leads to inhibited exit of lipid from the cell, provided lipid is available in normal or increased amounts. The defect in protein synthesis may be quantitative or qualitative, may be in the glycosylation of the protein needed to afford movement across membranes, or in the assembly of the VLDL from the lipid and apoprotein component (Fig. 3).

3. Experimental Models

There are several experimental models each of which illustrates the various possible mechanisms for cytotoxic, indirect hepatotoxicity. Ethionine, for example, produces hepatic injury by competing for ATP with methionine [140, 141, 143] (Fig. 3). In this example of "lethal synthesis" as PETERS [405] has called the *in-vitro* formation of toxic counterfeit compounds, S-adenosyl-ethionine (SAE) is formed instead of S-adenosyl-methionine (SAM) [140, 141]. The depletion of cellular ATP and perhaps the involvement of SAE in the reactions that normally utilize SAM appear to be responsible directly for the deficient synthesis of protein and indirectly by interfering with synthesis of RNA, needed to direct protein synthesis properly [140, 141]. This and the disaggregation of polysomes induced by ethionine leads to deficient synthesis of the apoprotein moiety and defective assembly of the lipoprotein needed to transport lipid from the liver, and results in steatosis [141].

Puromycin, an antibiotic of interest in experimental pathology and of clinical interest in the treatment of cancer, leads to a form of steatosis that resembles that produced by ethionine [141]. Puromycin also interferes with protein synthesis and leads to breakdown of polysomes [141]. The mechanism by which it inhibits protein synthesis appears to be attachment of the ribosome at the "P" site, supplanting the activated tRNA that would normally be attached. This leads to termination of the peptide molecule and formation of abnormal and incomplete proteins containing a terminal puromycin molecule [141].

Tetracyline (and its congeners) are antibiotics, which also are indirect, cytotoxic hepatotoxins [639]. These agents in high doses lead to a diffuse vacuolization of hepatocytes that consists of tiny droplets of lipid and non-lipid material [639, 54, 307]. This lesion occurs as a dose-related phenomenon, reproducible in experimental animals. It appears as a clinically important lesion in humans only when large doses are given parenterally and blood levels of the antibiotics are presumably high.

The mechanism has been shown [638, 54] to be inhibition of transport of lipid from the liver. The precise site of the defect remains unknown; conceivably it is related to the known [553] ability of tetracyline to inhibit protein synthesis by binding of tRNA *in vitro* systems; although other sites of injury to the lipid-transport system of the whole animal may be relevant.

Albitocin is a triterpinoid glycoside which can produce hepatic injury in rats [258]. Intraperitoneal injection into male rats was found by KERR [257] to lead to coagulation necrosis, basophilic bodies and steatosis in the periportal area of the lobule by 24 hrs. Ultrastructural changes in the hepatocyte include dilatation of the cisterna of the ER resembling those of pyrrolidyene alkaloids, and swelling and dense granulation of mitochondria [257]. Albitocin appears to be categorizable as an indirect hepatotoxin with its mode of toxicity presumably related to the mechanism of its other biologic properties.

Ethanol produces hepatic steatosis by mechanisms which appear to differ from those described for other hepatotoxins. The acute steatosis of large single doses of ethanol appears to be mainly the result of excess mobilization of lipid from the depots [227]. Chronic administration seems to be steatogenic by leading to increased synthesis, decreased oxidation, increased absorption and perhaps decreased exit of lipid [308]. A role for peroxidation of membrane lipids by ethanol and its metabolism has been proposed [120] and rejected [63] as a factor in the pathogenesis of alcoholgeneous hepatic injury. Recent studies by RUBIN and LIEBER [476] have demonstrated the ability of chronic administration of ethanol to primates to produce the gamut of hepatic injury observed in alcoholic humans. Alcoholic hepatitis with necrosis, "alcoholic hyaline", steatosis and cirrhosis all can be produced [476].

The mechanism for the induction of necrosis by the indirect hepatotoxins is obscure, as in the case of the direct. As cited above, a number of agents that produce specific metabolic defects in the cell produce necrosis or necrosis and steatosis. *Thioacetamide* produces central necrosis which, by light microscopy, resembles that of CCl_4 toxicity [348]. It also produces striking nuclear abnormalities [555], however, that suggest selective alterations of RNA. The dialkylnitrosamines produce necrosis and steatosis, presumably related to alkylation of purine and pyrimidene components of nucleic acids [325]. The manner in which the specific metabolic defects introduced by these agents leads to necrosis is quite unclear, but it seems reasonable to infer the metabolic lesion to be responsible for the tissue damage.

Brombenzene (and a number of other halobenzene derivatives) produces a dramatic centrizonal necrosis, accompanied by little or no steatosis [56, 274]. The extensive studies of BRODIE, GILLETTE and their coworkers have clarified to a considerable degree the mechanism for hepatic injury [169, 56]. In the course of these studies they have developed enormously potent models for the study of other hepatotoxic phenomena [368], the role of glutathione depletion and covalent binding to macromolecules, and have provided extremely important insight into mechanisms of hepatic injury produced by therapeutic agents [368].

The toxicity of bromobenzene appears to be mediated by its metabolic conversion by a cytochrome P-450 enzyme system to an epoxide which binds covalently to macromolecules [169, 56]. Glutathione traps the epoxide and only when the available glutathione is depleted does the binding of the epoxide to macromolecules occur. It is the latter that is presumably responsible for the manifest hepatic injury, although the manner in which it does so remains unclear.

Galactosamine produces hepatic necrosis which is not zonal and is accompanied by some hepatic steatosis [113]. The biochemical mechanism for toxicity resembles that of ethionine somewhat, in that GALN leads to a relative insufficiency of UTP, analogous to the insufficiency of ATP induced by ethionine [113]. The hepatic injury induced in the rat by these two compounds, however, differs. These differences and similarities may provide useful tools for examination of the role of the nucleotides in the maintenance of integrity of the hepatocyte.

The character and apparent pathogenesis of hepatic injury of a few of the indirect cytotoxic hepatotoxins is discussed at greater length in the following pages. Selected for inclusion are ethionine, thioacetamide, the dialkylnitrosamines, tannic acid, the aflatoxins, pyrrolidizine alkaloids, hepatotoxic mushrooms, galactosamine and orotic acid. Other agents that we believe to belong to this category are listed in Table 10.

4. Ethionine

The ethyl analogue of methionine (Fig. 4) has provided an excellent model for the study of experimental hepatic steatosis, cirrhosis and carcinoma [139, 140]. Toxic for the liver of many species [139, 140], the adverse effects seem attributable to a selective metabolic lesion [141, 142, 143]. Accordingly it is a prototype of *indirect, cytotoxic* hepatotoxins [638]. Ethionine was synthesized by DYER [129] in 1938 during the investigation of methionine metabolism and shown by her to be toxic to animals. Subsequently, FARBER *et al.* [275, 139] demonstrated that this agent could produce a fatty liver in rats. Extensive studies by FARBER and his associates, and by many others, during the past quarter-century have unravelled the remarkable biochemical phenomena associated with the induction by ethionine of hepatic injury [139, 613].

a) Significance

The chief importance of ethionine is the provision of an experimental model of a form of hepatotoxicity and hepatocarcinogenicity. It produces hepatic steatosis,

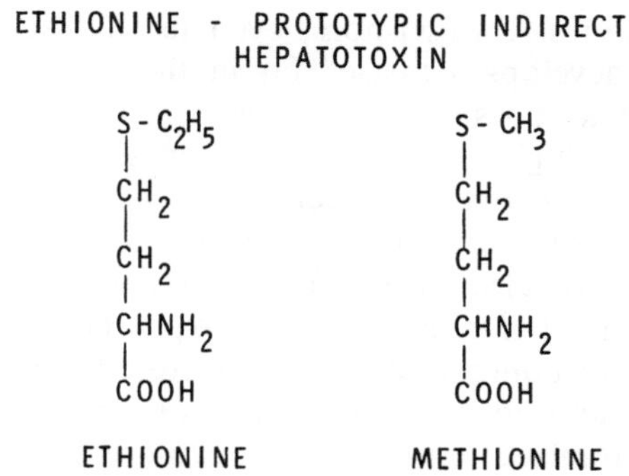

Fig. 4. Structure of ethionine and methionine

which in the rat is accompanied by little or no necrosis [610]. Prolonged administration can lead to cirrhosis and carcinoma [476, 417, 251, 593]. There is no evidence of disease in humans attributable to ethionine toxicity, other than the observation of hepatic injury during the one reported [608] effort to employ the compound in cancer chemotherapy. It is of interest, however, that there are several species of bacteria that produce ethionine [263]. One (a strain of E. coli) is a normal member of intestinal flora of mammals [139] and the possibility remains that ethionine might be an enterogenous hepatotoxin.

b) Chemical Properties

The chemical and physical properties of ethionine are very similar to those of methionine [139], to which it is an antimetabolite. The similarity of chemical reactivity accounts for the similarity of metabolic disposition in a wide variety of biological systems. Ethionine can serve as substrate for enzyme systems that act on methionine. Both optical isomers and the racemic form of ethionine are toxic, although L-ethionine is somewhat more potent. Presumably conversion of the D- to the L-isomer is accomplished by the D-amino oxidase of the tissues [139].

c) Factors in Susceptibility

Species. Most studies have employed rats [139, 140]. Other species with demonstrated susceptibility include mice, dogs, cats, guinea pigs, chickens, pigeons, rabbits and monkeys. Although there are important differences between these species in the type of response [139, 140], all exhibit some vulnerability to the hepatic injury. A variety of microorganisms show inhibition of metabolism and growth when exposed to ethionine [139].

Endocrine. Female rats are more susceptible than males to the hepatic injury [140]. The relative resistance of males depends on androgenic function; since it is lost after orchidectomy and provided to the female by administration of androgens [140]. The difference between males and females is not observed, or is not as striking, in other species. Furthermore, even in the rat careful studies have revealed that the male develops increased fat in the liver after ethionine, albeit to a much lesser degree than does the female. Increased susceptibility of the female has been ascribed to the higher activity of the enzyme that converts ethionine to S-adenosylethionine in females (see mechanism), a view that has recently been challenged [172]. The status of adrenal and anterior pituitary function also modifies ethionine effects [140]. Adrenalectomized female rats develop less hepatic steatosis than do females with intact adrenal function. Apparently replacement of both medullary and cortical hormones is required to restore the usual steatogenic effect of ethionine. The role of anterior pituitary function in the ethionine-induced injury is unclear. Hypophysectomized animals develop more hepatic steatosis than do intact animals; Somatotopin inhibits the ethionine effect, while ACTH and glucocorticoids increase it. Glucocorticoids inhibit the proliferation of ductular cells but not the hepatocarcinogenesis of chronic ethionine toxicity [139].

Age. Observations on the effect of age on ethionine toxicity are limited. Nevertheless, it is apparent that newborn as well as mature animals develop hepatic steatosis when given the agent [139, 140].

Diet. The effects of dietary ethionine is, of course, counteracted by supplementing the diet with methionine. Addition of large amounts of carbohydrate, especially as glucose [75, 424], can prevent the fat accumulation and the ultrastructural abnormalities of the nucleus, despite the fact that some of the biochemical abnormalities that result from ethionine are not presented. The mechanism by which glucose inhibits some of the adverse effects of ethionine is unclear. RAICH *et al.* [424] have suggested that insulin output provoked by glucose may enhance protein synthesis.

d) Form of Hepatic Injury

Single or repeated doses rapidly lead to hepatic steatosis in a variety of species [140]. In the rat no, or only focal, necrosis is produced [140]; while in the dog and rabbit [9] there is both fat and necrosis induced by repeated doses. Prolonged administration can lead to a curious ductular cell and bile duct proliferation [583], cirrhosis [251] and carcinoma [139].

Acute Effects. A single large dose (1.23 μMol) given to an adult female rat by injection or gastric intubation, is followed by a lag phase of 3 or 4 hrs. By 4 hrs there is a slight increase in hepatic triglycerides. Thereafter, there is a linear increase which reaches a peak at 24 to 48 hrs. By 6 hrs lipid values are 4 times the normal; and by 12 hrs fat content is 10-fold increased over control values. By 24 to 48 hrs, the hepatic fat content is increased 15 to 20 times the normal. These values, after a single dose, drop rapidly from the peak to reach the normal range by 72 to 100 hrs [140].

The histologic changes consist of accumulation of fat in relatively small droplets, first in the periportal hepatocytes and subsequently with progression centrally. (This order of development is the reverse of the steatosis of choline deficiency, which begins centrally and progresses peripherally.) The fat can first be seen by light microscopy by 6 to 7 hrs and by electron microscopy by 3 to 4 hrs [140].

Necrosis is minimal [129] or absent [140] in rats as reported by most [140] but not all [263] investigators. Dogs and rabbits develop degeneration and necrosis of hepatocytes, usually focal and at times diffuse [9, 595]. Conversely, fatty liver in these species is more variable in severity than in the rat.

Ultrastructural studies show the lipid to accumulate first in the vesicles of the SER and RER [140]. At first, the fat appears as small membrane-bound droplets at the sinusoidal pole of the hepatocyte. As the lesion progresses, the droplets are scattered throughout the cell and later fuse to form larger droplets, no longer membrane-bound. Lipid does not appear in the nucleus, although liposomes may be found within the double nuclear membrane [140].

The lipid which accumulates in the liver is virtually all triglyceride. The disproportionate increase in oleic and linoleic acids among the fatty acids of the TG fraction suggests the source to be depot fat [140].

Nuclear changes begin within 1 hr, with the appearance of small electron-dense spherules within the nucleolemma and at the periphery of the nucleoli [542]. Aggregates of interchromatin material surrounded by a zone of lighter density are prominent by 1 to 2 hrs. Between 4 and 6 hrs, distinction between fibrillar and granular zones becomes conspicuous and by 12 hrs there is dissociation of the fibrillar from the granular component of the nucleoplasm. By 24 hrs, the nuclear contour has become irregular; some cells show dilatation of the perinuclear space and there is condensation of chromatin along the nuclear membrane and around nucleoli. At this time there is also fragmentation of nucleoli, with dispersion of their structural elements interspersed with dense aggregates [513]. *Macrosegregation* and *nuclear* capping, such as occurs with DMN and several other toxins is not seen [555].

Disorganization of cytoplasmic organelles begins by 2 to 3 hrs and reaches a peak at 24 to 36 hrs after a single dose [513]. There is loss of parallel arrangement of the ER, disruption of the RER with an approximately 70% loss of polysomes and a corresponding accumulation of dispersed ribosome monomers, and dilatation of cisternal spaces. Progressive accumulation of lipid appears as increasing numbers of small and large lipid bodies with and without membranes [513].

By 36 hrs, reformation of polysomes appears despite the continued presence of multiple remnants of the disrupted RER, accompanied by proliferation of the SER often with concentric arrays of particle-free membranes "whorls" ("fingerprints"). By 48 hrs, the normal nucleolar morphology is usually restored. By 96 hrs, the cytoplasmic ultrastructure is restored to normal [369].

Chronic Effects. Bile duct proliferation and coarse, nodular cirrhosis develop in several species fed or injected chronically with ethionine [583, 251, 593], Curious, regenerative nodules, which develop in the rat after prolonged feeding, consist of areas of proliferation of bile ducts surrounded by fibrous tissue ("chologiofibrosis") [139]. Cancer of the liver, usually of the hepatocellular type and rarely cholangio-cellular carcinoma, occurs after prolonged (8 to 9 months) feeding of a diet containing 0.25% ethionine [139].

Chronic administration also produces distortion of lobular architecture as the result of proliferation of ductulor cells.

Cirrhosis. Prolonged administration of ethionine (0.5% DL-ethionine in the diet) to female rats leads to bile duct proliferation and "coarse nodular cirrhosis"

[555, 139, 583, 542, 251, 593, 513] within two months. The cirrhosis is preceded by fatty liver, focal necrosis and a striking proliferation of cells of ductular origin. Within one to three weeks of starting ethionine the small, round, ductular cells begin to accumulate in the periportal zone and gradually extend into the lobule. By two months the process has become extensive with two-thirds of the cells of the liver of ductular origin. The ductular cells appear to grow along sinuisoids, in the space of Disse and, by encircling individual or small clusters of hepatocyte, lead to dissociation and distortion of the structure of the liver. Some of the remaining hepatocytes, which at this stage compose only approximately 10% of the cells of the liver, undergo atrophy. Others become hypertrophic with large single or multiple hyperchromatic nuclei and an abundant easinophilic cytoplasm.

Carcinoma. Rats maintained on this diet for eight months or longer develop hepatocellular carcinoma [139]. In some animals the carcinoma develops as early as five months, and there are appreciable strain-differences in susceptibility. The HOLTZMAN strain of rats has seemed to be somewhat more resistant than Wistar or Fisher strains. Male and female rats, in contrast to the differential susceptibility to the acute effects of ethionine, are both susceptible to the hepatocarcinogenic effects. Diets ranging in composition between 0.2% and 1.0% ethionine have proved to be carcinoginic. Feeding the ethionine-containing diet for 8 or 9 months leads to carcinoma and cirrhosis in the non-cancerous liver, while feeding the ethionine diet for 5 months and then restoring a normal diet leads to an equal incidence of cancer but accompanied by relatively little cirrhosis. Administration of methionine can reverse the chronic hepatic injury if instituted prior to 4 months after starting ethionine administration, but not if given after 5 months [476].

Metabolic and Biochemical Effects. The metabolic effects of ethionine have been studied most extensively in the rat but also have been demonstrated in a number of other species [140, 476]. They include the production of deficiency of ATP, inhibition of synthesis of proteins, ethylation of several types of RNA and of several other cellular proteins, blockade of methylation of RNA and other cellular components, substitution of ethionine for the methionine of proteins and the formation of abnormal proteins (Figs. 3, 5) [141].

Impaired protein synthesis is demonstrable within 2 hrs after ethionine by the defective incorporation of labelled amino acid into protein in the whole animal or in separated hepatic ribosomes [141, 142, 143]. This defect is also apparent in impaired synthesis of plasma proteins, especially clotting factors, in the depressed hepatic levels of phosphorylase [515], urocanase [279] and ornithine carbamoylase [354] as well as in the prevention by ethionine of the increased hepatic enzyme content induced by diet, polycyclic hydrocarbons, hormones or regenerative activity [133]. Accompanying the fatty liver of acute ethionine toxicity is the depression of serum levels of triglycerides, phospholipids, cholesterol, cholesterol esters, lipoproteins and glucose [140, 476].

Other changes in hepatic function induced by ethionine include impaired excretion of BSP, mild elevation of serum bilirubin levels and depressed levels of plasma proteins [133, 613]. Serum enzyme levels are minimally elevated [640]. Very modest (50 m.i.u.) levels of SGOT and even lower values of SGPT are noted. Depressed hepatic production of bile can be demonstrated within 16 hrs of a single dose of ethionine [24]. Ethionine has a curious biphasic effect on iron metabolism

[270, 262]. During the first 6 weeks of ethionine administration intestinal absorption of iron, hepatocyte affinity for iron and liver stores of iron all are increased. Subsequently, this propensity to iron overload disappears. The significance of these changes is obscure, although during the period of increased hepatocyte avidity for iron, a PAS-positive, diastase-resistant material appears in hepatocytes at sites that correspond to the loci of increased iron stores [262].

Mechanism of Toxicity. The pathogenesis of the chief, acute histologic abnormality in the rat has been clarified to a considerable degree by the extensive studies of FARBER and his associates and by other workers [139, 140, 141, 143]. There is compelling evidence that ethionine rapidly leads to ATP deficiency and that many of the adverse effects of ethionine are traceable to the ATP deficiency [141, 143].

Deficiency of ATP is clearly the result of the trapping of adenosyl moieties as S-adenosylethionine (SAE). Since, in the rat, SAE turns over more slowly than the normal counterpart S-adenosylmethionine (SAM), levels of available ATP decrease sharply and may reach values lower than 20% of the normal. In response to this phenomenon the rate of generation of ATP increases, but not sufficiently to maintain the normal level. FARBER and his associates and others have developed considerable evidence in support of the view that the ATP deficiency leads to the fatty liver, the inhibition of synthesis of phospholipid, protein and RNA and the ultrastructural abnormalities of nucleoli, nuclei and the cytoplasmic orgonelles [141, 143]. All of these adverse effects are reversed by the administration of ATP, precursors of ATP such as adenine, inosine, or 4-imidazole-carboxamide, or by methionine. Deficiency of ATP appears responsible for the deficient synthesis of proteins including the apoprotein of the lipoprotein complex required for movement of triglyceride from the liver, and accordingly for the production of fatty liver and depressed plasma lipids and lipoproteins. While the inhibition of formation of RNA-protein or the production of abnormal ethylated RNA might, thru deficiency of mRNA, contribute to impaired protein syntheses, the available evidence suggests this to be less important than the induced ATP deficiency in the production

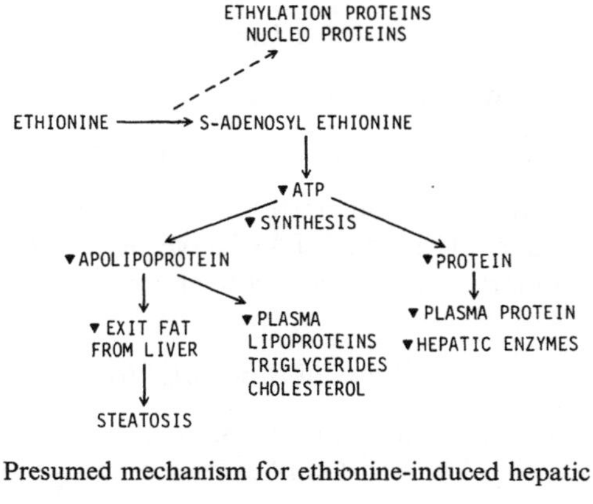

Fig. 5. Presumed mechanism for ethionine-induced hepatic injury

of the fatty liver [141]. Inhibition of RNA production, presumably through the inhibition by ethionine of RNA polymerase, appears, from circumstantial evidence, to be responsible for the nucleolar abnormalities and presumably for the hepatocarcinogenesis [143]. While the evidence for the importance of ATP-trapping in the genesis of hepatic steatosis is convincing, GLASER and MAGER have recently suggested that the deficiency of glutathione, induced by ethionine, might be relevant to the hepatic injury and, indeed, would correlate with the observed effect of sex on susceptibility of rats to ethionine [172]. The relevance of ATP depletion to nuclear changes remains uncertain [176] and the involvement of ethylation of macromolecules, substitution of ethionine for methionine in proteins [141] in the genesis of tissue injury remains to be clarified (Fig. 5).

5. Thioacetamide

Thioacetamide (TAA) first aroused interest in 1945, when it was considered for use as a fungicide to control decay of oranges [88]. The resultant presence of the agent in orange juice posed a potential health hazard which prompted FITZHUGH and NELSON [148] and AMBROSE *et al.* [10, 11] to study its toxicity. In 1949 these workers reported that a single dose of the compound produced centrizonal hepatic necrosis [10] and that chronic administration led to cirrhosis and carcinoma [148, 10, 11]. Subsequent studies have defined the character of the acute and chronic hepatic injury and have demonstrated the hepatocarcinogenic property of this agent [429, 184, 160, 271, 272, 567, 26, 19, 174, 219, 545, 265, 373, 27, 436, 166, 33, 335, 480, 467, 8, 55, 485, 486, 408, 471, 246, 247, 549, 285, 39, 266, 516, 462, 248, 511, 630, 185, 312, 179, 250, 249, 528, 266].

a) Significance

Recognition of the toxicity of thioacetamide led to its removal from use in circumstances permitting toxicity for humans. There has been great interest, however, in this compound as a model toxin for the study of hepatotoxicity [348, 160], hepatocarcinogenicity and cellular response to injury [26]. It has also been a useful chemical probe to study the metabolic function of the nucleolus [383].

b) Chemical Characteristics

Thioacetamide is a white, crystalline, simple, organic compound with the formula $CH_3-C\begin{smallmatrix}\nearrow NH\\ \searrow SH\end{smallmatrix}$. It is soluble in water and in absolute alcohol. It is unstable in acid or alkaline solution undergoing decomposition to liberate H_2S. Studies employing S^{35}- and H^3-labeled TAA have demonstrated that it is rapidly metabolized after administration [55] with conversion to acetate via the acetamide pathway [391, 438].

c) Factors in Susceptibility

Species. There are no systematic studies of *species* differences in susceptibility to the necrogenic effects of TAA. Most studies have employed rats as the experimental model [26]. Mice [630], guinea pigs [516], and dogs [462] also are vulnerable. Indeed, dogs appear to be much more susceptible than rats [462].

Endocrine. There appear to be no striking sex differences in vulnerability. GUPTA [184] described males to be more susceptible to TAA hepatotoxicity, but others [26] describe males and females to be equally vulnerable. Furthermore, gonadectomy does not seem to modify susceptibility to TAA—induced hepatic necrosis. Adrenalectomy appears to reduce it, but other endocrine—altering manouvers have relatively little effect [26].

Age. The neonatal rat is resistant [26]. Susceptibility to the necrogenic effects does not appear until the age of 3 weeks [82]—several weeks later than the development of susceptibility to CCl_4 toxicity. During the phase of stimulated DNA synthesis of the *regenerating* rat liver, after partial resection, susceptibility to TAA-mitotic injury seems enhanced [272, 26].

Diet. Studies on the effects of dietary manipulations on TAA hepatotoxicity are limited. HRUBAN *et al.* [219] have demonstrated that low, moderate and high protein diets all permit essentially the same degree of chronic hepatic injury from the agent. They found that administration of supplemental casein hydrolysate, methionine or guanosine failed to modify the hepatic injury; although it did reduce markedly the renal toxicity of the agent.

d) Experimental Toxicity

Administration of TAA by gastric intubation, or by subcutaneous, intramuscular, intravenous, intraperitoneal or intraportal administration can produce toxic changes. For rats the LD_{50} dose may be estimated from the studies of AMBROSE *et al.* [10, 11] and GUPTA [184], to be approximately 200 mg/Kg. This dose produces zonal hepatic necrosis, renal tublar necrosis and thymic injury, but little injury to other organs, despite the demonstration that the agent reaches many other organs in equivalent concentrations [26]. Although this is the dose that is customarily employed to produce acute injury, smaller doses can produce necrosis, acutely, and cirrhosis and hepatic carcinoma when given chronically [55].

Acute Effects. A single large dose (200 mg/Kg) is followed by degenerative changes in 6 to 8 hrs. By 12 hrs this dose in rats leads to centrizonal necrosis, which by 24—30 hrs is maximal [26]. The prenecrotic changes include loss of glycogen by 6 hrs, and acidophilic degeneration of cells in the central zone by 8 hrs. This is accompanied by dilatation of sinusoids to form pathways ("edema channels") between the central veins of contiguous lobules [184]. By 9 hrs hepatocytes of the central zone contain a few lipid droplets. At 24 hrs the necrosis involves the inner 25 to 50% of the lobule, and there is a mononuclear inflammatory response. Repair begins at 36 hrs, and the liver has returned to normal by 7 days [184].

Necrosis in the dog differs somewhat [462]. According to RODRIGUEZ-OLLEROS *et al.* [462], the brunt of the injury is periportal rather than centrizonal; and there is some injury in all parts of the lobule.

Fat accumulation after thioacetamide is much less striking than after CCl_4 administration. Indeed, JUDAH and his associates [348, 240] have focused considerable attention on the necrosis without steatosis observed by them in thioacetamide poisoning, and have considered this as evidence of the separate pathogenesis of necrosis and steatosis in hepatotoxic states. Nevertheless, several reports [545, 335, 485, 486, 528] have recorded fatty change in TAA toxicity, although clearly of much lesser magnitude than that of CCl_4 toxicity.

Ultrastructural changes resemble those of CCl_4 poisoning [472, 555, 567, 26, 19], but do not develop as rapidly. There is disorganization of the ER, loss of parallel array of membranes, formation of vacuoles, loss of ribosomes from the RER and disaggregation of polysomes similar to that induced by CCl_4. The membrane and ribosome injury is first apparent by 5 hrs [26, 19, 545], later than that induced by CCl_4. This is also evident in the biochemical manifestations of injury. Protein synthesis is impaired and 80S ribosomes are dissociated by 5 to 6 hrs [26, 19], a phenomenon held responsible for the demonstrable inhibition of hepatocyte respiration and mitochondrial function. The accumulation of calcium and sodium as well as loss of potassium and magnesium from hepatocytes [160] has been attributed to an adverse effect of thioacetamide on permeability of the plasma membrane of the cell, a deduction based on the preventability of this change by pretreatment with "membrane stabilizers" [238].

Injury to the membranes of the ER differ from that induced by CCl_4 *qualitatively* as well as quantitatively. While that induced by CCl_4 appears to involve general destruction of the SER and the RER with impairment of multiple measure functions of these organelles, that produced by TAA is more selective. Significant injury to the SER is not seen by electron microscopy until 12 [26] or even 24 [26] hrs. At that time the levels of the membrane-associated cytochromes first begin to decline, "as though their integrity is maintained by association with the membrane" [27]. The concentration of cytochrome P-450 and b_5 and the metabolic functions that are P-450-dependent also decrease at approximately 24 hrs [26]. Furthermore, there is distinct dissociation of reactions dependent on the electron-transport system, with early marked depression of demethylation, while NADPH-neotrazolium reduction is depressed relatively little [26]. CASTRO *et al.* [82] also point out that TAA, in contrast to CCl_4 does not lead to lipid peroxidation. These differences from the behavior of CCl_4 toxicity indicate that the TAA effect involves selective injury to key sites. These observations also have provided insight into pathways of drug metabolism in the normal liver.

Dramatic nuclear changes are observed by 24 hrs. There is marked enlargement of nuclei and nucleoli; indeed nucleoli become gigantic. This may be accompanied by extrusion of the nucleolus into the cytoplasm and even out of the cell into the sinusoids [246, 247]. Nuclei often contain droplets of fat, which appear to have originated in the cytoplasm and to have been incorporated into the nucleus as inclusions of cytoplasm [528].

Chronic administration leads to even more profound changes. After two weeks of ingestion of a diet containing 0.04% thioacetamide, the volume of the nucleus is enlarged two-fold and that of the nucleolus may be enlarged 14-fold. The RNA content of the nucleus is increased three-fold and that of the gigantic nucleolus is increased up to 13-fold. The rate of cytidine incorporation into RNA is increased 30 times, while cytoplasmic volume is increased only slightly (20%). Increase of the granular component of the nucleolus and segregation of it into small clumps leads to the pattern of *microsegregation* and "nucleolar capping" [555].

Density gradient centrifugation shows that nucleolar RNA is altered to yield disproportionate amounts of higher molecular weight ribosomal type. These changes, accompanied by decreased incorporation of C^{14} orotate into cytoplasmic RNA [361] have been interpreted to indicate inhibition of the polysome-forming mechanism.

Chronic Toxicity. The daily administration of a diet containing 50 mg/Kg body weight of TAA (rats) also leads to centrizonal necrosis. When continued for 12 weeks this regimen leads to cirrhosis. A dose, one-fourth, as great leads to similar changes in the dog. Diets containing 0.032% of TAA, and TAA administered in drinking water (30 mg/100 ml) also lead to cirrhosis and ultimately to hepatic carcinoma. Even smaller doses [249, 250, 528], however, can lead to carcinoma without an intervening cirrhosis.

Cirrhosis occurs by 3 months in virtually all rats which receive high doses (200 mg/kg) [55] and in 3 to 6 months in those receiving smaller (30 – 50 mg/kg) doses. Smaller doses (25 mg/kg on alternate days) leads to cirrhosis by 30 days in dogs [462].

The cirrhosis is characterized by irregular fibrosis, bile duct multiplication, nodular regeneration of the parenchyma and cytoplasmic, hyalinized, eosinophilic bodies, which, in dogs, are described [462] to resemble MALLORY [371] bodies.

Carcinoma of the liver was first demonstrated to be produced by feeding of TAA to rats by FITZHUGH and NELSON [148]. Since that time this agent has become one of the standard experimental hepatocarcinogens [555], usually requiring up to 1 year of administration. Cirrhosis is not an obligate precursor of the carcinoma. While most studies have show cirrhosis to precede the hepatic carcinoma [148, 185], the dose of TAA may be kept so small that carcinoma develops without cirrhosis [250].

e) Mechanism of Injury

The striking nucleolar changes induced by TAA have led to the hypothesis [26] that it interferes with movement of RNA from nucleus to cytoplasm. The relevance of this change to the genesis of necrosis is, however, unclear. The demonstration that "membrane-stabilizing" compounds (e.g. antihistamines) can protect against the necrosis, suggests that TAA may have an adverse effect on the cell membrane, leading to necrosis by distortion of the cellular ionic environment [238]. There is good evidence that a metabolite of TAA is responsible for the hepatic injury [119]. The metabolite appears to be formed by a non-P-450-dependent enzyme system [119].

6. Dialkylnitrosamines

This group of compounds includes a number of potent hepatotoxins and hepatocarcinogens [327]. Dimethylnitrosamine (DMN), the first to be studied, drew attention 20 years ago [29] as an industrial poison suspected of having caused liver disease in exposed workers. Its acute effects include centrizonal necrosis and fatty change in the liver, and its chronic effects include cirrhosis and carcinoma [327].

a) Significance

Dimethylnitrosamine and its congeners are important to the experimental pathologist as models of hepatotoxicity [348, 325] and as carcinogens for the liver and other organs [327]. The recent demonstration that some preserved foods contain DMN [483, 155, 136], and that dialkylnitrosamines can be formed in the intestinal tract of mammals when secondary amines and nitrates are ingested [18, 507, 273] has raised DMN to the rank of an hepatotoxin of relevance to human and veterinary medicine [309, 631].

b) Chemical Characteristics

Dimethylnitrosamine is a simple, water-soluble compound. It is chemically very similar to cycasin (Fig. 6) [498], a hepatotoxin of botanical origin (nut of the cycad tree) which also produces hepatic lesions similar to those induced by DMN [164]. The biological (and chemical) properties of dialkylnitrosamines depend on the length and shape of the alkyl groups [199]. In compounds with symmetrical alkyl groups the hepatotoxic and hepatocarcinogenic potency diminishes with increasing length of the chain [199]. Hydroxylation of one of the alkyl groups appears to destroy the toxic potential and introduction of branched alkyl groups (e.g. di-isopropylnitrosamine) to decrease it markedly [199]. The nitrosamine portion of the molecule appears to be important for the hepatotoxic effects, since dimethylformamide is much less toxic [199].

$(CH_3)_2N{-}N{=}O$	$CH_3{-}N{=}N{-}CH_2{-}O{-}$Glucose
Dimethylnitrosamine	Cycasin

Fig. 6. Structure of DMN and cycasin

c) Factors in Susceptibility

Species. A large number of species are susceptible. Rats, mice, dogs, rabbits, guinea pigs, hamsters, duckling, sheep, pigs and fish [418, 483, 80, 29, 494, 536], are vulnerable. Mink [80] seem particularly susceptible.

Age. Effects of age are somewhat similar to those observed with CCl_4. The newborn rat is resistant, but by the age of one week becomes susceptible [324]. Nevertheless, administration of DMN to the newborn animal will prevent development of SER and acquisition of its normal complement of enzymes [418].

Endocrine. There is no demonstrable *sex* difference in susceptibility. While data are scanty, both males and females have been found to shows similar response to DMN.

Diet. Dietary manipulation modifies DMN toxicity. A diet deficient in protein decreases the hepatic injury and lethality of the agent [349, 557, 346], but appears to increase the late hepatocarcinogenic effect and the carcinogenicity for other tissues (kidney) [557, 346]. The LD_{50} for rats is almost doubled by a protein-deficient diet, which also decreases the ability of the liver to metabolize DMN by about 60% [557]. It is of interest that, in contrast to CCl_4 toxicity, phenobarbitol does not alter the inhibitory effects of a protein-deficient diet, while benzo-α-pyrine reverses it [557, 346]. These apparent characteristics of the enzyme system involved in conversion of DMN to its toxic metabolite differs from that responsible for metabolizing CCl_4 to its toxic produce [324].

d) Toxic Effects

The potency of the dialkylnitrosamines varies with the nature of the alkyl groups and the species, age and diet of the animal. In the rat, DMN is a potent toxin, approximately as hepatotoxic as CCl_4.

The acute toxicity of DMN is expressed as hemorrhagic necrosis and steatosis [348, 325, 18, 483, 29]. The necrosis is centrizonal in all species except mink [80]. Fat is seen at the periphery of the necrotic zone. Mink, the most sensitive species studied, develop diffuse, panlobular necrosis [80]. Accompanying the necrosis in several species there is injury to the central veins and sublobular branches of the hepatic veins [350], with occlusion and a lesion resembling that of the pyrrolidiozines.

Light microscopy reveals changes by 12 to 18 hrs after a single doze [324, 325]. In the rat a dose of 30 mg/kg yields extensive necrosis after 24 hrs [29, 346]. By 72 hrs the central zone consists only of blood-filled spaces and debris of necrotic hepatocytes. At this time the endothelial lining of the central veins appears swollen and abnormal. By day 7, the necrotic tissue has been removed and the central zone appears collapsed. The central veins within the collapsed, scarred areas appear distorted; and, occasional ones are occluded by thrombus. Nevertheless, the hepatic architecture of animals which survive the acute injury returns to normal, although some animals develop cirrhosis [350, 320].

Prior to the development of necrosis, hepatocytes in the central zone show loss of glycogen, acidophilic degeneration and fat accumulation. Cells in the mid- and peripheral zones of the lobule become vacuolated, and some form "free" acidophilic bodies [290].

Ultrastructural studies reveal ribosomal disaggregation within 3 hrs of the first dose followed by fragmentation and vesicle formation of the RER. By 5 to 6 hrs RER has largely disappeared, and only scattered detached ribosomes are seen [135, 381]. Lysozomal changes are apparent by 16 hrs, and precede the necrosis [205]. Damage to mitochondria is apparent by 20 hrs [205]; but serum enzyme levels and ultrastructural studies suggest mitochondrial injury to be a relatively minor component of the lesion.

Injury to the plasma membrane may be inferred from the observation, at 24 hrs, of numerous coated, circular (60 mμ) vesicles apparently arising from it. Other vesicles, perhaps detached, are also seen in the interior of the hepatocyte [555].

Nuclear changes include prominent *microsegregation* of the nucleolus [555]. Multiple small, aggregated condensations of the fibrillar componant are diposed within the granular component. At 24 hrs there are dense plaques at the periphery ("nucleolar capping") and by 48 hrs the granular interior of the nucleolus is surrounded by stellate aggregates of mixed granules and fibrils [555, 289].

Chronic changes induced by prolonged administration of DMN include the development of cirrhosis, veno-occlusive disease with ascites and portal hypertension, and neoplasms [44, 418, 324, 495, 563, 635, 561, 91]. In most species, the usual tumor is hepatocellular carcinoma [635]. Less commonly cholangiocarcinoma develops [561]; occasionally sarcomas are produced [91]. In mice the usual tumor is hemangioendothelioma [91].

Cirrhosis develops after weeks to months of administration of doses of 2 to 6 mg/kg/day. Within this range, the larger doses lead to earlier development of cirrhosis. Susceptibility to cirrhosis seems greater with large species (dogs, pigs) than with small ones (guinea pigs, rats) [494, 495].

During the course of chronic administration some hepatocytes and their nuclei become gigantic and the nuclei become hyperchromatic and multiple-nucleolated. Centrolobular cells develop varying degrees of acidophilic degeneration and moderate degrees of fatty change. Ultrastructural studies reveal patchy loss of glycogen, injury of the RER with slight detachment of ribosomes, vesicular changes in the SER, and dilatation and emptiness of the GOLGI apparatus. The lysosomes become dark and shrunken and there is an increase in microbodies. In the *nucleus* there develop multiple clumped condensations of the fibrillar component with microsegregation. All of these chronic ultrastructural abnormalities are similar to those produced by several other hepatocarcinogens [555] and are not specific to DMN [555].

Biochemical changes in the serum include elevated levels of SDH, ICDH, F-1-aldolase GPT, GOT, OCT, MDH and LDH. Of this group [284] SDH seems most sensitive in providing a quantitative reflection of injury.

e) Metabolism of DMN and Mechanism of Injury

After administration of DMN, it is quickly and evenly distributed throughout body water [324]. Within 24 hrs in the rat, and by 4 hrs in the mouse, it has been removed by the liver, where it is metabolized by microsomal N-demethylase [324]. MAGEE and his associates [324] have suggested that it is metabolized according to the scheme shown in Fig. 7. The toxicity has been attributed to the diazomethane or perhaps the monomethylnitrosamine, both powerful alkylating agents. Studies cited above suggest that the enzymes that metabolize DMN differ from those involved in the conversion of CCl_4 to its toxic metabolite.

Studies cited above and others, have demonstrated that the toxic effects of DMN are those of a metabolite [418, 240, 324]. Inhibition of metabolism by dietary protein deprivation [557, 346], or administration of aminoacetonitrile [151] decreases the hepatotoxicity, while restoration of metabolizing activity (by administration of benzo-δ-pyrine) restores the hepatotoxicity [346]. The demonstration that dietary manipulation which decreases hepatotoxicity increases the carcinogenicity for the kidney has been attributed to the prolonged survival in the circulation of DMN with opportunity to exert its adverse effect on the kidney, denied when DMN is metabolized by the liver [240, 557].

The hepatotoxicity seems to be related to the alkylation of cellular constituents essential to hepatocyte viability [324]. Introduction of a methyl group into the guanine (C-7 position) moiety of DNA and RNA and into the histidine of proteins has been demonstrated. These changes can be held accountable for the carcinogenic potential and, with alterations in RNA, could lead to deficient protein synthesis.

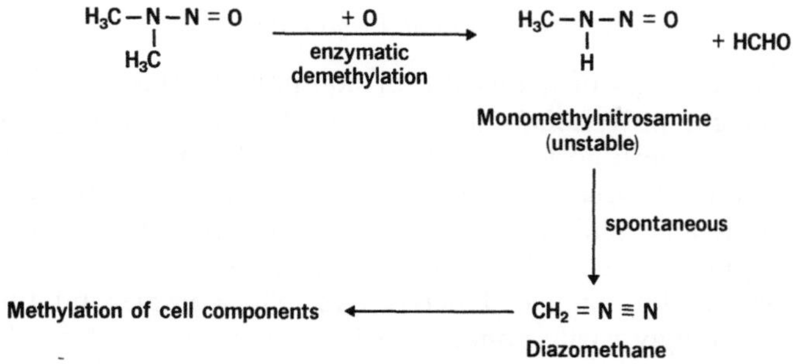

Fig. 7. Metabolism of DMN with production of presumed toxic metabolites. (From McLean *et al.* [348] with permission of authors and publisher)

Within 3 hrs of a dose, there is a block in incorporation of labelled amino acid into rat liver protein [324]. Presumably, alkylation of proteins or other adverse effects of metabolites of DMN also are responsible for injury of the ER and other cytoplasmic organelles. While the manner in which this leads to necrosis is unclear, the damage by metabolites to the active biosynthetic apparatus and of the hepatocytes and injury to mitochondria and even lysosomes presumably contribute.

Categorization of DMN and its congeners as *indirect hepatotoxins* in our classification is predicated on the *selective* injury to the RNA and DNA which has been demonstrated. This precision and specificity seems more in the category of specific block to the metabolic machinery than direct injury to the structural basis [164].

7. Tannic Acid

The toxicity of tannic acid for humans and for a number of other animal species has been of interest for over three decades. First suspected of being hepatotoxic during World Ward II [601, 30], almost two decades after its introduction for the treatment of burns, it has since been demonstrated convincingly to have the property of producing acute and chronic hepatic injury [472, 269, 195, 555, 23, 283, 156].

a) Significance

The importance of tannic acid as a hepatotoxin includes its role in iatrogenic hepatic injury [601, 30, 283, 156, 337, 315, 130], as a hazard to grazing animals [422], as a *theoretical* cause of hepatic damage in humans who take tannic-acid containing beverages [282, 189] and as an experimental hepatotoxin [13] and hepatocarcinogen [282]. Acute injury includes centrizonal, hemorrhagic necrosis and fatty metamorphosis [13]. Prolonged administration to rats leads to cirrhosis and carcinoma [282]. While the mechanism for injury is unclear, the evidence that tannic acid appears to interfere selectively with transcription at the level of the DNA-RNA axis leads [435] us to categorize it as an indirect hepatotoxin.

b) Chemical Properties

"Tannic acid" consists of a mixture of compounds produced in plants from low-molecular weight polyphenals as a result of tissue injury [287]. These are presumed to serve an antibiotic role that protects the plants from infection, by the tanning of invading virus and fungi [50]. "Tannic acid" preparations consist mainly of 3-galloyl-gallic acid (usually referred to as "pure tannic acid"). In addition, tannic acid mixtures contain various amounts of gallic acid, pyrogallal and other polyhydric alcohols and acid derivatives. The complex mixture is soluble in water and accordingly easily administered to experimental animals by various routes. The gallotanin (the active component), however, according to BLUMENBERG and KESSLER, is developed in the intestine by enzyme action [45].

c) Injury in Humans

Humans have developed hepatic necrosis in several circumstances. During the 4th and 5th decades of this century the use of tannic acid for local treatment of burns was attended by the development of severe hepatic necrosis [601, 30]. The experimental demonstration of the hepatotoxicity of this agent led to abandoment of its use in burn therapy [73, 95]. Two decades later, however, instances of hepatic necrosis in patients who had received diagnostic barium enemas containing tannic acid led to a re-awareness of the hepatotoxic potential of even this exposure [156, 337]. There is no evidence of hepatotoxicity of tannic acid taken in wines or tea and, indeed, the absorption of orally administered tannic acid in solution has been discounted [189]. However, the studies of KORPASSY [282] suggest that tannic acid can be absorbed even after oral administration and provoke hepatic injury. The demonstration that animals grazing on or fed plants rich in tannic acid develop hepatic injury [422], also indicates the potential hepatotoxicity of ingested tannic acid.

d) Experimental Toxicity

Toxic effects of tannic acid have been demonstrated by ingestion of plant products [422], of tannic acid solutions [282], rectal instillation [564], subcutaneous injection [13] or intraperitoneal [13] administration. A number of authors have reported no toxic effects from oral administration, presumably because of conversion of the toxic gallotannin to the non-toxic products in the duodenum [189, 45, 46]. KORPASSY [282], however, has demonstrated appreciable blood levels of tannins and hepatic injury after oral administration and the demonstration of hepatotoxicity from ingestion of plants [422] supports this view. There is general agreement, however, that rectal administration is more potentially toxic and parenteral administration is even more toxic.

e) Factors in Susceptibility

A number of species have been shown to be susceptible to tannic acid hepatotoxicity. Rats, guinea pigs, rabbits, cattle, sheep and humans all develop the same type of acute hepatic injury [23, 131]. Data on the effects of sex, diet, and age are sparse but presumably these factors play a relatively slight modifying role. KORPASSY [282] has described the male rat to be more sensitive than the female to tannic acid toxicity. Many reports, however, have been based on studies of animals of both sexes and have not distinguished a sex difference in susceptibility.

f) Acute Injury

Tannic acid leads to hemorrhagic centrizonal necrosis within 48 hrs of administration [13]. By 4 hrs fatty metamorphosis is apparent, and by 12 hrs it is prominent. By 24 hrs there is early necrosis which by 48 hrs is marked. Early changes seen by 1 hr with EM include a marked decrease in hepatic glycogen, decreased prominence and degranulation of the RER, with freed ribosomes scattered throughout the cytoplasm, and moderate dilation of cisternae. By 4 hrs the RER is distinctly decreased in amount, the remaining cisternae are seen to be curled around mitochondria; there is overt loss of ribosomes, the SER is prominent with many profiles which are directly continuous with the remaining SER. There also are small (100—200 μ) dense bodies in the sinusoids and spaces of disse. Similar bodies in the hepatocyte coalesce to form larger, recognizably lipid granules [473].

Fatty change which is severe by 12 hrs [13] is accompanied by prominent cytoplasmic degeneration and formation of acidophilic bodies [13]. Necrosis, which reaches a peak by 48 hrs, is centrizonal. It may be hemorrhagic especially when very large subcutaneous doses (1 200 mg/kg) are given. In the hepatocytes peripheral to the necrotic areas large hyperchromatic nuclei and mitoses are prominent. Restoration to normal liver occurs by 7 days after a single, non-fatal dose [13].

Nuclear changes, seen by EM, include a relatively unique form of *macrosegregation* [555]. The nucleolus appears to shrink and shows condensation of compact RNP granules into one or more dark zones, which are surrounded by light areas made up of RNP granules and fibrils [423]. This form of macrosegregation is reversible and differs from that of aflatoxin, and lasiocarpine in that the areas of RNP condensation remain within the interior of the nucleolus rather than as a peripheral "nucleolar cap" [555].

g) Chronic Toxicity

Prolonged administration of TA leads to cirrhosis and carcinoma [282]. Doses in excess of 100 mg/kg, given subcutaneously to rats leads to a diffuse, micronodular cirrhosis by 3 to 4 months. Hepatocellular carcinoma has been demonstrated by KORPASSY [282] in over 50% of rats on this regimen.

Ultrastructural changes include dilation and detachment of ribosomes, some increase in SER, dilated and empty vesicles of the GOLGI apparatus and changes in the nuclei [555]. The latter consist of increase in interchromatin granules and the presence of iron-containing inclusions and macrosegregation in the nucleoli with the formation of nucleolar "capping" [555].

h) Mechanism of Injury

Interference with protein synthesis may be inferred to be responsible for the hepatic injury, but support for this view is sparse. The character of the nuclear and nucleolar changes suggest an important site of injury to be in the synthesis or release of RNA from the nucleus [555].

8. Aflatoxins

The aflatoxins have been studied with enormous intensity during the 14 years that have elapsed since the discovery of the phenomenon of aflatoxicosis [498, 472, 348, 286, 175, 68, 403, 626, 627, 628]. First recognized in 1960 as the cause of an epidemic of acute hepatic necrosis in turkey poults ("Turkey × disease"), ducklings and young phesants in England [558] [181], this group of compounds has been found to contain several extremely potent hepatotoxic and hepatocarcinogenic agents [68, 628]. The early studies quickly demonstrated the hepatic injury to be caused by metabolites of the fungus, *Aspergillus flavus* found in the peanut meal fed to the fowl [68]. Retrospective analysis of prior epidemics of hepatic disease in laboratory and domestic animals (rats, guinea pigs, hamsters, dogs) has led to the inference that these might have represented aflatoxin poisoning [628].

a) Significance

Interest in this group of compounds has derived from their great toxic and carcinogenic potency and the speculation that hepatic disease in humans, especially carcinoma, may be the result of ingestion of aflatoxins or other mycotoxins [286, 68, 626, 385]. This implicit practical importance for human health; the relevance to animal husbandry and veterinary medicine of aflatoxin-contamination of feeds; and the intrinsic biologic and biochemical interest of this group of compounds has provided the impetus for an explosive increase in knowledge of the toxicity of aflatoxins and to intensive study of many other mycotoxins [286, 175, 68, 626, 627, 628, 385]. Studies have led to a rapid isolation of a family of compounds (Fig. 8) from cultures of *A. flavus* and of their metabolites; determination of environmental and cultural conditions that affect production of the compounds by the fungus, and recognition of the relative hepatotoxicity of the individual compounds [175, 68].

b) Chemical Characteristics

The aflatoxins (AF) are a group of furano coumarins. At least 13 have been identified (Fig. 8). Six of these (AFB_1, AFG_1, AFB_2, AFG_2, AFB_{2a}, and AFG_{2a}), are found in cultures of *Aspergillus flavus*. The others have been synthesized or are metabolites of the native compounds. All are lactones or lactams. Their toxic properties appear to be related to their high reactivity to electrophilic agents and potential action as alkylating agents. WOGAN [627] has categorized the compounds with the aflatoxin configuration into two groups according to their structural relationship to the first two identified compounds of this series, aflatoxin B_1, (AFB_1) and G_1 (AFG_1).

AFB_1 is an extremely important substance, not only as the parent compound of one series, but also as the major component of toxic mixtures produced in

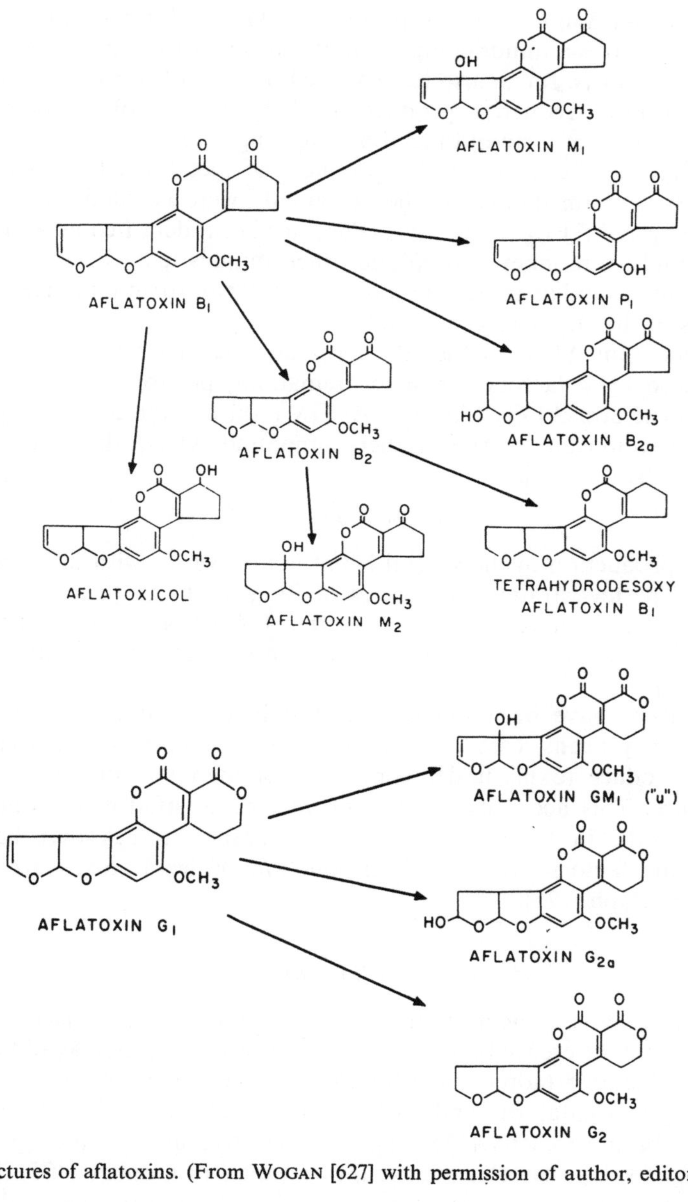

Fig. 8. Structures of aflatoxins. (From WOGAN [627] with permission of author, editors and publisher)

natural media, by practically all aflatoxin-producing fungi [627]. It is the most potent hepatotoxic and hepatocarcinogenic member of the aflatoxins [627]. Indeed, in the following description of toxic properties, lesions produced and mechanism of injury, of the aflatoxins, attention will be focused on AFB_1; and qualitative differences, from the effects of AFB_1, of the other members of the group will be presented.

AFB_2 (dihydro AFB_1), a reduction product of AFB, is formed only by special strains of the fungus. It is a minor component of the hepatotoxic mixtures extracted from cultures of *A. flavus*. It can also be produced by controlled catalytic reduction of AFB_1 [627]. Another reduction product of AFB_1, aflatoxicol can be produced by the action on AFB_1 of a steroid metabolizing fungus [627].

AFM_1 and AFM_2 are, respectively, products of metabolic hydroxolation of AFB_1 and AFB_2, so named because they originally were isolated from the milk of cows, fed AFB_1 and AFB_2. However, AFM_1 has been identified as a metabolite in other body fluids of monkeys, sheep and other animals fed AFB_1. Both AFM_1 and AFM_2 also are found as minor components of hepatotoxic mixtures produced by some strains of the *A. flavus* group [627].

AFG_1 differs from AFB_1 in that the terminal five membered ring of AFB_1 has been replaced by a lactone while the remaining portion of the compound has the same structure. AFG_2, AFG_{2a}, $AFGM_1$ (also referred to as AF "u") have the same relationship to the mother compound AFG_1 that the respective derivatives of AFB_1 do [627].

c) Sources

The relative production of the several hepatotoxins varies with different strains of fungi [175]. The few strains and species of fungi that can produce aflatoxins are widely distributed in nature. Members of the *A. flavus* group have the greatest capacity for aflatoxin production and are the most important source of these toxic agents [175].

These organisms have been found to contaminate a variety of nuts, wheat, corn, rice, oats, soy beans, cassava, cottonseed and other substances [175], and to be able to produce toxins under conditions of high moisture and relatively high temperature. This accounts for the prevalence of aflatoxin production in contaminated foods, in tropical areas. The extensive studies that have been conducted on the factors that modify production of hepatotoxin are reported in a recent monograph [175].

d) Factors in Susceptibility

Species. An analysis of acute toxicity in several species reveals that there is over a hundred-fold difference between the most susceptible (one-day old duckling) and the least vulnerable (adult mice) [68, 627]. Duckling, rainbow trout, guinea pig, rabbit, dog, neonatal rat and turkey poult seem to be highly susceptible to acute and subacute toxicity [175, 68]. Less sensitive are the pig, growing rat (weanling to six weeks), hamster, chicken, pheasant and monkey [175]. Mice and sheep are among the most resistant species [627]. Even for sheep which have been described to be completely resistant to AF-contaminated food and to resist any adverse effect from several years of taking 1 mg/kg/day, however, AFB_1 must be regarded as a potent hepatotoxin; since according to ARMBRECHT *et al.*, the LD_{50} for the ewe is 2.0 mg/kg of AFB, and large single doses can kill sheep with acute central necrosis [15].

Even within related species an interestingly wide range of susceptibility prevails. Rainbow trout are among the most sensitive species (LD_{50}, 0.5 mg/kg) to acute effects and, on chronic dosing, develop hepatic carcinoma. Coho salmon are at least 10 times, and channel catfish at least 30 times, as resistant to the acute effects and are refractory to the carcinogenic one [187]. Among poultry, ducklings and turkey are very sensitive, pheasants and quail moderately resistant, and chickens very resistant to the effects of aflatoxins [627].

Age. Newborn and young animals of a number of species studied appear to be more susceptible than older animals of the respective species. The weanling rat (LD_{50} of 5.5–7.4 mg/kg) is approximately one-tenth as susceptible to the acute toxicity of AFB_1, as the neonate (LD_{50}, 0.5 mg/kg) [68]. Hamsters at 30 days of ge have an LD_{50} 10.2 mg/kg twice that of 21-day old hamsters [625].

Female rats appear to be more resistant than male [68]. The acute LD_{50} of the female is much higher than that of the male; and carcinoma of the liver develops after a longer latent period in the female than in the male rat. Curiously, pregnancy (especially late pregnancy) enhances susceptibility in rats [68].

Diet. ROGERS and NEWBERNE [463, 464] and MADHAVEN *et al.* [355, 321, 322] have studied the effect of diet on the toxicity of aflatoxins. Reduced protein intake appears to increase the susceptibility of rats [464] and monkeys [322] to the acute toxic, and rats [463, 321] to the carcinogenic, effects of the aflatoxin mixtures. A diet marginally deficient in choline appears to reduce the acute toxicity of single doses [464] but to increase toxicity and carcinogenicity of repeated doses [463] for the rat; while a diet sufficiently deficient to produce cirrhosis, does not enhance carcinogenesis [464]. These data have been interpreted [464] as consistent with other observations that suggest that 1. metabolic products of AFB_1, are involved in both acute toxicity and carcinogenicity and 2. the metabolites responsible for the acute injury and carcinogenesis differ [403, 626]. Others [240] have deduced that AFB_1 is itself an acutely toxic molecule and that a metabolite is responsible for carcinogenesis.

e) Hepatic Injury

The aflatoxins are powerful, toxic agents for all species of animal thus far studied. The effects are dose-related and show species, age, and, to some degree, sex-dependence [175, 68, 403, 626]. Comparison of these factors requires separation of the effects of acute from chronic toxicity [175].

The liver is the chief and most dramatically affected organ in acute and chronic aflatoxin injury [68, 626]. Depending on the species, age, dose of AFB_1 or aflatoxin mixture, varying degrees of hepatocellular change including necrosis and steatosis, bile duct multiplication, vascular abnormalities and inflammatory response are seen [175, 68, 626]. Sequelae and chronic changes include fibrosis and cirrhosis in many species. Only in the duckling, trout, rat, and ferret [68, 626] can hepatic carcinoma be induced.

Acute Injury. Single doses in the lethal range (Table 11) lead to hepatic necrosis in many but not all species studied. The location of the necrosis also varies with different species. In the duckling, turkey poult, rat, and the cat it is mainly *periportal* [68, 4, 323]. In the pig, dog, guinea pig, ferret and sheep it is mainly *central* [68, 386, 15]. In the rabbit necrosis while not marked, is mainly *midzonal* [681, 386], with scattered centrizonal injury; while in the monkey it is variably central,

Table 11. Lesions Produced by Aflatoxin B_1 in Various Species[a]

Species	Necrosis	Fat	Bile Duct Multip.	V.O.D.[b]	Ca[c]	Rel. Susc.[i] (acute)
Ducks	PZ	+	+	−	+	100
Turkeys	PZ	+	+	−	−	60
Chickens	F or Dg	+[d]	+	−	−	70
Trout	CZ	+	+	−	+	80
Salmon	Df	?	?	?	−	5
Rats	PZ	+	±	−	+	6
Mice	−	−	−	−	[e]	7
G. Pigs	CZ	+	+	−	−	40
Rabbits	MZ	+	+	−	−	80
Dogs	CZ	+	+	−	−	80
Cats	PZ	+	+	−	−	70
Ferrets	CZ	+	+	−	+	40
Pigs	CZ	+	+	+	−	70
Cattle	F or Dg	+	+	+	−	2
Sheep	CZ[f]	−	−	−	[h]	1
Monkeys	CZ, PZ	+	+	−	[h]	11
Humans	[g]	[g]	?	?	[g]	?

[a] Based on data in references 286, 175, 68, 386, 15, 187, 625, 463, 322, 321, 4, 5, 323, 6. Changes described refer to adults with exception of fowl. PZ=Peripheral necrosis; CZ=Central necrosis; MZ=Midzonal necrosis; F=Focal necrosis; Df=Diffuse necrosis; Dg=Degeneration; + =occurs; − =Reported not to occur; ?=Insufficient data.
[b] V.O.D. =Veno-occlusive changes.
[c] Ca=Hepatic Carcinome.
[d] Fat present as lakes.
[e] Tumors reported in mice but apparently not carcinoma.
[f] Sheep are resistant but necrosis has been reported.
[g] Aflatoxin-related lesions inferred from circumstantial evidence.
[h] Only 1 instance reported.
[i] Estimated from published LD_{50} data.

midzonal or focal [4, 323, 6]. In the rainbow trout it is *central* or *massive* [187] and in the Soho salmon it is *diffuse* [188]. The chicken and cow show degeneration but not necrosis [323, 6].

Fat appears mainly as scattered lakes (duckling) or in portal zones in the guinea pig, in the dog and in the monkey [175]; indeed in the monkey it may occupy almost the entire liver [509]. The chicken does develop a periportal accumulation of fat [386].

Chronic Injury. Cirrhosis has been produced in cattle, pigs, ducklings (slight), chicken, rats, guinea pigs, cats rabbits and monkeys [323]. It is relatively mild in the rat. Curiously in some species (cattle) veno-occlusive lesions are produced that resemble closely the lesions of the pyrrolidizine alkaloids [6].

Megalocytosis, like the large cells induced by the pyrrolidizine alkaloids, can be produced in cattle, pigs and the rat [4]. Characteristically, increase and great variability in size of nuclei is produced in a number of species [175].

In most species studied there is little inflammatory infiltration accompanying the parenchymal injury; although, in the chicken, which shows relatively slight degeneration and almost no necrosis, inflammatory response may be marked. In that species, large lymphoid follicles appear in the areas of fatty fibrosis [4].

Bile duct proliferation, which can be striking, is an early lesion in many species (Table 11). Indeed, it is prominent in almost all species, except the rat. The day-old duckling responds to AFB_1 with bile duct proliferation so promptly and sensitivity that it has been proposed as a model for bio-assay of the toxin [175, 68, 4].

Subacute toxicity i.e. that which develops after 7 to 10 days of oral administration includes hemorrhagic necrosis, fibrosis, bile duct hyperplasia, veno-occlusive disease (cattle) and megalocytosis [175, 68, 626, 4]. In monkeys, a form of "biliary cirrhosis" has been described [578, 427].

Ultrastructural changes include injury to the RER with detachment and dispersal of ribosomes, development of fat droplets, loss of glycogen and swelling of metachondria. The nucleus develops, rapidly, nucleolar microsegregation [555, 628].

Carcinoma. The carcinogenic potential of AF derivatives is perhaps the most important aspect of their hepatotoxicity. Indeed, AFB_1 is the most potent hepatocarcinogen for the rat known [326]. Only a few species are susceptible, however. These include the trout, rat, duckling and ferret [68]. Evidence that sheep are vulnerable is unconvincing [68]. One instance of carcinoma in a non-human primate [2] attributed to aflatoxin has been reported. Circumstantial epidemiologic evidence for the possible role of aflatoxins in humans has been offered [500].

Carcinogenesis has been studied most intensively in the rat. Administration of diets containing as little AFB_1 as 15 ppb for 60 to 80 weeks or a total dose 0.4 mg per animal given in 10 daily, divided doses yields a high incidence of hepatic carcinoma [629]. Even survivors of a single LD_{50} dose, given to the weanling rat, develop carcinoma [68]. In the rat and in the rainbow trout, AFG_1, is a less potent hepatocarcinogen, but is more likely to produce renal carcinoma than AFB_1 [627]. AFB_2 is hepatocarcinogenic only at a dose 150 times that at which AFB_1 produces carcinoma [626].

The rainbow trout is even more sensitive to the carcinogenic effect of AFB_1 [627]. Doses ranging from 1/150 to 1/4 those that produce carcinoma in the rat are effective in the rainbow trout. Aflatoxins other than AFB_1 and AFG_1 do not appear to produce carcinoma in this species, although AFM_1 is a potent cocarcinogen when fed with cyclopropenoid fatty acids [627].

Ducklings appear to be somewhat less sensitive than rats to aflatoxin-carcinogenesis. Doses twice those that affect the rat are required to produce hepatic cancer in the duckling [625]. Ferrets have been reported to develop hepatic tumors after ingesting aflatoxin-contaminated peanut meal for three years [627].

All other species tested have appeared to be resistant to hepatocarcinogenesis, despite sensitivity to the acute effects (Table 11).

f) Mechanism of Hepatic Injury

Most of the studies relating to the biochemical basis for the hepatic injury have been conducted in the rat or rat tissues. Both *in-vivo* and *in-vitro* studies strongly support the view that the genesis of the hepatic lesions is related to impairment of nucleic acid synthesis [628]. The administration of AFB_1 leads to a rapid inhibition of synthesis of nucleic acid; within 15 min of a lethal dose of the toxin there is 90% inhibition of incorporation of precursor into RNA, especially by the nucleus [629]. This is attributable to the equally rapid depression of activity of the DNA-dependent RNA polymerase activity [416]. The ultrastructural parallel of microsegregation of fibrillar and granular elements of the nucleolus at 15 min, and the macrosegregation ("nuclear capping") observed at one hour supports the relevance of the importance of the inhibition of RNA polymerase activity [416]. Also the observation that there was a close correlation between the relative toxicity and ability to inhibit the RNA polymerase for several aflatoxins supports the view that the inhibition of the activity of this critical enzyme is the biochemical basis for the hepatotoxicity [489, 407]. The physiochemical basis for the inhibition of polymerase activity is less clear. While binding of DNA by aflatoxins has been demonstrated and, at first, was postulated to be responsible by way of template alteration for the inhibition of polymerase, the further demonstration of WOGAN that the ability of an AF derivative to bind DNA was not correlatable with hepatotoxicity has led him to discount that theory. He has concluded that the inhibition of polymerase is probably central to the hepatic injury, but that the adverse effect of the AF is the result of interaction with nuclear chromatin rather than directly on the enzyme [628].

Inhibition of synthesis of protein is demonstrable by 3 hrs. There is also some inhibition of lipid and cholesterol synthesis. Fat accumulation as with many other toxins seems ascribable to impairment of exit of fat from the liver—perhaps secondary to impaired protein synthesis.

9. Pyrrolidizine Alkaloids

The toxicity of Senecio plants and related species has been of interest [352, 60] and the subject of experimentation for almost a century. At the turn of the century they were suspected of causing disease in grazing domestic animals. Within a few years this suspicion was confirmed by a series of studies which have been reviewed recently in the excellent publications of BULL *et al.* [60] and of McLEAN [352]. The toxic principles (pyrrolidizine alkaloids) have been identified, their presence in over 200 species of plants has been established and the characteristics of the hepatic injury they produce has been defined [352, 60].

The pyrrolidizine alkaloids (PAs) produce, acutely, centrizonal hepatic necrosis, minor degrees of fat accumulation and injury with occlusion of the small branches of the hepatic veins [352, 60]. Chronic changes include the development of "megalocytes", a congestive type of cirrhosis which resembles "cardiac cirrhosis" and hepatocellular carcinoma [60]. The mechanism of injury is uncertain but presumably [352] involves the injury by a pyrrole derivative of the hepatic vasculature and reaction of the pyrrole derivative with nuclear DNA and RNA [352].

a) Significance

The PAs are of great importance as the cause of a curious form of chronic hepatic disease in humans ("venoocclusive disease", "VOD") and as an example of the extremely important group of botanical hepatotoxins that constitute hazards to man and domestic animals [498]. As experimental tools to assist in the elucidation of mechanisms of hepatotoxicity, they have provided models that permit exploration of relationship of chemical structure to hepatic injury [500]. As hepatocarcinogens in experimental animals and perhaps in man, they also have provided useful tools for the exploration of hepatocarcinogenesis [500].

b) Chemical Characteristics

All of the PAs contain the core structure of pyrrolidizine (Fig. 9) which consists of 2 fused 5-membered rings with a nitrogen atom at position 4, one of the 2 points of fusion. The hepatotoxic derivatives (Fig. 9) are esters of 1-hydroxymethyl-1, 2-dehydro-7-hydroxy pyrrolidizine. Requirements for toxicity apparently include the 1−2 unsaturation and the esterification with a branched-chain acid [352, 60, 500]. Solubility of the alkaloids in aqueous solvents is low at a neutral pH, and is enhanced by acidification [60]. Reliable methods for chemical identification are available [352].

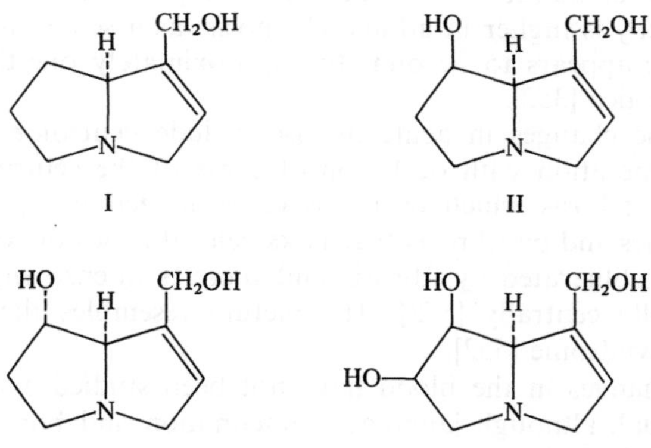

Fig. 9a. Chemical structures of the basic moieties of hepatotoxic pyrrolizidine alkaloids, the necins: I, Supinidine, 1-hydroxymethyl-1,2-dehydro-8α-pyrrolizidine; II, Retronecine, 1-hydroxymethyl-1,2-dehydro-7β-hydroxy-8α-pyrrolizidine; III, Heliotridine, 1-hydroxymethyl-1,2-dehydro-7α-hydroxy-8α-pyrrolizidine; IV, Crotanecine, 1-hydroxymethyl-1,2-dehydro-6β,7β-dihydroxy-8α-pyrrolizidine

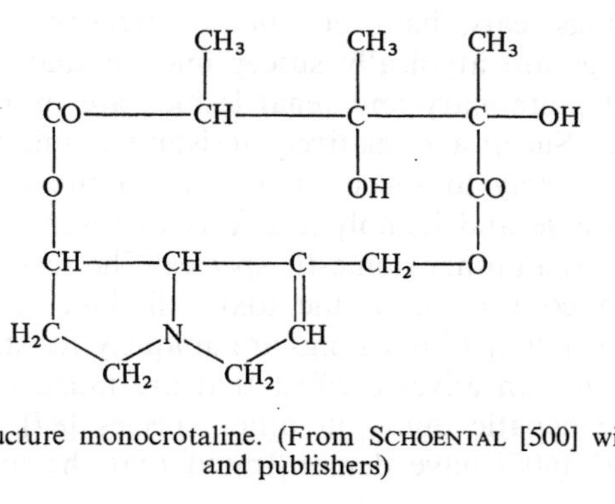

Fig. 9b. The chemical structure monocrotaline. (From SCHOENTAL [500] with permission of author and publishers)

c) Injury in Humans

Clearly documented outbreaks of acute hepatic injury from PAs have been reported from various parts of the world, particularly the West Indies where pyrrolidizine-induced disease is endemic [352]. Exposure to the PAs in Jamaica is usually the result of drinking "bush tea" for medicinal purposes [352]. Bush tea is a hot water infusion of *Crotolaria fulva* or of other plants that contain PAs. In other parts of the world exposure to PAs has usually resulted from the ingestion of contaminated bread or grains [352].

Clinical features of acute injury include the rapid development of ascites, hepatomegaly and splenomegaly and slight fever. In children death from liver failure occurs in this acute phase in 20% of patients; the illness may progress to a full clinical picture of cirrhosis including portal hypertension with esophageal varices in approximately 30%. One third of those who develop this subacute or chronic phase die, while the remainder recover. Thus, the illness is followed by complete recovery in about half of the patients [552]. The mortality of acute pyrrolidizine toxicity is higher in adults. Cirrhosis, as a sequel to the hepatotoxic effects of the PAs appears to account for approximately one-third of the cases of cirrhosis in Jamaica [352].

Histopathologic changes in acute disease include centrolobular hemorrhagic necrosis and degeneration with occlusion of some of the central and sublobular veins [552]. The cirrhosis which occurs is characterized by spared portal areas and periportal zones and by fibrosis that links central zones of contiguous lobules. Central veins are obliterated by fibrosis and there is intense engorgement of the sinusoids, especially centrally [552]. The picture resembles that of the liver in the Budd-Chiari syndrome [552].

Biochemical changes in the blood have not been studied extensively. Hepatic dysfunction is usual, although jaundice is uncommon and bilirubin levels mildly elevated or normal [352, 552]. Hypoalbuminemia and hypoprothrombinemia occur. Values for GOT and GPT, described in only a few patients, are modestly increased [58].

d) Factors in Susceptibility

Species. Species susceptible to the hepatotoxic effects of PAs include sheep, pigs, rats, rabbits, dogs, cats, hamsters, mice, chickens, turkeys, monkeys and humans [352, 60]. Pigs are atypically susceptible, in that liver damage may be less pronounced, but pulmonary and renal lesions are more marked than those of other species [352]. Sheep are relatively resistant requiring longer or repeated exposure and are less likely to succumb to liver failure and more likely to die of combined liver disease and hemolytic effects of severe copper overload or of ammonia intoxication than other domestic species. The relative resistance of sheep may be the result of conversion of the toxic alkaloid to nontoxic metabolites by bacteria of the rumen [60]. Guinea pigs are uniquely resistant to PA hepatotoxicity, requiring doses for an adverse effect that are much (50 times) greater than those which produce hepatic injury in other species [87]. CHESNEY and ALLEN [87] and WHITE *et al.* [607] have demonstrated that the apparent refractionness of guinea pigs to PA hepatotoxicity is paralleled by, and presumably the result of, relative inability of guinea pig microsomes to convert the PA to the toxic metabolite (pyrrole). Canaries are resistant to PA hepatotoxicity while, curiously, chickens and turkeys are susceptible. The metabolic basis for these phenomena remains to be understood.

Sex. There appears to be no consistent difference between the sexes in vulnerability to the hepatotoxic effects of PA [60]. Some differences emerge with studies involving different alkaloids. Female rats are much more susceptible to the immediate "peracute" lethality of lasiocarpene-n-oxide, but approximately equal with males in susceptibility to the hepatic necrogenic effects [60], and are less susceptible than males to the hepatic effects of retrorsine.

Age. Susceptibility to PA hepatotoxicity remains uniform in rats beyond the age of 30 days. A number of reports described young animals to be more sensitive than adults, but the validity of these observations has been questioned [352]. The fetal rat develops severe hepatic injury from administration to its mother of doses of a PA (lasiocarpine) too small to hurt the mother [384]. Suckling rats are more sensitive than weanlings [556]. The evidence that weanlings are more susceptible than rats beyond the age of 30 days [300] has been questioned by McLean [352].

Diet. Relatively few studies on the effects of manipulation of the diet on susceptibility to PA toxicity have been reported. Low protein diets do not enhance the toxicity for rats of a PA (retrorsine). Indeed choline-deficient diets seem to decrease the vulnerability somewhat to the acute effects of monocrotaline but not to the toxicity of a pyrrole metabolite presumed to be the proximate toxin [387]. Fetal rats and their mothers, however, show increased vulnerability to the PA hepatotoxicity [384]. Efforts to relate these effects to the presumed mechanism of toxicity remain speculative, although they are consistent with the view that a metabolite of the PA may be the proximate toxin [352, 60, 332].

e) Experimental Toxicity

Oral administration of whole plants, extracts, or pure alkaloids, or parenteral administration (subcutaneously, intravenously, intraperitineally) of pure alkaloids is effective in producing hepatic injury. Large* doses produce acute, severe, centrizonal necrosis and death, probably as the result of hepatic and extrahepatic injury. Smaller** doses given for a more prolonged period yield cirrhosis and carcinoma [60]. Several of the PAs are very potent hepatotoxins [60, 500].

Acute Injury. Administration of an LD_{50} dose of one of the hepatotoxic PAs (Fig. 9) leads to death from liver failure in 3 to 4 days [352]. (Larger doses can lead to earlier death by mechanisms unrelated to hepatic injury [352].) The liver shows severe hemorrhagic necrosis, which reaches its peak by 24 hrs [352, 60, 61]. It is characteristically centrizonal in the rat, cat, rabbit, hamster, mouse and chicken, but some of the alkaloids can lead to periportal localization of the necrosis in mice, monkeys and hamsters [352]. Studies in the rat show changes to begin with loss of basophilia after 1 hr, and of glycogen by 4 hrs. Necrosis becomes

* For rats 40 to 300 mg/Kg depending on the alkaloid (see Ref. 352).
** For rats 4 to 3 mg/Kg depending on the alkaloid (see Ref. 352).

apparent between 12 and 20 hrs and involves the entire middle and central third of the lobule by 20 hrs [60, 61]. At this time the sinusoids are strikingly congested and their walls destroyed [60, 61]. The necrosis, as a consequence, is massively hemorrhagic in character. Necrotic cells disappear rapidly with little inflammatory response [60]. Prior to the development of necrosis minor fatty change in the centrolobular cells is observed [60]. These changes are characteristic for all of the toxic alkaloids, although the necrosis is more likely to be midzonal after administration of lasiocarpine [61].

Vascular changes are a prominent component of injury induced by PAs and are considered by some [352] but not all [60, 556] to be the primary lesion. Degeneration and lysis of the endothelium of the central and sublobular veins, followed by fibrotic occlusion is the characteristic lesion [352].

Ultrastructural changes include the prompt development of nuclear and nucleolar abnormalities followed by changes in the ER and liposomes [352, 555, 556, 60]. Within 30 min there is *microsegregation* of the fibrillar and granular components of the nucleosus and by 4 to 8 hrs macrosegregation had occurred [556]. These changes had disappeared with reversion of the nucleolus to normal appearance by 72 hrs, in surviving rats. The earliest (1 hr) cytoplasmic change is vacuolization of the RER with severe polysome disaggregation [352]. By 3 hrs centrolobular cells show loss of glycogen; by 9 hrs mitochondria appear abnormal, and by 12 hrs there is evidence of increased lysosomal activity. KERR [255] has described the presence by 24 hrs of large, spherical lysosomes, most numerous in the vicinity of the most severely damaged cells, and has emphasized the similarity to changes in the liver induced by ischemia.

The *biochemical* reflections of injury include an almost immediate (15 min) severe decrease in cytoplasmic protein synthesis [352, 192]. This is accompanied by a sharp drop in DNA-dependent RNA synthesis and demonstrably decreased RNA polymerase activity [597]. Changes in the blood include the usual elevated levels of several serum enzymes that reflect necrosis.

Chronic Injury. Delayed effects of a single dose or prolonged administration of the toxic PAs leads to a curious change in hepatocytes, megalocytosis [352, 60].

Other evidences of chronic injury are induced in the adult by chronic administration of PAs or in the weanling rat [501, 388] as a delayed effect of a single dose. These include hepatocyte degeneration, fatty change, bile duct proliferation, nodular hyperplasia and cirrhosis [352, 60]. The "megalocyte" is an enormously enlarged (10 to 30 times normal) cell containing a huge nucleus and markedly increased amounts of RER, loss of normal organization of cytoplasmic organelles and multiple centrioles [229]. These cells have been interpreted [352, 229] to represent ability to grow but not to divide, a phenomenon consistent with the known antimitotic effects of PAs. Cirrhosis may resemble the cardiac type with bridging between central veins [552], or may be macronodular in type [388]. Small doses administered over a long period of time lead to fibrosis and bile duct multiplication that may progress to bridging between portal areas and an appearance [277] that resembles biliary cirrhosis.

Carcinoma. The potential of the PAs to produce carcinoma remains controversial. SCHOENTAL [500], MAGEE [326] and WARWICK [597] consider these agents carcinogenic. McLean [352] and Bull *et al.* [60] believe the evidence to be equivocal and the carcinogenic potential of these agents unproved.

f) Mechanism of Injury

The evidence that the hepatotoxic effects of the PAs are effected by toxic metabolites is compelling. The effects of dietary manipulation [344], age [352], and enzyme induction [607, 344] on the toxicity, however, have been more complicated than in the case of CCl_4 toxicity [432]. The neonatal animal which, lacking drug metabolizing-enzymatic equipment, is resistant to CCl_4 toxicity, is at least as sensitive as the adult to hepatotoxic effects of the PAs [352]. A low protein diet, which depresses the metabolism of CCl_4 and inhibits its toxicity [344] also depresses the metabolism of retrorsine without affecting its toxicity [344]; and enzyme induction with DDT which enhances CCl_4 toxicity does not affect retrorsine toxicity [344]. Nevertheless, the studies of Maddocks [332], Chesney and Martin [87] and Newberne and his associates [384, 387] provide convincing evidence that a pyrrolic metabolite of the PA is responsible for the hepatotoxicity (and presumably carcinogeneity). Presumably, some of the paradoxical responses to manipulation of microsomal enzyme function reflects a balance between one metabolic pathway to a toxic pyrrole and another to a non-toxic, hydroxylated, pyrrolidizine ring [344]. Presumably the pyrrole alkylates macromolecules [597] to produce the inhibition of RNA production and the nucleolar changes, and, perhaps cytoplasmic components to lead to the pathologic changes. As in the case of all other toxins the mechanism for the necrosis is unknown.

10. Hepatotoxic Principles of Mushrooms

Poisonous mushrooms have been known for several millenia [638]. Studies on toxicity of *Amanita phalloides* have been underway for almost two centuries [611] and of its toxic components for almost 100 years [612]. There are a number of species of hepatotoxic mushrooms and several toxic peptides in each (Fig. 10) [612]. A description of the various species is beyond the scope of this review but the thorough ones of T. Wieland [612] and others [261, 591] are available. *A. phalloides* and *A. verna,* which produce the same or closely related toxic principles are responsible for most of the cases of fatal mushroom poisoning [612]. The character of the toxic principles has been elucidated by the work of the Wielands [319, 609] and their associates, Fiume [150] and other investigators [158, 503].

a) Significance

The hepatotoxic components of poisonous mushrooms are important with respect to the instances of human intoxication that occur and to the provision of experimental models that permit studies of therapy. These agents also provide models of hepatotoxicity characterized by an exquisite correlation between structural features and toxicity and which have made important contributions to molecular biology [150].

b) Chemical Characteristics of Toxic Principles

The elegant studies of T. WIELAND and his associates [611, 612] preceded by the observations of LYNEN and U. WIELAND [319] and of H. WIELAND and HALLEWUNGEN [609] have identified and defined the chemical structure of toxic compounds isolated from poisonous species. They have demonstrated two types of toxins, the *phallotoxins* and the *amatoxins*. The phallotoxins are heptapeptides which are rapidly (hours) lethal in mice; while the amatoxins are octapeptides which are much more (10 to 20 times) potently hepatotoxic than the phallotoxins, but express their lethality more slowly, over a few days. Each of these groups contain several related agents [611, 612]. The best studied of the phallotoxins is *phalloidin* and of the amatoxins is *α-amanitin*.

Recent studies by COURTILLET and STARIN [107] suggest that the toxic peptides isolated from mushrooms are artefactual and probably fragments of much larger and more complex molecules. They have demonstrated differential toxicity of various larger (M.W. 10–80,000) molecules which contain, as easily dissociable fragments, the peptides heretofore considered the toxins of the poisonous mushrooms [107]. Since the extensive literature on hepatotoxicity of peptides of mushrooms comprises an important and fascinating chapter in experimental hepatotoxicity and the relationship of these observations to the recently demonstrated larger molecules remains to be elucidated, the following account focuses on the traditional views of hepatotoxic cyclopeptides rather than on the newly described [310] larger, more complex molecules.

The toxic peptides are all cyclic (Fig. 10) with a molecular weight in the vicinity of 1,000. They all contain a gamma-hydroxylated amino acid and a thioether bridge derived from a cysteine residue. Both phallo- and amatoxins lose their toxicity with destruction of the thioether bridge [610]. Removal of the gamma hydroxyl group of the side chain of phalloidin does not destroy the toxicity. α-Amanitin, however, loses its toxicity with removal of the gamma hydroxyl from its side chain [612].

c) Factors in Susceptibility

A variety of animals are susceptible to the mushroom toxins. These include guinea pigs, rabbits, mice, horses, goats, sheep, monkeys, and pigeons [611]; and, of course, humans are very vulnerable. Amphibians are much less sensitive, requiring doses many times greater than those lethal for mammals and birds [611]. WIELAND [611] has attributed this lesser susceptibility to the "sluggish metabolism" of poikilotherms. Invertebrates (*Helix pomotia* and *Limax arborium*) are resistant to the toxic effects of phalloidin, but are susceptible to those of α-amanitin [611].

The rat is much more resistant to the hepatotoxic effects of amanitin than is the mouse, dog, guinea pig or rabbit [150]. Nevertheless, this agent leads to ultrastructural evidence of hepatic injury even in the rat. The relative resistance of rats to mushroom toxicity has been hypothetically attributed to the rapid elimination by that species of the amanitin in the urine [150].

Both males and females are susceptible, although female mice are somewhat more susceptible [573]. Administration of androgenic steroids enhances the resis-

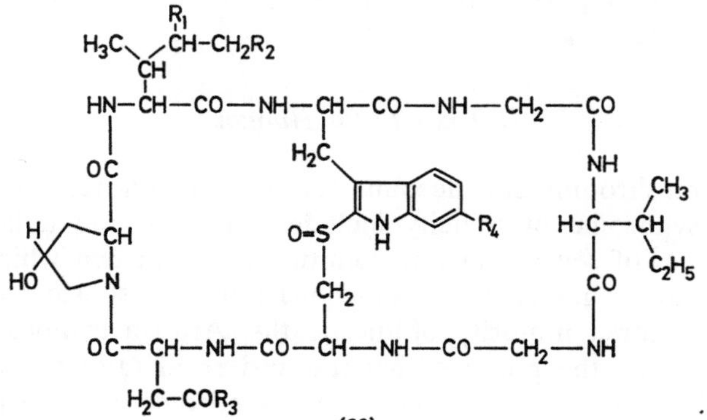

(32)

	R_1	R_2	R_3	R_4
a α-Amanitin	OH	OH	NH_2	OH
b β-Amanitin	OH	OH	OH	OH
c γ-Amanitin	H	OH	NH_2	OH
d Amanin	OH	OH	OH	H
e Amanullin	H	H	NH_2	OH

(a)

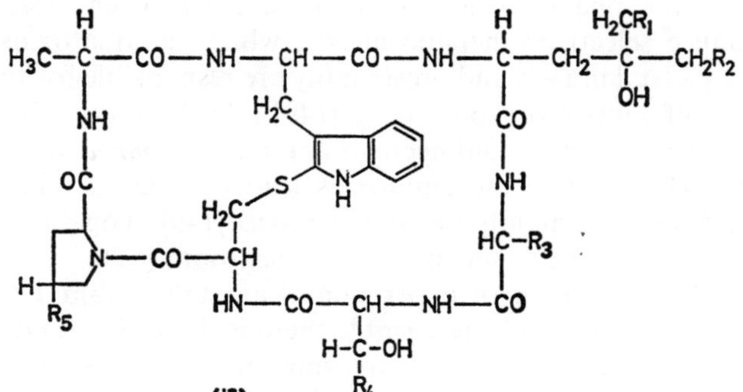

(17)

	R_1	R_2	R_3	R_4	R_5
a Phalloidin	OH	H	CH_3	CH_3	OH
b Phalloin	H	H	CH_3	CH_3	OH
c Phallisin	OH	OH	CH_3	CH_3	OH
d Phallicidin	OH	H	$CH(CH_3)_2$	CO_2H	OH
e Phallin B (tentatively)	H	H	$CH_2C_6H_5$	CH_3	H

(b)

Fig. 10a and b. Structure of amatoxins (a) and phallotoxins (b). (From WIELAND [612] with permission of author and publisher) tance of females [573]. Neonatal animals are resistant to phalloidin, but apparently susceptible to amanitin [149]. The regenerating rat liver is somewhat resistant to phalloidin injury [576].

d) Toxicity for Humans

Hepatotoxic mushrooms still account for several hundred world deaths per year [150]. The syndrome of toxicity includes an early and a late phase. The early phase consists of severe nausea, vomiting and diarrhea which begin 10 to 20 hrs after ingestion. This gastrointestinal phase usually subsides quite promptly and is responsible for a minority of the deaths. After a symptom-free interval of three to four days, the phase of hepatic and renal failure, which is mainly responsible for the high mortality (30%) of the syndrome, appears [132].

The *histopathologic* changes include hemorrhagic, centrizonal, hepatic necrosis and steatosis. Renal damage consists of tubular fat and necrosis [401, 193, 365].

Biochemical changes reflect the severe hepatic injury. There are striking elevations of serum levels of the transaminases (and other serum enzymes) [193] and of bilirubin, and depressed plasma levels of a number of clotting factors [358]. Early in the course there may be hyperglycemia. Later severe hypoglycemia accompanied by elevated lactic acid levels is characteristic [611].

e) Experimental Studies

The toxicity of the phallotoxins and amatoxins has been clearly separated. Phallotoxins produce selectively hepatic injury; while the amatoxins injure liver, kidney, heart and skeletal muscle and presumably are responsible for the myocardial and muscle injury of mushroom poisoning [149]. Furthermore, the phallotoxins produce centrizonal hemorrhage and necrosis and almost *immediate* injury to cytoplasmic organelles [149]; while the amatoxins lead to *delayed* injury focused on the nucleolus, and produce mainly hepatic steatosis [149]. Together they produce necrosis and steatosis, as do extracts of whole mushroom [611].

Phalloidin can lead to death of experimental animals within 1 to 2 hrs [149]. By 15 min after administration of the agent*, there is dilatation, and vacuolization of the ER [612]. By 1 hr injury to the plasma membrane is apparent. Within 2 hrs after administration to the rat, hepatic glycogen virtually disappears, fat droplets appear and mitochondria appear abnormal. Hemorrhagic necrosis and striking sinusoidal dilatation with engorgement are apparent within 2 to 4 hrs [577].

α-Amanitin usually does not lead to death for two or three days. Even with the highest doses** employed, death does not occur before 15 hrs. Histologic abnormalities by light microscopy also are delayed for 12 to 24 hrs [149]. By EM, however, nuclear and nucleolar changes are apparent within 15 min after administration of α-amanitin [149, 359]. Chromatin begins to collect in dense compact masses and to condense at the inner membrane of the nucleus; while the nuclear

* For the mouse a dose of 2 mg/kg.
** For the mouse doses in excess of 0.1 mg/kg.

sap begins to become clearer and more homogeneous, changes that lead to a "vesicle-like" [150] appearance of the nuclei by LM. In parallel with this nuclear change, chromatin condensation within the nucleoli leads to loss of reticular appearance with the segregation of granules from fibrils and formation of round or oval fragments each containing mainly granules or fibrils. By 15 hrs, only fragments of the nucleoli are apparent, and, by 24 hrs, these fragments contain only indistinct remnants of RNP fibrils [150].

Prominent hepatocyte changes seen by LM follow the nucleolar changes. Fat accumulates, first in the periportal cells and, ultimately, may include the entire liver. Necrosis is variable; when it occurs, it is centrizonal.

f) Mechanism of Injury

The phallotoxins and amatoxins have independent toxic effects. Phalloidin, the prototype of the phallotoxins, has an almost immediate adverse effect on membranes of the cell, especially the ER but also, importantly, on the plasma membrane. "Weakening" of the plasma membrane presumably accounts for the development of blebs on the surface of the hepatocyte within 10 min of administration of phalloidin [577]. A considerable amount of circumstantial evidence suggests that phalloidin must be metabolized to express its toxic effects. The resistance to phalloidin toxicity of the newborn animal, the regenerating liver and the animal pretreated with other hepatotoxic agents supports the view that a metabolite of phalloidin is the ultimate toxic principle [612]. Attachment of the phalloidin to membranes clearly is an essentially feature of its toxicity [316]. The possible relationship of the toxicity to glutathione-binding would seem to warrant exploration, in view of the similarity of the lesion to that [368] of acetominophen, the metabolic conversion of the latter to a toxic metabolite [368], which binds glutathione [368], and the recorded glutathione depletion in mushroom [425] and acetominophen [368] poisoning.

α-Amanitin leads to decreased nucleolar content of RNA, the basis for the altered EM pattern of the nucleoli. Studies with a variety of experimental models (rat liver, sea urchin, calf thymus, influenze virus) have demonstrated that this agent inhibits RNA polymerase. Specifically, it is the DNA-dependent RNA polymerase II, responsible for synthesis of the RNA, which is inhibited by amanitin. The inhibition has been ascribed to a specific interaction of amanitin with the polymerase or with a complex of DNA and polymerase. Inhibition of synthesis of ribosomal RNA (and perhaps other biochemical defects) is presumably responsible for inhibition of synthesis of protein by the hepatocyte [150].

g) Prevention of Toxicity

A number of agents have been described to prevent or even reverse the toxic effects of α-amanitin or of whole extracts of poisonous mushrooms [154]. Some are presumed to act by inhibiting the conversion of phalloidin to its toxic metabolic product. Others are described as effective against α-amanitin, perhaps by displacing it from binding sites and accelerating its excretion. The most effective is described to be cytochrome C [154]. Cytochrome C has been shown to reverse the toxic effects and prevent death in *female mice* given amanitin as long as eight hours before the cytochrome C [154]. The curious ineffectiveness in males and in rats of either sex remains unexplained and may have an important bearing on the mechanism of injury. Thioctic acid also has been reputed to be effective in preventing and reversing experimental α-amanitine toxicity and therapeutically effect in human poisoning, observations which have been challenged by FLOERSHEIM [154]. The mechanism of action of cytochrome C remains to be explained.

11. Galactosamine

Galactosamine (GALN) is a recent arrival on the scene of experimental hepatotoxicity. First reported by KEPPLER *et al.* in 1968 [252] as a cause of acute hepatocellular injury, it has been subjected to intensive study by that [113] and several other groups [356, 241, 278, 448, 301, 330, 374, 482, 204, 412, 47, 304, 12, 362, 493, 277] as a useful experimental model of hepatic injury.

Single or a few repeated doses of the agent cause acute hepatic necrosis [113]. Prolonged administration leads to cirrhosis [304]. The relationship of the parenchymal injury to the metabolism of galactosamine appears to have been clarified by series of elegant studies of KEPPLER and his associates [252, 113, 556, 192], SHINOZUKA *et al.* [412], and KOFF and his co-workers [277, 278].

a) Significance

Galactosamine-induced hepatic injury is an extremely interesting model of hepatic injury, KEPPLER and his associates have been impressed by its similarity to the lesion of viral hepatitis [252]. Their observations of the similarity of hepatitis appear valid with regard to the form of hepatocyte damage observed by light microscopy and the inflammatory response. The ultrastructural studies suggest however, a different fundamental lesion; particularly the accumulation of fat [356, 277] which is a feature not characteristic of viral hepatitis. Nevertheless, it is of interest that galactosamine-hepatic injury is a model that appears to resemble galactosemia of humans which may serve to study the relationship between key defects in this area of metabolism and the development of hepatic disease [113]. The enormous information on the specific injury induced by galactosamine developed by the studies of DECKER and KEPPLER [113] and others [356, 241, 278, 448, 301, 330, 374, 482, 204, 412, 47, 304, 12, 362, 493, 277] in a short time is an important achievement.

b) Chemical Characteristics

Galactosamine is a simple water soluble amino sugar. In the N-acetylated form it is a component of the glycoproteins and mucopolysaccharides of many tissues. It is not found in tissues as the free aminosugar. A specific method for identification of its metabolites is available [113].

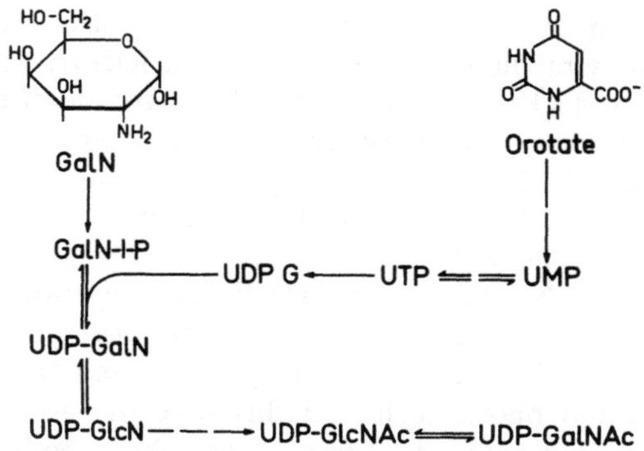

Fig. 11. Metabolism of GALN. (From DECKER and KEPPLER [113] with permission of authors, editors and publisher)

c) Factors in Susceptibility

Species. There have not been extensive studies of differences between species in susceptibility. Rats, rabbits, guinea pigs, mice, marmoset monkeys and trout all appear to be vulnerable to the agent [113]. Guinea pigs seem unusually susceptible and mice unusually resistent.

Age and Stage of Development. SHINOZUKA *et al.* [512] have reported that the liver of fetal and neonatal rats, the regenerating liver and Morris hepatoma cells are resistant. LEINWEBER *et al.* [301], however, have described in baby rats a lesion resembling giant-cell hepatitis of infants when given Gal-N, metabolized by an adult liver. Curiously, human fetal hepatocytes in tissue culture are injured by GALN [276]. Aging rats are somewhat more susceptible than young but mature ones [113].

Endocrine and Other Factors. There appears to be little sex difference in susceptibility [113]. Adrenalectomy seems to enhance the toxic effects of small but not of large doses [64], and glucocorticoids in large doses seem to protect against GALN toxicity [180].

Blockade of the RES leads to increased susceptibility, while RES activation decreases vulnerability to injury [183]. Administration of GALN simultaneously with intravenous carbon particles enhances vulnerability strikingly, while administration of GALN 8 days after the RES blockade (time of RES activation) enhances resistance [183].

d) Experimental Hepatotoxicity

Administration of doses greater than 100 mg/kg of body weight by various routes (I.P., I.V., or SC) rapidly produces hepatocellular injury [113]. This amount may be given as a single dose or divided into multiple doses during a 24-hr period. The effects of Gal-N are clearly dose-related. A dose of 100 mg/kg produces only slight hepatic injury in rats; one twice that leads to areas of necrosis, and a dose of 400 mg leads to extensive necrosis [113].

The lesion consists mainly of hepatocyte injury. KEPPLER and his associates

[113] describe the lesion to be diffuse and multi-focal necrosis and believe it to resemble the lesion of viral hepatitis of humans sufficiently to provide a useful experimental counterpart. KOFF *et al.* [278] also have described focal necrosis with inflammatory response but consider the lesion, which also includes lipid accumulation, to resemble other toxic injury more than it does viral hepatitis. They [277] as well as MEDLINE *et al.* [356] have found the ultrastructural changes to be unlike those of viral hepatitis.

A single dose of GALN leads to acidophilic degeneration in four hours and necrosis of individual cells in six hours. By 24 hrs, disseminated focal areas of necrosis have developed, often accompanied by an inflammatory response of neutrophils, lymphocytes and plasma cells. At this time the non-necrotic cells show prominent acidophilic degeneration, "free" acidophilic bodies and ballooning. Many cells show accumulations of fat. Kupfer cells show evidence of enlargement and increase in number by 6 hrs; these changes become prominent by 24 hrs. The hepatocyte injury is non-zonal, being disseminated throughout the lobule. The injury reaches a maximum 48 hrs after administration of the agent; at this time there is marked dissociation of cell plates and extensive areas of necrosis. Portal areas show edema, inflammatory infiltration and bile ductular proliferation at the peak of the injury. Restitution of normal structure begins in surviving animals after 48 hrs [305]. By 7 to 12 days, the liver has regained a normal appearance [113].

The repeated administration of GALN over a six-month period leads to cirrhosis, which from the published photomicrographs appears to be micronodular [304]. DECKER and KEPPLER [113] describe it as "chronic hepatitis" followed by cirrhosis.

Ultrastructural studies [356, 277] demonstrate the injury to involve all of the hepatocytes. It includes membrane-bound autophagic vacuoles, which contain remnants of mitochondria, glycogen, and granular and fibrillar debris; reduction of glycogen particles, and hypertrophy of the SER. These changes are seen by 2 [113] to 6 [277] hrs in some hepatocytes. By 24 hrs, all of the hepatocytes show some degree of abnormality which includes collections of amorphous cellular debris, subcellular organelles in varying stages of degeneration and virtual disappearance of glycogen. There is dilatation of the RER with the attendant increase in free ribosomes and hyperplasia of the SER. The mitochondria show little change after low doses (1.8 mMole/kg) but abnormal size and shape after larger doses. Nuclei show condensation of chromatin; and nucleoli are fragmented and dispersed within 4 hrs [356, 277].

By 48 hrs the remaining SER consists only of irregularly dilated vesicles. Fat droplets are prominent and mitochondrial injury (crenation of outer and invagination of inner membrane) is more obvious.

Fat, both membrane-bound and free is seen by 3 hrs [277]. Nuclear changes, best observed after repeated doses, includes fragmentation and dispersal of the RNA. Kupfer cells are seen to contain hepatocyte debris including acidophilic bodies.

Biochemical manifestations in the blood of the hepatic injury include 10-to-20-fold elevations of levels of GOT, GPT, SDH, and glutamate dehydrogenase. Alkaline phosphatase levels are elevated approximately 4-fold and bilirubin levels are usually only moderately increased [113].

e) *Mechanism of Injury*

Galactosamine is a relatively simple molecule found in the glycoproteins and mucopolysaccharides of many animal tissues; but it is not found as the free amino sugar. There is no evidence that endogenous galactosamine ever leads to spontaneous disease in humans or animals [113]; although KOFF [277] has drawn attention to the similarity of the galactosamine-induced hepatic injury to the disease galactosemia. When administered as a pure compound to experimental animals galactosamine induces hepatic injury related to its metabolism in the liver and the consequent effect on nucleic acid metabolism [113].

Promptly after administration of the amino sugar, it is taken up by the liver. Within 3 hrs, one-fifth of an injected dose of Gal-N can be recovered from the liver. In the liver its initial metabolic fate is along the pathway for galactose metabolism, after which there are two hypothetical alternative pathways for galactosamine metabolism (Fig. 11); both lead to the production of UDP-glucosamine. The latter compound, in contrast to UDP-glucose, which is normally produced in the metabolism of galactose, apparently does not serve as a uridylate donor in the uridyltransferase reaction. Accordingly, UDP-hexosamine formation from galactosamine leads to the trapping of uridylate [253, 254]. Other hexosamines that can also be derived from galactosamine are UDP-N-acetylgalactosamine and UDP-N-acety-glucosamine which accumulate after galactosamine administration [113].

The rate of trapping of uridylate by the metabolism of Gal-N, when toxic doses of the latter are given, exceeds the synthetic capacity for uridylic acid in the adult rat liver. Accordingly, the metabolism of galactosamine by hepatocytes is associated with a striking decrease in the concentration of UDP-glucose, UDP-galactose, UTP, UDP, UMP, and UDP-glucuronate [113]. This occurs despite the increased synthesis of uridylic acid that is provoked by the galactosamine metabolism. Galactosamine toxicity thus appears to be a form of "high output failure" of uridylate biosynthesis provoked by the galactosamine metabolism, and recovery from the initial biochemical impact of galactosamine is marked by increased levels of uracil nucleotides. KEPPLER and his associates [113] have pointed out that there is a critical level or threshold below which deficient hepatic UTP levels can lead to hepatic injury. Specifically, they suggest that a decrease in concentration of UTP to a level below 25–30% of the normal, that persists for several hours, leads to subsequent signs of liver damage [113].

In support of their view that the hepatic injury induced by Gal-N is a result of uridylate trapping, and a subsequent decrease in UTP, KEPPLER *et al.* [113, 281] have shown that the administration of 2-deoxy-galactose to guinea pigs or of D-galactose to guinea pigs or of D-galactose plus 6-azauridine to adult rats can provoke a deficit of uridylate. Prolongation of the uridylate deficit by repeated injections of this combination, leads to biochemical and histologic changes that are almost identical with those observed after Gal-N administration.

DECKER and KEPPLER [113] have drawn the interesting analogy of galactosamine hepatotoxicity with its dependence on trapping of UTP, to ethionine toxicity which produces hepatic injury by trapping of ATP. Just as ethionine toxicity can be inhibited to an important degree by the administration of ATP precursors so can galactosamine toxicity be inhibited by the administration of uridine or by the administration of orotate which increases the uridylic biosynthesis (Fig. 11). Indeed, circumstances that lead to more rapid uridylic biosynthesis, as is seen in the rapidly growing liver, lead to lesser susceptibility to galastosamine toxicity. Examples of this phenomenon are provided by neonatal rats and adult rats with livers regenerating after partial hepatectomy. Similarly, animals may be relatively refractory to galactosamine treatment after 3 months of exposure; at this time there appears to be an enhanced activity of uridylate biosynthesis.

It has also been suggested that differences between species in susceptibility may be explained by differences in rate of uridylate synthesis. Guinea pigs which have a relatively low rate of uridylate formation are much more susceptible to hepatic injury than mice which have a high rate of uridylate synthesis [113].

The toxicity of Gal-N can not be related to an immediate adverse effect of the agent or of a metabolite, but appears to be an indirect result of loss of a key metabolite to a metabolic cul-de-sac. DECKER and KEPPLER [113] have suggested that galactosamine behaves as an indirect toxin by our classification.

The impact of the biochemical lesions of UTP depletion appears to be expressed in functional defects and in the ultimate structural ones. Functional defects include depression of the uracil nucleotide-dependent synthesis of nucleic acids, and a presumably consequent lack of synthesis of protein, membrane structures, glucose, lipids and glycogen [113, 434]. Depression of nucleic acid synthesis would primarily involve inhibited formation of RNA since UTP is incorporated into RNA; but also may include DNA, since uridylate is also a precursor of TTP [113]. There is also inhibited hepatic formation of plasma glycoproteins which include α-lipoprotein, lecithin-cholesterol-acyl-transferase and coagulation factors [113]. Impaired coagulation, however, is also in part the result of D.I.C. [382]. The inhibition of protein synthesis also appears to be expressed in impaired synthesis of hepatic enzymes of the gluconeogenetic pathway and presumably is responsible for impaired synthesis of glycogen. Impaired protein synthesis is apparent by 2 hrs [113] and at its peak at 6 hrs.

The inhibition of protein synthesis may be inferred to be responsible for or to contribute to the accumulation of fat in the hepatocytes, as in a number of other forms of toxin-induced fatty liver. It presumably results from impaired exit of lipid from the liver because of lack of lipid carrier protein or because of changes in the cell membrane.

12. Orotic Acid

Orotic acid has been of interest as a precursor of uridine and other pyrimidines, as a biochemical marker of distorted pyrimidine metabolism, and as a possible but unproved therapeutic agent for a number of conditions. One of the properties of this compound that has attracted considerable interest [421, 239, 405, 397, 535, 257, 258, 120, 63, 244, 518, 519, 590, 616, 426, 465, 620, 621, 622, 112, 230, 617, 390, 159, 264, 559, 585, 215, 487, 63, 245] is its ability to produce fatty liver in the rat.

a) Significance

The chief importance of the orotic acid-induced fatty liver is the provision of a model system for the study of lipid transport from the liver [539]. Indeed, studies of the mechanism for the orotic acid effect have thrown important light on the pathogenesis of fatty liver [539].

b) Chemical Characteristics

Orotic acid (6-carboxyuracil) is a pyrimidine which is readily synthesized in the body of animals. A precursor of the pyrimidines of nucleic acid, it is first converted to orotidylic acid, subsequently decarboxylated to form uridylic acid, which is further converted to other nucleotides. The initial step in the metabolism of orotic acid, reaction with PP-ribose-P to form orotidylic acid, is considered the pivotal step in the production of the fatty liver (Fig. 12).

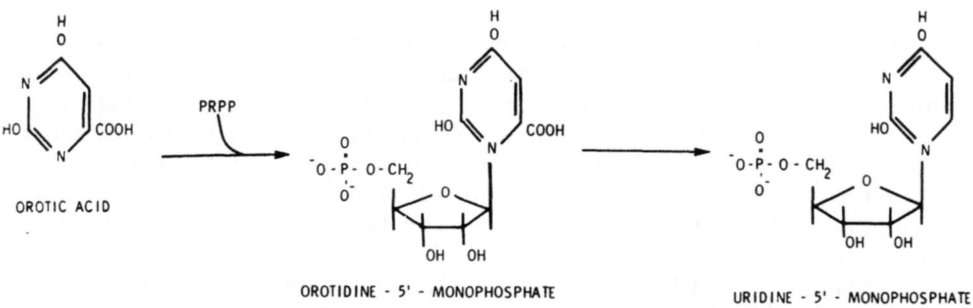

Fig. 12. Structure and metabolic pathway of orotic acid

c) Factors in Susceptibility

Species. Only the rat has proven to develp hepatic abnormality when given orotic acid. Rabbits, hamsters, guinea pigs, mice, chickens [147], monkeys [585] and man [245] appear to be resistant.

Sex. Females appear to be more susceptible to the steatogenic effects [518] but less susceptible to the effects of the fatty liver on microsomal enzymes [215]. SIDRANSKY [518] found that females developed a more severe fatty liver than males. By castration and hormone replacement studies he demonstrated androgens to be protective. Curiously, HOLTZMAN and GILLETTE [215] found that the orotic acid-induced fatty liver of the male rat had a sharply reduced aniline hydroxylase activity and P-450 content; while the fatty liver of the female had no significant reduction in these parameters.

Diet. The effects of diet on the orotic acid fatty liver remain unclear. Animals which are starved, forced-fed casein hydrolysate, or given a diet enriched with lactose do not develop fatty liver, while those force-fed a normal diet do. Diet, according to SARMA and SIDRANSKY, may be important for the maintenance of sufficiently adequate fat synthesis for the steatogenic effect of orotic acid to be expressed [487].

d) Experimental Injury

Administration of a force-fed diet containing 1% orotic acid leads to a fatty liver in 3 to 4 days [619, 519]. The fat is deposited first or mainly in the periportal zone [519, 426]. Chemical measurement shows a 2- to 4-fold increase in triglycerides. No changes other than steatosis are seen by L.M.

Ultrastructural abnormalities include dilatation and fragmentation of the ER by 4 days. Lipid droplets and increased activity in the GOLGI apparatus which contain electron opaque material also appear [230].

Biochemical changes in the blood are slight. Serum levels of GOT are doubled and of GPT are increased slightly [603]. Levels of VLDL are depressed [619]. Functional changes with regard to metabolism of drug [215] and endogenous steroids [603] have been demonstrated and inferred respectively.

e) Mechanism of Injury

The evidence is compelling that the steatogenic effects of orotic acid relate to the relative deficiency of ATP consequent to the acceleration of pyrimidine synthesis [244, 590, 465]. Increase in uridine synthesis and decrease in hepatocyte ATP precede the accumulation of lipid. Administration of adenine [616] and of 5-amino-imidazole-carboxamide [244] which elevate hepatic ATP content can prevent or reverse the fatty liver. Reaction of orotic acid with P-R-PP is the first step in the pathway to depletion of the ATP [590, 616, 465, 621]. Inhibition of pyrimidine synthesis can prevent the fatty liver [618].

The steatosis is clearly the result of striking reduction in transport from the liver [619, 616, 622, 245] providing that normal lipid synthesis continues [539]. Demonstration of depressed plasma VLDL [619, 622, 147] and studies with the perfused liver [622] demonstrate decreased secretion of lipoprotein with its lipid load to be responsible for the steatosis. The defect, however, is not in the synthesis of the apoprotein [465, 112] but appears to be in its glycosylization. Presumably, the abnormal protein cannot form the complex with the lipid for transport or be secreted [539]. The report [264] that peroxidation occurs in the orotic acid fatty liver has been challenged [63].

II. Cholestatic Indirect Hepatotoxins

A number of agents produce hepatic injury characterized mainly or exclusively by arrested bile flow with little or no injury to the hepatic parenchyma [472, 269, 638, 523, 202]. Some drugs produce cholestatic injury in humans who are uniquely susceptible because of hypersensitivity or other form of idiosyncrasy [638, 639, 547]. These idiosyncratic reactions are beyond the scope of this review. There are other agents, however, which can produce selectively, cholestatic injury as a dose-related phenomenon [523, 202, 62]. These are accordingly categorizable as cholestatic *indirect* hepatotoxins [638]. The prototype is *icterogenin* (Fig. 13), an agent found in Lippia rehmanni and several other plants [62, 453]. Also in this category are the C-17-alkylated anabolic [638, 14] and contraceptive [201] steroids, estrogenic steroids [162], dinitrophenol [522], dinitrodiphenymethane [280], manganese ion [624], flavaspidic acid [216] rifampicin [1], and ANIT [481]. The interruption of bile flow may be the result of selective interference with uptake of bilirubin by the hepatocyte [498], selective interference with bile secretion, or

Structures of C_{17}-alkylated anabolic and contraceptive steroids, icterogenin and rehmannic acid

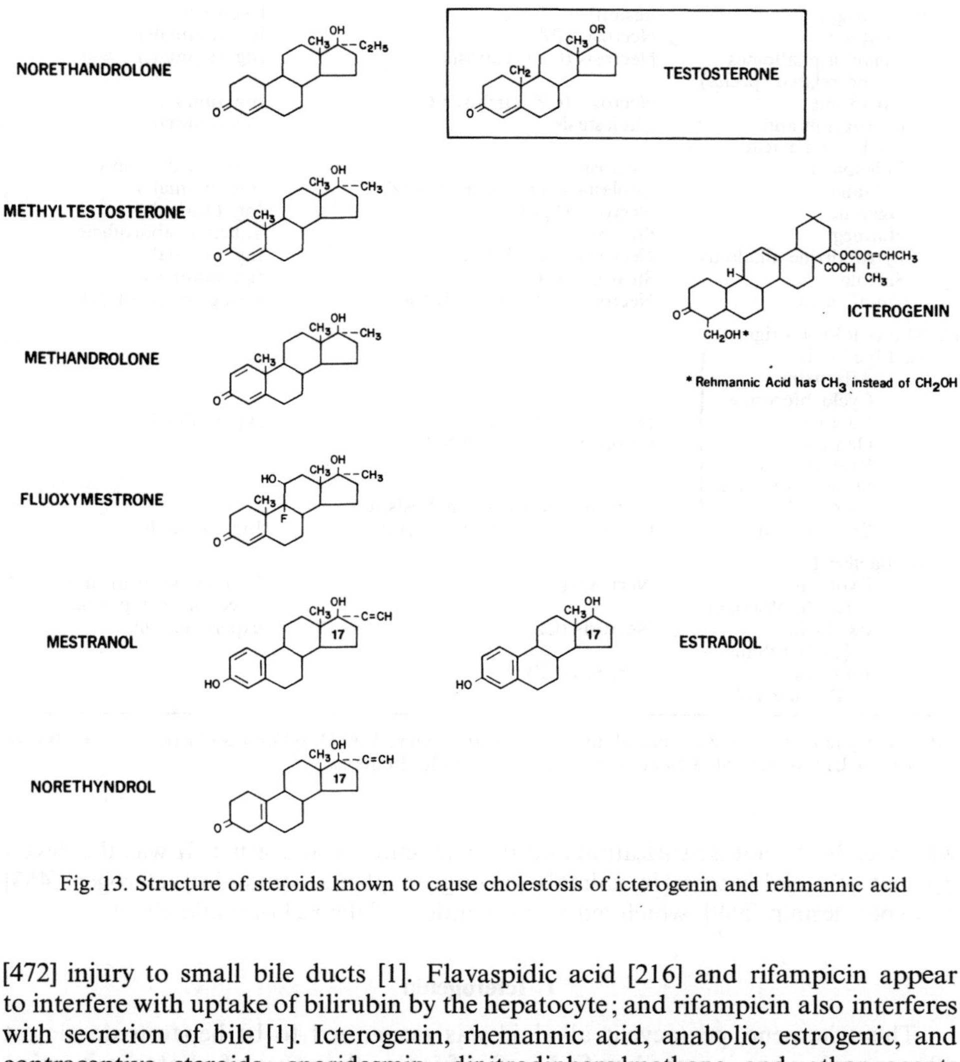

Fig. 13. Structure of steroids known to cause cholestosis of icterogenin and rehmannic acid

[472] injury to small bile ducts [1]. Flavaspidic acid [216] and rifampicin appear to interfere with uptake of bilirubin by the hepatocyte; and rifampicin also interferes with secretion of bile [1]. Icterogenin, rhemannic acid, anabolic, estrogenic, and contraceptive steroids, sporidesmin, dinitrodiphenylmethane and other agents shown in Table 12, interfere selectively with bile excretion, either by apparent canalicular injury (icterogenin [62]) or by interfering with the cellular function (ATP levels [522]) required for bile secretion. Cholestasis as a result of bile duct injury is characteristic of ANIT toxicity. Some of these agents (sporidesmin [62], ANIT [378]) produce varying degrees of overt cellular injury in addition to or instead of cholestasis in some species.

A curious phenomenon, of particular veterinary interest, has led to the recognition of several of the agents in this group [62, 93]. Facial eczema in ruminants may result from cholestasis [93]. Arrest of bile flow leads to accumulation in the blood and tissues of a product of chlorophyll degradation, phylloerytherin,

Table 12. Natural hepatotoxins to which domestic exposure is known or potential

	Lesion[a]	Exposure
I. Plant origin		
Albitocin	Necrosis (PZ)	Ing. (animals)
Amanita phalloides (and related species)	Necrosis (CZ) steatosis	Ing. (animals)
Cycad nut	Necrosis (CZ) cirrhosis Ca	Ing. (animals)
Icterogenin and rehmannic acid	Cholestasis	Ing. (animals)
Indospicine	Steatosis	Experimental only
Lantana	Cholestasis plus necrosis (PZ)	Ing. (animals)
Ngaione	Necrosis (MZ)	Ing. (animals)
Nutmeg	Steatosis	Taken as abortifacient
Pyrrolidizine alkaloids	Necrosis (CZ), V.O.D., Ca	Ing. (animals)
Safrole	Steatosis, Ca	Ing. (animals)
Tannic acid	Necrosis (CZ), steatosis Ca	Iatrogenic (see text)
II. Microbiologic origin		
A. Mycotoxins		
Aflatoxins, Cyclochlorotine, Luteoskyrin, Ochratoxins, Rubratoxins, Sterigmatocystins	Necrosis, steatosis Cirrhosis (Some lead to Ca)	Ing. (animals)
Griseofulvin	Necrosis, steatosis, Cirrhosis, Ca	
Sporidesmin	Cholestasis plus Necrosis (PZ)	Ing. (animals)
B. Bacterial		
Exotoxin (C. diphtheriae)	Necrosis (CZ)	Lesions occur during infection or reproduced experimentally
Exotoxin (Cl. botulinus)	Necrosis (CZ)	
Endotoxin (Pr. vulgaris)	Necrosis (PZ)	

[a] PZ = Peripheral zone; CZ = Central zone; Ca = Carcinoma; V.O.D. = Veno-occlusive disease; Ing. = Ingestion. Unless stipulated as animals, exposure includes humans.

which leads to photosensitization and the resultant facial eczema. It was the development of facial eczema in animals grazing on plants containing icterogen [453] and sporidesmin [569], which led to recognition of their cholestatic effect.

1. Icterogenin

This triterpene, pentacyclic alkaloid was recognized to be hepatotoxic almost 40 years ago when it was identified in S. Africa as the cause of photosensitization and facial eczema in grazing sheep which had ingested the plant *Lippia rehmanni* [453]. Subsequent studies have demonstrated the cholestatic effects of icterogenin [62]. Icterogenin is chiefly of interest as a model of almost pure cholestasis, as a prototype of disease of veterinary importance and as an interesting chemical and physiologic analogue of the steroids that produce cholestasis [14].

a) Chemical Properties

The chemical structure of icterogenin, shown in Fig. 13, resembles that of the cholestasis-producing steroids. Indeed, the cholestatic properties have a striking relationship to chemical structure [59]. A nonpolar compound, icterogenin is almost totally insoluble in water, a property which has hampered efforts to test quantitative aspects of its toxicity [62]. BULLOCK *et al.* [62] have found solution in small amounts of ethanol useful in preparing injectable icterogenin.

Several analogues of icterogenin that are even more potent in producing cholestasis have been described [59]. The apparent molecular requirements have been demonstrated by BROWN [59].

b) Experimental Models

Intact animals [18, 453, 59], animals with the bile duct cannulated [14] and the *ex vivo* perfused liver [62] have been employed in the study of the effects of icterogenin. The intact herbiverous animal has served to demonstrate the direct cholestatic effects, i.e. the hyperbilirubineninia and the indirect effect, i.e. the photosensitization that results from retention of phylloerythrin [202].

The animal with bile duct cannulated has served to compare the cholestatic effect of various agents and to study the mechanism [14]. Quantitation of the effect of the icterogenin, however, has been hampered by the uncertain absorption attendant on the poor solubility in aqueous solvents [62]. The employment of the *ex vivo* perfused liver has circumvented this problem and has permitted definition [62] of the concentration of the agent that reaches the liver and studies of the mechanism for its cholestatic effect.

c) Factors in Susceptibility

Species. Sheep, cattle, rats and rabbits all have been found to be vulnerable [62]. Indeed, no refractory species has been reported. We are aware of no studies of the effect of age, endocrine status or sex on the response to icterogenin. Male and female seem equally vulnerable. Efforts to demonstrate the adverse effects of this agent, however, have been handicapped by the problems of solubility.

d) Toxic Effects

The effect on the liver seems almost purely cholestatic. Interference with bile flow occurs within 30 min of introduction* into the perfused liver [62]. Although variable, it seems to develop rapidly in the whole animal, and to reach its peak in 24 to 48 hrs [202]. The parenchyma seems intact [202], but there are changes in the canalicular membrane [62]. Material is extruded into the canalicular space and there is loss of canalicular microvilli [62]. The striking cholestatic effect occurs without diminution of ATP content of the cell sap [522]. The suggestion of SLATER and DELANEY [522] that the icterogenin-induced cholestasis is the result of inhibition of canalicular ATPase has found support in the studies of BULLOCK and his associates [62].

---

* 4 mg of icterogenin in 120 ml of perfusate.

2. Sporidesmin

This fungal toxin, derived from *Pithomyces chartarum*, was first discovered to cause cholestasis when it was found to be responsible for facial eczema in sheep [569] grazing on pasture contaminated with the fungus. Administration of sporidesmin to rabbits, guinea pigs and rats leads to cholestasis [379, 94, 632, 524, 525]. In the rat there is very little parenchymal injury [524, 525]; but in sheep there is periportal, parenchymal necrosis [379]. The canaliculi show a striking loss of microvilli and the adjacent hepatocytes show numerous lipozome-like structures [62].

Sporidesmin appears to have a striking ability to produce membrane injury. It leads to increased capillary fragility which is said to be responsible for the development of ascites and pleural effusion in the rat [62]. The membrane injury has been attributed to the interaction of the disulfide bridge of sporidesmin with the membrane-bound sulfhydryl groups. It appears to involve membrane of intracellular organelles as well as of the canaliculi: injury to the canalicular microvilli is considered by BULLOCK *et al.* to be responsible for the cholestatic lesion [62].

3. α-Naphthylisothiocyanate (ANIT)

This agent has evoked considerable interest among students of hepatotoxicity during the past several decades. First reported a quarter century ago in rats by MAZZANTI *et al.* [72, 313, 336] to produce a striking bile duct proliferation, it has since been studied extensively as an apparent model for the production of intrahepatic cholestasis [584, 474, 36, 97, 413, 491] and of a form of experimental biliary cirrhosis [409, 353, 72].

Administered acutely as a single dose, ANIT leads in the rat to necrosis of portal bile ducts and ductules, inflammation of portal areas and varying degrees of parenchymal injury [491, 177]. In several species, ANIT leads to hyperbilirubinemia and other biochemical reflections of cholestasis [409, 77, 223]. Long term intoxication with this agent leads to proliferation of bile ducts, chronic parenchymal injury and cirrhosis [313, 409, 353, 72]. In some species hepatocellular injury is prominent and bile duct injury is trivial [409, 77, 223].

a) Significance

The importance of ANIT is mainly as an experimental tool for the production of a distinctive form of cholestasis and of acute and chronic bile duct injury and for the study of the histogenesis of ducts in hepatic disease [43]. There is no evidence of human exposure to the toxic effects of this agent, and there remains considerable question regarding its use as a model for either intrahepatic cholestasis or extrahepatic obstruction [491]. Indeed, the apparent cholestasis is now generally recognized to be accompanied by significant parenchymal injury.

b) Chemical Characteristics

Hepatotoxicity of the isothiocyanates depends on precise and specific structural features. Of 17 compounds tested by BECKER and PLAA [38] only the α-naphtyhyl-, and the phenylisothiocyanate produced hepatic injury. The β-naphthylisothiocyanate, all of the alkyl-isothiocyanates, several thiocyanates and isocyanates all failed to produce hepatic damage or hyperbilirubinemia [38]. BECKER and PLAA deduced that an *aryl* compound of *planar* configuration with a substitute radical containing N, C and S are probably chemical requirements for the production of the hepatic lesion. Since ANIT, a non-polar molecule, is insoluble in water it must be given in sesame oil or appropriate solvents.

c) Experimental Models

Almost all of the studies conducted with ANIT have employed the intact animal, most often rats or mice. A few have evaluated the effects of the agent on guinea pigs [313, 409, 353], hamsters [223], rabbits [353], dogs [223], sheep [178] and cattle [178]. Observations made have included histological and histochemical changes, biochemical reflections of hepatic injury, and studies on the modification of toxic effects by various manipulations. A few studies have utilized animals with cannulated bile ducts; others have studied the metabolic properties of liver homogenates from animals which had received ANIT [413]. In all studies the agents have been administered enterally either by intragastric instillation or mixed with the food. *In vitro* observations of the direct effects of ANIT on isolated ribosomes also have been conducted [415, 454].

d) Factors in Susceptibility

Rats and mice are the most sensitive, of the species studied [409, 223], to bile duct injury. They develop marked hyperbilirubinemia and cholestasis after a single dose, with mice described to be somewhat more susceptible than rats [223]. Guinea pigs are less sensitive, and hamsters and rabbits are even more resistant, developing mild hepatic injury but no jaundice even after large doses [409, 223]. Dogs [223], sheep and cows [178] develop parenchymal injury but little or no bile duct injury and no cholestasis when given ANIT. Furthermore, doses required to produce injury are 2 to 4 times as great as those which produce the cholestatic lesion in more susceptible species. Species differences and susceptibility have been attributed [223] to the requirement for conversion of ANIT to a toxic metabolite in order to produce the hepatobiliary injury and to the demonstrated [77] species differences in the metabolism of this compound. Young rats, however, seem more susceptible than mature animals, a paradoxical feature. No sex difference in susceptibility is apparent.

e) Toxic Effects

Acute Injury. Single doses of 50 to 150 mg/kg given orally to rats rapidly lead to biochemical and histologic abnormalities. Initial changes can be seen as early as 6 hrs; by 48 hrs the effects are maximal and then gradually subside with return to normal of all parameters by the third or fourth week. Although there are minor differences in the details described by various authors [584, 313, 491, 409, 353, 72, 177, 134, 538] the following account reflects the consensus.

Histologic abnormalities are apparent by 12 to 24 hrs. Administration of 50 to 150 mg/kg to rats leads to swelling, vacuolization and necrosis of the epithelium of interlobular portal bile ducts, with desquamation of the necrotic debris into the lumens and apparent occlusion. Surrounding the necrotic ducts are edematous portal spaces containing a prominent infiltration of neutrophilic leukocytes, some of which invade the duct walls. By 48 hrs the portal bile ducts and lobular ductules show signs of proliferation; and inflammation surrounds the small *intra* lobular bile ducts, many of which contain plugs of mucous with or without desquamated cells. Ductular proliferation is maximal on day 4. Between the fourth and seventh days, the bile ducts have assumed an almost normal appearance with restitution of the epithelium; subsidence of the inflammation, and with only some residual irregularity of luminal diameter, portal edema and prominence of fibroblasts.

Minor parenchymal abnormalities are seen in the rat by LM. Focal necrosis, described as mainly *periportal* by ELIAKIM *et al.* [134] and by GOLDFARB and his associates [177] and as *mid-* and *centrizonal* by MCLEAN and REES [353], is maximal between days 2 and 4. Restitution of normal liver structure begins by the end of the first week and is generally complete by 21 days.

In guinea pigs *parenchymal* injury including focal necrosis is more characteristic and bile duct injury less prominent than in the rat [409]. In sheep and cows, acute doses of ANIT lead mainly to parenchymal injury [178]. A dose as high as 400 mg/kg leads to very little evidence of injury of bile ducts, but does produce histochemical evidence of hepatocyte damage. Cells in the periportal zone show loss of glycogen, tinctorial changes and loss of mitochondrial enzymes.

Evidence of canalicular injury is apparent in all species. Canalicular ectasia, tortuosity and side-branching are seen in guinea pigs and rats [409]. Side-branching has been presumed to reflect intracellular invagination of the canaliculi. In these species, as well as in ruminants, increased canalicular staining for ATPase, alkaline phosphatase and 5-nucleotidase is observed, especially in the periportal zone [116].

Studies by EM [409, 538, 541] reveal injury to mitochondria of periportal hepatocytes and of bile duct epithelium, maximal at 24–48 hrs but, apparent as early as 3 hrs after a single dose of ANIT. Other significant changes include dilatation of the GOLGI apparatus, especially in centrizonal hepatocytes as early as 3 hrs. In the periportal zone, dilatation of canaliculi with loss of microvilli is seen by 24 hrs. At 24 to 48 hrs depletion of glycogen and increased prominence of the SER is seen in hepatocytes in all portions of the lobule, while apparent decrease in RER is noted in the cells of the periportal zone. Injury to the plasma membrane at both the canalicular and sinusoidal poles of hepatocytes and the luminal pole of ductal epithelium is apparent at 24 hrs [538, 541].

Biochemical abnormalities that occur after single, acute doses include hyperbilirubinemia, elevated alkaline phosphatase levels and hypercholesterolemia in the rat and mouse [134, 458, 37, 461]. Hyperbilirubinemia appears to result from cholestasis (both impaired excretion and impaired uptake from the blood), and, to a varying degree, hepatocellular dysfunction [36, 457, 412, 459]. This is augmented by the increased bilirubin production of ANIT-induced hemolysis [459] and destruction of non-heme compounds (e.g. P-450) by the toxin. Elevated levels of alkaline phosphatase and cholesterol reflect the cholestatic response and resemble the values observed in extrahepatic obstruction [134]. Bilirubin levels are dose-

and species-related [223]. Despite the convincing evidence for increased production of bilirubin, the blood bilirubin is almost entirely in the conjugated form [458]. Alkaline phosphatase levels in the rat are 2- to 5-fold elevated and cholesterol levels usually less than 2-fold increased [134].

To a varying degree single doses of ANIT lead to biochemical manifestations of hepatic injury. Increased blood levels of GOT, GPT, and vitamin B_{12} all appear to reflect necrosis [377]. In sheep and cattle increased blood levels of glutamate dehydrogenase, a mitochondrial enzyme, corresponds to the microscopic evidence of mitochondrial injury [178].

Other abnormalities include impaired excretion of BSP and prolongation of narcotic effects of pentobarbital [37]. Homogenates of liver, after single doses of ANIT, show impaired ability to metabolize hexobarbital, aniline, and aminopyrine but not chlorpromazine [415, 454].

Chronic Toxicity. Prolonged administration of ANIT leads to a "massive" proliferation of bile ducts and ductules accompanied by increased fibrosis [409, 353, 72, 177] and the production of a lesion that has been called [409, 353, 72] biliary cirrhosis. This effect has been dubbed by McLean and Rees [353] a "primary cholangioplastic" one to denote the lack of its dependence on biliary obstruction.

During the first two weeks of feeding of ANIT bile duct lesions and focal necrosis similar to the injury seen acutely after large single doses develop. These lesions are noted after one week and begin to subside after the second week. Thereafter the epithelium of portal bile ducts appears normal; while focal necrosis and portal inflammation remain until 4 weeks of feeding ANIT have elapsed [177]. Bile ductule proliferation and fibrosis continue, however; and by 7 weeks a lesion that Goldfarb *et al.* [177] have defined as biliary cirrhosis is seen.

By LM the chief adverse effect of chronic administration of ANIT on hepatocytes appears to be the disorganization of the lobule imposed by the ductular proliferation. Studies by EM, however, have demonstrated profound changes in the hepatocytes. The RER becomes disorganized; the ribosomes are shed; the degranulated membranes become arranged in "fingerprints" and SER becomes hypertrophied and compacted. These changes become progressively more severe with continued feeding [409].

Biochemical manifestation of chronic ANIT toxicity are surprisingly scant. At two weeks, the time of peak ductal injury, jaudice and cholestasis are prominent [177]. Jaundice then subsides and, thereafter, hyperbilirubinemia is mild or even absent [177]. In agreement with this observation is the disappearance of the inhibition of bile flow seen at the peak of the lesion; even some degree of increased bile secretion is observed at this stage [177].

f) Mechanism of Injury

Injury induced by ANIT, although assumed to be mainly cholestatic, clearly includes hepatocellular damage [36]. Impaired uptake and excretion of bilirubin, impaired excretion of BSP *prior* to any evidence of cholestasis, impairment of drug metabolism at a dose of ANIT too small to lead to cholestasis all demonstrate hepatocellular injury [413]. Nevertheless, frank cholestasis and outspoken duct injury are characteristic of the lesion in rats and mice. Recent studies suggest that the cholestatic effect is partially independent of the hepatocyte injury [225].

The cholestatic injury has been shown by PLAA and his associates be dependent on metabolism of ANIT [455, 571]. Agents that enhance drug metabolism (phenobarbital) enhance the cholestatic effect on rats [455]. SKF 525A initially (2 hrs) inhibits and later (24 hrs) enhances the cholestatic effect, a phenomenon consistent with the effects of SKF 525A on drug metabolism [455]. Agents that inhibit protein synthesis (actinomycin D, cycloheximide, ethionine) inhibit the cholestatic effect [456, 76]. These observations are consistent with the view that ANIT must be converted to a metabolite in order to lead to cholestasis [455]. They also would appear to explain the greater susceptibility of rats and mice, which metabolize ANIT to a greater degree, than that of other species [77]. PLAA and his associtеs [224] have shown that hepatocellular, in contrast to cholestatic, injury does not appear to depend on metabolism of ANIT. One might speculate that sheep and cattle, which develop hepatocellular injury but no cholestasis [178], are unable to convert ANIT to the metabolite that leads to the cholestatic effect, but are sensitive to the native compound or to an hepatocyte-damaging metabolite. Rabbits which develop neither hepatic injury nor cholestasis may be presumed not to metabolize the ANIT, and also perhaps to have some other reason for refractoriness.

K. Concluding Comments

The foregoing discussion has reviewed the general aspects of hepatotoxicity and means of investigating the phenomena; has offered a classification of hepatotoxic agents based on presumed mechanism and type of injury; and has analyzed the characteristics of a few specific agents. An additional focus on the phenomenology of hepatotoxicity is provided by arranging toxic agents according to source, chemical category and circumstances of human exposure (Tables 12, 13). For a more complete listing of hepatotoxic agents, the extensive reviews of ROUILLER [472] and KLATSKIN [269] should be consulted.

Toxic agents may derive from a living (Table 12) or non-living (Table 13) source. Hepatotoxic agents of non-living origin are mostly synthetic or extracted from minerals, and may be inorganic or organic. Exposure of humans may be domestic, occupational iatrogenic (Table 12).

I. Toxins of Living Origin

Plants are the source of a number of hepatotoxic substances. The *Amanitae* and other toxic mushrooms (toodstools), the several hundred species of plants that yield PAs, the plants that contain tannic acid, and those that contain icterogenin and rehmannic acid already have received comment. These and a few other botanical hepatotoxins are listed in Table 12. With the exception of the cholestasis-producing icterogenin and its congeners, hepatotoxins of plant origin are cytotoxic-able to produce necrosis, steatosis and, in some instances, hepatic carcinoma.

Table 13. Synthetic and other non-living hepatotoxins

Inorganic	Lesion	Circumstances of exposure[a]
Antimony	Steatosis	I, D-A, O
Arsenic	Steatosis, Necrosis (CZ)	I, D-A, O
Barium	Steatosis	Exp
Borates	Steatosis	D-A, O
Bismuth	Steatosis	I, Exp
Cadmium	Necrosis	D-A, O
Cerium	Steatosis	Exp, O
Chromates	Steatosis	O
Ferrous salts	Necrosis (PZ)	D-A
Lanthanum	Steatosis	Exp, O
Lead	Necrosis (CZ)	D-A, Exp. O
Manganese	Necrosis (CZ)	O, Exp
Neodymium	Steatosis	Exp, O
Phosphorous	Steatosis, Necrosis (PZ)	D-A
Praseodymiun	Steatosis	Exp, O
Thallium	Steatosis	D-A, O
Hydrazine	Steatosis, CA	O
Organic		
Variety of aliphatic aromatic, polycyclic, heterocyclic, azo compounds, nitrosamines, etc. employed as occupational reagents	Steatosis, or Necrosis, or cirrhosis, or Ca, or cholestasis produced by respective agents	O or D-F or D-A
Insecticides		O or D-F or D-A
Medicinals	Steatosis, necrosis, cholestasis	I or D-A

[a] I = Iatrogenic; D-A = Domestic accident; D-F = Food contamination; O = Occupational exposure; Exp = Experimental.

Microbiologic sources of hepatotoxic agents include several species of fungi, and several bacteria (Table 12). Among the mycotoxins, those produced by Aspergilli have commanded the most interest during the past decade [586]; although luteoskysin, islanditoxin, and sporidesmin also have received attention [370]. These mycotoxins are cytotoxic. Sporidesmin, produced by Pithomyces Chartarum is cholestatic. Several bacteria yield substances that produce centrizonal (exotoxins of C. diphtheriae and Cl. botulinus) or peripheral (endotoxin of Pr. vulgaris) necrosis. An additional cytotoxic agent of bacterial origin is ethionine; produced by some strains of E. coli. Work in progress in our laboratory (unpublished data) suggests that the endotoxin of E. coli has a cholestatic effect.

II. Toxins of Non-Living Origin

A number of inorganic elements and compounds have hepatotoxic properties. Elemental phosphorous and inorganic arsenicals produce steatosis with or without necrosis. Some toxic only in large doses (salts of cadmium, copper, iron, lead) produce degeneration and at times hepatic necrosis. Inorganic compounds of antimony, barium, thallium, and cerium (and other low atomic-number rare earths) produce hepatic steatosis. Hydrazine, borates and chromates, also produce fatty liver (Table 13).

The number of synthetic organic compounds that are hepatotoxic is vast [472] and beyond presentation or chemical categorization. They include the haloalkanes, haloalkenes, and various other derivatives of aliphatic compounds. These substances and others including benzene derivatives and various azo compounds, heterocyclic and polycyclic substances and other chemical types are employed widely in industry where they constitute potential threats.

Domestic exposures to some of the industrial hepatotoxins (e.g. CCl_4) may be accidental or suicidal (Table 13). Ingestion of food contaminated by toxic organic chemicals or mycotoxins, or of toxic substances in ignorance of their toxicity (poisnous mushrooms, pyrrolidizine alkaloids) may lead to hepatotoxicity in a domestic setting (Table 12).

Insecticides include chlorinated hydrocarbons and other compounds some of which are toxic for experimental animals. Exposure of humans to insecticides is widespread by way of the "food-chain", occupational experience and at times accidental ingestion. Nevertheless, only rare instances of human hepatotoxicity have been observed.

Many medicinal agents can cause hepatic injury; some lead to liver damage because of hypersensitivity to the agent; others produce injury because they are converted to toxic metabolites by the abnormal metabolism of the susceptible patient, and other drugs produce injury when given as a large therapeutic dose (tetracycline) or taken with suicidal intent (acetaminophen) [639].

The goals which experimental hepatotoxicity should meet are two-fold. The studies should provide information useful for the understanding of disease. More importantly and specifically, they should lead to identification of toxic agents, mechanism of injury, circumstances of exposure and means of prevention in order to permit the benefits of use of the many chemicals without the cost of injury.

Appendix

Meaning of Abbreviations

AF	Aflatoxin
ALD	Aldolase
ANIT	α-Naphthylisothiocyanate
ATP	Adenosine triphosphate
BSP	Sulfobromophthalein
DMN	Dimethylnitrosamine
DNA	Usual meaning
EM	Electron microscopy
ER	Endoplasmic reticulum
F-I-P-ALD	Aldolase the substrate of which is Fructose-1-phosphate
F-I-P-Aldolase	F-I-P ALD
GALN	D-galactosamine
GOT	Glutamic-oxalacetic transaminase (Aspartate aminotransferase)
GPT	Glutamic-pyruvic transaminase (Alanine aminotransferase)
ICDH	Isocitric dehydrogenase

IP	Intraperitoneal
IV	Intravenous
LDH	Lactic dehydrogenase
LDH_5	Slowest-migrating isoenzyme of LDH, at pH 8.6
LD_{50}	Usual toxicologic meaning
LM	Light microscopy
MDH	Malic dehydrogenase
3-MeDAB	3-Methyldiaminoazobenzene
NADPH	(TPNH) Reduced form nicotinamide-adenine-dinucleotide phosphate
mRNA	Messenger RNA
OCT	ornithine-carbamoyltransaminase
P-450	Cytochrome P-450
PAs	Pyrrolidizine alkaloids
PHI	Phosphohexoisomerase
P/O	Mols inorganic phosphorous taken up for each mol O_2 consumed; measure of oxidative phosphorylation
ppb	Parts per billion
Pr-R-P	5-Phosphoribosylpyrophosphate
RER	Rough endoplasmic reticulum
RES	Reticuloendothelial system
RNA	Usual meaning
RNP	Ribonucleoprotein
SAE	S-Adenosylethionine
SAM	S-Adenosylmethionine
SC	Subcutaneous
SDH	Sorbitol dehydrogenase
SER	Smooth endoplasmic reticulum
SKF 525	2-2-Diethylaminoethyl 2,2-diphenylvalerate; inhibitor of drug metabolism
TA	Tannic acid
TAA	Thioacetamide
tRNA	Transfer RNA
UDP	Uridine diphosphate
UTP	Uridine triphosphate
VLDL	Very low density lipoproteins

References

1. Acocella, G., Nicolis, F.B., Tenconi, L.T.: The effect of an intravenous infusion of rifamycin SV on the excretion of bilirubin, bromsulphalein, and indocyanine green in man. Gastroenterology **49**, 521 (1965).
2. Adamson, R.H., Correa, P., Dalgord, D.W.: Occurrence of a primary liver carcinoma in a Rhesus monkey fed aflatoxin B_1. J. nat. Cancer Inst. **50**, 549 (1973).
3. Aiken, D.E., Byard, E.H.L.: Histological changes in lobsters (Homarus americanus) exposed to yellow phosphorous. Science **176**, 1434 (1972).
4. Allcroft, R.: Aflatoxicosis in farm animals. In: Aflatoxin Scientific Background Control and Implications, p. 237—264. New York: Academic Press 1969.

5. ALLEN, J.R., LALICH, J., SCHMITTLE, S.C.: Crotolaria spectrabilis-induced cirrhosis in turkeys. Lab. Invest. **12**, 512 (1963).
6. ALPERT, E., SERCK-HANSSEN, A., RAJAGOPOLEN, B.: Aflatoxin-induced hepatic injury in the African monkey. Arch. environm. Hlth **20**, 723 (1970).
7. ALTHAUSAN, T.L., THOENES, E.: Influence on carbohydrate metabolism of experimentally induced hepatic changes. II. Phosphorous poisoning. Arch. intern. Med. **50**, 58 (1932).
8. ALTMANN, H.-W., OSTERLAND, U.: Über cytoplasmatische Wirbelbildungen in den Leberzellen der Ratte bei chronischer Thioacetamidvergiftung. Beitr. path. Anat. **124**, 1 (1961).
9. ALVIZOURI, M., CORTES, J.: Effect of DL-ethionine on the liver of dog and rabbit. Arch. Path. **77**, 57 (1964).
10. AMBROSE, A.M., DE EDS, F., RATHER, L.J.: Toxicity of thioacetamide in rats. J. industr. Hyg. Toxicol. **31**, 158 (1949).
11. AMBROSE, A.M., DE EDS, F., RATHER, L.J.: Further studies on toxicity of thioacetamide in rats. Proc. Soc. exp. Biol. (N.Y.) **74**, 132 (1950).
12. ANUKARAHANONTA, T., SHINOZUKA, H., FARBER, E.: Inhibition of Protein synthesis in Rat Liver by D-Galactosamin. Res. Comm. Chem. Path. Pharmacol. **5**, 481 (1973).
13. ARHELGER, R.B., BROOM, J.S., BOLER, R.K.: Ultrastructural hepatic alterations following tannic acid administration to rabbits. Amer. J. Path. **46**, 409 (1965).
14. ARIAS, I.M.: Effects of a plant acid (icterogenin) and certain anabolic steroids on the hepatic metabolism of bilirubin and sulfobromophthalein. Ann. N.Y. Acad. Sci. **104**, 1014 (1963).
15. ARMBRECHT, B.H., SHALKOP, W.T., ROLLINS, L.D., POHLAND, A.E., STALKOFF, L.: Acute toxicity of aflatoxin B_1 in Wethers. Nature (Lond.) **225**, 1062 (1970).
16. ASADA, M.: Transaminase activity in liver damage. I. Study on experimental liver damage. Med. J. Osaka Univ. **9**, 45 (1958).
17. ASADA, M., GALAMBOS, T.J.: Sorbitol dehydrogenase and hepatocellular injury: an experimental and clinical study. Gastroenterology **44**, 578 (1963).
18. ASAHINA, S., FRIEDMAN, N.A., ARNOLD, E., MILLAR, G.N., NISHKIN, N., BISHOP, Y., EPSTEIN, S.S.: Acute synergistic toxicity and hepatic necrosis following oral administration of sodium nitrite and secondary amines to mice. Cancer Res. **31**, 1201 (1971).
19. ASHWORTH, C.T., WERNER, D.J., GLASS, M.D., ARNOLD, N.J.: Spectrum of fine structural changes in hepatocellular injury due to thioacetamide. Amer. J. Path. **47**, 917 (1965).
20. ATERMAN, K.: Studies in fibrosis of the liver induced by carbon tetrachloride. I. Relation between hepatocellular injury and new formation of fibrous tissue. Arch. Path. **57**, 1 (1954).
21. ATERMAN, K.: Studies in fibrosis of the liver induced by carbon tetrachloride. II. A quantitive study of the effects of cortisone on fibrosis of the liver in rats. Arch. Path. **57**, 12 (1954).
22. BAHOR, R.E.: The Role of Liver Lipid in the Potentiation of Carbon Tetrachloride Toxicity. Doctoral Dissertation. University of Michigan, Ann Arbor, Michigan, 1966.
23. BAKER, R.D., HANDLER, P.: Animal experiments with tannic acid suggested by the tannic acid treatment of burns. Ann. Surg. **118**, 417 (1943).
24. BALAZS, T., GRICE, H.C.: The relationship between liver necrosis and pentobarbital sleeping time. Toxicol. appl. Pharmacol. **5**, 387 (1963).
25. BARKA, T.: Lysozomes and regulation of cell proliferation. In: The Liver and Its Disease (SCHAFFNER, F., SHERLOCK, S., LEEVY, C.M., eds.), p. 19–33. New York: Intercontinental Book Corp. 1974.
26. BARKER, E.A.: Cytotoxicity of Thioacetamide. Ph.D. Dissertation. University Microfilms, Ann Arbor, Mich., 1970.
27. BARKER, E.Z., SMUCHLER, E.A.: Altered microsome function during acute thioacetamide poisoning. Molec. Pharmacol. **8**, 318 (1972).
28. BARNES, J.M.: Mechanisms of toxicity: Introduction. Brit. med. Bull. **25**, 219 (1969).
29. BARNES, J.M., MAGEE, P.N.: Some toxic properties of dimethyl nitrosamine. Brit. J. industr. Med. **11**, 167 (1954).
30. BARNES, J.M., ROSSITER, R.J.: Toxicity of tannic acid. Lancet **1943 II**, 218.
31. BARONE, P., BATELO, D.: Modificazioni della vascolarizzazione epitica e istogenesi della cirrhosi sperimentale de tetacloruro di carbonio. Biol. lat. (Milano) **11**, 503 (1958).
32. BARONE, C., CITTADINI, A., GALEOTTI, T., TERRANOVA, T.: The effect of intoxication induced in rat liver by carbon tetrachloride, ethionine and white phosphorous on the level of microsomal cytochromes b_5 and P 450. Experientia (Basel) **29**, 73 (1973).
33. BARTSOKAS, ST.K., PAPADIMITRIOU, D.G., PAPACHARALAMPOUS, N.X., KATAPOTI, Z., KANNAS, D.: Heparinoids—a new inhibitor of experimental liver necrosis in rats. Acta hepato-gastroent. **21**, 253 (1974).
34. BASSAN, H., KENDLER, J., ZIMMERMAN, H.J.: Effect of ethionine and ethanol on the function of the perfused rat liver. Proc. Soc. exp. Biol. (N.Y.) **137**, 852 (1971).
35. BAUER, C., BACHMANN, W., REUTTER, W.: Determination of galactosamine in the developing rat liver. Hoppe-Seylers Z. physiol. Chem. **353**, 1053 (1972).
36. BECKER, B.A., PLAA, G.L.: The nature of α-naphthyl-isothiocyanate-induced cholestases. Toxicol. appl. Pharmacol. **7**, 680 (1965).

37. Becker, B.A., Plaa, G.L.: Quantitative and temporal delineation of various parameters of liver dysfunction due to naphthylisothiocyanate. Toxicol. appl. Pharmacol. **7**, 708 (1965).
38. Becker, B.A., Plaa, G.L.: Hepatotoxicity of α-naphthylisothiocyanate congeners with particular emphasis on phenylisothiocyanate. Toxicol. appl. Pharmacol. **7**, 804 (1965).
39. Becker, U., Walter, W.: Die Wirkung von Thioacetylverbindungen auf das Leberparenchym im Tierexperiment. Acta hepato-splenol. (Stuttg.) **12**, 129 (1965).
40. Bernard, C.: La science experimentale, p. 237. Paris: Bailliere 1878. Cit. by Stoner and Magee, ref. 63, and by Farber, ref. 64.
41. Berry, M.N., Friend, D.S.: High yield preparations of isolated rat liver parenchymal cells: as biochemical and fine structural study. J. Cell Biol. **43**, 506 (1969).
42. Best, C.H., MacLean, D.L., Ridout, J.H.: Choline and liver fat in phosphorous poisoning. J. Physiol. (Lond.) **83**, 275 (1935).
43. Bhathal, P.S., Christie, G.S.: A fluorescence microscopic study of bile duct proliferation induced in guinea pigs by α-naphthylisothiocyanate. Lab. Invest. **20**, 480 (1969).
44. Bhathal, P.S., Hurley, J.V.: An electron microscope study of the production of ascites in acute dimethylnitrosamine (DMN)-induced liver injury. J. Path. **111**, 103 (1973).
45. Blumenberg, F.W., Enneker, C., Kessler, F.J.: On the question of the hepatotoxic effect of orally administered tannins and their galloyl components. Arzneimittel-Forsch. **10**, 223 (1960).
46. Blumenberg, F.W., Kessler, F.J.: Absorption of orally administered tannin. Arzneimittel-Forsch. **10**, 742 (1960).
47. Boelcke, G., Poser, W., Michelssenm, A., Erdmann, W.D.: Cholinesteraseaktivität im Plasma nach schwerem Leberschaden durch D-Galaktosamin-HCl an Kaninchen. Arch. Toxicol. **28**, 192 (1971).
48. Bonesch, H., Cornelius, C.E.: Indocyanine green clearance; a liver function test for the dog. Amer. J. vet. Res. **25**, 254 (1964).
49. Bouvier, C.A., Maurice, P.A.: Liver and blood coagulation. In: The Liver. Rouiller, Ch. (ed.), vol. II, p. 197. New York: Academic Press 1964.
50. Boyd, E.M., Bereczky, K., Godi, I.: The acute toxicity of tannic acid administered intragastrically. Canad. med. Ass. J. **92**, 1292 (1965).
51. Boyd, J.W.: Glutamate-oxaloacetate transaminase isoenzymes in rat serum. Clin. chim. Acta **7**, 424 (1962).
52. Brauer, R.W. (ed.): Liver Function: A Symposium on Approaches to the Quantitative Description of Liver Function: A.I.B.S., Washington, D.C., 1958.
53. Brauer, R.W., Leong, G.F., Holloway, R.J.: Liver injury in isolated perfused rat liver preparation exposed to chloroform. Amer. J. Physiol. **200**, 548 (1961).
54. Breen, K., Schenher, S., Heimberg, M.: The effect of tetracycline on the hepatic secretion of triglyceride. Biochim. biophys. Acta (Amst.) **270**, 74 (1972).
55. Brodehl, J.: Thioacetamid in der experimentellen Leberforschung. Klin. Wschr. **39**, 956 (1961).
56. Brodie, B.B., Reid, W.D., Cho, A.K., Sipes, G., Krishna, G., Gillette, J.R.: Possible mechanism of liver necrosis caused by aromatic organic compounds. Proc. nat. Acad. Sci. (Wash.) **68**, 160 (1971).
57. Brody, T.M., Calvert, D.N., Schneider, A.F.: Alterations of carbon-tetrachloride-induced pathological changes in the rat by spinal transection, adrenalectomy and adrenergic blocking agents. J. Pharmacol. exp. Ther. **131**, 341 (1961).
58. Brooks, S.E.W., Miller, C.G., McKenzie, K., Audreloch, J.J., Bras, G.: Acute veno-occlusive disease of the liver. Arch. Path. **89**, 507 (1970).
59. Brown, J.M.M., Remington, C., Sawyer, B.C.: Studies on biliary excretion in the rabbit. Proc. roy. Soc. B **157**, 473 (1963).
60. Bull, L.B., Culvenor, C.C.J., Dick, A.T.: The Pyrrolidizine Alkaloids. New York: John Wiley and Sons, Inc. 1968.
61. Bull, L.B., Dick, A.T., Keast, J.C., Edgar, G.: The acute toxic effects of heliotrine and lasiocarpine and their N-oxides on the rat. J. Path. Bact. **75**, 17 (1958).
62. Bullock, G., Eakins, M.N., Sawyer, B.C., Slater, T.F.: Studies on bile secretion with the aid of the isolated perfused liver. I. Inhibitory action of sporidesmin and icterogenin. Proc. roy. Soc. B **186**, 333 (1974).
63. Bunyan, J., Cawthorne, M.A., Diplock, A.T., Green, J.: Vitamin E and hepatotoxic agents. II. Lipid peroxidation and poisoning with orotic acid, ethanol and thioacetamide in rats. Brit. J. Nutr. **23**, 309 (1969).
64. Burns, J.J.: Application of metabolic and disposition studies. In: Fundamentals of Drug Metabolism and Disposition (B.N. LaDue, H.G. Mandel and E.L. Way, eds.), p. 340–366. Baltimore: Williams and Wilkins 1971.
65. Busch, H., Adams, H., Muramatsu, M.: Effects of alkylating agents and thioacetamide on nuclear metabolism. Fed. Proc. **21**, 1093 (1962).
66. Busuttil, A., Alston, W.C., Horne, C.H.W., MacSween, R.N.M.: Effect of the production of experimental cirrhosis in rats on serum aminotransferase levels. Europ. J. clin. biol. Res. **27**, 979 (1972).

67. BUTLER, T.C.: Reduction of carbon tetrachloride in vivo and reduction of carbon tetrachloride and chloroform in vitro by tissues and tissue constituents. J. Pharmacol. exp. Ther. **134**, 311 (1961).
68. BUTLER, W.H.: Liver injury induced by aflatoxin. In: Progress in Liver Disease, vol. III (H. POPPER and F. SCHAFFNER, eds.), p. 408–418. New York: Grune and Stratton, Inc. 1970.
69. CALVERT, D.N., BRODY, T.M.: Role of the sympathetic nervous system in carbon tetrachloride hepatotoxicity. Amer. J. Physiol. **198**, 669 (1960).
70. CAMERON, G.R., KARUNARATNE, W.A.E.: Carbon tetrachloride cirrhosis in relation to liver degeneration. J. Path. Bact. **42**, 1 (1936).
71. CAMERON, G.R., KARUNARATUE, W.A.E., THOMAS, J.E.: Massive necrosis ("toxic infarction") of the liver following intra-portal administration of poisons. J. Path. Bact. **44**, 297 (1937).
72. CAMERON, G.R., MCLEAN, M.R., PROSAD, L.B.G.: Recovery from the bile duct hyperplasma induced by feeding alpha-naphthylisothiocyanate to rats. J. Path. Bact. **80**, 137 (1960).
73. CAMERON, G.R., MILTON, R.F., ALLEN, J.W.: Toxicity of tannic acid; an experimental investigation. Lancet **1943II**, 179.
74. CAMERON, R., SPECTOR, W.G.: The Chemistry of the Injured Cell. Springfield, Ill.: Charles C. Thomas 1961.
75. CAMPONARI-VISCONTI, L., CAMPONARI, F., KOCH-WESER, D.: Inhibition by glucose of the ethionine induced fatty liver. Proc. Soc. exp. Biol. (N.Y.) **111**, 479 (1962).
76. CAPIZZO, F., ROBERTS, R.J.: Effect of phenobarbital, chlorpromazine, actinomycin D and chronic-naphthylisothiocyanate administration on α-naphthylisothiocyanate-^{14}C disposition and α-naphthylisothiocyanate-induced hyperbilirubinemia. J. Pharmacol. exp. Ther. **179**, 455 (1971).
77. CAPIZZO, F., ROBERTS, R.J.: α-naphthylisothiocyanate (ANIT)-induced hepatotoxicity and disposition in various species. Toxicol. appl. Pharmacol. **19**, 176 (1971).
78. CARGILL, C.F., SHIELDS, R.P.: Plasma arginase as a liver function test. J. comp. Path. **81**, 447 (1971).
79. CARLSON, G.P., FULLER, G.C., FAUSTO, N.: Effect of spironolactone on carbon tetrachloride hepatotoxicity. Proc. Soc. exp. Biol. (N.Y.) **145**, 182 (1974).
80. CARTER, R.L., PERCIVAL, W.H., ROE, F.J.C.: Exceptional sensitivity of mink to the hepatotoxic effects of dimethyl nitrosamine. J. Path. **97**, 79 (1969).
81. CASPER, J.L.: Drei neue Fälle von Chloroformtod. Wschr. ges. Heilk. **16**, 273 (1850). Cit. by DRILL ref. 1.
82. CASTRO, J.A., D'ACOSTA, N., DE FERREYRA, E.C., DE CASTRO, C.R., DIAZ GIMEZ, M.I., DE FENOS, O.M.: Studies on thioacematide-induced liver necrosis. Toxicol. appl. Pharmacol. **30**, 79 (1974).
83. CASTRO, J.A., DE FERREYRA, E.C., DE CASTRO, C.R., DE FENOS, O.M.: Prevention of carbon tetrachloride-induced necrosis by inhibitors of drug metabolism—further studies on their mechanism of action. Biochem. Pharmacol. **23**, 295 (1974).
84. CAWTHORNE, M.A., PALMER, E.D., GREEN, J.: Effect of 6-ethoxy 2,2,4-trimethyl-1,2-dihydro-quinoline (ethoxyquin) on carbon tetrachloride metabolism in the rat. Biochem. Pharmacol. **22**, 783 (1973).
85. CHALIFOUX, A.: L'activité serique de l'ornithine transcarbamylase (OCT) lors d'hepatopathies canines expérimentales. Canad. J. comp. Med. **34**, 289 (1970).
86. CHEDID, A., NAIR, V.: Diurnal rhythm in endoplasmic reticulum of rat liver. Science **175**, 176 (1972).
87. CHESNEY, C.F., ALLEN, J.R.: Resistance of the guinea pig to pyrrolidizine intoxication. Toxicol. appl. Pharmacol. **26**, 385 (1973).
88. CHILDS, J.F., SIGLER, E.A.: Controlling orange decay. Industr. Engin. Chem. **38**, 82 (1946).
89. CHOPRA, P., ROY, S., RAMALINGSWANU, V., NAYAK, N.C.: Mechanism of carbon tetrachloride hepatotoxicity: an *in vivo* study of its molecular basis in rats and monkeys. Lab. Invest. **26**, 716 (1972).
90. CHRISTOPHERSON, B.D.: The inhibitory effect of reduced glutathione on the lipid peroxidation of the microsomal fraction and mitochondria. Biochem. J. **106**, 515 (1968).
91. CLAPP, N.K., CRAIG, A.W., TOYA SR., R.E.: Pulmonary and hepatic oncogenesis during treatment of male RF mice with dimethylnitrosamine. J. nat. Cancer Inst. **41**, 1213 (1968).
92. CLARA, M.: Über den Bau der Leber beim Kaninchen und die Regenerationserscheinungen an diesem Gewebe bei experimenteller Phosphorvergiftung. Z. mikr.-anat. Forsch. **26**, 45 (1931).
93. CLARE, N.T.: Photosenitization in Diseases of Domestic Animals. Farnham Royals, Bucks, England: Commonwealth Agricultural Bureau 1952.
94. CLARE, N.T.: Photosensitivity diseases in New Zealand. N.Z.J. agric. Res. **2**, 1249 (1959).
95. CLARK, E.J., ROSSITER, R.J.: Liver function in rabbits after injections of tannic acid. Lancet **1943II**, 222.
96. CLEVELAND, P.D., SMUCKLER, E.A.: Effect of CCl_4, dimethyl and thioacetamide on hepatic DPNH and TPNH Cytochrome C Reductase. Proc. Soc. exp. Biol. (N.Y.) **120**, 808 (1965).
97. CLODI, P.H., STEFENELLI, N.: Gallenfluß, Gallendruck und Bromsulphophaleinausscheidung bei der experimentellen intrahepatischen Cholestase der Ratte. Z. ges. exp. Med. **142**, 1 (1967).

98. COMBES, B.: Excretory Function of the Liver. In: The Liver (CH. ROUILLER, ed.), vol. II, p. 1–35. New York: Academic Press 1964.

99. CONNEY, A.H.: Pharmacological implications of microsomal enzyme induction. Pharmacol. Rev. **19**, 317 (1967).

100. CORNELIUS, C.E., BISHOP, J., SWITZER, J., RHODE, E.A.: Serum and tissue transaminase activities in domestic animals. Cornell Vet. **19**, 16 (1959).

101. CORNISH, H.H.: Problems posed by observation of serum enzyme changes in toxicology. CRC Crit. Rev. Toxicol. **1**, 1–32 (1971).

102. CORNISH, H., ADEFUIN, J.: Potentiation of carbon tetrachloride toxicity by aliphatic alcohols. Arch. environm. Hlth **14**, 447 (1967).

103. CORNISH, H.H., BARTH, M.L., DODSON, V.N.: Isozyme profiles and protein patterns in specific organ damage. Toxicol. appl. Pharmacol. **16**, 411 (1970).

104. CORNISH, H.M., BLOCK, W.D.: A study of carbon tetrachloride II. The effect of carbon tetrachloride inhalation on serum and tissue enzymes. Arch. environm. Hlth **1**, 96 (1960).

105. CORNISH, H.H., RYAN, R.C.: A study of carbon tetrachloride VI. Aminoaciduria in response to carbon tetrachloride inhalation. Toxicol. appl. Pharmacol. **6**, 96 (1964).

106. CORSSEN, G., SWEET, R.B., CHENOWETH, M.B.: Effects of chloroform, halothane and methoxyfluorane on human liver cells *in vitro*. Anesthesiology **27**, 155 (1966).

107. COURTILLET, M., STARON, T.: Toxic amanitae, Amanita virosa. Rev. Path. Comp. Med. Exp. **7**, 141 (1970).

108. CURTIS, S.J., MORITZ, M., SNODGRASS, P.: Serum enzymes derived from liver cell fractions. I. The response of carbon tetrachloride intoxication in rats. Gastroenterology **62**, 84 (1972).

109. CZOK, R.: The behavior of plasma enzymes in toxicological experiments. Proc. Europ. Soc. Study Drug Tox. **5**, 68 (1965).

110. DAIKUHARA, Y., ICHIHARA, A., TANIOKA, H., TAKEDA, Y.: Secretion of lipid from dispersed rat liver cells. J. Biochem. **60**, 322 (1966).

111. DAVIS, D.C., HASHIMOTO, M., GILLETTE, J.R.: Effects of brombenzene and carbon tetrachloride on the synthesis and release of proteins by perfused rat liver. Biochem. Pharmacol. **22**, 1989 (1973).

112. DEAMER, D.W., KRUGER, F.A., CORNWELL, D.G.: Total liver protein and amino acid incorporation into liver protein in orotic acid-induced fatty liver. Biochim. biophys. Acta (Amst.) **97**, 147 (1965).

113. DECKER, K., KEPPLER, D.: Galactosamine induced liver injury. In: Progress in Liver Disease (H. POPPER and F. SCHAFFNER, eds.), vol. IV, p. 183–199. New York: Grune and Stratton, Inc. 1972.

114. DE DUVE, C., WATTIAUX, R., WIBO, M.L.: Effects of fat-soluble compounds on lysosomes *in vitro*. Biochem. Pharm. **9**, 97 (1962).

115. DE RITIS, F., COLTORTI, M., GIUSTI, G.: Le attivita, transaminasche del siero in fisiopatologie ed in clinica. Recenti Progr. Med. **20**, 533 (1956).

116. DESMET, V.J., KRSTULOVIC, B., VAN DAMME, B.: Histochemical study of rat liver in alpha-naphthyl isothiocyanate (ANIT). Amer. J. Path. **52**, 401 (1968).

117. DESQUEYROUX, J.: Sur les troubles des échanges azatés dans l'intoxication phosphorée aigue expérimentale. C.R. Soc. Biol. (Paris) **86**, 143 (1922).

118. DIAZ-RIVERA, R.S., CALLAZO, J.P., PONS, E.R., TORREGROSA, M.V.: Acute phosphorous poisoning in man; a study of 56 cases. Medicine (Baltimore) **29**, 269 (1950).

119. DI LUZIO, N.R.: Influences of intravenously administered hexahydrocoenzyme Q_4 on liver injury. Life Sci. **5**, 1467 (1966).

120. DI LUZIO, N.R.: Prevention of the acute ethanol-induced fatty liver by the simultaneous administration of antioxidants. Life Sci. **3**, 113 (1964).

121. DI LUZIO, N.R., COSTALES, F.: Inhibition of the ethanol and carbon tetrachloride induced fatty liver by antioxidants. Exp. molec. Path. **4**, 141 (1965).

122. DINMAN, B.D., BERNSTEIN, I.A.: Acute carbon tetrachloride hepatotoxicity IV. Liver and serum enzyme activity during the acute damage phase. Arch. environm. Hlth **16**, 770 (1968).

123. DINMAN, B.D., FOX, C.F., FRAJOLA, W.J., RABOR, A.: Serum enzyme and B_{12} changes in CCl_4 hepatotoxicity. Arch. environm. Hlth **4**, 168 (1962).

124. DOLJANSKI, L., ROSIN, A.: Studies on the early changes in the livers of rats treated with various toxic agents, with special reference to the vascular lesions; the histology of the rat's liver in urethane poisoning. Amer. J. Path. **20**, 945 (1944).

125. DOMINIS, M., SOLTER, D., DAMJANOV, I.: Aspiration cytological and cytochemical study of changes induced in rat liver cells by carbon tetrachloride (CCl_4). Beitr. Path. Bd. **150**, 132 (1973).

126. DRILL, V.A.: Hepatotoxic agents: mechanism of action and dietary interrelationship. Pharmacol. Rev. **4**, 1 (1952).

127. DUJOVNE, C.A., SHOEMAN, D., BIANCHINE, J., LASAGNA, L.: Experimental basis for the different hepatotoxicity of erythromycin preparations in man. J. Lab. clin. Med. **79**, 832 (1972).

128. DURST, A., DISHON, T., ROSENMANN, E., BOSS, J.H.: Urinary excretion of liver antigens in experimental hepatic diseases of the rat. Lab. Invest. **25**, 35 (1971).

129. DYER, H.M.: Evidence of the physiological specificity of methionine in regard to the methylthiol group: the synthesis of s-ethylhomocysteine (ethionine) and a study of its availability for growth. J. biol. Chem. **124**, 519 (1938).
130. Editorial: Deadly enemas. New Engl. J. Med. **270**, 209 (1964).
131. Editorial: Toxicity of tannic acid. Lancet **1966 II**, 34.
132. Edit.: Death cap poisoning. Lancet **1972 I**, 1320.
133. ELIAKIM, M., EISNER, M., UNGAR, H.: Correlation between morphologic changes in the liver and liver function tests in rabbits following administration of ethionine. Bull. Res. Coun. Israel E **7**, 189 (1958).
134. ELIAKIM, M., EISNER, M., UNGAR, H.: Experimental intra-hepatic obstructive jaundice following ingestion of alpha-naphthyl-iso-thiocyanate. Bull. Res. Counc. E **8**, 7 (1959).
135. EMMELOT, P., BENEDETTI, E.L.: Changes in the fine structure of rat liver cells brought about by dimethylnitrosamine. J. biophys. biochem. Cytol. **7**, 393 (1960).
136. ENDER, F., HAVRE, G.N., MADSEN, R., CĚH, L., HELGEBOSTAD, A.: Studies on conditions under which N-nitrosodimethylamine is formed in herring meal produced from nitrite-preserved herring. The risk of using nitrite uncritically as a preservative agent. Z. Tierphysiol. Tierernähr. Futtermittelk. **22**, 181 (1967).
137. ESPINOSA, E., INSUNZA, I.: Hepatic antigens in the blood of rats with toxic liver damage. Proc. Soc. exp. Biol. (N.Y.) **111**, 174 (1962).
138. FAL, H., PURI, G.C.: Impairment of hepatic drug metabolism by carbon tetrachloride inhalation. Tox. appl. Pharmacol. **16**, 35 (1970).
139. FARBER, E.: Ethionine carcinogenesis. Advanc. Cancer Res. **7**, 383 (1963).
140. FARBER, E.: Ethionine fatty liver. Advanc. Lipid Res. **5**, 119 (1967).
141. FARBER, E.: Biochemical Pathology. Ann. Rev. Pharmacol. **11**, 71 (1971).
142. FARBER, E. (ed.): The Biochemistry of Disease, vol. 2. The Pathology of Transcription and Translation. New York: Marcel Dekker 1972.
143. FARBER, E.: The pathology of translation. In: Biochemistry of Disease, vol. 2 (E. FARBER, ed.), p. 123–158. New York: Marcel Dekker, Inc. 1972.
144. FARBER, E., SIMPSON, M.V., FARNER, H.: Studies on ethionine. II. The interference with lipide metabolism. J. biol. Chem. **182**, 91 (1950).
145. FAVARGER, P.: The liver and lipid metabolism. In: The Liver (CH. ROUILLER, ed.), vol. I, p. 549–604. New York: Academic Press 1964.
146. FEINMAN, L., RUBIN, E., LIEBER, C.S.: Adaptation of the liver to drugs. In: Liver and Drugs (F. ORLANDI and A.M. JEZEQUEL, eds.), p. 41–83. New York: Academic Press 1972.
147. FEO, C., GARCON, E.: Study of steatosis induced in the rat by orotic acid. Biomedicine **19**, 61 (1973).
148. FITZHUGH, O.G., NELSON, A.A.: Liver tumors in rats fed thiourea or thioacetamide. Science **108**, 626 (1948).
149. FIUME, L.: Mechanism of action of phalloidin. Lancet **1965 I**, 1284.
150. FIUME, L.: Pathogenesis of the cellular lesions produced by α-amanitin. In: The Pathology of Transcription and Translation (E. FARBER, ed.), p. 105–122. New York: Marcel Dekker, Inc. 1972.
151. FIUME, L., ROFFIA, S.: Inhibition by amino-acetonitrile of dimethylnitrosamine metabolism in the rat's liver. Nature (Lond.) **206**, 4989 (1965).
152. FLEISCHER, G.A., WAKIM, K.G.: Presence of two glutamic oxalacetic transaminases in serum of dogs following acute injury of the liver. Proc. Soc. exp. Biol. (N.Y.) **106**, 283 (1959).
153. FLETCHER, G.F., GALAMBOS, J.T.: Phosphorous poisoning in humans. Arch. intern. Med. **112**, 846 (1963).
154. FLORSHEIM, G.L.: Curative potencies against α-amanitin poisoning by Cytochrome C. Science **171**, 808 (1972).
155. FONG, Y.Y., WALSH, E.O.F.: Carcinogenic nitrosamines in Cantonese dried fish. Lancet **1971 II**, 1032.
156. FORBES, J.C., EVANS, E.I.: Tannic acid and liver necrosis. Surg. Gynec. Obstet. **76**, 612 (1943).
157. FOX, C.F., DINMAN, B.D., FRAJOLA, W.J.: CCl_4 poisoning II. Serum enzymes, free fatty acids and liver pathology: effects of phenoxybenzamine and phenergan. Proc. Sci. exp. Biol. Med. III, 731 (1962).
158. FRIMMER, M.: Toxic cyclipeptides of the toadstool Amanita phalloides and related species. Arch. Pharmacol. **269**, 152 (1971).
159. GAJDOS, A., GAJDOS-TOROK, M., PALMA-CARLOS, A., PALMA-CARLOS, L.: Porphyria induced in rats by orotic acid and the effect of adenine-5′-monophosphoric acid. Nature (Lond.) **211**, 974 (1966).
160. GALLAGHER, C.H., GUPTA, D.N., JUDAH, J.D., REES, K.R.: Biochemical changes in liver in acute thioacetamide intoxication. J. Path. Bact. **72**, 193 (1956).
161. GALLAGHER, G.H.: The effect of antioxidants on poisoning by carbon tetrachloride. Aust. J. exp. Biol. med. Sci. **40**, 241 (1962).

162. Gallagher, T.F., Mueller, M.N., Kappas, A.: Estrogen pharmacology. IV. Studies on the structural basis for estrogen-induced impairment of liver function. Medicine (Baltimore) **45**, 471 (1966).
163. Ganote, C.E., Otis, J.B.: Characteristic lesions of yellow phosphorous-induced liver damage. Lab. Invest. **21**, 207 (1969).
164. Ganote, C.E., Rosenthal, E.S.: Characteristic lesions of methyl-azoxyl-methanol-induced liver damage. A comparative ultrastructural study with dimethylnitrosamine, hydrazine sulfate and carbon tetrachloride. Lab. Invest. **19**, 382 (1968).
165. Gardner, George H., Grove, R.C., Gustafson, R.K., Maire, E.D., Thompson, M.J., Wells, H.S., Paul D. Lamson: Studies on the pathological histology of experimental carbon tetrachloride poisoning. Bull. Johns Hopk. Hosp. **46**, 107 (1925).
166. Georgii, A., Mehnert, H.: Über Leberveränderungen durch Thioacetamid bei gleichzeitiger Belastung mit blutzuckersenkende Substanzen. Beitr. path. Anat. **124**, 278 (1961).
167. Ghoshal, A.K., Porta, E.A., Hartroft, W.S.: The role of lipoperoxidation in the pathogenesis of fatty liver induced by phosphorous poisoning in rats. Amer. J. Path. **54**, 275 (1969).
168. Ghoshal, A.K., Porta, E.A., Hartroft, W.S.: Isotopic studies on the absorption and tissue distribution of white phosphorous in rats. Exp. molec. Path. **14**, 212 (1971).
169. Gillette, J.R.: A perspective on the role of chemically reactive metabolites of foreign compounds in toxicity I. Correlation of changes in covalent binding of reactivity metabolites with changes in the incidence and severity of toxicity. Biochem. Pharmacol. **23**, 2785 (1974).
170. Gilruth, J.A.: 11th Ann. Rept. Agr. N.Z., Div. Vet. Sci. 1903, p. 228–278.
171. Giusti, G., Galanti, B., Mancini, A.: Serum guanase activity in viral hepatitis and some other hepatic and extrahepatic diseases. Enzymologia **38**, 373 (1970).
172. Glaser, G., Mager, J.: Biochemical studies on the mechanism of action of liver poisons. III. Depletion of liver glutathione in ethionine poisoning. Biochem. biophys. Acta (Amst.) **372**, 237 (1974).
173. Glynn, L.E., Himsworth, H.P.: Intralobular circulation in acute liver injury by carbon tetrachloride. Clin. Sci. **19**, 63 (1948).
174. Gmaz-Nikulin, E., Stern, P.: The protective effect of E-aminocaproic acid on the liver cirrhosis of rat. Atti Accad. med. lombarda **20**, 20 (1965).
175. Goldblatt, L.A. (ed.): Aflatoxin—Scientific Background Control and Implications. New York: Academic Press, Inc. 1969.
176. Goldblatt, P.J., Sullivan, R.J., Farber, E.: Induction of partial nucleolar segregation in hepatic parenchymal cells by Actinomycin D following inhibition of ribonucleic acid synthesis by ethionine. Lab. Invest. **20**, 283 (1969).
177. Goldfarb, S., Singer, K., Popper, H.: Experimental cholangitis due to alpha-naphthyl-isothiocyanate (ANIT). Amer. J. Path. **40**, 685 (1962).
178. Gopinath, C., Ford, E.J.H.: The effect of alpha-naphthyl isothiocyanate on the liver of sheep and calves. J. Path. **100**, 269 (1970).
179. Grant, H.C., Rees, K.R.: The precancerous liver; correlatives of histological and biochemical changes in rats during prolonged administration of thioacetamide and butter yellow. Proc. roy. Soc. 13, **148**, 117 (1958).
180. Grases, P.J., Reutter, W., Lesch, R.: Protective role of prednisolone upon galactosamine-induced hepatitis in rats. G.E.N. Organo de la Sociedad **27**, 197 (1972).
181. Grice, H.C., Barth, M.L., Cornish, H.H., Foster, G.V., Gray, R.H.: Correlation between serum enzymes, isoenzyme patterns and histologically detectable organ damage. Food Cosmetic Toxic. **9**, 847 (1971).
182. Grice, H.C.: The changing role of pathology in modern safety evaluation. CRC Crit. Rev. Toxicol. **1**, 119 (1972).
183. Grun, M., Liehr, H., Grun, W., Rasenack, U., Brunswig, D.: Influence of liver-RES on toxic liver damage due to galactosamine. Acta Hepato-Gastroenterol. **21**, 5 (1974).
184. Gupta, D.N.: Acute changes in the liver after administration of thioacetamide. J. Path. Bact. **72**, 183 (1956).
185. Gupta, D.N.: Nodular cirrhosis and metastasizing tumors produced in the liver of rats by prolonged feeding with thioacetamide. J. Path. Bact. **72**, 415 (1956).
186. Habig, W.H., Pabst, M.J., Fleischner, G., Gatmaitan, Z., Arias, I.M., Jakoby, W.B.: The identity of glutathione S-transferase B with ligandin, a major binding protein. Proc. nat. Acad. Sci. (Wash.) **71**, 3879 (1974).
187. Halver, J.E.: Aflatoxicosis and trout hepatoma. In: Aflatoxin—Scientific Background Control and Implications, p. 265–306. New York: Academic Press 1969.
188. Halver, J.E., Ashley, L.M., Smith, R.R.: Aflatoxicosis in Coho salmon. Nat. Cancer Inst. Monogr. **31**, 141 (1969).
189. Handler, P., Baker, R.D.: The toxicity of orally administered tannic acid. Science **99**, 393 (1944).
190. Hargreaves, T.: The Liver and Bile Metabolism. New York: Appleton-Century-Crofts 1968.
191. Hargreaves, T.: The Liver and Bile Metabolism, p. 123–159. New York: Appleton-Century-Crofts 1968.

192. HARRIS, C., REDDY, J., CHIGA, M., SVOBODA, D.: Polyribosomal disaggregation by lasiocarpine. Biochim. biophys. Acta (Amst.) **180**, 587 (1969).
193. HARRISON, D.C., COGGINS, C.H., WELLAND, F.H., NELSON, S.: Mushroom poisoning in five patients. Amer. J. Med. **38**, 787 (1965).
194. HARTROFT, W.S.: Experimental hepatic injury. In: Diseases of the Liver (L. SCHIFF, ed.), p. 92–124. Philadelphia: Lippincott 1956.
195. HARTROFT, S.W.: Experimental Cirrhosis. In: The Liver (CH. ROUILLER, ed.), vol. II, p. 477–514. New York: Academic Press 1964.
196. HASE, T.: Hepatic microcirculatory changes in acute and chronic carbon tetrachloride poisoning in rats. Amer. J. Path. **49**, 1069 (1966).
197. HASE, T.: Development of porto-hepatic venous shunts and cirrhosis in carbon tetrachloride poisoning in rats. Amer. J. Path. **53**, 83 (1968).
198. HAUFF, V.: Tödliche Vergiftung durch Phosphorpaste. Med. Cor-Bl. Würtemb. Arzel. Ver. (Stuttg.) **30**, 265 (1860).
199. HEATH, D.F., MAGEE, P.N.: Toxic properties of dialkylnihosamines and some related compounds. Brit. J. industr. Med. **19**, 276 (1962).
200. HEBERT, S., GERVAIS, P., ROU, F., RICHSHOPPER, N.: Cultures de tissue hepatique en toxicologie experimentale. Europ. J. Toxicol. **4**, 175 (1971).
201. HEIKAL, T.A.J., LATHE, G.H.: The effect of oral contraceptive steroids in bile secretion and bilirubin in rats. Brit. J. Pharmacol. **38**, 593 (1970).
202. HEIKEL, T., KNIGHT, B.C., RIMINGTON, C.: Studies on biliary excretion in the rabbit. I. The effect of icterogenic and rehmannic acid on bile flow and the excretion of bilirubin, phyloerythrin, coproporphyrin, alkaline phosphatase and bromsulphthalein. Proc. roy. Soc. B **153**, 47 (1960).
203. HEIMBERG, M., WATKINS, M.L., TOOKER, R.: Carbon tetrachloride hepatotoxicity: the direct action of CCl_4 on the liver. J. Pharmacol. exp. Ther. **145**, 92 (1969).
204. HEISSMEYER, H., STEIN, U.: Funktion lysosoma-Enzyme bei der Galaktosaminhepatitis. Verh. dtsch. Ges. inn. Med. **78**, 1377 (1972).
205. HENDY, R., GRASSO, P.: Autophagy in acute liver damage produced in the rat by dimethylnitrosamine. Chem. Biol. Interact. **5**, 401 (1972).
206. HESS, B.: Enzymes in Blood Plasma. New York: Academic Press 1963.
207. HESS, B.: Biochemistry and biology of plasma enzymes. Proc. Europ. Soc. Study Drug Tox. **5**, 37 (1965).
208. HICKENBOTTOM, R.S., HORNBROOK, K.R.: Effects of carbon tetrachloride on the metabolism of liver glycogen in the rat. J. Pharmacol. exp. Ther. **178**, 383 (1971).
209. HIMSWORTH, H.P.: The Liver and its Diseases, p. 32–34. Cambridge, Massachusetts: Harvard University Press 1947.
210. HINSHAW, L.B., REINS, D.A., HILL, R.J.: Response of isolated liver to endotoxin. Canad. J. Physiol. Pharmacol. **44**, 529 (1966).
211. HIRAYAMA, C.: Hepatic fibrosis: biochemical considerations. In: The Liver and its Diseases (SCHAFFNER, F., SHERLOCK, S. and LEEVY, C.M., eds.), p. 273–282. New York: Intercontinental Medical Book Corp. 1974.
212. HIRAYAMA, C., HIROSHOGA, K., MASAYA, T.: Hepatic collagenolytic activity in rats after carbon tetrachloride poisoning. Biochem. J. **118**, 229 (1972).
213. HIRAYAMA, C., MOROTOMI, I., HIROSLUGE, K.: Quantitative and metabolic changes of hepatic collagens in rats after carbon tetrachloride poisoning. Biochem. J. **118**, 229 (1970).
214. HOFFMAN, J., HINES, M.B., LAPAN, S., RISZKI, R., POST, J.: Effects of acute carbon tetrachloride poisoning. Arch. Path. **59**, 429 (1955).
215. HOLTZMAN, J.L., GILLETTE, J.R.: Effect of dietary orotic acid and adenine sulfate on hepatic microsomal enzymes in male and female rats. Biochem. Pharmacol. **18**, 1927 (1969).
216. HOMMAKER, L., SCHMID, R.: Interference with bile pigment uptake in the liver by flavospidic acid. Gastroenterology **53**, 31 (1967).
217. HORNE, C.H.W., SCOTT, C.A., BUSUTTI, A., MACSWEEN, R.N.M.: Effect of the production of experimental cirrhosis in rats on serum protein levels. Biomedicine **19**, 3 (1973).
218. HOWLAND, J., RICHARDS, A.N.: An experimental study of the metabolism and pathology of delayed chloroform poisoning. J. exp. Med. **11**, 344 (1909).
219. HRUBAN, Z., GRADMAN, W., SLESERS, A., LUBRAN, M.B.: Toxicity of thioacetamide. Lab. Invest. **15**, 1748 (1966).
220. HURWITZ, A.: Effects of microsomal enzyme inducers on animals poisoned with hepatotoxins. Toxical. appl. Pharmacol. **22**, 339 (1972).
221. HUTTERER, F., SCHAFFNER, F., KLION, F.M., POPPER, H.: Hypertrophic hypoactive smooth endoplasmic reticulum: A sensitive indicator of hepatotoxicity exemplified by dieldrin. Science **161**, 1017 (1968).
222. IDEO, G., DEL NINNO, E., DE FRANCHIS, R.: Behavior of some enzymes and isoenzymes in plasma liver and bile of rats treated with carbon tetrachloride. Enzyme **12**, 242 (1971).

223. INDACOCHEA-REDMOND, N., PLAA, G.L.: Functional effects of α-naphthylisothiocyanate in various species. Toxicol. appl. Pharmacol. **19**, 71 (1971).
224. INDACOCHEA-REDMOND, N., WITSCHI, H., PLAA, G.L.: Effect of inhibitors of protein and ribonucleic acid synthesis on the hyperbilirubinemia and cholestasis on the hyperbilirubinemia and cholestasis produced by α-naphthylisothiocyanate. J. Pharmacol. exp. Ther. **184**, 780 (1973).
225. INDACOCHEA-REDMOND, N., WITSCHI, H., PLAA, G.L.: Effects of inhibitors of protein and ribonucleic acid synthesis on α-naphthylisothiocyanate-induced hyperbilirubinemia, sulfobromophthalein retention and prolongation of pentobarbital hypnosis. J. Pharmacol. exp. Ther. **189**, 278 (1974).
226. International Agency for Research on Cancer. W.H.O. Liver Cancer: Proceedings of a Working Conference held at the Chester Beatty Research Institute, London, Eng. IARC Scientific Publ. No. 1. Lyon, France 1971.
227. ISSELBACHER, K.J., ALPERS, D.H.: Fatty liver: biochemical and clinical aspects. In: Diseases of the Liver (L. SCHIFF, ed.), p. 672–688. Philadelphia: J.B. Lippincott Co. 1969.
228. JACKSON, S.H.: The metabolic effects of nonvolatile anesthetics on mammalian hepatoma cells in vitro: II. Inhibition of macromolecular precursor incorporation. Anesthesiology **35**, 268 (1971).
229. JAGO, M.V.: The development of the hepatic megalocytosis of chronic pyrrolidizine poisoning. Amer. J. Path. **56**, 405 (1969).
230. JATLOW, P., ADAMS, W.R., HANDSCHUMACHER, R.E.: Pathogenesis of orotic acid induced fatty change in the rat liver; light and electron microscope studies. Amer. J. Path. **47**, 125 (1965).
231. JEZEQUEL, A.-M.: Les effects de l'intoxication aigue au phosphore sur le foie de rat. Etude au microscopie electronique. Ann. Anat. path. **3**, 512 (1958).
232. JENNINGS, R.B.: Fatal fulminant acute carbon tetrachloride poisoning. Arch. Path. **55**, 269 (1955).
233. JOB, C.K.: Portal venous pressure in acute hepatic necrosis and early cirrhosis due to carbon tetrachloride. J. Path. Bact. **89**, 397 (1965).
234. JOHN, D.W., MILLER, L.L.: Influence of actinomycin D. and puromycin on net synthesis of plasma albumin and fibrinogen by the isolated perfused liver. J. biol. Chem. **241**, 4817 (1966).
235. JUDAH, J.D.: Discussion, in: Cellular Injury (A.V.S. DE REUCK and J. KNIGHT, eds.), p. 117–118. Boston: Little, Brown Co. 1964.
236. JUDAH, J.D.: Biochemical disturbances in liver injury. Brit. med. Bull. **25**, 274 (1969).
237. JUDAH, J.D., AHMED, K., MCLEAN, A.E.M.: Possible role of ion shifts in liver injury. In: Cellular Injury (A.V.S. DE REUCK and J. KNIGHT, eds.), p. 187–208. Boston: Little Brown Co. 1964.
238. JUDAH, J.D., AHMED, H.J.Z., MCLEAN, A.E.M.: Protection provided against carbon tetrachloride and thioacetamide poisoning by strophanthin G. J. Path. Bact. **89**, 619 (1965).
239. JUDAH, J.D., AHMED, K., MCLEAN, A.E.M., CHRISTIE, G.S.: Ion transport in ethionine intoxication. Lab. Invest. **15**, 167 (1966).
240. JUDAH, J.D., MCLEAN, A.E.M., MCLEAN, E.K.: Biochemical mechanisms of drug injury. Amer. J. Med. **49**, 609 (1970).
241. KALTERMANN, R., ACHELIS, R., WOLFRUM, D.I.: Leberschaden und Lipidstoffwechsel. III. Lipidstoffwechsel bei der experimentellen Hepatitis an der Ratte. Acta hepato-splenol. (Stuttg.) **18**, 153 (1971).
242. KASCHNITZ, R., MITTERMEYER, K.: Reversible inhibition of bile secretion during isolated liver perfusion. Experientia (Basel) **26**, 765 (1970).
243. KATO, N., MURAKAMI, S.: The effect of experimental hepatic necrosis on the vitamin B_{12} content in serum and liver. J. Lab. clin. Med. **54**, 365 (1959).
244. KAYANO, K., TSUBONE, T., AZUMA, I., YAMAMURA, U.: The prevention of orotic acid fatty liver by the administration of 5-aminoimidazole-carboxamide. J. Biochem. **52**, 379 (1962).
245. KELLEY, W.N., GREENE, M.L., FOX, I.H., ROSENBLOOM, F.M., LEVY, R.I., SEEGMITLER, J.E.L.: Effects of orotic acid on purine and lipoprotein metabolism in man. Metabolism **19**, 1025 (1970).
246. KENDRY, G.: Über das Verhalten und Schicksal der Nukleolen von Leberzellen bei Thioazetamidvergiftung. Naturwissenschaften **51**, 42 (1964).
247. KENDRY, G.: Über das Verhalten der Nucleolen von Leberzellen bei Thioazetamidvergiftung. Vorläufige Mitteilung. Acta morph. Acad. Sci. hung. **12**, 407 (1964).
248. KENDREY, V.G.: Thioacetamide induced liver cirrhosis in rats. I. Light microscopic observations. Exp. Path. **2**, 295 (1968).
249. KENDRY, G.: Structure and importance of intra-nuclear inclusions in thio-acetamide (Hepatocarcinogenesis). Acta morph. Acad. Sci. hung. **16**, 53 (1968).
250. KENDREY, G., NEMETH, K.: Histogenesis of thioacetamide-induced liver carcinoma. Arch. Geschwulstforsch. **26**, 1 (1965).
251. KENT, G., POPPER, H., DUBIN, A., BRUCE, C.: The spleen in ethionine-induced cirrhosis. Its role in γ-globulin elevation. Arch. Path. **64**, 398 (1957).
252. KEPPLER, D., LESCH, R., REUTTER, W., DEKKER, K.: Experimental hepatitis induced by D-galactosome. Exp. molec. Path. **9**, 279 (1968).
253. KEPPLER, D.O.R., PAUSCH, J., DECKER, K.: Selective uridine triphosphate deficiency induced by D-galactosamine in liver and reversed by pyrimidine nucleotide precursors. J. biol. Chem. **249**, 211 (1974).

254. KEPPLER, D.O.R., SMITH, D.F.: Nucleotide contents of ascites hepatoma cells and their changes induced by D-Galactosamine. Cancer Res. **34**, 705 (1974).
255. KERR, J.F.R.: Lysosome change in acute liver injury due to heliotrine. J. Path. Bact. **93**, 167 (1967).
256. KERR, J.F.R.: An electron microscope study of liver cell necrosis due to heliotrine. J. Path. **97**, 557 (1970).
257. KERR, J.F.R.: Liver cell defaecation: an electron-microscope study of the discharge of liposomal residual bodies into the intercellular space. J. Path. **100**, 99 (1970).
258. KERR, J.F.R., POUND, A.W.: Acute liver injury due to albitocin. Aust. J. exp. Med. **44**, 197 (1966).
259. KERSHENOBICH, D., FIERRO, F.J., ROJKIND, M.: The relationship between the free pool of proline and collagen content in human liver cirrhosis. J. clin. Invest. **49**, 2246 (1970).
260. KHANNA, J.M., KALAUT, H., LIN, G., BUSTOS, G.O.: Effect of carbon tetrachloride treatment on ethanol metabolism. Biochem. Pharmacol. **20**, 3269 (1971).
261. KINGSBURY, J.J.: Poisonous Plants of the United States and Canada, 3rd ed. Engelwood Cliffs, N.J.: Prentice-Hall Inc. 1964.
262. KINNEY, T.D., KAUFMAN, N., KLAVINS, J.V.: Disposition of iron in association with a periodic acid-schiff (PAS)-positive material in the liver of ethionine-treated rats. Lab. Invest. **12**, 978 (1963).
263. KINNEY, T.D., KAUFMAN, A., KLAVINS, J.V.: Centrilobular cirrhosis carried by ethionine. Arch. Path. **79**, 34 (1965).
264. KINSELLA, J.E.: Protein and lipoperoxide levels in orotic acid-induced fatty livers. Canad. J. Biochem. **45**, 1206 (1967).
265. KIZER, D.E., HOWELL, B.A., CLOUSE, J.A., SHIRLEY, B.C.: Studies on the relationship between increased adenylic acid deaminase activity and changes in nuclear RNA Metabolism in rat liver caused by thioacetamide. Cancer Res. **26**, 1376 (1966).
266. KIZER, D.E., SHIRLEY, B.C., COX, B., HOWELL, B.A.: Effect of thioacetamide on adenylic acid deaminase activity and nuclear ribonucleic acid metabolism in rat liver. Cancer Res. **25**, 596 (1965).
267. KLAASSEN, C.D., PLAA, G.G.: Relative effects of various chlorinated hydrocarbons on liver, and kidney function in man. Toxicol. appl. Pharmacol. **10**, 119 (1967).
268. KLAASSEN, C.D., PLAA, G.L.: Effect of carbon tetrachloride on the metabolism, storage and excretion of sulfobromophthalein. Toxicol. appl. Pharmacol. **12**, 132 (1968).
269. KLATSKIN, G.: Toxic and drug-induced hepatitis. In: Diseases of the Liver, 3rd ed. (L. SCHIFF, ed.), p. 498–601. Philadelphia: J.B. Lippincott Co. 1969.
270. KLAVINS, J.V., KINNEY, T.D., KAUFMAN, N.: Changes in affinity of liver for iron and loss of liver iron during prolonged ethionine administration. Amer. J. Path. **46**, 969 (1965).
271. KLEINFELD, R.G.: Early changes in rat liver and kidney cells induced by thioacetamide. Cancer Res. **17**, 954 (1957).
272. KLEINFELD, R.G., VON HAAM, E.: Effect of thioacetamide on rat liver regeneration. II. Nuclear RNA in mitosis. J. biophys. biochem. Cytol. **6**, 393 (1959).
273. KLUBES, P., JONDORF, W.R.: Dimethylnitrosamine formation from sodium nitrite and dimethylamine by bacterial flora of rat intestine. Res. Com. Chem. Path. Pharmacol. **2**, 24 (1971).
274. KOCH-WESER, D., DE LA HUERGA, J., POPPER, H.: Hẹpatic necrosis due to brombenzene and its dependence upon available sulfur amino acids. Proc. Soc. exp. Biol. (N.Y.) **79**, 196 (1952).
275. KOCH-WESER, D., FARBER, E., SZANTO, P.B., POPPER, H.: Histological and biochemical changes in fatty livers with and without necrosis. Fed. Proc. **9**, 336 (1950).
276. KOFF, R.S.: Acute toxic effects of D-galactosamine on human embryo cells in tissue culture. Europ. J. clin. Biol. Res. **17**, 69 (1972).
277. KOFF, R.S., DAVIDSON, L.J., GORDON, G., SABESIN, S.M.: D-Galactosamine Hepatotoxicity III. Normactive Smooth endoplasmic reticulum and modification by phenobarbital. Exp. molec. Path. **19**, 168 (1973).
278. KOFF, R.S., GORDON, G., SABESIN, S.M.: D-Galactosamine hepatitis I. Hepatocellular injury and fatty liver following a single dose. Proc. Soc. exp. Biol. (N.Y.) **137**, 696 (1971).
279. KOLENBRANDER, H.M.: A comparison of the effect of diet and of ethionine on rat liver histidine deaminase and urocanase. Canad. J. Biochem. **47**, 437 (1969).
280. KOPELMAN, H., SCHEUER, P.J., WILLIAMS, R.: The liver lesion of the Epping jaundice. Quart. J. Med. **35**, 553 (1966).
281. KEPPLER, D.O.R., HUBNER, G.: Liver injury induced by 2-Deoxy-D-Galactose. Exp. molec. Path. **19**, 365 (1973).
282. KORPASSY, B., KOVACS, K., SZTANAJEVITS, A.: The influence of sex and dietary casein content upon lethal and liver injurious effect of tannic acid. Acta physiol. Acad. Sci. hung. **3**, 233 (1952).
283. KORPASSY, B.: The hepatocarcinogenicity of tannic acid. Cancer Res. **19**, 501 (1959).
284. KORSRUD, G.O., GRICE, H.G., GOODMAN, T.K., KNIPFIL, J.E., MCLAUGHLIN, J.M.: Sensitivity of several serum enzymes for the detection of thioacetamide, dimethylnitrosanine and diethanolanine-induced liver damage in rats. Toxicol. appl. Pharmacol. **26**, 299 (1973).

285. KOULISH, S., KLEINFELD, R.G.: The role of the nucleolus. I. Tritiated cytidine activity in liver parenchymal cells of thioacetamide-treated rats. J. Cell Biol. **23**, 39 (1964).
286. KRAYBILL, H.F.: The toxicology and epidemology of natural hepatotoxin exposure. Israel J. med. Sci. **10**, 416 (1974).
287. KREZANOSKI, J.Z.: Tannic acid: chemistry, analysis, and toxicology. Radiology **87**, 655 (1966).
288. KROKER, R., HEGNER, D.: Solubilization of phalloidin binding sites from rat liver hepatocytes and plasma membranes by trypsin. Naunyn-Schmiedeberg's Arch. Pharmacol. **279**, 339 (1973).
289. KUME, F.: Acute nucleolar morphological change produced by dimethyl-nitrosamine in mouse hepatic parenchymal cells. Gann **59**, 151 (1968).
290. KUSTER, G.R., WOODS, J.E., LUDWIG, J.: Pathology of liver necrosis and regeneration after administration of dimethylnitrosamine in massive doses. J. Surg. **5**, 9 (1973).
291. LADUE, B.N., KALLOW, W. (eds.): Pharmacogenetics. Ann. N.Y. Acad. Sci. **151**, 691 (1968).
292. LADUE, B.N., MANDEL, H.G., WAY, E.L. (eds.): Fundamentals of Drug Metabolism and Disposition. Baltimore: Williams and Wilkins 1971.
293. LADUE, J.S., SCHENKEN, J.R., KUKER, L.H.: Phosphorous poisoning; a report of sixteen cases with repeated liver biopsies in a recovered case. Amer. J. med. Sci. **208**, 223 (1944).
294. LAMBERT, S.M.: Carbon tetrachloride in the treatment of hookworm disease. J. Amer. med. Ass. **53**, 526 (1923).
295. LAQUET, A.M.: Experimental pathology of the liver. VIII Effects of carbon tetrachloride on the normal and on the restored liver after partial hepatectomy. Arch. Path. **14**, 164 (1932).
296. LARSON, R.E., PLAA, G.L.: A correlation of the effects of cervical cordotomy, hypothermia and catecholamines on carbon tetrachloride induced hepatic necrosis. J. Pharmacol. exp. Ther. **147**, 103 (1965).
297. LAWRENCE, J., HOFFMAN, M.M.: Fatty changes in the Kupfer cells in the liver of the guinea pig in phosphorous poisoning. Arch. Path. **7**, 809 (1929).
298. LEDUC, E.H.: Regeneration of the liver. In: The Liver (CH. ROUILLER, ed.), vol. II, p. 76–78. New York: Academic Press 1964.
299. LEEVY, C.M.: Dye extraction by the liver. In: Progress in Liver Diseases, vol. I (H. POPPER and F. SCHAFFNER, eds.), p. 174–186. New York: Grune and Stratton, Inc. 1961.
300. LEINWEBER, B.: Galactosamine-hepatitis and anti-cholestasis. Fortschr. Medicin **91**, 792 (1973).
301. LEINWEBER, D., PLATT, D.: Tierexperimentelle Untersuchungen zur Frage der Galaktosaminschadung bei Babyratten. Beitr. path. Anat. **142**, 345 (1971).
302. LE PAGE, R.N., DORLING, P.R.: Plasma membranes in acute liver injury; biochemical changes induced by carbon tetrachloride. Aust. J. exp. Biol. **49**, 345 (1971).
303. LESCH, R., DEUS, B., REULTER, W.: Die Beeinflussung der akuten Galatosaminschädigung der Ratte durch bilaterale Adrenalektomie. Dtsch. Ges. inn. Med. **70**, 1380 (1972).
304. LESCH, R., KEPPLER, D., REUTTER, W., RUDIGIER, J., OEHLERT, W., DECKER, K.: Entwicklung einer experimentellen Leberzirrhose durch D-Galaktosamin. Histologische, biochemische und autoradiographische Untersuchungen an Ratten. Virchows Arch. Abt. B **6**, 57 (1970).
305. LESCH, R., REUTTER, W., KEPPLER, D., DECKER, K.: Liver restitution after acute galactosamine hepatis: Autoradiographic and biochemical studies in rats. Exp. molec. Path. **12**, 58 (1970).
306. LEWIS, N.B., IZUMO, S.: The influence of hydrazine and its derivatives on metabolism. II. Changes in the non-protein nitrogen constituents of the blood in the metabolism of injected glycine in hydrazine intoxication. J. biol. Chem. **71**, 33 (1926).
307. LEWIS, M., SCHENKER, S., COMBES, B.: Studies on the pathogenesis of tetracycline-induced fatty liver. Amer. J. dig. Dis. **12**, 429 (1967).
308. LIEBER, C.S.: Hepatic and metabolic effects of alcohol (1966–1973). Gastroenterology **65**, 821 (1973).
309. LIJINSKY, W., EPSTEIN, S.: Nitrosamines as environmental carcinogens. Nature (Lond.) **225**, 21 (1970).
310. LITTON, W.: The most poisonous mushrooms. Sci. Amer. **232**, 90 (1975).
311. LOMBARDI, B., RECKNAGEL, R.O.: Interference with secretion of triglycerides by the liver as a common factor in toxic hepatic injury; with some observations on choline deficiency fatty liver. Amer. J. Path. **40**, 571 (1962).
312. LOPEZ, M.: Proliferazioni iperplastiche e neoplastiche delle vie bilifere intrahepatiche da thioacetamide. Experentia (Basel) **12**, 185 (1956).
313. LOPEZ, M., MAZZANTI, L.: Experimental investigation on alpha-naphthyl-isothiocyanate as a hyperplastic agent of the biliary ducts in the rat. J. Path. Bact. **69**, 243 (1955).
314. LOYKE, H.F.: Experimental hypertension treated with CCl_4: measurement of adrenal function, vascular responsiveness, angiotensinase and converting enzyme. Proc. Soc. exp. Biol. (N.Y.) **115**, 1035 (1964).
315. LUCKE, H.H., HODGE, K.E., PATT, N.L.: Fatal liver damage after barium enemas containing tannic acid. Canad. med. Ass. J. **89**, 1111 (1963).
316. LUTZ, F., GLOSSMAN, H., FRIMMER, M.: Binding of ^{3}H-desmethylphalloin to isolated plasma membranes from rat liver. Naunyn-Schmiedberg's Arch. Pharmacol. **273**, 341 (1972).

317. Lyachovich, V.V., Mishin, V.M., Dolgov, A.V., Jakobson, G.S., Panov, A.V., Tsyrlov, I.B.: Functional and structural changes in liver mitochondria of rats due to CCl_4 intoxication II. Respiratory chain and ion transport. Biochem. Pharmacol. **20**, 1443 (1971).
318. Lyachovich, V.V., Mishin, V.M., Dolgov, A.V., Tsyrlov, I.B.: Functional and structural changes in liver mitochondria of rats due to CCl_4 Intoxication I. Studies on state of electron transport chain. Biochem. Pharmacol. **20**, 1437 (1971).
319. Lynen, F., Wieland, U.: Über die Giftstoffe des Knollenblätterpilzes IV. Justus Liebigs Ann. Chem. **533**, 93 (1937).
320. Madden, J.W., Gertman, P.M., Peacock, E.E., Jr.: Dimethylnitrosamine-induced hepatic cirrhosis: a new canine model of an ancient human disease. Surgery **68**, 260 (1970).
321. Madhaven, T.T., Gopalen, C.: The effect of dietary protein on carcinogenesis of aflatoxin. Arch. Path. **85**, 133 (1968).
322. Madhaven, T.T., Rao, S.K., Tulpule, P.G.: Effect of dietary protein level on susceptibility of monkeys to aflatoxin liver injury. Indian J. med. Res. **53**, 984 (1965).
323. Madhaven, T.T., Tultpule, P.G., Gopalen, C.: Aflatoxin-induced hepatic fibrosis in Rhesus monkeys. Arch. Path. **79**, 466 (1965).
324. Magee, P.N.: Cellular injury and alkylation of cell components. CIBA Foundation Symposium in Cellular Injury, 1965 (N.V.S. de Reuck and J. Knight, eds.), p. 1–22. Boston: Little, Brown and Company 1964.
325. Magee, P.N.: Toxic liver necroses. Lab. Invest. **15**, 111 (1966).
326. Magee, P.N.: Liver Carcinogens in the human environment. In: Liver Cancer: Proceedings of a Working Conference Held at the Chester Bealty Research Institute, London, Eng. IARC Scientificist Publ. No. 1, Lyon, France, 1971, p. 110–120.
327. Magee, P.N., Swann, P.F.: Nitroso compounds. Brit. med. Bull. **25**, 240 (1969).
328. Majno, B.: Death of liver tissues: A review of cell death, necrosis and autolysis. In: The Liver (Rouiller, Ch., ed.), vol. II, p. 267–313. New York: Academic Press 1964.
329. Maki, Y., Takeshita, M., Miyata, S., Tanaka, S.: Observations on enzymes in carbon tetrachloride fatty liver. Kumanota med. J. **17**, 153 (1969).
330. Maley, F., Tarentino, A.L., McGarrahan, J.F., del Giacco, R.: The metabolism of D-galactosamine and N-acetyl-D-galactosamine in rat liver. Biochem. J. **107**, 637 (1968).
331. Mallory, F.B.: Phosphorous poisoining and alcoholic cirrhosis. Amer. J. Path. **9**, 557 (1933).
332. Mattocks, A.R.: Acute hepatotoxicity and pyrrolic metabolites in rats dosed with pyrrolidizine alkaloids. Chem. Biol. Interact. **5**, 227 (1972).
333. Mayes, P.A., Felts, J.M.: Liver function studied by liver perfusion. Proc. Europ. Soc. Study Drug Tox. **7**, 16 (1966).
334. Mazel, P.: General Principles and Procedures for Drug Metabolism *in vitro*. In: Fundamentals of Drug Metabolism and Disposition (B.N. La Due, H.G. Mandel, and E.L. Way, eds.), p. 527–545. Baltimore: Williams and Wilkins 1971.
335. Mazzanti, L.: Biological effects of thioacetamide and dimethylamino-azobenzene in rats on a lipogenic diet. Arch. ital. Sci. Farmacol. **10**, 289 (1960).
336. Mazzanti, L., Lopez, M.: In terma di epatopatie sperimentali sui rapporti tra lesione epitehale e proliferazione mesenchimale nella fibrosi da alfanaftilisotiocianato. Arch. De Vecchi Anat. pat. **17**, 825 (1952).
337. McAlister, W.H., Anderson, M.S., Bloomberg, G.R., Margulis, A.: Lethal effects of tannic acid in the barium enema. Radiology **80**, 765 (1963).
338. McCloskey, J.F., Mc Gehee, E.H.: Effect of subcutaneous and intraoral administration of carbon tetrachloride on the liver of the rat. Arch. Path. **49**, 200 (1950).
339. McGee, J. O'D., Patrick, R.S.: The synthesis of sulfated mucopolysaccharides in mouse liver following carbon tetrachloride poisoning. I. Autoradiographic studies. Brit. J. exp. Path. **40**, 46 (1969).
340. McGee, J. O'D., Patrick, R.S.: The role of perisinusoidal cells in hepatic fibrogenesis: An electron microscopic study of acute carbon tetrachloride liver injury. Lab. Invest. **26**, 429 (1972).
341. McGill, C.M.: Death and illness from use of carbon tetrachloride. Northw. Med. (Seattle) **45**, 169 (1946).
342. McIntyre, N., Sherlock, S. (eds.): Therapeutic Agents and the Liver. Philadelphia: F.A. Davies 1965.
343. McLean, A.E.M.: The effect of diet and vitamin E on liver injury due to carbon tetrachloride. Brit. J. exp. Path. **48**, C32 (1967).
344. McLean, A.E.M.: The effect of protein deficiency and microsomal enzyme induction by DDT and phenobarbitone in the acute toxicity of chloroform and a pyrrolidizine alkaloid, retrorsine. Brit. J. exp. Path. **51**, 317 (1970).
345. McLean, A.E.M.: Determinants of toxicity. Biochem. Pharmacol. **20**, 1019 (1971).
346. McLean, A.E.M., Magee, P.N.: Increased renal carcinogenesis by dimethyl nitrosamine in protein deficient rats. Brit. J. exp. Path. **51**, 587 (1970).
347. McLean, A.E.M., McLean, E.K.: Diet and toxicity. Brit. med. Bull. **25**, 278 (1969).
348. McLean, A.E.M., McLean, E., Judah, J.D.: Cellular necrosis in the liver induced and modified by drugs. Int. Rev. exp. Path. **4**, 127 (1965).

349. McLean, A.E.M., Verschuddoren, H.G.: Effect of diet and microsomal enzyme induction on the toxicity of dimethytritrosamines. Brit. J. exp. Path. **50**, 22 (1969).
350. McLean, E., Bras, G., McLean, A.E.M.: Venous occlusions in the liver following dimethylnitrosamine. Brit. J. exp. Path. **46**, 36 (1965).
351. McLean, E.L., McLean, A.E.M., Sutton, P.M.: "Instant cirrhosis." An improved method for introducing cirrhosis of the liver in rats by simultaneous administration of carbon tetrachloride and phenobarbitone. Brit. J. exp. Path. **50**, 502 (1969).
352. McLean, E.R.: The toxic actions of pyrrolidizine (senecio) alkaloids. Pharmacol. Rev. **22**, 429 (1970).
353. McLean, M.R., Rees, K.R.: Hyperplasia of bile ducts induced by alpha-naphthyl-iso-thiocyanate: experimental biliary cirrhosis free from biliary obstruction. J. Path. Bact. **76**, 175 (1958).
354. McLean, P.: Effect of ethionine treatment on the activity of enzymes concerned with urea synthesis in the rat liver. Biochem. J. **99**, 776 (1966).
355. Madhaven, T.T., Gopalen, C.: Effect of dietary protein on aflatoxin liver injury in weanling rats. Arch. Path. **80**, 123 (1965).
356. Medline, A., Schaffner, F., Popper, H.: Ultrastructural features in galactosamine-induced hepatitis. Exp. molec. Path. **12**, 201 (1970).
357. Mehrota, R.M.L., Chaturvedi, U.C.: Age as a modifying factor of acute hepatic injury in albino rats. Indian J. Path. Bact. **9**, 182—187 (1966).
358. Meili, E.D., Frick, P.G., Straub, P.W.: Coagulation changes during massive hepatic necrosis due to Amanita phalloides poisoning; with special reference to antihemophilic globulin. Helv. med. Acta **35**, 309 (1969/70).
359. Meldolisi, J., Pelosi, G., Brunelli, A., Genovese, E.: Electron microscopic studies on the effect of amanitin in mice; liver and heart lesions. Virchows Arch. path. Anat. **342**, 221 (1967).
360. Meyer, J., Pessoa, S.B.: A study of the toxicity of carbon tetrachloride. Amer. J. trop. Med. **3**, 177 (1923).
361. Meyer, J.G.: Über RNS-Veränderungen in der Rattenleber unter Thioacetamid-Applikation. Z. Naturforsch. **21** B, 342 (1966).
362. Meyer-Burg, J., Hirner, A.: Elektronenoptische Untersuchungen zur Galactosamin-Schädigung der Rattenleber. Klin. Wschr. **49**, 1240 (1971).
363. Michael, U.F., Barenberg, R.L., Levi, D., Pardo, V., Chavez, R., Popper, S.: Abnormal sodium regulation in rats following chronic intermittent exposure to carbon tetrachloride. Proc. Soc. exp. Biol. (N.Y.) **138**, 796 (1971).
364. Michaelis, L.: Das Wesen der chronischen Phosphorwirkung und der Phosphornekrose. Arch. Gewerbepath. Gewerbehyg. **7**, 477 (1936).
365. Michon, P., Larcon, A., Lamarche, M., Grignion, G., Huriet, C., Vicarim, F.: Les nephropathies phalloidiennes. Presse méd. **69**, 1327 (1961).
366. Miller, E.C., Miller, J.A.: Mechanisms of chemical carcinogenesis, nature of proximate carcinogens and interactions with macromolecules. Pharmacol. Rev. **18**, 805 (1966).
367. Miller, J.A.: Carcinogenesis by chemicals: an overview. Cancer Res. **30**, 559 (1970).
368. Mitchell, J.R., Jollow, D.J., Gillette, J.R., Brodie, B.B.: Drug metabolism as a cause of drug toxicity. Drug. Met. and Disp. **1**, 418 (1973).
369. Miyai, K., Ritchies, A.C.: Natural resolution of hepatic ultrastructure changes induced by ethionine. Amer. J. Path. **61**, 211 (1970).
370. Miyake, M., Saito, M.: Liver injury and liver tumors induced by toxins of Penicillium islandandicium Sopp growing on yellowed rice. In: Mycotoxins in Foodstuffs (G.N. Wogan, ed.), p. 133—146. Cambridge: M.I.T. Press 1965.
371. Mjassnikow, A.K.: Über die Rolle der Leber im Cholesterinstoffwechsel. Klin. Wschr. **11**, 1910 (1932).
372. Molander, D.W., Wroblewski, F., laDue, J.S.: Transaminase compared with cholinesterase and alkaline phosphatase as an index of hepatocellular integrity. Clin. Res. Proc. **3**, 20 (1955).
373. Molnár, Z.: The effect of hypothermia on thioacetamide-induced hepatic damage. Acta physiol. Acad. Sci. hung. **34**, 95 (1968).
374. Monier, D., Wagle, S.R.: Studies on gluconeogenesis in galactosamine hepatitis. Fed. Proc. **30**, 1186 (1971).
375. Moon, H.D.: The pathology of fatal carbon tetrachloride poisoning with special reference to the histogenesis of the hepatic and renal lesions. Amer. J. Path. **26**, 1041 (1950).
376. Moon, V.H.: Experimental cirrhosis in relation to human cirrhosis. Arch. Path. **18**, 381 (1934).
377. Moran, E., Eliakim, M., Suchowalshi, A., Ungar, H.: Serum vitamin B_{12} and glutannic oxalaretic transaminase in experimental intrahepatic obstructive jaundice. Gastroenterology **40**, 408 (1961).
378. Moran, E., Ungar, H.: The effect of intermittent administration of alpha-naphthyl isothiocyanate to rats. Amer. J. Path. **49**, 947 (1964).
379. Mortimore, P.H., Taylor, A.: The experimental intoxication of sheep with sporidesmin, a metabolic product of Pithomyces chartarum. Res. Vet. Sci. **3**, 147 (1962).

380. MOSSBERG, S.M., ROSS, C., BERKOWITZ, J.: Glucose-6-phosphatase activity in human serum. Amer. J. med. Sci. **244**, 97 (1962).
381. MUKHERJEE, T., GUSTAFSSON, R.G., AFZELIUS, B.A., ARRHENIUS, E.: Effects of carcinogenic amines on amino acid incorporation by liver systems. II. A morphological and biochemical study on the effect of dimethylnitrosamine. Cancer Res. **23**, 944 (1963).
382. MÜLLER-BERGHANS, G., REUTER, C.: Disseminated intravascular coagulation in galactosamine-induced experimental hepatitis. Thrombosis Res. **1**, 473 (1972).
383. MURAMATSU, M., BUSCH, H.: Effects of thioacetamide on metabolism of proteins of normal and regenerating liver. Cancer Res. **22**, 1100 (1962).
384. NEWBERNE, P.: The influence of a low lipotrope diet on response of maternal and fetal rats to lasiocarpine. Cancer Res. **28**, 2327 (1968).
385. NEWBERNE, P.M.: Chronic aflatoxicosis. J. Amer. vet. med. Ass. **163**, 1262 (1973).
386. NEWBERNE, P.M., BULTER, W.H.: Acute and chronic effects of aflatoxin on the liver of domestic and laboratory animals; a review. Cancer Res. **29**, 236 (1969).
387. NEWBERNE, P.M., WILSON, R., ROGERS, A.E.: Effects of a low-lipotrope diet on the response of young male rats to the pyrrolidizine alkaloid, monocrotaline. Toxicol. appl. Pharmacol. **18**, 387 (1971).
388. NOLAN, J.P., SCHEIG, R.L., KLATSKIN, G.: Delayed hepatitis and cirrhosis in weanling rats following a single small dose of the Senerio alkaloid, lasiocarpine. Amer. J. Path. **49**, 129 (1966).
389. NOTHNAGEL: Die fettige Degeneration der Organe bei Äther und Chloroformvergiftung. Berl. klin. Wschr. **3**, 31 (1866). Cit. by DRILL ref. 1.
390. NOVIKOFF, A.B., ROHEIM, P.S., QUENTANA, N.: Changes in rat liver induced by orotic acid feeding. Lab. Invest. **15**, 27 (1966).
391. NYGAARD, O., ELDJARN, L., NAKKEN, K.F.: Studies on the metabolism of thioacetamide-S in the intact rat. Cancer Res. **14**, 625 (1954).
392. OBERLIN, CH., ROUILLIER, CH.: Les effects de l'intoxiation aigue au tetrachlorure de carbone sur le foie de rat. Etude au microscope electronique. Ann. Anat. path. **1**, 401 (1956).
393. OETTINGEN, W.F. VON: Poisoning, 2nd ed. Philadelphia: W.B. Saunders Co. 1958.
394. OETTINGEN, W.F. VON: The Halogenated Hydrocarbons of Industrial and Toxicological Importance. Amsterdam: Elsevier 1964.
395. OPIE, E.L., ALFROD, L.B.: The influence of diet upon necrosis caused by hepatic and renal porisons. I. Diet and hepatic lesions of chloroform, phosphorous, or alcohol. J. exp. Med. **21**, 1 (1915).
396. OSTERTAG, R.: Die todtliche Nachwirkung des Chloroforms. Virchows Arch. **118**, 250 (1889).
397. O'SULLIVAN, W.J.O.: Orotic acid. Aust. N.Z.J. Med. **3**, 417 (1973).
398. PALMER, W.L., WOODALL, P.S., WANG, K.C.: Cincophen and toxic neuroses of the liver: a survey of the problem. Trans. Ass. Phycns **51**, 381 (1936).
399. PANAHANDEH, J.: High sodium intake and the production of ascites during chronic liver intoxication. J. Path. Bact. **83**, 491 (1962).
400. PANI, P., GRAVELLA, E., MAZZARINO, C., BURDINO, E.: On the mechanism of fatty liver in white phosphorous poisoned rats. Exp. molec. Path. **16**, 201 (1972).
401. PANNER, B.J., HANSS, R.J.: Hepatic injury in mushroom poisoning; electron microscopic observations on two nonfatal cases. Arch. Path. **87**, 35 (1969).
402. PARKE, D.V., WILLIAMS, R.T.: Metabolism of toxic substances. Brit. med. Bull. **25**, 256 (1969).
403. PATTERSON, D.S.P., ALLCROFT, R.: Metabolism of Aflatoxin in susceptible and resistant animal species. Food Cosmet. Toxicol. **8**, 43 (1970).
404. PETERS, J.P., VAN SLYKE, D.D.: Quantitative Clinical Chemistry: Interpretations, 2nd ed., vol. I, p. 344, 345. Baltimore: Williams and Wilkins Co. 1946.
405. PETERS, R.A.: Biochemical Lesions and Lethal Synthesis. Oxford: Pergamon Press 1963.
406. PETHICK, W.H.: Special report on Picton cattle disease. Health of Animals. Department of Agriculture of Canada, Ottawa, 1906.
407. PETOUT, M.J., MCGEE, H.A., SCHABORT, J.C.: The effect of aflatoxin B_1, aflatoxin B_2 and sterigmatocyotion on nuclear desoxyribonucleases from rat and mouse livers. Chem. Biol. Interact. **3**, 353 (1971).
408. PETZOLD, H., SCHAUER, L.: Die Wirkung von Magnesium-Thiosulfat auf die durch Thioacetamid geschädigte Rattenleber. Dtsch. Z. Verdau.- u. Stoffwechselkr. **23**, 37 (1963).
409. PHILLIPS, M.J., STEINER, J.W.: Comparative study of α-naphthylisothiocyanate-induced liver injury. Lab. Invest. **13**, 779 (1964).
410. PITOT, H.C.: Recent advances in the mechanism of hepatic carcinogenesis. In: Progress in Liver Disease, vol. III (H. POPPER and F. SCHAFFNER, eds.), p. 77–88. New York: Grune and Stratton 1970.
411. PLAA, G.L.: Evaluation of liver function methodology. In: Medical Research Series (A. BURGER, ed.), vol. III, p. 255–288. New York: Marcel Dekker, Inc. 1968.
412. PLAA, G.L.: Functional aspects of the cholestatic response indicated by α-naphthylisothiocyanate in mice and rats. Agente Actions **1**, 22 (1969).

413. Plaa, G.L.: Hyperbilirubinemia and cholestases, a different form of liver injury produced in animals. Essays Toxicol. **2**, 137 (1970).
414. Plaa, G.L., Evans, E.A., Hine, C.H.: Relative hepatotoxicity of seven balogenated hydrocarbons. J. Pharmacol. exp. Ther. **123**, 224 (1958).
415. Plaa, G.L., Rogers, L.A., Fouts, J.R.: Effects of acute alpha-naphthylisothiocyanate administration on hepatic microsomal drug metabolism in the mouse. Proc. Soc. exp. Biol. (N.Y.) **119**, 1045 (1965).
416. Pong, R.S., Wogan, G.N.: Time course and dose-response characteristics of aflatoxin B_1 effects on rat liver RNA polymerase and ultrastructure. Cancer Res. **30**, 299 (1970).
417. Popper, H.: Coarse nodular cirrhosis produced by ethionine. Amer. J. Path. **31**, 594 (1955).
418. Popper, H., Rubin, E., Gardoil, D., Schaffner, F., Paronetto, F.: Drug-induced liver disease. Arch. intern. Med. **115**, 128 (1965).
419. Popper, H., Udenfriend, S.: Hepatic fibrosis: correlation of biochemical and morphologic investigations. Amer. J. Med. **49**, 707 (1970).
420. Post, J., Himes, M.B., Klein, A., Hoffman, J.: Responses of the liver to injury. Arch. Path. **64**, 284 (1957).
421. Pottenger, L.A., Getz, G.S.: Serum lipoprotein accumulation in the livers of orotic acid-fed rats. J. Lipid. Res. **12**, 450 (1971).
422. Pryor, W.J., McDonald, W.J.F., Seawright, A.A.: Supplejack (Ventilago viminalis) feeding of sheep; nutritional and toxicological investigations. Austr. vet. J. **48**, 339 (1972).
423. Racela, A., Grady, H., Svoboda, D.: Ultrastructural nuclear changes due to tannic acid. Cancer Res. **27**, 1658 (1967).
424. Raich, A.N., Narayanan, S., Ritchie, A.C.: Effect of glucose on the biochemical changes in rat liver in acute ethionine intoxication. Exp. molec. Path. **14**, 176 (1971).
425. Raisfeld, I.H.: Models of liver injury. In: The Liver (F.F. Becker, ed.), p. 217. New York: Marcel Dekker, Inc. 1974.
426. Rajalhakshmir, S., Sarma, D.S.R., Sriramachow, S., Sarma, R.S.: Periportal fatty liver in the rat induced by high protein orotic acid diets. Indian J. med. Res. **52**, 1183 (1964).
427. Rao, M.G., Dayal, Y., Ramalinyaswami, V.: Aflatoxins and liver injury in the Rhesus monkey. J. Path. **101**, 47 (1970).
428. Rappaport, A.M.: Acinar units and pathophysiology of the liver. In: The Liver (Ch. Rouiller, ed.), vol. I, p. 265–328. New York: Academic Press 1963.
429. Rather, L.J.: Experimental alteration of nuclear and cytoplasmic components of the liver cell with thioacetamide. I. Early onset and reversibility of volume changes of the nucleolus, nucleus and cytoplasm. Bull. Johns Hopk. Hosp. **88**, 38 (1951).
430. Recknagel, R.O.: Carbon tetrachloride hepatotoxicity. Pharmacol. Rev. **19**, 145 (1967).
431. Recknagel, R.O., Ghoshal, A.K.: Quantitative estimation of peroxidative degeneration of rat liver microsomal and mitochondrial lipids after carbon tetrachloride poisoning. Exp. molec. Path. **5**, 413 (1966).
432. Recknagel, R.O., Glinde, E.A.: Carbon tetrachloride hepatotoxicity: an example of lethal cleavage. C.R.C. Crit. Rev. Toxicol. **2**, 263 (1973).
433. Recknagel, R.D., Lombardi, B.: Studies on the biochemical changes in subcellular particles from rat liver and their relationship to a new hypothesis regarding the pathogenesis of CCl_4 fat accumulation. J. biol. Chem. **236**, 564 (1961).
434. Record, C.O., Alberti, K.G.: Glucose tolerance and blood metabolite changes in galactosamine hepatitis and obstructive jaundice in the rat. Europ. J. clin. Invest. **3**, 130 (1973).
435. Reddy, J.K., Chiga, M., Harris, C.C., Svoboda, D.J.: Polyribosome disaggregation in rat liver following administration of tannic acid. Cancer Res. **30**, 58 (1970).
436. Reddy, J., Chiga, M., Sroboda, D.: Initiation of the division cycle of rat hepatocytes following a single injection of thioacetamide. Lat. Invest. **20**, 405 (1969).
437. Reddy, D.G., Krishnamurthy, K.R., Bhaskard, G.R.: Carbon tetrachloride cirrhosis in rats. 1. The influence of age, sex and gonadectomy. 2. The changes in the livers of fetuses born to mothers exposed to carbon tetrachloride. Arch. Path. **74**, 73 (1962).
438. Rees, K., Rowland, G., Varcoe, J.: The metabolism of tritiated thymidine in the rat. Int. J. Cancer **1**, 197 (1966).
439. Rees, K.R., Shotlander, V.L.: Fat accumulation in accute liver injury. Proc. roy. Soc. B **157**, 517 (1963).
440. Rees, K.R., Sinha, K.P.: Blood enzymes in liver injury. J. Path. Bact. **80**, 297 (1960).
441. Rees, K.R., Tarlow, M.J.: The hepatotoxication of allyl formate. Biochem.J. **104** 757 (1967).
442. Reissman, K.R., Boley, J., Christianson, J.F., Delp, M.H.: The serum iron in experimental hepatocellular rencrosis. J. Lab. clin. Med. **43**, 572 (1954).
443. Reuber, M.D.: Effect of 3-methylcholanthrene on hyperplastic and early neoplastic hepatic lesions induced in rats by carbon tetrachloride. J. nat. Cancer Inst. **45**, 1237 (1970).
444. Reuber, M.D., Glover, E.L.: Hyperplastic and early neoplastic lesions of the liver in Buffalo shain rats of various ages given subcutaneous carbon tetrachloride. J. nat. Cancer Inst. **38**, 891 (1967).

445. Reuber, M.D., Glover, E.L.: Thrombosis of hepatic veins accompanying carbon tetrachloride induced cirrhosis. Arch. Path. **83**, 267 (1967).
446. Reuber, M.D., Glover, E.L.: Carbon tetrachloride induced cirrhoses, effect of age and sex. Arch. Path. **85**, 275 (1968).
447. Reuber, M.D., Glover, E.L.: Cirrhosis and carcinoma of the liver in male rats given subcutaneous carbon tetrachloride. J. nat. Cancer Inst. **44**, 419 (1970).
448. Reutter, W., Bauer, Ch., Lesch, R.: On the mechanism of action of galactosamine; different response to galactosamine during development. Naturwissenschaften **57**, 674 (1970).
449. Reynolds, E.S., Ree, H.J.: Liver parenchymal cell injury VII. Membrane denaturation following carbon tetrachloride. Lab. Invest. **25**, 269 (1971).
450. Reynolds, E.S., Ree, H.J., Moslen, M.T.: Liver parenchymal injury. IX. Phenobarbital potentiation of endoplasmic reticulum denaturation following carbon tetrachloride. Lab. Invest. **26**, 290 (1972).
451. Reynolds, E.S., Thiers, R.E., Vallee, B.L.: Mitochondrial function and metal content in carbon tetrachloride poisoning. J. biol. Chem. **237**, 3546 (1962).
452. Rice, A.J., Plaa, G.L.: The role of triglyceride accumulation and of necrosis in the hemodynamics responses of the isolated perfused rat liver after administration of carbon tetrachloride. Toxicol. appl. Pharmacol. **14**, 151 (1969).
453. Rimington, C., Quin, J.I., Roets, G.C.S.: Studies on the photosensitization of animals in South Africa. The ictogeneric factor in geeldikkop. Isolation of the active principle from Lippia rehmanni. Onderstepoort. J. vet. Sci. **9**, 225 (1937).
454. Roberts, R.J.: Microsomal metabolism of the hepatotoxin α-naphthylisothiocyanate (ANIT) following phenobarbital, chlorpromazine or actinomycin D treatment. Proc. Soc. exp. Biol. (N.Y.) **142**, 365 (1973).
455. Roberts, R.J., Plaa, G.L.: Potentiation and inhibition of α-naphthylisothiocyanate-induced hyperbilirubinemia and cholestasis. J. Pharmacol. exp. Ther. **150**, 499 (1965).
456. Roberts, R.J., Plaa, G.L.: Effect of norethandroline, acetohexamide, and enovid on α-naphthylisothiocyanate-induced hyperbilirubinemia and cholestasis. Biochem. Pharmacol. **15**, 333 (1966).
457. Roberts, R.J., Plaa, G.L.: Alteration of the plasma disappearance and biliary excretion patterns of exogenously administered bilirubin by α-naphthylisothiocyanate. J. Pharmacol. exp. Ther. **155**, 330 (1967).
458. Roberts, R.J., Plaa, G.L.: Alteration of the plasma disappearance and biliary excretion patterns of exogenously administered bilirubin by α-naphthylisothiocyanate. J. Pharmacol. exp. Ther. **155**, 330 (1967).
459. Roberts, R.J., Plaa, G.L.: Alteration in biliary bilirubin content and nonerythropoietically derived bilirubin synthesis in rats after α-naphthylisothiocyanate administration. J. Pharmacol. exp. Ther. **161**, 382 (1968).
460. Robinson, D.S., Seakins, A.: The development in the rat of fatty livers associated with reduced plasma-lipoprotein synthesis. Biochim. biophys. Acta (Amst.) **62**, 163 (1962).
461. Rodriguez Garay, E.A., Piccaluga, A., Perez, V., Royer, M., Listrani, J.: Acute cholestasis in the rat. Acta hepato-splenol. (Stuttg.) **16**, 221 (1969).
462. Rodriguez-Olleros, A., Taveras, J.E., Delanoy, A.A.: Thioacetamide research in dogs. I. Hepatic cirrhosis. Scand. J. Gastroent. **3**, 65 (1968).
463. Rogers, A.E., Newberne, P.M.: Aflatoxin B_1 carcinogenesis in lipotrope deficient rats. Cancer Res. **29**, 1965 (1969).
464. Rogers, A.E., Newberne, P.N.: Diet and aflatoxin B_1 toxicity in rats. Toxicol. appl. Pharmacol. **20**, 113 (1971).
465. Roheim, P.S., Switzer, S., Girard, A., Eder, H.A.: The mechanism of inhibitor of lipoprotein synthesis by orotic acid. Biochem. biophys. Res. Commun. **20**, 416 (1965).
466. Rojkind, M.: Inhibition of liver fibrosis by L-Azetidine-2-carboxylic and in rats treated with carbon tetrachloride. J. clin. Invest. **52**, 2451 (1973).
467. Rondez, R., Ruttner, J.R.: Die Bedeutung der Kuppfferzellen bei der Thioacetamid induzierten Leberzirrhose der Ratte. Med. Exp. **3**, 189 (1960).
468. Rondez, R., Ruttner, J.R.: Zur Pathologie des Ikterus. Fermenthistochemische Untersuchungen über das Verhalten der Gallenkapillaren nach experimenteller, ikterogener Leberschädigung. Path. et Microbiol. (Basel) **26**, 784 (1963).
469. Rosenbaum, F.: Kohlehydratbestand nach acuten Intoxicationen. Naunyn-Schmiedebergs Arch. exp. Path. Pharmakol. **15**, 450 (1882).
470. Rosenthal, S.M.: Some effects of alcohol upon the normal and damaged liver. J. Pharmacol. exp. Ther. **38**, 291 (1930).
471. Röttger, P., Nolite, F., Kuhn, H.A., Creutzfeldt, W.: Untersuchungen über die therapeutische Beeinflußbarkeit experimenteller Lebercirrhosen bei der Ratte. Z. ges. exp. Med. **136**, 486 (1963).
472. Rouiller, C.: Experimental toxic injury of the liver. In: The Liver (C. Rouiller, ed.), vol. II, p. 335—476. New York: Academic Press 1964.

473. Rubetskoli, L.S., Korotkina, R.N.: A method of production of cirrhosis of the liver with splenomegaly and ascites in rabbits by means of carbon tetrachloride. Bull. exp. Biol. Med. **50**, 757 (1961).
474. Rubin, E., Goldfarb, S., Schaffner, F.: Two sites of intrahepatic cholestase. Fed. Proc. **21**, 303 (1962).
475. Rubin, E., Hutterer, F., Popper, H.: Cell proliferation and fiber formation in carbon tetrachloride poisoning. Amer. J. Path. **42**, 715 (1963).
476. Rubin, E., Lieber, C.S.: Fatty liver, alcoholic hepatitis and cirrhosis produced by alcohol in primates. New Eng. J. Med. **290**, 128 (1974).
477. Rubitsky, H.J., Myerson, R.M.: Acute phosphorous poisoning. Arch. intern. Med. **83**, 164 (1949).
478. Rueber, M.D., Glover, E.L., Dove, L.F.: Hepatic lesions in aged rats given carbon tetrachloride. Gerontologia **15**, 7 (1969).
479. Ruggiero, G., Utili, R., Izzo, E.: Enzyme Changes during Phalloidin Poisoning on the Isolated Rat Liver (I. Bartosek, A. Guartami and L. Miller, eds.), p. 135–138. New York: Raven Press 1973.
480. Rüttner, J.R., Rondez, R.: Zur formalen Genese der Thioacetamide-zirrhose der Ratte. Path. et Microbiol. (Basel) **23**, 113 (1960).
481. Rüttner, J.R., Spycher, M.A., Kuenzle, C.: Zur Pathologie des Ikterus. Der ANIT-induzierte Ikterus der Ratte, ein Modell einer durch Zellmembranschädigung bedingten toxischen Hepatose. Path. et Microbiol. (Basel) **27**, 403 (1964).
482. St.-Arneault, G., Walter, L., Bekesi, J.G.: Cytotoxic effects of exogenous D-galactosamine on experimental tumors. Int. J. Cancer **7**, 483 (1971).
483. Sakshaug, J., Sognen, E., Hansen, M.A., Koppang, N.: Dimethylnitrosamine: its hepatotoxic effect in sheep and its occurence in toxic batches of herring meal. Nature (Lond.) **206**, 1261 (1965).
484. Salfelder, K., Doehnert, H.R., Doehnert, R., Sauerteng, E., deLiscano, T.R., Fabrega, E.: Fatal phosphorous poisoning: a study of forty-five autopsy cases. Beitr. Path. Bd. **147**, 321 (1972).
485. Salomon, J.C.: Modifications des cellules du parenchyme-hepatique du rat sous l'effet de la thioacetamide. J. Ultrastruct. Res. **7**, 293 (1962).
486. Salomon, J.C., Salomon, M., Bernhard, W.: Modifications des cellules du parenchyme hepatique du rat sous l'effet de la thioacetamide. Bull. Ass. franç. Cancer **49**, 139 (1962).
487. Sarma, D.S.R., Sidransky, H.: Studies on orotic acid fatty liver in rats; factors influencing the induction of fatty livers. J. Nutr. **98**, 33 (1969).
488. Sartoni, P., Bellodi, G., Bottarelli, E., Poma, C.: Changes of destribution of the vascular system in the course of hepatic cirrhosis induced experimentally by CCl_4 prior to and following subtotal hepatectomy. Fegato **12**, 175 (1966).
489. Schabort, J.C., Petout, M.J.: The relationship between the chemical structure of aflatoxins and their effect on bovine pancreas desozyribonuclease. Euzymologin **41**, 201 (1971).
490. Schaffner, F., Raisfeld, I.H.: Drugs and the liver: a review of metabolism and adverse reactions. Advan. intern. Med. **15**, 221 (1969).
491. Schaffner, F., Scharnbeck, H.H., Hutterer, F., Denk, H., Greim, H.A., Popper, H.: Mechanism of cholestasis. VII. α-Naphthylisothiocyanate-induced jaundice. Lab. Invest. **28**, 321 (1973).
492. Schaffrir, E., Khassis, S.: Role of enhanced fat mobilization in liver triglyceride accumulation in carbon tetrachloride-induced liver injury. Israel J. med. Sci. **5**, 975 (1969).
493. Scharnbeck, H., Schaffner, F., Keppler, D., Decker, K.: Ultrastructural Studies on the Effect of Choline.
494. Schmahl, D., Osswald, H., Mohr, U.: Hepatotoxische und cancerogene Wirkung von Diäthylnitrosamin bei Schweinen. Naturwissenschaften **54**, 341 (1967).
495. Schmahl, D., Thomas, C., Sattler, W.: Hepatotoxische und zirrhogene von Diäthylnitrosamin bei Hunden. Arzneimittel-Forsch. **14**, 73 (1964).
496. Schmidt, F.H.: Experience with enzyme determination in toxicity studies. Proc. Europ. Soc. Study Drug Tox. **5**, 97 (1965).
497. Schmid, R.: Cutaneous porphyria in Turkey. New Engl. J. Med. **263**, 397 (1960).
498. Schoental, E.: Liver disease and "natural" hepatotoxins. Bull. Wld Hlth Org. **29**, 823 (1963).
499. Schoental, R.: Liver lesions in young rats suckled by mothers treated with pyrrolidizine alkaloids lasiocarpine and retrorsine. J. Path. Bact. **77**, 485 (1959).
500. Schoental, R.: Toxicology and carcinogenic action of pyrrolidizine alkaloids. Cancer Res. **28**, 2237 (1968).
501. Schoental, R., Magee, P.N.: Chronic liver changes in rats after a single dose of lasiocarpine a pyrrolidizine (Senerio) alkaloid. J. Path. Bact. **74**, 305 (1957).
502. Schwarzmann, V.: Les hépatites toxiques experimentales. Rev. int. Hépat. **7**, 387 (1957).
503. Schweitzer, C.H.: Pilzgifte und Pilzvergiftungen. Münch. med. Wschr. **112**, 1085 (1970).
504. Schwetz, B.A., Plaa, G.L.: Catecholamine potentiation of carbon tetrachloride-induced hepatotoxicity in mice. Toxicol. appl. Pharmacol. **14**, 495 (1969).

505. SEAKINS, A., ROBINSON, D.S.: Changes associated with the production of fatty livers by white phosphorous and by ethanol in the rat. Biochem. J. **92**, 308 (1964).
506. SELL, D.A., REYNOLDS, E.S.: Liver parenchymal injury: VII. Lesions of membranous cellular components following iodoform. J. Cell Biol. **41**, 736 (1969).
507. SEN, N.P., SMITH, D.C., SCHURINGHAMER, L.: Formation of N-nitrosamines from secondary amines and nitrite in human and animal gastric juice. Fd. Cosmet. Toxicol. **7**, 301 (1969).
508. SENEVIRATNE, R.D.: Physiological and pathological responses in blood vessels of liver. Quart. J. exp. Physiol. **35**, 77 (1949).
509. SHANH, R.C., JOHNSEN, D.O., TANTICHOROENYOS, P., WOODING, W.L., BOURGEOIS, C.H.: Acute toxicity of aflatoxin B_1 in the Macaque monkey. Toxicol. appl. Pharmacol. **20**, 227 (1971).
510. SHAUER, B.A., LUKACS, L., ZIMMERMAN, H.J.: Biochemical indices of tetracyline hepatic injury in rats. Proc. Soc. exp. Biol. (N.Y.) **147**, 868 (1974).
511. SHEA, S.M., MANSEAU, E.J.: Experimental toxic cirrhosis in the rat. II. Kinetics of hepatocyte proliferation during intermittent thioacetamide intoxication. Amer. J. Path. **52**, 55 (1968).
512. SHINOZUKA, H., FARBER, J.L., KONISHI, Y., ANUDARAHANONTA, T.: D-Galactosamine and acute liver cell injury. Fed. Proc. **32**, 1515 (1973).
513. SHINOZUKA, H., GOLDBLATT, P.J., FARBER, E.: The disorganization of hepatic cell nucleoli induced by ethionine and its reversal by adenine. J. Cell Biol. **36**, 313 (1968).
514. SHINOZUKA, H., LOMBARDI, B., FARBER, E.: Dynamics of injury and repair in hepatic cells: Association of membranes with lipid during recovery from ethionine-induced fatty liver. Amer. J. Path. **63**, 161 (1971).
515. SHULL, K.H., MCCONOMY, J., VOGT, M., CASTILLO, A., FARBER, E.: On the mechanism of induction of hepatic adenosine triphosphate deficiency by ethimine. J. biol. Chem. **241**, 5060 (1966).
516. SICKINGER, K., WINTER, H., WOLF, H.P., CREUTZFELDT, W.: The influence of a relative vitamin C deficiency on the development of thioacetamide-liver fibrosis in guinea pigs. Z. ges. exp. Med. **141**, 21 (1966).
517. SICOT, C., BISMUTH, C., FREJAVILLE, J.P., BERTHELOT, P., RUEFF, B., BENHAMOU, J.P.: Les hepatites toxique. Rev. franç. Étud. clin. biol. **14**, 192 (1969).
518. SIDRANSKY, H.: Sex difference in induction of fatty liver in the rat by dietary orotic acid. Endocrinology **72**, 709 (1963).
519. SIDRANSKY, H., VERNEY, E., LOMBARDI, B.: Factors influencing the induction of fatty liver by orotic acid. J. Nutr. **81**, 348 (1963).
520. SLATER, T.F.: Necrogenic action of carbon tetrachloride in the rat; a speculative mechanism based on activation. Nature (Lond.) **209**, 36 (1966).
521. SLATER, T.F.: Toxic agents and liver cell lysosomes. Proc. Europ. Soc. Study Drug. Tox. **7**, 30 (1966).
522. SLATER, T.F., DELANEY, V.B.: Liver adenosine triphosphate content and bile flow rate in the rat. Biochem. J. **116**, 303 (1970).
523. SLATER, T.F., DELANEY, V.B.: The effects of various drugs and toxic agents on the liver. Toxicol. appl. Pharmacol. **20**, 157 (1971).
524. SLATER, T.F., GRIFFITHS, D.B.: Effects of sporidesmin on bile flow rate and composition in the rat. Biochem. J. **88**, 60 (1963).
525. SLATER, T.F., STRÄULI, U.D., SAWYER, B.C.: Sporidesmin poisoning in the rat. Res. vet. Sci. **5**, 450 (1964).
526. SMETANA, H.: Nephrosis due to carbon tetrachloride. Arch. intern. Med. **63**, 760 (1939).
527. SMILLIE, W.G., PESSOA, S.B.: Treatment of hookworm disease with carbon tetrachloride. Amer. J. Hyg. **3**, 35 (1923).
528. SMITH, E.B., NOSANCHUK, J.S., SCHNITZER, B., SWARM, R.L.: Fatty inclusions and microcysts: thioacetamide induced fatty inclusions in nuclei of mouse liver cells and hepatoma cells. Arch. Path. **85**, 175 (1968).
529. SMITH, K.M.: "Disease" of turkey poults. Vet. Rec. **72**, 652 (1960).
530. SMUCKLER, E.A.: Studies on carbon tetrachloride intoxication. IV. Effect of carbon tetrachloride on liver slices and isolated organelles in vitro. Lab. Invest. **15**, 157 (1966).
531. SMUCKLER, E.A., ARCASOY, M.: Structural and functional changes of the endoplasmic reticulum of hepatic parenchymal cells. Int. Rev. exp. Path. **7**, 305 (1969).
532. SMUCKLER, E.A., BARKER, E.A.: Ribosomal changes in thioacetamide and CCl_4 poisoned liver and absence of changes in yellow phosphorous poisoning. Fed. Proc. **23**, 335 (1964).
533. SMUCKLER, E.A., BARKER, E.A.: Effects of drugs on amino acid incorporation in the liver. Europ. Soc. Study Drug Tox. **7**, 83 (1966).
534. SNIDER, I.S., AGARWAL, M.K., BERRY, L.J.: Influence of carbon tetrachloride on inducible liver enzymes and response to endotoxin in mice. J. Bact. **94**, 1817 (1967).
535. STANDERFER, S.B., HANDLER, P.: Fatty liver induced by orotic acid feeding. Proc. Soc. exp. Biol. (N.Y.) **90**, 270 (1955).
536. STANTON, M.F.: Diethylnitrosamine-induced hepatic degeneration and neoplasia in the aquarium fish, Brachydenio Rerio. J. nat. Cancer Inst. **34**, 117 (1965).

537. STATO, N., OTA, N., ABARA, K.: Metabolism *in vitro* of 14C-testosterone by liver homogenates of normal and carbon tetrachloride injured rats. Tokoka J. exp. Med. **98**, 281 (1969).
538. STEFENELLI, N., HOLZNER, J.H., POINTER, H., STOCKINGER, L.: Strukturelle und mikrozirkulatorische Veränderungen in der Rattenleber nach intermittierender Gabe von Alpha-Naphthyl-isothiocyanat (ANIT) über 12 Monate. Virchows Arch. Abt. A **353**, 302 (1971).
539. STEIN, O., BAR-ON, H., STEIN, Y.: Lipoproteins and the liver. In: Progress in Liver Disease, vol. IV (H. POPPER and F. SCHAFFNER, eds.), p. 45–62. New York: Grune and Stratton 1972.
540. STEIN, O., STEIN, Y., ARONOVITCH, J., GROSSOWICZ, N., ROCHMILEVITZ, M.: Effect of liver damage and regeneration on vitamin B_{12} concentration in rat liver. J. Lab. clin. Med. **54**, 545 (1959).
541. STEINER, J.W., BAGLIO, C.M.: Electron microscopy of the cytoplasm of parenchymal liver cells in α-naphthyl isothiocyanate-induced cirrhosis. Lab. Invest. **12**, 765 (1963).
542. STEINER, J.W., MIYAI, K., PHILLIPS, M.J.: Electron microscopy of membrane-particle arrays in liver cells of ethionine-intoxicated rats. Amer. J. Path. **44**, 169 (1964).
543. STENGER, R.J.: Hepatic sinusoids in carbon tetrachloride-induced cirrhosis; an electron microscopic study. Arch. Path. **81**, 439 (1966).
544. STENGER, R.J.: Organelle pathology of the liver: The endoplasmic reticulum. Gastroenterology **58**, 554 (1970).
545. STEPLEWSKI, Z., KRGYZOWSKA-GRUCA, I.: The effect of thioacetamide on the rat liver parenchyma cells. Folia histochem. cytochem. **4**, 7 (1966).
546. STEWART, R.D., BOETTNER, E.A., SOUTHWORTH, R.R., CERNY, J.C.: Acute carbon tetrachloride intoxication. J. Amer. med. Ass. **183**, 98 (1963).
547. STILES, MCDONALD: Scot. med. Soc. J. **15**, 97 (1909). Cit. by WHIPPLE and SPERRY.
548. STIRPE, F., FIUM, L.: Studies on the pathogenesis of liver necrosis by alpha-amanitin. Effect of alpha-amanitin on ribonucleic acid synthesis and on ribonucleic acid polymerase in mouse liver nuclei. Biochem. J. **105**, 779 (1967).
549. STOCKER, E.: Autoradiographische Untersuchungen zur funktionellen und pathologischen Kernschwellung in der Rattenleber nach Fütterung von Thioazetamid. Z. Zellforsch. **62**, 70 (1964).
550. STONER, H.B.: The mechanism of toxic hepatic necrosis. Brit. J. exp. Path. **37**, 176 (1956).
551. STONER, H.B., MAGEE, P.N.: Experimental studies on toxic liver injury. Brit. med. Bull. **13**, 102–106 (1957).
552. STUART, K.L., BRAS, G.: Veno-occlusive disease of the liver. Quart. J. Med. **26**, 291 (1957).
553. SUAREZ, G., NATHANS, D.: Inhibition of aminoacyl-s RNA binding to ribosomes by tetracyline. Biochem. biophys. Res. Commun. **18**, 743 (1965).
554. SVIRBELY, J.L., MONACO, A.R., ALFORD, W.C.: The comparative efficiency of various liver function tests in detecting hepatic damage produced in dogs by xylidine. J. Lab. clin. Med. **31**, 1133 (1946).
555. SVOBODA, D., HIGGINSON, J.: A Comparison of ultrastructural changes in rat liver due to chemical carcinogens. Cancer Res. **28**, 1703 (1968).
556. SVOBODA, D., SOGA, J.: Early effects of pyrrolidizine alkaloids on the fine structure of rat liver cells. Amer. J. Path. **48**, 347 (1966).
557. SWANN, P.F., MCLEAN, A.E.M.: The effect of diet on the toxic and carcinogenic actions of dimethyl nitrosamine. Biochem. J. **107**, 14 (1968).
558. SWARBRICK, O.: Disease of turkey poults. Vet. Rec. **72**, 671 (1960).
559. SZELENYI, I., PUCOOK, J., NEMESANSZKY, E., SOS, J.: Pathophisiologische Untersuchungen zum Lipoidmetabolismus der Leber und Magnesium Orotat. Arzneimittel-Forsch. (Drug Res.) **21**, 777 (1971).
560. TAKEUCHI, J., KUBO, T., YOSHIDA, H., KITAGAWA, T., TONE, T.: Hemodynamics in the dog liver after carbon tetrachloride injury. J. appl. Physiol. **32**, 320 (1972).
561. TAKYAMA, S., OOTA, K.: Malignant tumors induced in mice fed with N-nitrosodimethylamine. Gann **54**, 465 (1963).
562. TAMAO, H.: Experimental and clinical studies on the intrahepatic vascular changes in chronic liver injury. 1. Microscopic vital observations of the mouse liver in chronic carbon-tetrachloride intoxication. Jap. Circulat. J. **30**, 205 (1966).
563. TERRACINI, B., MAGEE, P.N., BARNES, J.M.: Hepatic pathology in rats on low dietary levels of dimethalnitrosamine. Brit. J. Cancer **21**, 559 (1967).
564. TEXL, A., KONECNY, M.: Hepatotoxic effect of tannic acid and rectobaryum in rats. Scr. med. Fac. Med. Brun. **41**, 301 (1968).
565. THIEM, C., FISCHER, P.: Über tödliche Nachwirkung des Chloroforms. Dtsch. med. Leitung **10**, 1111 (1889).
566. THOENES, W.: Fett im Nucleolus. J. Ultrastruct. Res. **10**, 194 (1964).
567. THOENES, W., BANNASCH, P.: Elektronen- und lichtmikroskopische Untersuchungen am Cytoplasma der Leberzellen nach akuter und chronischer Thioacetamidvergiftung. Virchows Arch. path. Anat. **335**, 556 (1962).
568. THOMAS, L.B., POPPER, H., SELIKOFF, I., KEY, M.: Vinyl chloride induced liver disease: from idiopathic portal hypertension (Bantis syndrome) to angiosarcoma. New Engl. J. Med. **292**, 17 (1975).

569. THORNTON, R.H., PERCIVAL, J.C.: A hepatotoxin from Sporidesmium bakeri capable of producing facial eczema disease in sheep. Nature (Lond.) **183**, 63 (1959).
570. TRAEGER, D.R., WRIGHT, R.: Studies on hepatic uptake of antigen. II. The effect of hepatotoxins on the immune response. Immunology **25**, 951 (1973).
571. TRAIGER, G.J., REPENTIGNY, L. DE, PLAA, G.L.: Effect of inhibitors of protein and ribonucleic acid synthesis on the alteration in biliary bilirubin excretion and non-erythropoietically derived bilirubin synthesis in rats after α-naphthylisothiocyanate administration. Biochem. Pharmacol. **23**, 2845 (1974).
572. TRAIGER, G.J., PLAA, G.L.: Differences in the potentiation of carbon tetrachloride in rats by ethanol and isopropanol pretreatment. Toxicol. appl. Pharmacol. **20**, 105 (1971).
573. TRUHAUT, RENE, CLAUDE, J.-R., THEVENIN, M.: Action protectrice de la testosterone et du phenylprionate de 19-nor-testosterene vis-a-vis de la steatose hepatique provoquee par l'Amanite Phalloide chez le Rat femelle. C.R. Acad. Sci. (Paris) **275**, 945 (1972).
574. TRUHAUT, R., CLAUDE, J.R., WARNET, J.M.: Etude cinétique dex la mobilization des lipides péripheriques chez le rat intoxiqué par le phosphore blanc. Europ. J. Toxicol. **5**, 357 (1972).
575. TRUHAUT, R., ROGER, R., WARNET, J.M.: Étude de l'incorporation de l'acid palmitique ^{3}H-9-10 dans les triglycerides et les lipoproteins du rat intoxiqué par le phosphore blanc. C.R. Acad. Sci. (Paris) **272**, 2400 (1971).
576. TUCHWEBER, B., KOVACS, K., KHANDEKAR, J.D., GORGE, B.D.: Prevention of phalloidin intoxication in rats by partial hepatecomy. Arch. Toxikol. **29**, 311 (1972).
577. TUCHWEBER, B., KOVACS, K., KHANDEHAR, J.D., GORG, B.D.: Peliosis-like changes induced by phalloidin in the rat liver; a light and electron microscopic study. J. Med. **4**, 327 (1973).
578. TULPULE, P.G., MADHAVEN, T.V., GOPALAN, C.: Effect of feeding aflatoxin to young monkeys. Lancet **1964 I**, 962.
579. TYGTAT, G.N., COLLEN, D., CLEI, L.D., VAN DAMME, B.: Fibrinogen metabolism in Realthy dogs and in dogs with CCl_4 induced liver damage and with portal vein occlusion. Thrombos. Diasthes. haemorrh. **28**, 320 (1972).
580. UMIKER, W., PEARCE, J.: Nature and genesis of pulmonary alterations in carbon tetrachloride poisoning. Arch. Path. **55**, 203 (1953).
581. UNGAR: Ueber tödtliche Nachwirkung der Chloroforminhalationen. Vjschr. gericht. Med. **47**, 98 (1887).
582. UNGAR, H.: Transformation of the hepatic vasculature of rats following protracted experimental poisoning with carbon tetrachloride; its possible relationship to the formation of urate calculi in the urinary tract. Amer. J. Path. **27**, 871 (1951).
583. UNGAR, H., GOLDBERG, M.G.: The nature of bile duct proliferations in the liver following ingestion of DL-ethionine. Lab. Invest. **8**, 1523 (1959).
584. UNGAR, H., MORAN, E., EISNER, M., ELIAKIM, M.: Rat intra-hepatic biliary tract lesions from alpha-naphthyl-isothiocyanate. Arch. Path. **73**, 427 (1962).
585. VALLI, E.A., SARMA, D.S.R., SARMA, P.S.: Species specificity in orotic acid induced fatty liver. Indian J. Biochem. **5**, 120 (1968).
586. VAN DER MERWE, K.J., STEYN, P.S., FOURIE, L., SCOTT, D.B., THERON, J.J.: Ochratoxin A, a toxic metabolite produced by Aspergillus ochraceus. Wilh. Nature (Lond.) **205**, 112 (1965).
587. VAN VLEET, J.F., ALBERTS, J.O.: Evalation of liver function tests and liver biopsy in experimental carbon tetrachloride intoxication. Amer. J. vet. Res. **29**, 2119 (1968).
588. VOGEN, E.E., BOKELMAN, O.L.: The influence of experimentally induced hepatotoxicity on the pressor sor responses to vasoactive substances in Beagle dogs. Toxicol. appl. Pharmacol. **20**, 291 (1971).
589. VOGIN, E., SHEGGS, H., BOKELMAN, D., MALTIS, P.: Liver function: postprandial urea nitrogen elevation and indocyanine green clearance in the dog. Toxic. appl. Pharmacol. **10**, 577 (1967).
590. VON EULER, L.H., RUBIN, R.J., HANDSCHUMACHER, R.E.: Fatty livers induced by orotic acid. II. Changes in nucleotide metabolism. J. biol. Chem. **238**, 2464 (1963).
591. VON FRIEDEN, L.: I Fungi De Tutti I Paesi. (Translated by R. STROM.) New York: Bobbs-Merrill 1969.
592. WACHSTEIN, M.: Cyto- and Histochemistry of the Liver. In: The Liver (ROUILLER, CH., ed.), vol. I, p. 146. New York: Academic Press 1964.
593. WACHSTEIN, M., MEISEL, E.: Enzymatic histochemistry of ethionine-induced liver cirrhosis and hepatoma. J. Histochem. Cytochem. **7**, 189 (1959).
594. WAHI, P.N., TANDON, H.D., BHARADWAJ, T.P.: Acute carbon tetrachloride hepatic injury. Acta path. **37**, 305 (1955).
595. WANG, C., STRAUSS, L., PARONETTO, F., ADLERSBERG, D.: Effects of ethionine administration in rabbits and dogs. II. Pathological studies. Arch. Path. **65**, 286 (1958).
596. WARREN, W.D., RESTROPO, J.E.: Portal circulation in experimental cirrhosis. Surg. Gynec. Obstet. **114**, 563 (1962).
597. WARWICK, G.P.: Metabolism of liver carcinogens and other factors influencing liver cancer induction. In: Liver Cancer: Proceedings of a Working Conference Held at the Chester Beatty Research Institute, London, Eng., 1969. IARC. Scientific Publication No. 1. Lyon, France, 1971, p. 121–157.

598. Wei, E., Wong, C.K., Hine, C.H.: Potentiation of carbon tetrachloride hepatotoxicity by ethanol and cold. Toxicol. appl. Pharmacol. **18**, 329 (1971).
599. Wei, E., Wong, L.C.K., Hine, C.H.: Selective potentiation of carbon tetrachloride toxicity by ethanol. Arch. intern. Pharmacol. **189**, 5 (1971).
600. Weldon, P.R., Rubenstein, B., Rubenstein, D.: The direct action of CCl_4 on the metabolism of liver slices. Canad. J. Biochem. **43**, 647 (1965).
601. Wells, D.B., Humphrey, H.D., Coll, J.J.: The relation of tannic acid to the liver necrosis occurring in burns. New Engl. J. Med. **226**, 629 (1942).
602. Wertham, F.: Central nervous system in acute phosphorous poisoning. Arch. Neurol. Psychiat. (Chic.) **28**, 319 (1932).
603. Wexler, B.C., Judd, J.T., Lutmer, R.F., Saroff, J.: Metabolic and histopathological consequences of a fatty liver during the acute stages of myocardial infarction in rats. Brit. J. exp. Path. **52**, 565 (1971).
604. Whipple, C.H.: Insusceptibility of pups to chloroform poisoning during the first three weeks of life. J. exp. Med. **15**, 259 (1912).
605. Whipple, C.H., Hurwitz, S.H.: Fibrinogen of the blood as influenced by the liver necrosis of chloroform poisoning. J. exp. Med. **13**, 136 (1911).
606. Whipple, C.H., Sperry, J.A.: Chloroform poisoning, liver necrosis and repair. Johns Hopk. Bull. **20**, 278 (1909).
607. White, I.N.H., Mattocks, A.R., Butter, W.H.: The conversion of the pyrrolidizine alkaloid retrorsine to pyrrolic derivatives *in vivo* and *in vitro* and its acute toxicity to various animal species. Chem. Biol. Interact. **6**, 207 (1973).
608. White, L.P., Shimkin, M.B.: Effects of D.-L. ethionine in six patients with neoplastic disease. Cancer (Philad.) **7**, 867 (1954).
609. Wieland, H., Hallermeyer, R.: Über die Giftstoffe des Knollenblätterpilzes VI. Amanitin, das Hauptgift des Knollenblätterpilzes. Justus Liebigs Ann. Chem. **548**, 1 (1941).
610. Wieland, O.: Changes in liver metabolism induced by the poisons of Amanita phalloides. Clin. Chem. **11**, 323 (1965).
611. Wieland, T., Wieland, O.: Chemistry and toxicology of the toxins of Amanita phalloides. Pharmacol. Rev. **11**, 87 (1959).
612. Wieland, Th.: Poisonous principles of mushrooms of the genus Amanita. Science **159**, 946 (1968).
613. Wille, L.E., Walaas, E.: Plasma pre-α-lipoproteins in ethionine induced fatty liver in rats. Experientia (Basel) **13**, 419 (1973).
614. Williams, R.T.: Species Variation in Drug Biotransformation. In: Fundamentals of Drug Metabolism and Drug Disposition (B.N. La Due, H.G. Mandel, and E.L. Way, eds.), pp. 187–205. Baltimore: Williams and Wilkins 1971.
615. Williams, R.T., Milburn, P., Smith, R.L.: The influence of enterohepatic circulation on toxicity of drug. Ann. N.Y. Acad. Sci. **123**, 110 (1965).
616. Windmueller, H.G.: An orotic acid-induced, adenine-reversed inhibition of hepatic lipoprotein secretion in the rat. J. biol. Chem. **239**, 530 (1964).
617. Windmueller, H.G.: Hepatic nucleotide levels and NAD-synthesis as influenced by dietary orotic acid and adenine. J. Nutr. **85**, 221 (1965).
618. Windmueller, H.G., Euler, L.H. von: Prevention of orotic acid-induced fatty liver with allopurinol. Proc. Soc. exp. Biol. (N.Y.) **136**, 98 (1971).
619. Windmueller, H.G., Levy, R.I.: Total inhibition of hepatic β-lipoprotein production in the rat by orotic acid. J. biol. Chem. **242**, 2246 (1969).
620. Windmueller, H.G., McDaniel, E.G., Spaeth, A.: Orotic acid-induced fatty liver; metabolic studies in conventional and germ-free rats. Arch. Biochem. **109**, 13 (1965).
621. Windmueller, H.G., Spaeth, A.E.: Stimulation of hepatic purine biosynthesis by orotic acid. J. biol. Chem. **240**, 4398 (1965).
622. Windmueller, H.G., Spaeth, A.E.: Perfusion *in situ* with tritium oxide to measure hepatic lipogenesis and lipid secretion. Normal and orotic acid-fed rats. J. biol. Chem. **241**, 2891 (1966).
623. Wirtschafter, Z.T., Cronyn, M.W.: Free radical mechanism for solvent toxicity. Arch. environm. Hlth **9**, 186 (1964).
624. Witzleben, C.L.: Physiologic and morphologic natural history of a model of intrahepatic cholestasis (Manganese-bilirubin overload). Amer. J. Path. **66**, 557 (1972).
625. Wogan, G.N.: Aflatoxin risks and control measures. Fed. Proc. **27**, 932 (1968).
626. Wogan, G.N.: Structure-activity relationships in toxicicity and carcinogenicity of aflatoxins and analogs. Cancer Res. **31**, 1936 (1971).
627. Wogan, G.N.: Mycotoxins and liver injury. In: The Liver (E.A. Gall and F.K. Mostofi, eds.), p. 161–181. Baltimore: Williams and Wilkins Co. 1973.
628. Wogan, G.N.: Biochemical effects of aflatoxins. Israel J. med. Sci. **10**, 441 (1974).
629. Wogan, G.N., Newberne, P.M.: Dose-response characteristics of aflatoxin B_1 carcinogenesis in the rat. Cancer Res. **27**, 2370 (1967).

630. WOHLRAB, F., BIENICK, C.: Study on the topography and histochemistry of oxidative enzymes in thioacetamide. Exp. Path. **9**, 101 (1970).
631. WOLFF, I.A., WASSERMAN, A.E.: Nitrates, nitrites and nitrosamines. Science **177**, 15 (1972).
632. WORKER, N.A., DODD, D.C.: Photosensitivity diseases in New Zealand. N.Z.J. agric. Res. **3**, 712 (1960).
633. WORSTER-DROUGHT, C.: Atophon poisoning. Brit. med. J. **1923 I**, 148.
634. WROBLEWSKI, F.: Clinical significance of alterations in transaminase activities in serum and other body fluids. Advanc. clin. Chem. **1**, 313 (1958).
635. YAMAMOTO, R.S., KROES, R., WEISBURGER, J.H.: Carcinogenicity of diethylnitrosamine in Mystromys albicaudatus. Proc. Soc. exp. Biol. (N.Y.) **140**, 890 (1972).
636. ZBINDEN, G.: Experimental and clinical aspects of drug toxicity. Advanc. Pharmacol. **2**, 1 (1963).
637. ZIEGLER, E., OBOLONSKY, N.: Experimentelle Untersuchungen über die Wirkung des Arseniks und des Phosphors auf die Leber und die Nieren. Hierzu Tafel XII und XIII. Beitr. path. Anat. **2**, 291 (1888).
638. ZIMMERMAN, H.J.: The spectrum of hepatotoxicity. Perspect. Biol. Med. **12**, 135 (1968).
639. ZIMMERMAN, H.J.: Hepatic injury caused by therapeutic agents. In: The Liver (F.F. BECKER, ed.), p. 225–302. New York: Marcel Dekker, Inc. 1974.
640. ZIMMERMAN, H.J.: Serum enzyme measurement in experimental hepatotoxicity. Israel J. med. Sci. **10**, 328 (1974).
641. ZIMMERMAN, H.J., DUJOVNE, C.A., LEVY, R.: The correlation of serum levels of two transaminases with tissue levels in six vertebrate species. Comp. Biochem. Physiol. **25**, 1081 (1968).
642. ZIMMERMAN, H.J., KENDLER, J.: Relationship between structure of phenothiazines and *in vitro* cytotoxicity. Proc. Soc. exp. Biol. (N.Y.) **135**, 201 (1970).
643. ZIMMERMAN, H.J., KENDLER, J., KOFF, R.S.: Intraperitoneal helothane administration: evidence of hepatic and muscle injury. Proc. Soc. exp. Biol. (N.Y.) **138**, 678 (1971).
644. ZIMMERMAN, H.J., KODERA, Y., WEST, M.: Rate of increase in plasma levels of cytoplasmic and mitochondrial enzymes in experimental carbon tetrachloride hepatotoxicity. J. Lab. clin. Med. **66**, 315–323 (1965).
645. ZIMMERMAN, H.J., MAO, R.: Cytotoxicity of carbon tetrachloride as measured by loss of cellular enzymes to surrounding media. Amer. J. med. Sci. **250**, 6 (1965).
646. ZIMMERMAN, H.J., MAO, R., ISROSENA, S.: Phenothiazine inhibition of carbon tetrachloride cytotoxicity *in vitro*. Proc. Soc. exp. Biol. (N.Y.) **123**, 893 (1966).
647. ZIMMERMAN, H.J., SEEFF, L.B.: Enzymes in hepatic disease. In: Diagnostic Enzymology (E.L. COODLEY, ed.), p. 1–38. Philadelphia: Lea and Fediger 1970.
648. ZUCKERMAN, A.J., BAKER, S.F., DUNKLEY, L.J.: The effect of tetracycline on human liver cells in culture. Brit. J. exp. Path. **49**, 20 (1968).
649. ZUCKERMAN, A.J., REES, K.R., ZUMAN, D.R., ROBB, I.A.: The effects of aflatoxin on human embryo liver cells in tissue culture. Brit. J. exp. Path. **49**, 20 (1968).

Liver Disease Due to Infection and Allergy*

IAN R. MACKAY

With 15 Figures

A. Introduction

This introduction will be addressed to some definitions and to the scope of this chapter. "Disease" is taken to refer to human disease, and references to diseases of animals will be mostly to illustrate how these pertain to human pathology. "Infection" will be taken to mean invasion and destruction of liver parenchyma by pathogenic organisms ranging in complexity from multicellular parasites to submicroscopic viruses. However recent research has not contributed substantially to knowledge of liver disease due to parasites or bacteria, and hence current knowledge concerning such infections will be rather briefly summarized with citation of contemporary reviews. On the other hand, there have been rapid advances in knowledge of liver disease due to viral infection, particularly that associated with the antigen particle known as Australia antigen or hepatitis B antigen (HBAg), and so this area will be dealt with in more detail.

In regard to allergy, some immunologists hold strongly to Von Pirquet's original concept of "allergy" as a state of altered reactivity consequent on prior exposure of the organism to any chemical or physical agent; in this sense, "allergy" would comprise the "normal" state of an augmented immune response upon secondary challenge with any microbial antigen, as well as the various "abnormal" states associated with hypersensitivity phenomena. Others use the term in the more restricted sense of an altered reaction essentially associated with damaging effects, and this usage takes in states of delayed hypersensitivity ("bacterial allergy"), and more particularly immediate hypersensitivity and anaphylaxis, and possibly also states of autoimmunity. There is an even further restriction of the term in Anglo-American usage to those diseases, such as hay fever, asthma, and certain dermatoses, attributable to reaginic antibody, now identified as IgE. Some modern immunologists might think that "allergy" is an anachronistic term best deleted from our vocabulary! At all events, "liver disease due to allergy" will be interpreted as including disease of the liver associated with evidence of autoimmune responses, and those associated with immunopathological responses to medicinal drugs.

* Publication No. 1999 from The Walter and Eliza Hall Institute of Medical Research, Victoria, Australia.

B. Liver Disease Due to Infection *

I. Multicellular Parasites

The multicellular parasites which can invade and reside in the human liver or biliary system include cestodes (tapeworms), trematodes (flukes) and nematodes (round worms). There is a current review by MARCIAL-ROJAS (1973).

1. Cestodes

Taenia Echinococcus. The liver is parasitized by cysts of cestode worms when animals function as the intermediate host. The only cestode for which man functions with any frequency as intermediate host is *Taenia echinococcus*. The classical reference monograph is that of DEW (1928). This short tapeworm lives in the intestine of the dog as the definitive host. The terminal segment of the worm contains some 500 ova, and these are discharged and ingested by grazing animals. The ova pass through the intestine via the portal vein and lodge in the liver to form cysts known as hydatid cysts. From the inner wall of these cysts there develop scolices which are new larval forms of the worm. The cycle is perpetuated when a dog ingests offal containing living cysts and the larvae mature in the dog's intestine. Humans can become infested as intermediate hosts, as do sheep and cattle, by ingesting larvae discharged by dogs, and cysts similarly develop in the liver and occasionally elsewhere. Echinococcal disease formerly was a considerable problem in various pastoral countries, Argentina, Australia, New Zealand and Iceland, but the incidence has declined considerably with measures for control, particularly treatment of infested dogs and supervised killing of livestock.

2. Trematodes (Flukes)

a) Schistosomiasis (Bilharziasis). The schistosome liver flukes are important hepatic pathogens in Afro-Asian areas causing schistosomiasis (bilharziasis). Both *S. mansoni* and *S. japonicum* can infest the liver, although the natural habitat of schistosomes are the mesenteric veins.

Adult worms may reside in mesenteric veins for 20—30 years and can produce some 300 eggs/worm-pair/day. The eggs of the adult worm penetrate the colon and are excreted in the feces and hatch out in still water, and release miracidia infective for fresh-water snails. In the snail host, miracidia develop into cercariae, and the free-swimming circariae can penetrate unbroken human skin, after which there is dissemination by the blood. The cercariae migrate to the lungs for a few days and then to the portal vein, and finally undergo maturation in mesenteric veins, so completing the cycle. The lateral-spined egg, and sometimes the adult worms, may be carried via the portal veins to the liver, there setting up an inflammatory granulomatous reaction in portal tracts. The specific histological lesion is a portal granuloma often containing an ovum (Fig. 1a—d). The appearances of

* Methods, see Vols. 16, Vols. 9—11 Infections.

the granulomata vary according to their stage of evolution, the terminal phase being a dense portal fibrous reaction. This produces Symmers "pipestem fibrosis", and a coarsely nodular cirrhosis may eventuate (ANDRADE, 1965) (Fig. 1e).

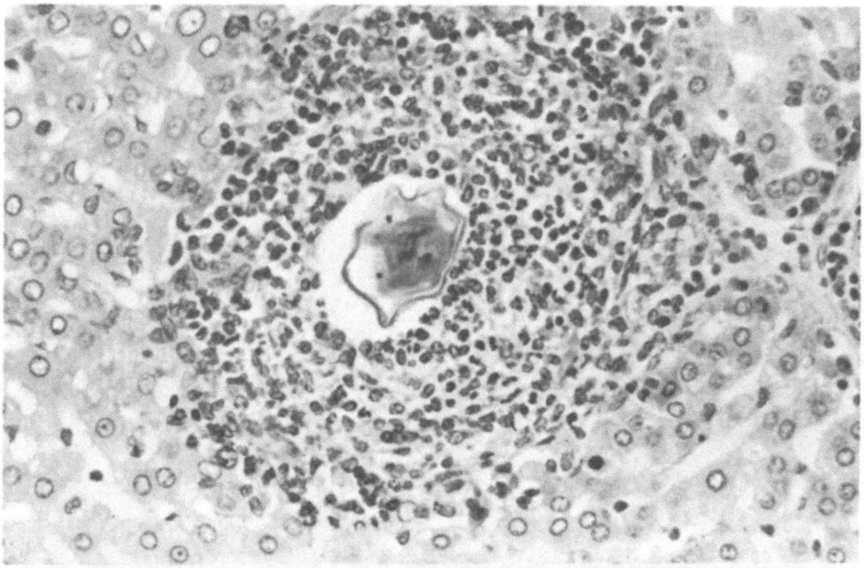
(a)

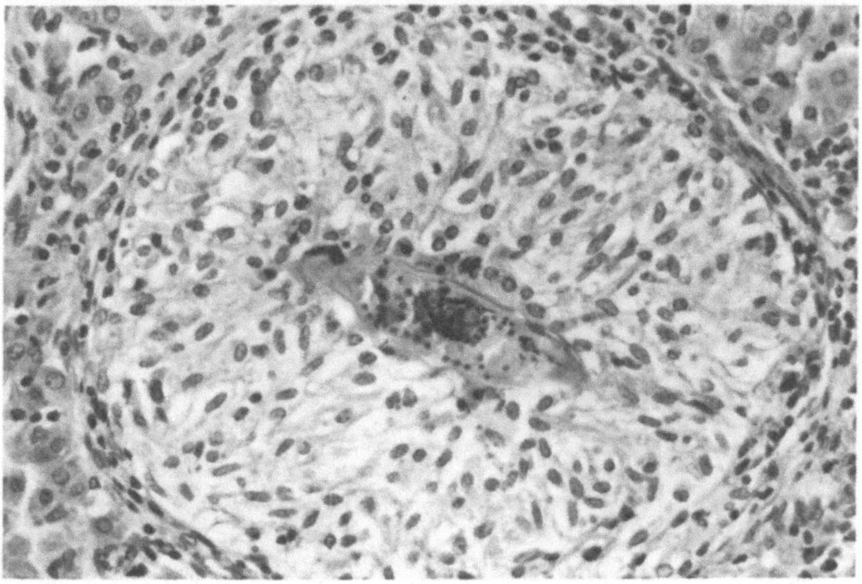
(b)

Fig. 1a and b. The schistosome lesion as seen microscopically in the liver of the experimentally infected hamster, the T cell depleted mouse and the naturally infected human. (a) Lesion 1 week after infection in liver of hamster: degenerating egg surrounded by a moderate inflammatory focus with numerous eosinophils. HE ×530. (b) Lesion 1 week after infection in liver of hamster: classic epithelioid granuloma bordered by fibroblasts and lymphoid cells. HE ×530. (Fig. 1a and b by courtesy of Dr. F. VON LICHTENBERG and Editor of American Journal of Pathology)

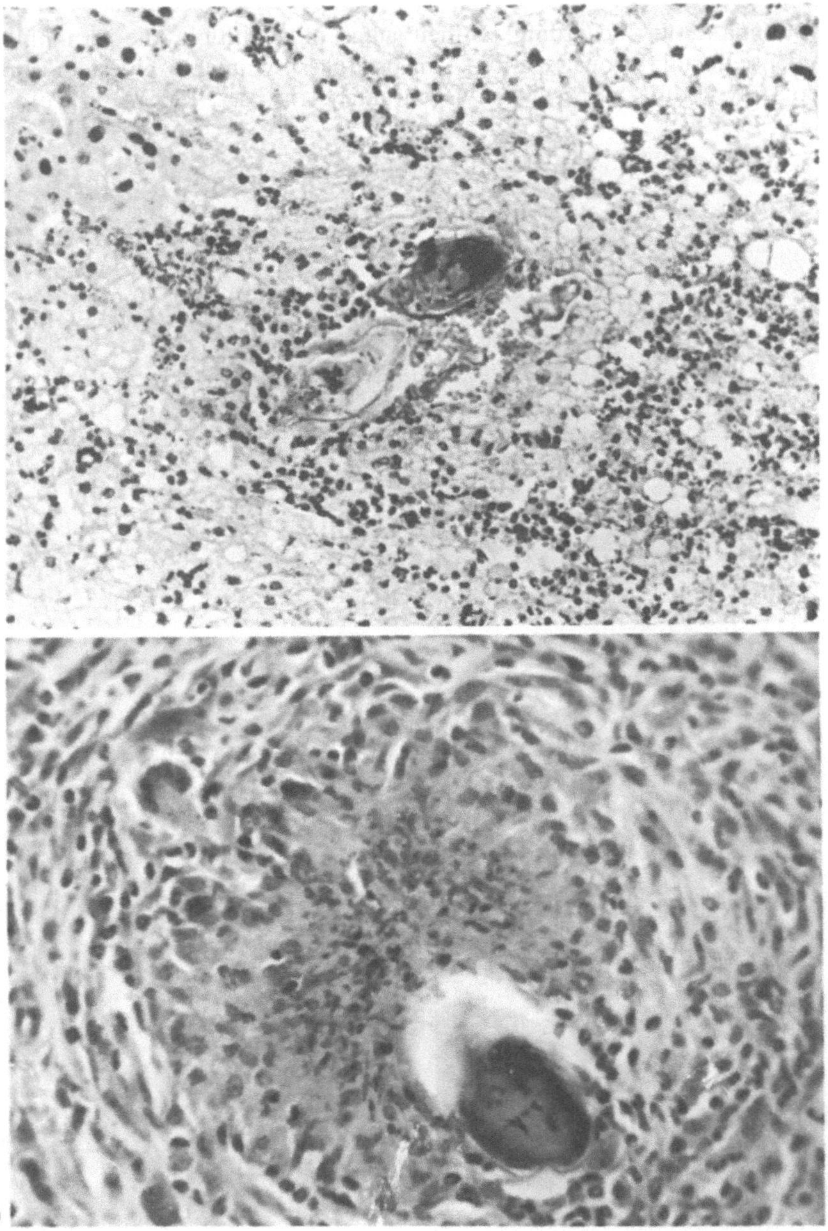

(c)

(d)

Fig. 1. (c) Lesions $7^1/_2$ weeks after infection in liver of mouse depleted of T cells by thymectomy and anti-thymocyte serum: failure of granuloma formation and extensive surrounding hepatic cell necrosis. HE ×640. (By courtesy of Dr. D.G. COLLEY and Editor of American Journal of Pathology.) (d) Lesion in liver of naturally infected human: typical schistosome granuloma with necrosis, lymphoid infiltrate and concentric fibrosis. HE ×500. (By courtesy of Dr. Z.A. ANDRADE)

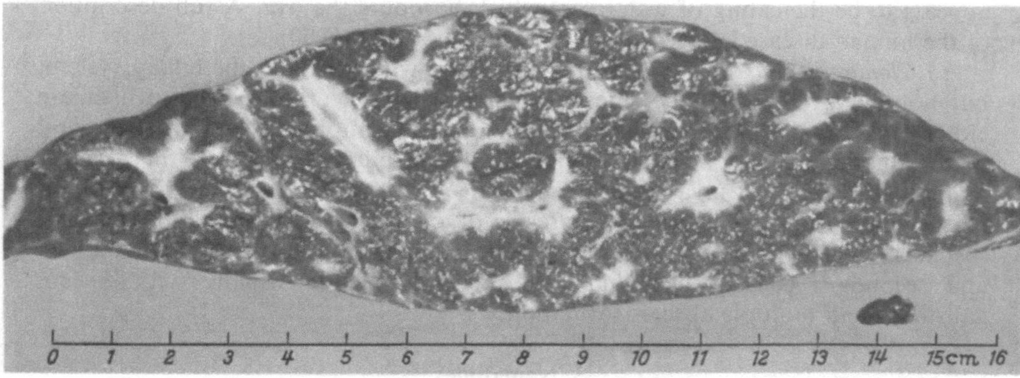

Fig. 1. (e) Liver as seen macroscopically in advanced schistosomiasis in man, showing dense portal fibrosis (Symmers liver). (By courtesy of Dr. Z.A. ANDRADE)

Tissue damage in schistosomiasis is attributable more to a host response than to toxic effects of ova. Thus schistosomal eggs, deposited experimentally in the mouse in liver sinusoids induced a cell-mediated granulomatous reaction (WARREN *et al.*, 1967), and this granulomatous reaction can be elicited also by a soluble antigen of the eggs (BOROS and WARREN, 1970). Whilst various immunosuppressive measures are known to suppress the granulomatous response to bilharzia ova, mice deprived of thymus-dependent responses are less resistant to experimental infection and develop necrotic rather than granulomatous lesions (BUCHANAN, FINE and COLLEY, 1973). The immunopathology of the schistosome granuloma was examined in the hamster by von LICHTENBERG *et al.* These authors attributed differing characteristics of schistosome lesions to the antigenic determinants of the ova, some being species specific and others shared, and the host immune response, with cell-mediated components (granulomatous reactions) and humoral components (plasma cell proliferation, vasculitis, amyloid) being identified.

In summary, schistosomal infection of the liver represents a fascinating parade of immunopathological events. The accidentally sequestered egg secretes soluble antigens through micropores of the shell. These initiate a cell mediated (T cell) response with secretion of lymphokines and a granulomatous reaction, and probably also a humoral (B cell) response, the sum of which is represented by varying patterns of liver damage. Later the process subsides with establishment of a "new immunologic equilibrium" (VON LICHTENBERG *et al.*, 1973), associated with "endogenous desensitization", "accelerated antigen sequestration" or "enhancing antibody".

b) Fascioliasis. Fasciola hepatica, the sheep liver fluke, is a common parasite of herbivores and has a world-wide distribution. However only a few hundred human infestations have been recorded, from areas including Cuba, France, Spain, Algeria, England and Australia (MANGOS and MENZIES, 1973). The life cycle of the parasite is similar to that of the schistomes except that the ingested cercariae burrow through the duodenal wall, cross the peritoneal cavity and enter the liver by penetrating Glisson's capsule. In the liver, the flukes can induce massive necrosis, known as "liver rot" of sheep, or areas of fibrosis. The source of human infestation appears to be the eating of watercress which harbours the ova. A full description of the human disease is given by FACEY and MARSDEN (1960).

c) Clonorchiasis. Clonorchis sinensis is a fluke which invades the biliary system, but not the liver itself. The intermediate hosts are cyprinoid fishes which are either eaten raw or improperly cooked, and thus transmit the fluke. Larvae develop in the duodenum and reach their habitat in the biliary passages either via the ampulla of Vater or by invasion of the liver through its peritoneal coat. Chlonorchis in the bile ducts, presumably as a result of obstruction, or for other reasons, results in recurrent bouts of severe febrile cholangitis (HOU and PANG, 1964), and secondary consequences include bacterial infection usually with *E. coli*, gallstones and multiple abscess formation.

3. Nematodes

a) Ascariasis. Ascaris lumbricoides, the common roundworm, is 10–20 cm in length and resides in the lumen of the small bowel. It can migrate into the biliary system via the ampulla of Vater and cause biliary obstruction; damage to the liver is usually secondary to obstructive cholangitis. Other complications include haemobilia and abscess formation (SHERLOCK, 1968). Hepatic granulomata associated with Ascaris infestation are attributed to a reaction to ova from the worms (ANSTEY, 1960).

b) Toxocariasis. Toxocara canis is a round worm which infests dogs, and very occasionally infests humans, mostly children, and enters the liver; the histological features include sarcoid-like lesions and eosinophilia (DRURY, 1962).

II. Protozoa

1. Malaria

The liver is affected in acute attacks of malaria, particularly due to *P. falciparum*, and changes revealed in a study by liver biopsy (CORCORAN *et al.*, 1953) included swelling of parenchymal cells, increased mitotic activity, compression of sinusoids, sinusoidal infiltration with mononuclear cells, focal necrosis, and pronounced hyperplasia of Kupffer cells: so-called malarial hepatitis. In chronic cases there is hemosiderosis, fibrosis and occasionally granulomas. HUTT (1971) described proliferation of lymphocytes and plasma cells in the liver in that form of malaria associated with tropical splenomegaly, this being a hyper-immune response to malarial antigens. "Malarial cirrhosis" is described in tropical areas, but it is doubtful whether this is an actual entity, in that malarial infection may coexist with other conditions in the tropics causing liver damage and cirrhosis without being causally related to the cirrhosis.

2. Amoebiasis

"Hepatic amoebiasis" is taken to include all forms of liver disease caused by *Entamoeba histolytica*. Hepatic amoebiasis is always a sequel to intestinal disease, and the only proven form of the disease is the distinct and circumscribed liver abscess. About 95% of amoebic abscesses are single, and are usually located in

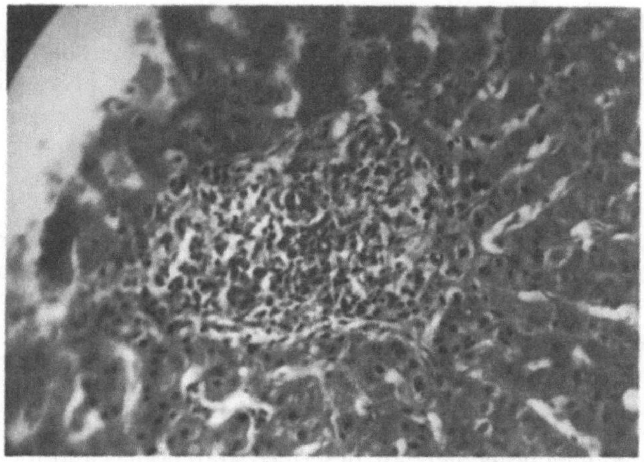

Fig. 2. Liver lesion in human amoebiasis showing focal collection of inflammatory cells (microabscess). (By courtesy of Dr. S. RAMACHANDRAN and Editor of Postgraduate Medical Journal)

the upper part of the right lobe of the liver. The earliest stages before significant liver necrosis occurs may be described as focal presuppurative hepatitis. Clinical features of liver disease were stated to occur in over 50% of cases of acute amoebic dysentery (RAMACHANDRAN *et al.*, 1973), and in these cases the liver microscopically showed a variety of changes in the category of non-specific reactive hepatitis including focal liver cell necrosis, lymphocyte infiltration in the parenchyma and/or portal tracts, granulomatous lesions, and fat (Fig. 2). These changes are presumably a reactive response in the liver to infection in the bowel, as amoebae were not demonstrable. The condition of "chronic diffuse amoebic hepatitis" is not considered to exist, nor is amoebiasis of the liver recognized as a precursor of cirrhosis (POWELL, 1969).

3. Toxoplasmosis

The two forms of infection with *Toxoplasma gondii* are the infantile, resulting from a presumed uterine infection, and the adult form. The infantile disease is usually fatal and, although there is clinical evidence of liver dysfunction, parenchymal damage is rare and the organism is seldom demonstrable in the liver (CALLAHAN *et al.*, 1946). Toxoplasmosis in the adult presents as an acute hepatitic illness associated with enlargement of the liver, spleen and lymph nodes; microscopically there is focal hepatocellular necrosis, and portal and parenchymal infiltrates with mononuclear cells; toxoplasma organisms were demonstrable in liver cells and Kupffer cells in two cases described by VISCHER *et al.* (1967).

III. Mycoses

1. Actinomycosis

Actinomycosis israeli infects the liver from the intestine, usually via the portal vein and less often via the hepatic artery. The source reference is the monograph of COPE (1952). Necrosis and fibrosis occur, and the eventual lesion is a multiloculated abscess with a dense fibrous wall containing pus and numerous organisms. Clinically, there is enlargement of the liver, systemic features of sepsis, and sinuses to the skin may develop.

2. Blastomycosis

There are two types infectious for man, *Blastomycis dermatitis* and *Paracoccidioides brasiliensis*, and both may infect the liver. The former and more important type produces suppurative or granulomatous lesions (MARTIN and SMITH, 1939) which later undergo fibrosis.

3. Coccidioidomycosis

In disseminated infections there are described granulomas and focal abscess-like areas in the liver (SCHWARTZ and MUTH, 1951).

4. Cryptococcosis

Cryptococcis neoformans, a yeast, is presumed to acquire pathogenicity as a result of impaired immune responsiveness. Very rarely, the liver is invaded, the resulting lesions being small granulomas or focal areas of necrosis (SABESIN *et al.*, 1963).

5. Histoplasmosis

Hepatomegaly and splenomegaly are stated to occur in more than half the cases of disseminated infection due to *Histoplasma capsulatum* (KLATSKIN, 1974). These features are presumably due to a toxic-reactive response, as liver disease is seldom a serious accompaniment of histoplasmosis. The high incidence of minor parenchymal lesions in an endemic area was shown in a necropsy study in which healed and calcified granulomata in the liver and spleen were frequently demonstrable, and *H. capsulatum* was identified in such lesions (OKUDAIRA *et al.*, 1961).

6. Candidiasis

The occasional occurrence of small abscesses in the liver in cases of disseminated moniliasis and aspergillosis is recorded (KLATSKIN, 1974). These are presumed to occur on the basis of debilitation and use of antibiotic drugs.

7. Mucormycosis

Organisms of the genus Rhizopus can be pathogenic in states of debilitation. A case is recorded (MCBRIDE *et al.*, 1960) of disseminated mucormycosis with necrotic liver lesions, presumed due to toxic injury.

IV. Bacteria

Liver damage can result from bacterial infection in various species, e.g. clostridia in dogs (*vide infra*), and vibrios in birds (HOFSTAD *et al.*, 1958; WHENHAM *et al.*, 1961), but attention will be confined to human diseases. Liver damage in man can result from several causes during the course of bacterial infections. Firstly, the most usual is toxic damage to liver cells manifested by mild abnormalities of the conventional "liver function tests". Secondly, there may be changes of "non-specific reactive hepatitis", a term introduced by SCHAFFNER and POPPER (1959) to describe mild liver injury and inflammatory changes as a response to a variety of disorders in extrahepatic sites. Thirdly, organisms may cause direct injury to liver cells, producing focal necrosis. Fourthly, more massive injury results in formation of an hepatic abscess, a contemporary review of which is given by LAZARCHICK *et al.* (1973).

1. Pneumococcus

Clinical evidence of liver dysfunction is usual in severe pneumococcal infection, and is attributed to toxic damage. There is acknowledged difficulty (KLATSKIN, 1974) in explaining the frequency of liver dysfunction and even jaundice in pneumococcal pneumonia on the basis of the histologically demonstrable liver lesions, which at most are those of non-specific reactive hepatitis.

2. Staphylococcus

Toxic damage occurs to the liver with extrahepatic staphylococcal infections, and the staphylococcus is a recognized cause of liver abscess (LAZARCHICK *et al.*, 1973).

3. Streptococcus

Two types of liver lesion are attributed to streptococcal infection, toxic and invasive, but this concept is based on old references dating back to 1931 and 1910 (KLATSKIN, 1974). "Streptococcal hepatitis" seems not to have been described since the antibiotic era, but streptococcal abscess still occurs (BATEMAN *et al.*, 1975).

4. Gonococcus

Toxic damage and abscess formation are cited (KLATSKIN, 1974) but gonococcal damage to the liver appears nowadays to be of little significance. Gonococcal perihepatitis was reported in the more recent literature by VICKERS and MALONEY (1964).

5. E. coli

Severe extrahepatic infections with *Escherichia coli* are usually accompanied by clinical evidence of hepatic dysfunction and histological evidence of non-specific reactive hepatitis. *E. coli* moreover is the most frequent cause of hepatic abscess (LAZARCHICK *et al.*, 1973). Also *E. coli* is one of the organisms whose invasion of the bloodstream is facilitated by the disorganized liver architecture associated with cirrhosis, leading to bacteraemic and septicaemic episodes. Chronic pericholangitis is known to accompany ulcerative colitis (MISTILIS, 1965), but whether recurrent seeding of *E. coli* to the liver via the portal circulation is the cause of this condition is uncertain.

6. Salmonellae

Extrahepatic infections with salmonella organisms cause no more than toxic or non-specific reactive changes in the liver. Septic liver lesions in typhoid fever are cited in the earlier literature (KLATSKIN, 1974) and, more recently, liver injury in typhoid fever is described by AYHAN *et al.* (1973).

7. Shigella

Shigella infections seem unimportant as a cause of liver injury except for their apparent coexistence in epidemic settings with hepatitis virus infections.

8. Brucella

Active brucellosis is frequently associated with granulomata in the liver, particularly infections with *Brucella abortus;* hence liver biopsy (with culture of the specimen) is an important diagnostic procedure in suspected cases, as living organisms are present in fresh lesions. The granulomata are of typical structure—epithelioid cells, giant cells and scanty lymphoid cells, with no features histologically characteristic of brucellosis (SPINK *et al.*, 1949). Necrosis occurs but there is no typical caseation, and eventually the lesions undergo fibrosis and even calcification. Similar granulomatous lesions occur in experimentally infected animals in which proliferation of epithelioid cells occurs as a response to intracellular growth of the organisms (KLATSKIN, 1974).

Healing of hepatic granulomata in brucellosis leads to hepatic scarring, and hence cirrhosis as a result of brucella infection of the liver is a possibility (McCULLOUGH and EISELE, 1951). Progression from fibrosis to cirrhosis was demonstrated in one study by serial biopsies (JOSKE and FINCKH, 1955).

9. Minor Gram-Negative Bacterial Pathogens

Five cases of liver abscess due to *Bacteroides fragilis* were described (FUTCH, ZIKRIA and NEU, 1973), the features being similar to those of hepatic abscess caused by more familiar organisms. A liver abscess due to infection with Aeromonas hydrophilia was reported by DEFRONZO, MURRAY and MADDREY (1973). There has been one reported case of disseminated granuloma inguinale with miliary abscesses in the liver (LYFORD *et al.*, 1946).

10. Clostridia

Clostridial invasion of the human liver is a rare terminal event, of uncertain pathogenesis, but possibly attributable to the presence of clostridia in the intestine: KLATSKIN (1974) noted that infarction of the liver is rapidly fatal in the dog because clostridia are normally present in the dog liver. Although this is not the case in man, the presence of clostridia in the intestine combined with liver injury or ischaemia could predispose to gas gangrene of the liver.

11. Tuberculosis

Tubercle bacilli are distributed to the liver by the blood, both in miliary tuberculosis and localized tuberculosis of the lungs. The characteristic lesion is the caseating miliary granuloma, but coalescence and spread of miliary lesions result in a large focal abscess—a tuberculoma. Early miliary lesions consist of epithelioid cells, giant cells and peripheral lymphocytes, and later lesions show central caseation; in surviving patients there is healing with or without scarring. The granulomata occur both within the parenchyma and in portal tracts. Demonstration in biopsy specimens of granulomata in which tubercle bacilli are present is important in the early diagnosis of miliary tuberculosis; culture of biopsy fragments is essential as bacteria are demonstrable microscopically in less than half the instances in which miliary granulomas are present in the liver (KORN *et al.*, 1959).

It has been claimed (HAEX and VAN BEEK, 1955) that assiduous study of liver biopsy material, including serial sectioning, will disclose tuberculous granulomata in over 90% of acute and chronic (non-miliary) cases of tuberculosis, but opinions differ on this (KLATSKIN, 1974). It is also stated that asymptomatic miliary lesions develop in the liver by haematogenous spread in primary tuberculosis infections, and these may even be susceptible to reactivation in later life. In "primary" miliary tuberculosis of the liver (TERRY and GUNNAR, 1957), in which tissues other than the liver are spared, infection is presumably distributed to the liver by the portal blood stream from an intestinal focus.

Tuberculous infection elsewhere in the body results in non-specific reactive lesions in the liver with portal infiltration and fibrosis, together with toxic changes and fatty infiltration, the incidence ranging from 34 to 42% in autopsy series (KLATSKIN, 1974). Cirrhosis is said to coexist in 1—6% of cases of general tuberculosis (KLATSKIN, 1974) but this is attributable to coexisting alcoholism rather than tuberculosis *per se*. Amyloidosis of the liver was a complication of the tuberculosis of previous times. Attention is drawn to granulomatous lesions in the liver as a consequence of immunotherapy of cancer with BCG vaccine (HUNT *et al.*, 1973; BODURTHA *et al.*, 1974).

12. Leprosy

Leprosy is a multisystem disease in which there are lesions in many viscera. Abnormalities of liver function are known to occur together with granulomatous lesions histologically; the latter are frequent in lepromatous leprosy but less common in tuberculoid leprosy. The study by KARAT *et al.* (1971) of biochemical and liver biopsy findings in 240 patients with leprosy indicated that leprosy exists in the liver, as elsewhere, as a disease spectrum ranging from pure or polar lepromatous leprosy, in which there is tissue destruction with bacilli readily demonstrable in lesions, to polar tuberculoid leprosy in which there are proliferative lesions with few or no bacilli demonstrable.

KARAT *et al.* (1971) found granulomatous lesions in the liver in 62% of patients with lepromatous leprosy and 21% with tuberculoid leprosy. Liver lesions tended to appear early, within a year of onset of disease, in both lepromatous and tuberculoid leprosy, presumably as a result of early bacillaemia. Alterations in biochemical indices of liver function correlated with the presence of granulomatous liver lesions, and these were more pronounced in lepromatous disease, in which there are more diffuse lesions. In lepromatous leprosy the presence of granulomata in the liver containing bacteria correlated with bacteria demonstrable in skin smears. However it was noteworthy that bacteria persisted in the liver in Kupffer cells long after they had disappeared from the skin, indicating the need for prolonged treatment to control such lesions.

13. Tularaemia

Focal hepatic necrosis or centrilobular caseation, or hepatic granulomata, may occur with infection with *Pasteurella tularensis.*

14. Leptospirosis

The five main hepatotropic strains of leptospirae comprise *L. icterohaemorrhica, L. canicola, L. pomona, L. griphotyphosa,* and *L. autumnalis.* All can produce acute hepatitis but classical Weil's disease is produced by *L. icterohaemorrhagica.* Leptospirae are spirillar organisms, $6-9\ \mu \times 0.25\ \mu$, and are demonstrable by the Giemsa stain in blood and silver stain in tissues. The main vector for man *L. icterohaemorrhagica* is the rat which excretes the organism in urine, and portals of entry include skin abrasions and mucosal surfaces. Formerly, workers at risk included those associated with sewers and docks where there was contact with rats, but today farmers and country recreationalists are vulnerable (TURNER, 1973). There are other animal vectors for the other strains of leptospirae, notably the dog for *L. canicola.* The incubation period after entry of the organism is 7—13 days, after which organisms invade the blood, become widely disseminated, and then vanish, persisting only in the kidney and liver. The epidemiology of Leptospirosis is reviewed in detail by FEIGIN and ANDERSON (1975).

Clinical evidence of liver damage tends to occur after the bacteraemic phase, in the second week of illness, when there is deep jaundice and hepatomegaly. The liver lesions are characterized histologically by intense disorganization and dissociation of liver cells, especially in centrilobular zones, relatively minor cytoplasmic change, intense regenerative activity, marked bile stasis, and cellular infiltration of portal tracts (AREAN, 1962), but it is not clear why jaundice is so pronounced with little frank necrosis of liver cells. It is also uncertain how leptospirae actually penetrate and damage liver cells, but presumably they can enter intact liver cells as they do renal tubular cells.

The diagnosis of Weil's disease of the liver depends on microscopic demonstration of the organisms in blood or urine using dark field examination, inoculation of guinea pigs or mice, and culture. However serological agglutination tests seem more convenient, and will identify the leptospiral strain involved (TURNER, 1973).

15. Syphilis

In congenital syphilis the liver can become infected in fetal life. Numerous spirochaetes are demonstrable in liver tissue and there is a diffuse hepatitis, after which there develops a fine pericellular fibrosis and lymphocytic infiltration, small granulomata and arteritis (FLEGEL, 1951).

Acute secondary syphilis with accompanying hepatitis was described by HAHN (1943), the incidence of hepatitis being 0.24%. The reported cases up to 1972 were reviewed by SOBEL and WOLF (1972) with varying liver lesions including pericholangitis, focal necrosis and mononuclear portal infiltrations; spirochaetes were present in the liver in two cases. Clear evidence for acute hepatitis in early syphilis was presented by FEHÉR *et al.* (1975).

In late tertiary syphilis the liver may be the site of a gumma, this being usually a granuloma with central necrosis and peripheral fibrosis. Numerous gummas may be present, and eventually heal by scarring, so producing the characteristic hepar lobatum which may superficially resemble a coarsely nodular cirrhosis. KLATSKIN (1974) cites reports of gummatous livers being associated with features of end-stage liver insufficiency—jaundice, ascites and portal hypertension; however SHERLOCK (1968) denies that syphilis can be classed as a cause of true cirrhosis, as coexisting causes of cirrhosis in subjects with usually cannot be excluded.

V. Rickettsia

Q Fever

Coxiella burneti, the causative organism of Q fever, is a well recognized cause of liver injury. *C. burneti* is carried by a cattle tick and hence Q fever is found endemically in areas where cattle are handled. The usual primary illness is a febrile pneumonitis and the hepatic lesions are secondary, but occasionally hepatitis is the major component of the illness (ALKAN *et al.*, 1965). The histological changes range from minor hepatic lesions—focal hepatocellular necrosis and portal cellularity—to epithelioid granulomata with giant cells, and even diffuse necrosis, as in one fatal case (TONGE and DERRICK, 1959). POWELL (1961) studied 72 consecutive cases of Q fever from the liver standpoint, and found hepatomegaly in 47, jaundice in 3 and abnormal tests of liver function in 61. Liver biopsy performed on 13 revealed focal hepatitic lesions, and more advanced lesions showed areas of frank necrosis; fatty change and granulomata were also seen. Notably, residual lesions could be demonstrated in the liver months after the onset of illness. DUPONT *et al.* (1971) reported on three cases, one naturally acquired, and two deliberately induced, in which serial liver biopsies were done; as early as day 8 after infection these showed discrete inflammatory foci in the liver parenchyma, with focal necrosis and histiocytic aggregates in portal tracts. It is likely that liver lesions are present in most cases of Q fever.

VI. Viruses (Excluding Classical Hepatitis Viruses A and B)

The liver is susceptible to various viruses other than those of classical infections and serum hepatitis (hepatitis viruses A and B). The list would include the Epstein-Barr virus of infectious mononucleosis, cytomegalovirus, herpes simplex virus, psittacosis virus, reovirus, rubella virus, adenovirus and coxsackie B virus. Usually these viruses of low pathogenicity (for man) cause hepatitis in infancy or in states of debilitation.

1. Infectious Mononucleosis

This disease is now identified causally with infections with the herpes-type Epstein-Barr virus (NIEDERMAN *et al.*, 1968). Studies reported between 1940 and 1950 (KLATSKIN, 1974) indicated that laboratory tests relating to "liver function" were abnormal in most if not all cases of infectious mononucleosis, although pronounced disturbance of liver function is quite infrequent. Jaundice occurs in less than 10% of cases and is seldom marked, and bilirubinaemia occurs in some 30% of cases (BENNETT *et al.*, 1950; JORDAN and ALBRIGHT, 1950); however a fatal case of hepatic necrosis was reported (ALLEN and BASS, 1963). The morphological changes resemble those of ordinary infectious hepatitis with marked portal and sinusoidal lymphoid inflammatory reactions, but only slight lobular necrosis, Kupffer cell hyperplasia and parenchymal regenerative activity. It is stated (KLATSKIN, 1974) that infectious mononucleosis hepatitis is never a precursor of chronic hepatitis or cirrhosis. HOLBOROW *et al.* (1973) reported a high incidence (81% of 120 subjects) for the occurrence of smooth muscle autoantibody in patients with recent Paul-Bunnell positive infectious mononucleosis, and a 38% incidence was obtained in subjects with a past history of mononucleosis; the Epstein-Barr virus may thus be a potent stimulus of this autoantibody.

2. Cytomegalovirus (CMV)

This virus belongs to the salivary gland virus group and is being recognized as an important pathogen, especially in infants and debilitated or immunosuppressed persons. Although most cases of neonatal hepatitis are claimed to be due to CMV infection (WELLER and HANSHAW, 1962), this has yet to be established. Most infections are presumably asymptomatic, as judged by the rising incidence of antibody throughout adolescence, but infections in infancy may be more serious. In an epidemiological study in London (STERN, 1968), 10% of children between 2 months and 5 years were excreting CMV in the throat and urine, and such infections were chronic; a high proportion had abnormal tests of liver function but biopsies of the liver were not available. However infantile excretors are said to show morphological evidence of hepatitis (ROWE *et al.*, 1958; HANSHAW *et al.*, 1965). Disseminated disease due to CMV in the newborn, acquired from the mother *in utero* (MEDEARIS, 1964), affects many tissues: the liver shows focal hepatocellular necrosis, giant cell transformation of hepatocytes and virus within liver cells. An adult patient with CMV infection showed granulomas in the liver (RELLER, 1973).

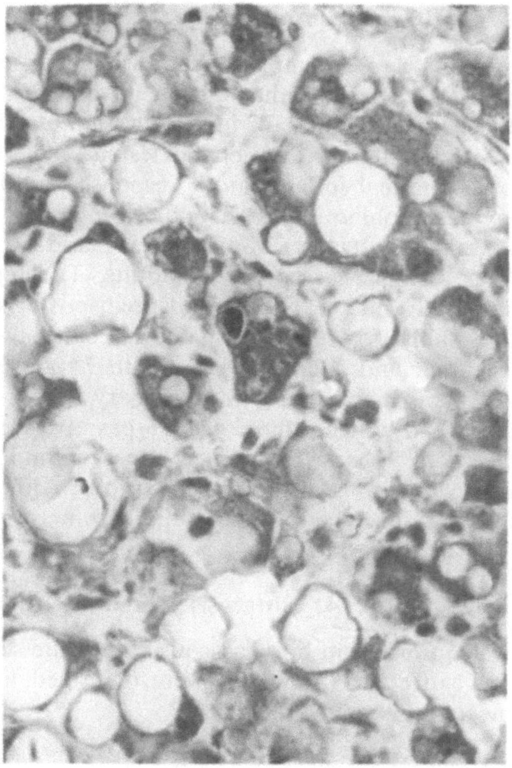

Fig. 3. Cytomegalovirus inclusion body in liver cells of immunosuppressed woman with lupoid hepatitis and terminal febrile illness: Cytomegalovirus in liver and other tissues attributed to opportunistic infection. HE ×270. (By courtesy of Editor of Australasian Annals of Medicine)

Pediatricians are familiar with types of liver injury ("giant-cell" hepatitis) in the neonate characterized by large multinucleate hepatocytes in the liver. Whilst some cases may be due to CMV infection, this condition is probably not a distinct aetiological entity, and may be more a manifestation of damage to the infant liver resulting from diverse forms of liver cell injury including viral infection, biliary obstruction and metabolic disturbance.

CMV infection in adults occurs usually in immunodepressed persons. One source of infection is by the transfusion of blood (STEVENS *et al.*, 1970). In symptomatic cases there is an acute illness resembling infectious mononucleosis with atypical monocytes in blood, but a negative Paul-Bunnell test; jaundice may supervene due to hepatocellular damage (LAMB and STERN, 1966; TOGHILL *et al.*, 1967). A case was described of a young woman with lupoid hepatitis who had received long-term immunosuppressive drugs and developed a fatal febrile illness; CMV was demonstrable in many organs including the cirrhotic liver (Fig. 3), but was considered to be an opportunistic infection (ROBSON and MACKAY, 1969).

3. Herpes Simplex

Damage to the liver by Herpes simplex virus occurs particularly in infancy. Herpes simplex hepatitis is acquired either during birth or neonatally in infants lacking maternally transferred antibody, or in infected infants in whom immunity to the virus is deficient. In infants, the hepatic lesions include focal or broad areas of bland necrosis, minimal inflammatory response, multinucleated hepatocytes and intranuclear eosinophilic inclusion bodies, and there are usually other visceral lesions (TUCKER and SCOFIELD, 1961; WILLIAMS and JACK, 1965).

Herpes hepatitis has also been recorded in adults. The reported cases were the subject of an Editorial Comment (1973), and predisposing debilitating conditions were prominent, notably hyperemesis gravidarum, extensive burns, prolonged steroid therapy for asthma, and coeliac disease with hypoproteinaemia. In the cases reviewed, hepatitis was associated with a primary herpes elsewhere, usually stomatitis, but in the burned patients there was herpes invasion of the skin. The condition was mostly fatal, with postmortem changes of multiple discrete areas of necrosis in the liver, with intranuclear viral inclusions. Although immune deficiency is a determinant of most cases in adults, this need not always be the case (JOSEPH and VOGT, 1974).

4. Psittacosis

Psittacosis virus is acquired from birds. It causes an acute severe febrile illness, the lungs being mainly affected. Two cases were described in which there was focal hepatocellular necrosis (YOW *et al.*, 1959).

5. Reovirus

Reovirus is rarely pathogenic in man and there are few reports of reovirus hepatitis. One report concerned three children with the "reovirus-enncephalitis syndrome" in which reovirus type 2 was detected in the faeces; in the one fatal case there were small focal necroses in the liver (JOSKE *et al.*, 1964). Reovirus isolated from sera in two cases of viral hepatitis was not considered aetiologically relevant by BARKER *et al.* (1969).

6. Rubella

Intrauterine infection with rubella virus may cause a congenital widely distributed multisystem disease which can include hepatomegaly and jaundice. The microscopic lesions range from a severe giant cell hepatitis to minimal hepatocellular necrosis (ESTERLY *et al.*, 1967).

7. Varicella

A case of chickenpox with hepatic lesions was reported by ESCHAR *et al.* (1973); these consisted of focal granulomatous areas, one showing central necrosis. A literature review disclosed several reports of varicella lesions in the liver associated with both chickenpox and herpes zoster, and it was held that varicella virus is capable of directly damaging liver cells (ESCHAR *et al.*, 1973).

8. Adenovirus

The adenoviruses comprise a group of 30 odd serologically related DNA viruses which are pathogenic for the respiratory tract of man. Adenoviruses have been repeatedly isolated from stools and blood of patients with infectious hepatitis, and hence have qualified as candidate hepatitis viruses. ZUCKERMAN (1970) reviewed the background of many of these claimed adenovirus isolations in infectious hepatitis, including the San Carlos agents (adeno types 1 and 3), adeno 5 from sporadic cases in Arizona, and also adeno types 16, 11 and 2, and untypable strains. Conceivably adenoviruses could account for some cases at least of sporadic infectious hepatitis in man, particularly since infectious canine hepatitis virus is an adenovirus. Alternatively, the isolations of adenovirus in cases of infectious hepatitis may be fortuitous, or represent activation of an unrelated latent adenovirus, and finally adenoviruses may act as "helper" viruses. ZUCKERMAN (1970) emphasized that whereas adenoviruses are readily identifiable by electron-microscopy, liver lesions from cases of typical infectious hepatitis never show evidence of the presence of such viruses by electron-microscopy.

9. Coxsackie Viruses

Coxsackie viruses belong to the picornavirus group and are small RNA viruses; they are divided into two groups, A and B. HERSEY and SHAW (1968) and KOFF and ISSELBACHER (1968) cite several reports of either Coxsackie virus A and B being isolated from patients regarded as having infectious hepatitis and so, like adenoviruses, these gained claims as candidate hepatitis viruses. Moreover a case is described of Coxsackie B infection with histological lesions in the liver consisting of portal and periportal inflammatory lesions (O'SHAUGHNESSEY and BUECHNER, 1962).

Work in mice shows that the liver is readily damaged by Coxsackie B1, as reported by BURCH *et al.* (1973). These authors cited previous studies in animals on Coxsackie B viral hepatitis, and showed that mice were readily susceptible to hepatitis after intraperitoneal inoculation of virus culture fluid. Neonatal and 14 day old mice developed necrotic lesions with fatal outcome, whereas adult mice had only mild lesions.

Whilst it can be accepted that hepatic damage can result from Coxsackie virus infection, particularly in young and debilitated subjects, such viruses cannot be implicated in "classical" human infectious hepatitis.

10. Yellow Fever

Yellow fever results from infection with a mosquito borne arbovirus; the dramatic history and heavy toll of life associated with this disease was reviewed by ZUCKERMAN (1970). Now, with effective prophylactic immunization, yellow fever is a disease of remote areas. The liver lesion is a diffuse severe midzonal necrosis of liver lobules in which dead liver cells appear as shrunken acidophilic masses, known as Councilman bodies; there are also fatty changes and haemorrhage. The lesions heal without fibrosis or scarring. Virus can be isolated from the blood early in the illness, and there are diagnostic serological tests.

There is a report by SMITH *et al.* (1973) that the hepatitis of yellow fever is associated with autoimmune-type antibodies, smooth muscle antibody and mitochondrial antibody, and these antibodies were demonstrable also in mice inoculated with yellow fever virus. It appears from this report that the anti-mitochondrial reactions in the human cases were not checked using human tissues as substrate (vide Section D.III.5.b), so that heterophil reactions may have been responsible.

11. "Marburg Virus" Disease

Marburg virus or green monkey disease was first recognized in 1967 when monkey handlers and laboratory workers in Marburg, Frankfurt and Belgrade developed a severe haemorrhagic fever; some 30 persons became severely ill and several died. The literature is reviewed and the pathology in man is described in detail in a paper by BECHTELSHEIMER *et al.* (1972) who had considerable experience in the investigation of this curious disease, and the pathology in monkeys is described by MURPHY *et al.* (1971).

The disease has been traced to direct contact with infected tissues of African green monkeys (*Cercopithicus aethiops*), originating from Uganda, and secondary transmissions occurred in hospital personnel via blood of infected persons. The agent proved transmissible by inoculation of infected blood to green monkeys, rhesus monkeys and guinea pigs, and all inoculated animals died; it was presumed that the infectious agent was contagious among monkeys and no vector appeared necessary (MAASS *et al.*, 1970). The clinical features of the disease included headache, vomiting, fever, rashes, haemorrhagic features and altered consciousness: clinical laboratory investigations gave results indicative of viral hepatitis, i.e. leucopenia and raised levels of serum enzymes, but there was minimal abnormality of serum bilirubin or excretion of bromsulphthalein.

Histologically, infected humans and experimentally infected animals including monkeys showed liver lesions consisting predominantly of focal bland necrotic lesions with haemorrhage and little reactive change. In milder lesions there was acidophilic necrosis of single liver cells, but necrosis usually involved larger areas with necrotic cells containing dense cytoplasmic inclusion bodies. Portal tracts contained lymphocytes showing marked transformation to plasma cells, and monocyte-like cells, and there was a pronounced Kupffer cell reaction. Fibrosis and cirrhosis never supervened.

The infecting agent, considered to be a virus, appears to represent a new type of agent hitherto not characterized. It has been visualized by electron microscopy as an elongated curled organism, 800—1000 nm length, with a periodic cross-striation along the surface. Its nature is still unknown.

12. "Candidate" Human Hepatitis Viruses

Search for the agent(s) of infectious hepatitis, and isolation of various viruses from man, has led to the proposal of many candidates for hepatitis virus; but most of these have no more than historical interest. The long saga of the search for "hepatitis virus" is well described in the comprehensive review by HERSEY and SHAW (1968) and reference can be made also to the review by KOFF and

ISSELBACHER (1968) and the monograph by ZUCKERMAN (1970). The list includes (a) known agents, as described earlier in this section, including Coxsackie virus A and B, echoviruses, adenoviruses, reoviruses, enteroviruses, myxovirus, paramyxovirus (DA virus) and O'Malley's A1 "virus" (a mycoplasma), and (b) various unidentified agents including Motol virus, Laszlo agent, K3 virus, Mitroui virus and various other dubious agents, including Chang's "lipovirus", Bolin's agent and "hemoviruses" grown on Detroit 6 cells.

A note might be made of the agents first described by Rightsel and colleagues from the Parke-Davis laboratories; these were isolated from sera and faeces of patients with hepatitis and grown on the cultured Detroit 6 epithelioid line, originally derived from human bone marrow (RIGHTSEL *et al.*, 1956; TAYLOR *et al.*, 1962). One virus strain cultured in this cell line, AR-17, induced hepatitis in humans inoculated with it. Independent confirmation of this work came from only two sources, Roumania and Australia. In Melbourne, Australia, a member of the original Parke-Davis group (R. COLE, 1965) obtained cytopathogenic effects on Detroit 6 cells using sera from cases of infectious hepatitis; however passage was effected with difficulty, and later in Melbourne the findings could not be repeated (FERRIS and COLE, 1966). Next, BOGGS *et al.* (1970) found that acute phase plasma from volunteers with induced type A hepatitis (from Krugman's MS 1 serum) induced cytopathogenic effects on cloned Detroit 6 cells. Plasma obtained from one infected volunteer, K, on the 30th day of illness (K-30 plasma), yielded a cytopathogenic isolate, and the agent was provisionally identified as a parvovirus by MELNICK and BOGGS (1972). This question now appears closed with the report of BERQUIST *et al.* (1972) that the K-30 virus belongs to the parvovirus group but is unrelated to hepatitis A as judged by absence of antibody to the K-30 agent in acute phase sera; these authors also state that currently available clones of Detroit 6 cells are no longer susceptible to the virus of hepatitis A.

VII. Granulomatous Liver Disease

A granuloma is a microscopic discrete inflammatory lesion containing macrophages, cells classed as "endothelioid", lymphocytes within and surrounding the lesion, and often multinucleated giant cells. Granulomata appear as a response to foreign agents and have an inflammatory and immunological component; in one sense, they represent an allergic response. The immune component is thought to be dependent essentially on a cell-mediated (thymus derived cell) response. In some cases granulomata can be part of an intrahepatic response to specific parasites or infectious agents in the liver, or to drugs; in others they are present as the hepatic component of the multisystem disease sarcoidosis; and in some 20–26% of cases there is no recognizable cause for hepatic granulomata (SIMON and WOLFE, 1973).

1. Granulomatous Response in Liver to Specific Infections

References have been made throughout Section B to organisms which elicit granulomatous reactions, these notably including parasites, e.g., schistosomes and ascaris, mycoses, bacteria particularly the organisms of tuberculosis, leprosy and brucellosis, and also viruses (see Section B.VI.2 and 7). The differential features of these of clinical relevance are tabulated in the monograph of SHERLOCK (1968,

p. 579). In a report by HUNT *et al.* (1973) on three instances of granulomatous hepatitis complicating immunotherapy for cancer with BCG, the question was raised as to whether the granulomata were due to infection in the liver or a hypersensitivity response to dead organisms.

2. Granulomatous Response in Liver in Drug Allergy

The granulomatous component of intrahepatic drug allergies is described in Section F.IV.

3. Sarcoidosis of the Liver

Sarcoid granulomata in the liver can be readily identified in the liver by the biopsy procedure (MATHER *et al.*, 1955), and subsequent literature on sarcoidosis of the liver, particularly as studied by liver biopsy, is described in full in the paper of MADDREY *et al.* (1970). Hepatic granulomata occur in some 65% of cases of sarcoidosis, mostly within portal triads. These are associated with a varying degree of fibrosis and inflammatory reaction, sufficient in some cases to result in architectural disorganization and cirrhosis, and even hepatocellular failure.

The nature of sarcoidosis, whether affecting the liver or body generally, is unknown. A relationship to tuberculous infection has long been suspected, but remains unproven. Subjects with sarcoidosis often show hyporeactivity to antigens known to elicit delayed hypersensitivity reactions, e.g., tuberculin, and one viewpoint is that the sarcoid reaction is an aberrant delayed hypersensitivity response, in subjects with a faulty cellular immune system, to a variety of extrinsic antigens, and possibly even intrinsic antigens.

4. Granulomatous Hepatitis of Unknown Origin

A series of 13 patients was described by SIMON and WOLFE (1973) exemplifying a syndrome of "granulomatous hepatitis and prolonged fever", and possibly representative of those cases of "hepatic granuloma of unknown cause" familiar to all hepatic histopathologists. In the above series the recognized causes of granulomata, notably sarcoidosis, infection, neoplasia and drug allergy were carefully excluded: improvement with treatment with corticosteroid drugs was a unifying feature in these patients. A similar series was described by ISRAEL and GOLDSTEIN (1973). It is likely that "idiopathic hepatic granulomatosis" is an allergic disorder, particularly as granulomata occur in the liver in many diseases with a suspected immunopathic basis. SIMON and WOLFE (1973) considered that the syndrome they described could result from an allergic host response either to an exogenous agent or to an autologous hepatic antigen as a type of autoimmune reaction.

C. Classical Human Viral Hepatitis

I. History

1. Infectious and Serum Hepatitis

Historical aspects of viral hepatitis, dating back to Hippocratic times, were reviewed by ZUCKERMAN (1970) including the numerous references to records of epidemic jaundice in military settings.

The modern history over the past 100 years extends from the erroneous concept of VIRCHOW (1865) of the disease as a "catarrhal jaundice" due to inflammatory blockage of the common bile duct through to the recent identification of the *Au antigen* particle as the infectious agent of serum hepatitis. MCDONALD (1908) first suggested that a virus might cause acute hepatitis, and EPPINGER (1908) recognized from autopsy studies that "catarrhal jaundice" was in reality a diffuse hepatitis. However the definitive evidence for this was derived in 1939 by means of aspiration biopsy of the liver (ROHOLM and IVERSEN, 1939; IVERSEN and ROHOLM, 1939).

The recognition of parenteral transmission of hepatitis by inoculation of blood products can be traced back to a description in shipyard workers in Bremen by LURMAN (1885). The historical background for serum hepatitis was presented by MACCALLUM (1972) with notations on various outbreaks of jaundice after mass inoculations with different vaccines, particularly measles and yellow fever. These events led to the use of the term "homologous serum jaundice" in 1943 in a British Ministry of Health Memorandum, and at that time also it was recognized that a similar agent caused the "syringe transmitted jaundice" seen particularly in venereal disease clinics.

The first observations on the transmission of hepatitis by the oral route appears to have been that of VOEGT (1942) who showed that typical clinical hepatitis could be induced in human volunteers fed with duodenal contents of patients with acute forms of the disease. The more definitive studies, cited by MACCALLUM (1972), were those done in 1944 in England by MACCALLUM and in America by HAVENS; these studies demonstrated the infectivity of suspensions of stools from patients with infectious hepatitis, given either orally or by subcutaneous inoculation of Seitz filtrates.

The above discoveries led to the realization that two forms of virus hepatitis existed (NEEFE, 1946). These were the naturally occurring epidemic type of disease, orally transmitted, of short (4 week) incubation period, and attributed to infectious hepatitis (IH) virus (hepatitis A), and homologous serum jaundice, parenterally transmitted and with a longer (12 week) incubation period, attributed to serum hepatitis (SH) virus (hepatitis B). These two disease types have held up subsequently, except for the recognition that hepatitis A may be transmitted parenterally, and hepatitis B orally. The agent of infectious hepatitis (virus A) is still not recognized, whereas the agent of serum hepatitis (virus B) has become identified with a characteristic antigenic particle in serum, known successively as Australia (Au) antigen, hepatitis associated antigen (HAA) and hepatitis B antigen (HBAg) (vide Section C.V).

2. The Willowbrook Studies—MS-1 and MS-2 Sera

The natural history of infectious hepatitis had been under investigation at the Willowbrook State School for mentally defective children, New York since 1956 (KRUGMAN *et al.*, 1962). In 1967 KRUGMAN and colleagues described the preparation of two sets of serum samples from a subject Mir who was considered to have had infectious hepatitis on one occasion, and serum hepatitis on a second occasion six months later; the respective samples were called MS-1 and MS-2

(KRUGMAN *et al.*, 1967). It was convincingly shown from inoculation studies that MS-1 induced type A hepatitis with a short incubation period of 30–38 days, a short period of raised transaminase (3–19 days) and a disease which was highly contagious. By contrast, MS-2 induced a type B hepatitis with a long incubation period of 41–108 days and a longer period of raised transaminase (41–108 days).

3. Hepatitis B Antigen

Substantial advances in knowledge relating to genetics, virology and hepatology have come from the fortuitous discovery in 1964 by B.S. BLUMBERG of the antigen associated with hepatitis B infection. According to BLUMBERG (BLUMBERG *et al.*, 1971a) a systematic survey was in progress to ascertain individual differences that might determine susceptibility to disease. The approach was to use the serum of frequently transfused persons as an antiserum, as this would be expected to contain antibodies to various antigens, both acquired and inherited, in the blood of the donors. The sera used were from patients with thalassaemia and haemophilia, and these were tested by double immunodiffusion against panels of sera, including panels from various parts of the world. First there was discovered a complex system of antigenic specificities on the low density lipoproteins, analogous to the red cell blood groups. Thereafter a new precipitin was found in the blood of an Australian aborigine, and hence the antigen, initially assumed to be an unusual lipoprotein, in the aborigine's serum was called "Australia antigen" (BLUMBERG *et al.*, 1965; ALTER and BLUMBERG, 1966) and later Au 1 (BLUMBERG *et al.*, 1966).

This antigen was not seen to appear or disappear from serum, and hence its presence was considered to be a fixed genetically determined trait. It was noted to have a prevalence of up to 10–20% in tropical populations, but to occur extremely rarely in healthy Americans, about 0.1%. In population studies in the U.S.A., a relatively high incidence of antigen (10%) was detected in subjects with leukaemia (BLUMBERG *et al.*, 1965), a disease known to be associated with abnormal chromosomes. Hence the antigen was next sought for, and detected, in Down's syndrome (30–35%); in the course of these studies on Down's syndrome, it was found that the antigen was acquired in serum in one patient during an episode of anicteric hepatitis, and another patient was found to have lost the antigen during convalescence from post-transfusion hepatitis, so that the possibility emerged of an association between the antigen and hepatitis virus (BLUMBERG *et al.*, 1967). As recounted by GRADY (1970), BLUMBERG sought the assistance of Prince for further identification and isolation of Australia antigen, and particles were found by electron microscopy to be associated with the presence of Au antigen. PRINCE (1968) demonstrated, in a patient developing post transfusion serum hepatitis, that there was an increase in titre of Au antigen reactive with a haemophilia serum, preceding the rise in transaminase; PRINCE (1968) therefore called the antigen SH antigen. At this point some controversy ensued, in that the antigen was associated with hepatitis of all types by BLUMBERG, whether or not transmitted parenterally and with short or long incubation period (BLUMBERG *et al.*, 1970) and the name "hepatitis antigen" was used (GOCKE and KAVEY, 1969). A compromise was attempted when another name was adopted, that of "hepatitis-associated-antigen" (HAA) (MCCOLLUM, 1969), and this term gained considerable currency.

4. Association of Hepatitis B Antigen with Serum Hepatitis

The identification of the hepatitis antigen with serum hepatitis (hepatitis B) infection followed from the studies of PRINCE *et al.* (1970) and GILES *et al.* (1969).

PRINCE *et al.* (1970) found a high incidence of positive tests for SH antigen (58—66%) in settings associated with Type B hepatitis as opposed to a low incidence (1%) in settings associated with Type A hepatitis. GILES *et al.* (1969) showed that the Au 1 (SH) antigen was not demonstrable in the MS-1 serum pool, but was regularly present in both the MS-2 pool and in sera of subjects infected from this pool, in some only transiently, but in others indefinitely. In a later study, KRUGMAN and GILES (1970) corroborated their earlier findings, using 25,000 serum specimens from more than 700 patients with hepatitis; the antigen was consistently present in sera from patients with MS-2 strain hepatitis but not MS-1 strain hepatitis. Moreover it was shown that both MS-1 and MS-2 strains induced hepatitis after either oral or parenteral exposure; the average incubation periods were 32 days for MS-1 infections, 65 days for MS-2 after parenteral exposure, and 98 days for MS-2 after oral exposure.

Therefore it appeared likely that the serum antigen was indeed specific for hepatitis type B and hence the most appropriate term would be hepatitis B antigen, with current usage being hepatitis B surface antigen (HBsAg).

5. Hepatitis A Antigen

The recognition of hepatitis B antigen in serum stimulated endeavours to identify a corresponding antigen for type A hepatitis. Claims were made from Milan for the existence of such an antigen in serum of patients with infectious hepatitis (DEL PRETE *et al.*, 1972; AJDUKIEWICZ *et al.*, 1972) but these claims have lapsed. The presence of a particle in feces associated with type A hepatitis was reported by FERRIS (1972), but this was not confirmed. A spherical 27 nanometer virus-like particle was visualized in feces of hepatitis A patients and serological studies indicated that this was the agent of hepatitis A (FEINSTONE *et al.*, 1973); an antibody response to this agent is regularly demonstrable in illness recognized as hepatitis A (PURCELL *et al.*, 1975).

II. Features of Viral Hepatitis, Types A and B

1. Clinical Features

Typical viral hepatitis is an illness of short duration with pre-icteric, icteric and post-icteric stages. In the pre-icteric stage, lasting from 5—10 days, there is anorexia and nausea, epigastric discomfort, headache, malaise and generalized myalgia. The icteric phase, lasting 2—3 weeks, begins with features of bile retention—dark urine, pale stools and jaundice. The post-icteric convalescent phase is of quite variable duration and can be marked by recurrences; there is poor appetite, malaise, loss of weight and ill-defined abdominal discomfort. The physical signs include jaundice, diffuse tender enlargement of the liver and moderate enlargement of the spleen.

Numerous clinical variants exist, particularly in adults. It is apparent during epidemics that there are many symptomatic but anicteric cases and there are even more cases in which there are no symptoms but only biochemical abnormalities of liver function on blood sampling; field surveys affirm that milder anicteric and asymptomatic cases outnumber icteric cases by up to ten to one (ZUCKERMAN, 1972, p. 28). HAVENS (1962) refers to four groups: A, "typical", with jaundice; B, "anicteric", with symptoms and signs, but no jaundice; C, "biochemical", with raised transaminases, but no clinical features; D, "non-hepatitic" with virus in blood or feces, but no other features; the disease may be more severe or even prostrating with jaundice persisting for several weeks, and in a small proportion of cases, less than 1%, there is a fulminant course with massive hepatic necrosis.

The more atypical and severe types of viral hepatitis occur with hepatitis B infections, usually in adults, in whom the degree of morbidity and particularly jaundice is usually greater, the course more protracted, with more likelihood of fulminant disease and death. It is uncertain whether hepatitis A ever progresses to a stage with fixed histological abnormalities in the liver, whereas it is now accepted that this does occur with hepatitis B.

2. Biochemical Features

The most useful biochemical test procedure is the measurement serially of the level of one or another of some 20 hepatocellular enzymes, e.g. aspartate (glutamic oxaloacetic, GOT) transaminase, or alanine (glutamic-pyruvic) transaminase, the latter being the more specific for liver injury. Peak levels of 1,000–2,000 units are reached in the pre-icteric stage, and drop quickly, but this index nonetheless is usually the last of the liver function indices to return to normal. The degree of increase in serum bilirubin reflects the degree of jaundice. In the occasional "cholestatic" type of viral hepatitis there occurs protracted elevation of serum bilirubin together with increase in serum alkaline phosphatase. Changes in serum protein levels are described below. The non-specific flocculation tests of "liver function" are still used in some centres, but these make little additional contribution to diagnosis. Informative studies on liver functional indices in acute hepatitis include those of KRUGMAN *et al.* (1962) in which indices were determined serially after inoculation of infective material under controlled conditions, ROZEN *et al.* (1970) in which interrelationships between tests were analysed by computer, and CONRAD (1972) on recurrent elevations of transaminase levels after attacks of endemic hepatitis in soldiers in Korea.

3. Immunological Features

a) Immunoglobulins. The changes in levels of immunoglobulins in viral hepatitis were described by WOLLHEIM (1968) and GILES and KRUGMAN (1969). In infectious hepatitis there is a marked and constant increase in IgM which occurs early, 3–4 days after the increase in levels of transaminase, whereas in serum hepatitis there is a less pronounced and less frequent rise in level of IgM. In both infectious and serum hepatitis there is an increase in IgG which occurs later and to a lesser degree than the rise in IgM, but persists longer. Small but significant increases in IgA occur, and there is no change in IgD. WOLLHEIM (1968) found a close correlation between the degree of thymol turbidity reaction and the level of IgM.

b) Non-Specific Immune Responses. There are various nonspecific components to the immunological response to hepatitis virus infection, some of which formerly were proposed as useful diagnostic adjuncts, but these hopes were not sustained.

Mention can be made of the capacity of sera for complement fixation using tissue homogenates (EATON *et al.*, 1944), agglutination of rhesus and chicken erythrocytes (McCOLLUM *et al.*, 1959), and the transient reactivity of sera with an antigen of smooth muscle (FARROW *et al.*, 1970).

c) Specific Immune Responses. There are specific immune responses to the antigens of hepatitis viruses, and the response is specific for Type A and Type B infections. For virus A infections, immunity is evidenced by (a) lasting protection against second attacks, and (b) the known effectiveness of immune globulin for passive prophylaxis; the availability of antigens of hepatitis A virus from the liver of infected marmosets has now allowed the development of specific antibody assays, immune adherence and complement fixation, for responses in man to infection with hepatitis A (PROVOST *et al.*, 1975; MILLER *et al.*, 1975; KRUGMAN *et al.*, 1975).

The specific humoral immune response to antigens of the hepatitis B virus can be assayed directly. Using sensitive radioimmunoassays, antibody to HBsAg was demonstrable in a United States study in 14% of voluntary blood donors, 23% of commercial blood donors, and in 83% of persons receiving multiple transfusions (LANDER *et al.*, 1971). Also, antibody can be raised by specific immunization of animals (MELARTIN and BLUMBERG, 1966). Specific cell-mediated immunity to HBAg, using HBAg positive serum as source of antigen, is claimed to be demonstrable by the *in vitro* techniques of lymphocyte transformation and leucocyte migration inhibition after acute virus B hepatitis, but not in persistent carriers (YEUNG *et al.*, 1973). Immune responses to HBsAg are described in more detail in section C.V.9.

d) Immunoprophylaxis. The effectiveness of human immune globulin in protecting vulnerable persons coming in contact with hepatitis A virus was first recognized in 1945 (see Co-operative Study, 1971), and subsequent studies have endorsed the value of passive immunization in outbreaks in family settings, schools and institutions (ROWLAND and SKONE, 1972); also administration of immune globulin to American soldiers on arrival in Korea was shown to reduce the frequency and severity (slightly) of attacks of hepatitis (Co-operative Study, 1971). The recommended dose of immune globulin varies, but 5 ml of a 16% concentration should be effective.

There is no consensus yet as to the effectiveness of gamma globulin administration (passive prophylaxis) in preventing hepatitis B infection. Gamma globulin appears to confer some protection against naturally acquired infection, at least in soldiers (Co-operative Study, 1971) and KRUGMAN *et al.* (1971) reported that specific immune serum globulin is protective against deliberate hepatitis B infection. Whether gamma globulin gives passive protection against post-transfusional hepatitis is doubtful (Co-operative Study, 1971) although there are claims that it does so (KATZ *et al.*, 1971); the content of antibody to hepatitis B in ordinary preparations of gamma globulin would not be high. Controlled studies in the United States support the use of hepatitis B immune globulin to prevent hepatitis B in "high-risk situations" (ALTER *et al.*, 1975) in protecting against serum hepatitis. Also, the possibility of active immunization against hepatitis B is under investigation (KRUGMAN and GILES, 1973). The current status of immunization against hepatitis B is presented in a WHO report on Viral Hepatitis (1975).

4. Histological Features

The histological changes in the liver in viral hepatitis are well described in the literature—the following summary is taken from descriptions by SMETANA (1954) and SCHEUER (1968). The early important changes are disruption of liver cell plates, and degeneration and necrosis of many single liver cells throughout the liver lobules, often leaving only an empty reticulum. Degenerative changes in liver cells are represented by vacuolar swelling, or acidophilic shrinkage and necrosis, forming the Councilman body. Monocytes accumulate in the vicinity of necrotic liver cells, and also in portal tracts together with a few neutrophil and eosinophilic granulocytes. Regenerative changes marked by multinucleate liver cells keep pace with necrosis. After 2—3 weeks of illness there is a tendency to focalization, with "spotty" necrosis and mononuclear aggregates within lobules, and persisting degenerative changes with acidophil bodies and regenerative activity. There is prominence of Kupffer cells which contain lipofuscin pigment. The portal infiltrate is the last lesion to resolve, usually after 6—8 weeks. Resolution is usually complete without residual pathological change. Sequelae of infectious hepatitis are discussed subsequently (Section C.I.1).

The histological features of hepatitis attributable to virus A and virus B are generally similar but a study (IWARSON *et al.*, 1972) of 165 cases separable into hepatitis A and B indicated that intrahepatic cholestasis was more prominent in hepatitis A and parenchymal cell damage and Kupffer cell reaction was more prominent in hepatitis B.

III. Epidemiology of Viral Hepatitis

1. General Aspects

Epidemiological differences between Type A and Type B hepatitis are in striking contrast to the similar clinical, biochemical and histological features of these two diseases. The earlier literature is reviewed by NEEFE (1946), and the more recent by MOSLEY (1972) and ROWLAND and SKONE (1972). Although hepatitis virus A is usually transmitted orally and virus B parenterally, this distinction is not absolute and the converse may occur. The incubation period, i.e. interval between infection and first evidence of disease differs, for virus A being 17—35 days and virus B 2—$4^1/_2$ months, and the onset of illness of virus A is more abrupt, with fever. Virus is demonstrable by transmission studies in the blood stream with both types of infection, and in the feces in virus A infections during the icteric phase of the disease. Recovery from infection is followed by resistance to infection with the original infecting agent, A or B, but there is no cross-resistance to the alternate type (NEEFE, 1946; KRUGMAN *et al.*, 1967); this resistance is known to be associated with a specific humoral immune response to antigens of the virus.

2. Modes of Spread

Patterns of community spread of hepatitis viruses were reviewed by MOSLEY (1972) and ROWLAND and SKONE (1972). Type A hepatitis is endemic in most communities, with highest attack rates amongst children aged 5–14 years, with a recent trend towards an increasing age. In addition, there are epidemic waves at intervals of 5–20 years. Local epidemics may be traced to fecal contamination of water supplies, exemplified by the massive epidemic in Delhi in 1955–56 (CHUTTANI *et al.*, 1966), and to contamination of foodstuffs, particularly shell-fish (KOFF *et al.*, 1967), and outbreaks due to food presumably contaminated by food handlers are described (DOUGHERTY and ALTMAN, 1962). Endemic infection may be predisposed to by crowding and poor hygiene and sanitation. It is uncertain to what degree virus A is transmitted parenterally but, if a shortness of incubation period is any guide, parenteral transmission of virus A by infected blood must be presumed to occur (ALTER *et al.*, 1972). SUTNICK *et al.* (1973a) claimed that no differences could be demonstrated for hepatitis occurring after transfusions of HBAg positive and HBAg negative blood, and co-identity of virus A and B was implied; apparent differences in hepatitis A and B would be explained by differences in host-response.

The association of Type B hepatitis with inoculations and blood transfusions was established over 25 years ago, and Type B hepatitis has been increasing in prevalence in recent years relative to Type A, partly as a result of increased parenteral use of addictive illicit drugs (CHERUBIN *et al.*, 1970). The most subtle form of parenteral transmission was that described in Scandinavian "track finders" who apparently acquired infection from scratches and abrasions during cross-country runs (RINGERZ and ZETTERBERG, 1967; GILLE *et al.*, 1967); such infections give strong testimony to the hardiness of the virus, the ubiquity of potential sources of infection, and the minute doses needed of infective material.

Non-parenteral infection with Type B virus can occur also, as was suggested from transmission by direct feeding of virus B (KRUGMAN *et al.*, 1967). It is known that hepatitis B virus spreads rapidly in institutions for the mentally retarded and within households, attributable to ingestion of virus-containing materials, minor skin abrasions and sexual contact (MOSLEY, 1972). Familial clustering of carriers of HBsAg is reported for various populations (BLUMBERG *et al.*, 1966; OHBAYASHI *et al.*, 1972; HELSKE and NEVANLINNA, 1973); this clustering could be indicative of both a genetic predisposition to the carrier state and the high transmissibility of the agent.

Particular importance is attached to the transmission of hepatitis B in association with haemodialysis for renal failure. A WHO Scientific Group (1973) reported a steadily increasing number of haemodialysis centres in operation and, in Europe, up to 43% of these had endemic hepatitis at any one time. Moreover, there was a rise in patients with hepatitis B antigen in such centres from 4.7% in 1966 to 11.5% in 1971; the mortality from hepatitis in such patients varies from 6% to 28%. Staff are also at risk, particularly dialysis technicians and nurses in whom the incidence of hepatitis B is around 4%. The likelihood of non-parenteral transmission of hepatitis B in haemodialysis centres is recognized, although the relative frequency of parenteral versus non-parenteral infection is uncertain. A household outbreak of hepatitis B, resulting from a haemorrhage at home by a haemodialysis patient, was reported by GARIBALDI *et al.* (1972) as exemplifying non-parenterally acquired hepatitis B infection.

The epidemiological importance of vertical transmission of hepatitis B infection, for certain populations at least, is illustrated by the frequency of antigenaemia

(63/158) in babies of carrier mothers in Taiwan; notable features were the demonstration in some of HBsAg in cord blood and the absence of manifest hepatitis in the affected babies (STEVENS *et al.*, 1975).

Non-parenteral hepatitis B infection is exemplified also by the epidemiological survey conducted by HEATHCOTE and SHERLOCK (1973). This was based on 67 patients with hepatitis B seen in two London Hospitals, and only 16 had likely parenteral exposure in the six months before becoming ill. This study pointed to transmission by infected sexual partners, including homosexual partners, but the exact route of infection could not be ascertained, i.e., whether through sexual activity *per se*, or by other routes in persons living in close association. These findings can be supplemented by the relatively high occurrence (1.39%) of hepatitis B carriers in 1650 patients attending a Venereal Disease Clinic in London, with particularly higher rates in homosexuals (3.8%) and non-European heterosexual patients (3.1%) (JEFFRIES *et al.*, 1973). It can be concluded that hepatitis B now rates as an important venereal disease.

Non-parenteral transmission was invoked also for the spread of HB virus in African populations. A report from Accra, Ghana, by MORROW *et al.* (1971) referred to the high carrier rates (1–6%) of HBsAg in Africa and the high proportion of cases of acute hepatitis with positive tests for HBsAg. The conclusion was that faecal-oral transmission occurred under the crowded unhygienic conditions of the African "shanty town". The role of "contact" transmission was discussed by BROTMAN *et al.* (1973) in relation to the high carrier rates of HBsAg in indigenous African populations. The findings of OGRA (1973) are relevant in that HBsAg was demonstrable for brief periods in hepatitis patients in urine and nasopharyngeal washings, and in faecal extracts for as long as four months after infection; replication of HBsAg in mucosal surfaces was postulated.

Another interesting epidemiological facet of hepatitis B transmission is the role of blood-sucking insect vectors. PRINCE *et al.* (1972) emphasized that the HBAg carrier state was 20–100 times more frequent in tropical than temperate regions, attributed by some to racial and genetic susceptibility. They presented findings on 187 pools of wild-caught mosquitoes in Kenya and Uganda; HBsAg was detected by radioimmunoassay in 28 pools, representing eight different species of mosquito. In a survey of this question, BROTMAN *et al.* (1973) concluded that replication of the hepatitis B virus did not occur in possible insect vectors, that transmission by such vectors may not be an important cause of the high carrier rates in indigenous Africans, but that insects may be important transmitters of hepatitis B to visitors to tropical regions.

3. Transfusion-Associated Hepatitis (Non A – Non B)

Hepatitis after transfusion of blood or blood products is particularly associated with hepatitis B and, as judged by "incubation period", with hepatitis A. However in a study of 22 patients with transfusion hepatitis after a short incubation period, there was no serological evidence of hepatitis A infection, and an as yet unidentified hepatitis agent was postulated (FEINSTONE *et al.*, 1975).

IV. Sequelae of Hepatitis

1. Differences for Type A and Type B Hepatitis

Infectious hepatitis is usually a short-duration illness with full recovery occurring within several weeks. The question of late sequelae of infectious hepatitis is one of considerable controversy. The viewpoint taken here, although by no means shared by all hepatologists (Lancet Editorial, 1973), is that whereas Type A virus infection may have a protracted course with recurrences, this virus does not cause progressive structural damage to the liver (post-hepatitic cirrhosis). Most of the evidence in regard to the non-chronicity of Type A, or presumed Type A, infections has come from follow-up reviews, usually after intervals of years, of victims of hepatitis epidemics, involving soldiers and civilians. These include, for example, the follow up studies on British soldiers (CULLINAN *et al.*, 1968), British civilians (BOTHWELL *et al.*, 1963), victims of the massive waterborne Delhi epidemic (CHUTTANI *et al.*, 1966), and American soldiers in Korea (CONRAD, 1972); a number of relevant studies are summarized in the review by FRANKEN *et al.* (1969). On the other hand Type B virus infection does have potential for chronicity, and progression to cirrhosis does occur. The possible outcomes after contact with hepatitis B are shown in Fig. 4 redrawn from SHERLOCK (1973).

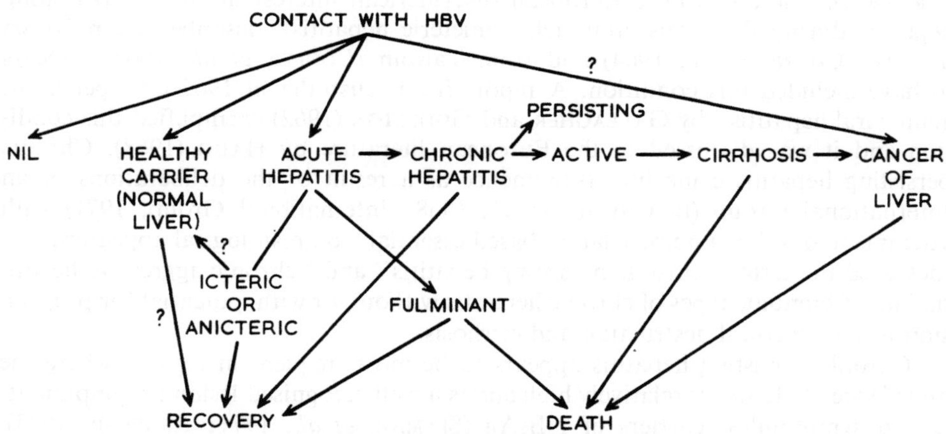

Fig. 4. Diagram showing possible outcomes of contact with hepatitis B virus (HBV). Doubtful pathways indicated by question mark (?). (Redrawn from SHERLOCK, 1973)

2. Mortality and Morbidity

The mortality rate for Type A infections is low, 0—1—0.2%, and that for Type B infection is higher; death is associated with the fulminant type of acute hepatitis. However the morbidity after type A hepatitis is substantial, particularly in adults. The reported rate of relapse, according to HAVENS (1962), is highly variable (1.5 to 18%), according to the frequency of observations and criteria used. Relapses with elevations of serum transaminase and biopsy changes of acute hepatitis were observed in 20% of cases in American servicemen during the year after the acute attack (CONRAD, 1972). The relationship of this relapsing course to "persistent hepatitis" is discussed subsequently. Persistence of the Type B hepatitis virus particle is known to occur in both serum and the liver, and to be associated with various types of histological lesions, in the liver and elsewhere (*vide infra*).

A severe sequel to infection with both hepatitis virus A and B is a lesion described clinically as subacute hepatitis, and histologically as submassive necrosis or subacute hepatic necrosis (SHN) by BOYER and KLATSKIN (1970). There is necrosis and disappearance of large groups of liver cells with intact reticulum, followed by collapse of the stroma, simulating scar formation, giving the appearance of "bridging" between portal tract and portal tract: this is said to be a forerunner of "post hepatitic cirrhosis". BOYER and KLATSKIN (1970) observed SHN with bridging after both Type A and Type B infections, but only in Type B infections was this lesion associated with progression to cirrhosis. Further discussion of liver lesions associated with chronic infection with hepatitis virus B follows in Section C.V, devoted to hepatitis B antigen.

3. Chronic Persisting Hepatitis

Chronic persisting hepatitis, first described by SMETANA (1954), refers to non-progressive forms of chronic hepatitis, and unresolved acute viral hepatitis (REDEKER, 1973). There was little European or American interest in chronic persisting hepatitis during the 1960s, although "anicteric hepatitis" described from Korea in 1964 (CHUNG *et al.*, 1964) and from Taiwan (COOPER *et al.*, 1966) appears to have included this condition. A report from Australia in 1962 on "persistent acute viral hepatitis" by GALLAGHER and GOULSTON (1962) exemplified this condition and it was discussed in the European literature by HAUG (1968). Chronic persisting hepatitis came into prominence as a result of the deliberations of an International Group (DE GROOTE *et al.*, 1968; International Group, 1971) with attempts to develop a nomenclature based essentially on histological appearances—they used the terms "chronic persisting hepatitis" and "chronic aggressive hepatitis" to differentiate types of chronic hepatitis without, or with, potential for progression to architectural destruction and cirrhosis.

Chronic persisting hepatitis appears to be most frequent in regions where the prevalence of HBsAg is relatively high and is a well recognised lesion in symptomatic and symptomless carriers of HBsAg (SELMAIR *et al.*, 1971; REDEKER, 1973). However chronic persisting hepatitis is described also in HBsAg negative subjects (BECKER *et al.*, 1970) and here could be attributed to the non-demonstrable hepatitis A virus, particularly in view of the frequency of protracted or relapsing illness in adults with epidemic Type A hepatitis (CONRAD, 1972).

V. Characteristics and Disease Associations of Hepatitis B Antigen (HBAg)

1. Serological Demonstration

HBsAg was first detected in serum by immunodiffusion in gel (BLUMBERG *et al.*, 1966) and this remained the standard technique for some years for demonstrating HBsAg. Immunodiffusion has now been replaced by other more rapid

Table 1. Techniques for measuring hepatitis B antigen and antibody. (By courtesy of World Health Organization)

Technique	Relative sensitivity for detecting[a] HBsAg	Relative sensitivity for detecting[a] anti HBs	Ease of performance[b]	Relative cost	Time required for completion (hrs)
Immunodiffusion[c]	1–5	1–10	simple	inexpensive	24–72
Counter-immunoelectrophoresis[d]	5–15	5–10	simple	moderate	2
Complement fixation[e]	15–20	5–10	moderate	inexpensive	2–24
Immune adherence[f]	20–2,000	50–150	moderate	inexpensive	2
Latex particle agglutination[g] (antibody-coated)	15–100	—	simple	inexpensive	0.1–0.2
Passive haemagglutination and inhibition[h]	15–20	10000	moderate	expensive	2
Radioimmunoassay[i]	2,000–10,000	10,000–1,000,000	complex	expensive	24–120
Immune electron microscopy[j]	1,000–2,000	—	complex	expensive	2–4

[a] Approximate reciprocal titre of an antigen or antibody arbitrarily assigned a titre of 1 when tested by the two-dimensional micro-Ouchterlony immunodiffusion technique. Range of sensitivity values obtained by various modifications of this basic technique.

[b] Including preparation of reagents.

[c] Highly specific; various modifications to improve sensitivity: use of templates, low concentration of agarose, radial diffusion, rheophoresis, staining of precipitin lines.

[d] Very useful for large-scale screening of sera but sensitivity is markedly influenced by quality of reagents and skill of technician in detecting faint precipitin lines.

[e] Usefulness of this method is limited by anticomplementary activity in a proportion of sera but it is useful for quantifying antigen and antibody. Prozones occur with high-titre sera and can result in false negative results unless sera are tested at several dilutions.

[f] Large prozones with high-titre antigen-positive sera can result in false negative results if serum is not tested at several dilutions. However, this technique combines sensitivity with speed for detecting antigen.

[g] Not fully evaluated but simplicity and speed make it potentially useful. Relatively high frequency of nonspecific agglutination makes it necessary to include appropriate controls.

[h] Comparable to complement fixation and counter-immunoelectrophoresis for detecting antigen. One of the most sensitive and useful techniques for detecting and quantifying antibody. High frequency of nonspeccfic agglutination makes it necessary to include appropriate controls.

[i] Several types of radioimmunoassay method are in use, including double-antibody and solidphase. One of the most expensive and elaborate of techniques, but the most sensitive for detecting antigen and antibody.

[j] Not suitable for large-scale testing and requires special skills and expensive equipment, but very valuable for identifying morphological types of antigen and antibody specific to them.

and increasingly sensitive technique (Taylor, 1972; Barker and Peterson, 1972) such as counter or "cross-over" immunoelectrophoresis which is the current "routine" test, complement fixation, haemagglutination, and the highly sensitive radioimmunoassay; these methods are discussed in the WHO Scientific Report (1973) from which Table 1 is taken.

It can be emphasized that the serologically demonstrable HB antigen, although undoubtedly infectious, cannot be equated with a conventional virus. For example, HBsAg is readily demonstrable in serum by the relatively insensitive immunodiffusion procedure and, in carriers at least, the more sensitive procedures for detection do not greatly increase the yield of positive tests—in only very few viral diseases, such as Rift Valley fever and avian erythromyeloblastosis, does the serum contain so many particles and sufficient antigen to give positive reactions by immunodiffusion. On the other hand SHULMAN (1970) emphasizes the observation that amounts of hepatitis B virus that can transmit hepatitis by inoculation is far below that detectable by sensitive immunological tests for HBsAg; thus a particular hepatitis-inducing plasma pool gave titre of 1:10, yet subclinical hepatitis was induced by 1 ml of this pool in dilutions as high as $1:10^6$.

2. Electron Microscopy

Immune aggregates derived from adding specific antiserum to serum samples containing HBsAg can be readily prepared for examination by electron microscopy (BAYER *et al.*, 1968; HIRSCHMAN *et al.*, 1969). The main constituents of such aggregates are pleomorphic spherical particles of varying size, and long tubular structures, classifiable as follows: (a) Small (22 nanometer, nm) particles, which are very pleomorphic, with no regular symmetry and existing as solid and empty forms. (b) Elongated particles, which are tubular structures, said to develop as a prolongation of the central cylinder of lipoprotein subunits, and extending in length up to 700 nm; they are part solid and part empty. (c) Large spherical particles (40–45 nm) also known as "Dane particles" (DANE *et al.*, 1970), which are virus-like, resembling virions with an inner core and an outer component (Fig. 5). The significance of the ultrastructural details in the particles is discussed by ZUCKERMAN (1972). The small (22 nm) particles and the tubules represent protein coat material of the virus. The "Dane particles" have been separated by detergents into an outer coat, presumably protein like the smaller 22 nm particles, and a 27 nm core component resembling a rhinovirus (ALMEIDA *et al.*, 1971). The core material generates an independent antibody response (HOOFNAGLE *et al.*, 1973), so that the surface material became known as HBsAg, and the core material as HBcAg.

NIELSEN *et al.* (1973) found that, whereas Dane particles were not demonstrable in "normal carriers" of HBsAg and rarely so in acute hepatitis, yet as many as 11 of 13 patients with antigenaemia together with chronic hepatitis had these particles.

3. Chemical Components of HBAg

It was generally claimed that the HBAg particle, despite its infectivity, was devoid of nucleic acids, although these may be lost as a result of nucleases in serum. There were earlier reports, cited by MACKAY and POPPER (1973), that small amounts of nucleic acid, particularly RNA, were demonstrable in the particles and that this nucleic acid could represent a DNA polymerase or reverse transcriptase. Later findings indicated that DNA polymerase activity was associated with Dane particles (KAPLAN *et al.*, 1973), that DNA polymerase activity was associated with the 27 nm core component of HBAg, and that there is DNA polymerase activity in serum in persons whose serum contains HBsAg.

The HBAg particle consists predominantly of complex polypeptides and lipoproteins (MILLMAN *et al.*, 1970; KIM, 1971; KIM and BISSELL, 1971; GERIN *et al.*, 1975), and also contains carbohydrate (BURRELL *et al.*, 1973). The proteins of

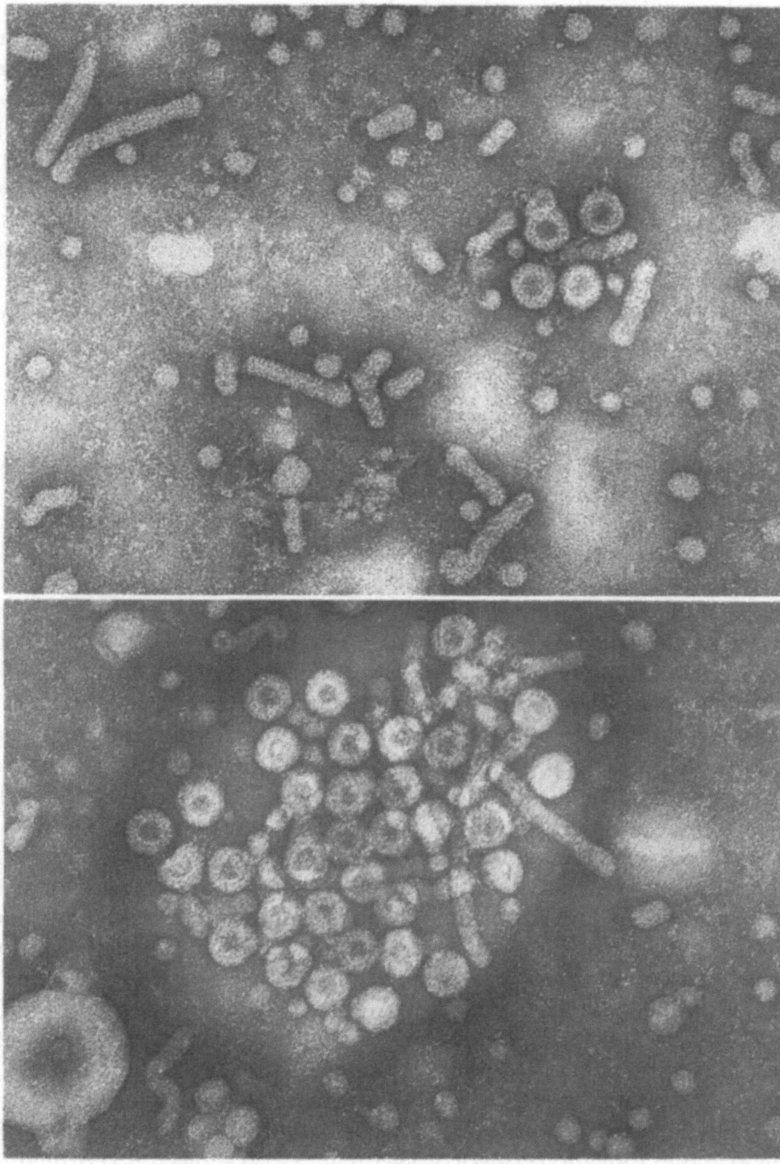

(a) (b)

Fig. 5a and b. Two electron micrographs of human serum pellet showing hepatitis B antigen particles. Three distinct morphological entities illustrated are (1) small pleomorphic spherical particles 20–22 nm in diameter, (2) tubular forms of varying length which display angularity, bulbous terminals and a regular transverse periodicity, and (3) large double-shelled spherical particles 42 nm in diameter (Dane particles). ×252,000. (By courtesy of Professor A.J. ZUCKERMAN, from "Hepatitis Associated Antigen and Viruses" and North Holland Publishing Co., Amsterdam) the particle were initially thought to include serum proteins or derivatives of plasma or organelle membranes of host origin, but improved techniques for purification yield HBsAg devoid of host components. Serological techniques, including immunofluorescence, specifically identify the proteins rather than other components of the complex. The proteins may be, as is the case with other viruses, specific newly formed antigens (capsides), or preformed host material from cell or organelle membranes as with influenza virus (HOLLAND and KIEHN, 1970), Epstein Barr virus (GERBER and GOLDSTEIN, 1970), or herpes virus (EDGINTON and RITT, 1970); or host lipids may be specifically incorporated as with certain RNA viruses (ROTT *et al.*, 1966). The heterogeneity of the protein component of HBsAg has been demonstrated chemically, immunologically and serologically (see MACKAY and POPPER, 1973).

4. Immunochemical Analyses—Subspecificities

There are variant antigenic subspecificities in HBsAg particles, recognizable by immunochemical means. There is a common specificity *a*, shared by all HBAg positive sera, and various mutually exclusive subspecificities. Subspecificities x, d, and y were described by LE BOUVIER (1971) and HOLLAND *et al.* (1972); *x* was present in most positive sera, and may be an immunogenic host component, whereas *d* and *y* were almost mutually exclusive and were held to reflect distinct genotypes of the infecting virus, D and Y (LE BOUVIER *et al.*, 1972). Subsequently additional determinants w and r were recognized (BANCROFT *et al.*, 1972). Thus HBsAg can be divided into four possible phenotypes, adw (D), adr (R), ayw (Y), and ayr, the latter being infrequent, and there are interesting geographical differences in prevalence of these subtypes (LE BOUVIER, 1973). Observations on disease transmission and localised outbreaks of Type B hepatitis established that these antigenic specificities were maintained. A further antigenic specificity e, unrelated to d and y, and w and r, was described by MAGNIUS and ESPMARK (1972).

The subtypes of HBsAg were claimed to have some correlation with disease, in that subtype ad appeared more common among blood donors and carriers, in whom it tended to be associated with normal liver function (IWARSON *et al.*, 1973), whereas subtype ay (the subtype of Willowbrook MS-2 serum) was more associated with acute serum hepatitis, outbreaks in dialysis units and hepatitis in drug addicts (Editorial Comment, 1973). In a Danish study (NIELSEN *et al.*, 1973a), the y subtype predominated in acute hepatitis (79%), and in HBAg associated chronic hepatitis; however healthy carriers and all 10 cirrhotic patients had the d subtype. On the other hand, cases studied in Los Angeles (GORDON *et al.*, 1972) and in England (PONS-ROMERO *et al.*, 1974) showed no correlation between a given form of hepatitis and a given antigenic determinant.

The present consensus is that there is no association of subtypes of HBsAg with clinical features, and apparent associations can be explained on an epidemiological basis. On the other hand, antigen e was associated with the presence in serum of Dane particles and with clinically progressive hepatitis (NIELSEN *et al.*, 1974), with antibody to e being present in healthy serum carriers of HBsAg without Dane particles; further data associating antigen e with progressive hepatitis appears in a Lancet Editorial (1975).

5. HBAg in the Liver

HBsAg has been demonstrated in liver tissues by electron-microscopy (Fig. 6) and immunofluorescence in several studies, cited by MACKAY and POPPER (1973). Virus-like particles were detected in hepatocytes by electron-microscopy in both

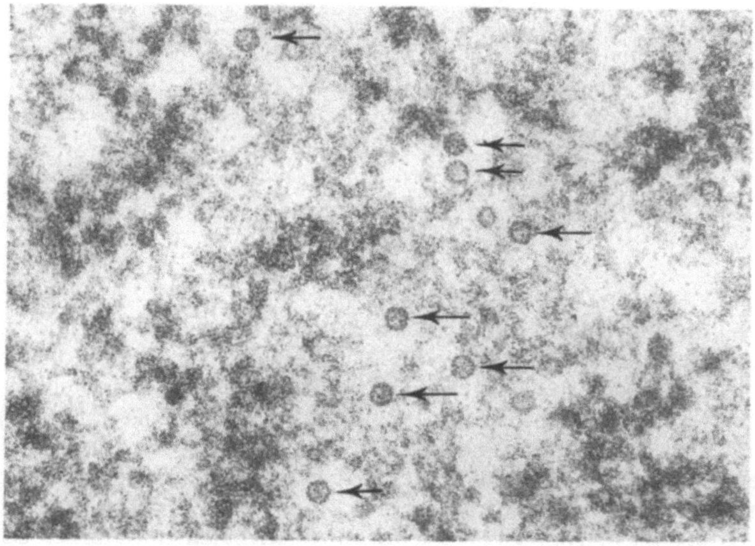

(a)

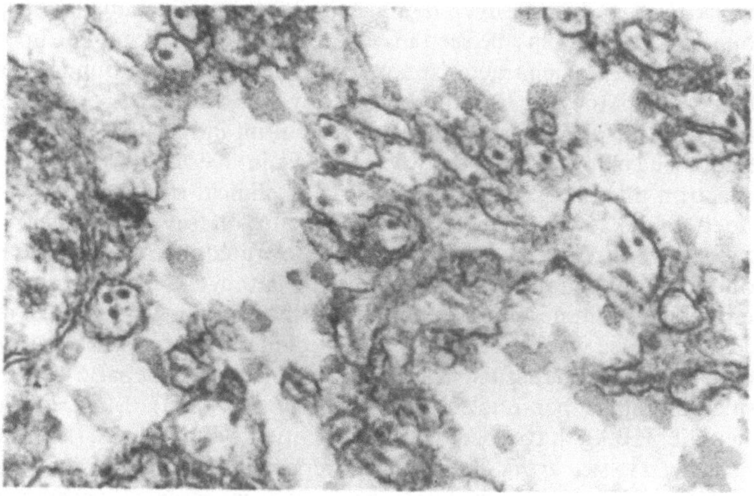

(b)

Fig. 6a—c. Hepatitis B particles in nucleus and cytoplasm of liver cells, as seen by electron microscopy, with suggested process of assembly of HBAg. (a) Virus particles (core structures) of 25 nm diameter in nucleoplasm of liver cell of 10 month infant. (By courtesy of Dr. R.L. PETERS and Dr. A.E.G. DUNN, and University Park Press, Baltimore.) (b) Particles of HBAg (coat structures) in cytoplasm of adult male with HBAg associated chronic hepatitis (see Fig. 7). ×100,000. (By courtesy of Dr. T. MANDEL.) (c) Diagram of liver cell showing presence in nucleus of core of hepatitis B virus and assembly in cytoplasm of "complete" (Dane) particles and production of excess coat material, with passage of this into serum. (Adapted from Figure published by Dr. R.H. PURCELL 1972)

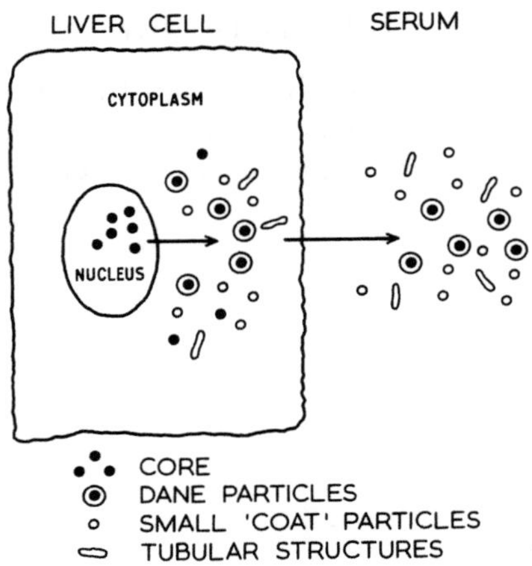

Fig. 6c

the nucleus and cytoplasm of hepatocytes, particularly close to and within the endoplasmic reticulum (STEIN *et al.*, 1972), where the "packing" of protein into the particles may take place. Aggregates of particles were demonstrated by immuno-electron-microscopy (GERBER *et al.*, 1972) and by fluorescence microscopy which demonstrated HBAg in hepatic cell nuclei in leukaemia (MILLMAN *et al.*, 1970), and in hepatic cell cytoplasm and in mesenchymal cells in viral hepatitis (EDGINTON and RITT, 1971).

In hepatitis the particles may be focally distributed and rather scanty, but in healthy carriers in whom liver damage is absent or minimal, conspicuously large amounts of HBsAg may be seen in hepatocytes by electron-microscopy (HADZIYANNIS *et al.*, 1972). A characteristic cytoplasmic change (ground-glass appearance) is seen in hepatocytes routine microscopy (HADZIYANNIS *et al.*, 1973), and is attributed to hyperplasia of endoplasmic reticulum induced by HBV.

Correlations have been sought between HBsAg in liver demonstrable by fluorescence or electron microscopy and histological or clinical evidence of liver disease. There tended to be fewer particles in hepatocytes in severe forms of hepatitis (KRAWCZYNSKI *et al.*, 1972), indicative of accelerated breakdown or decreased production of the antigen in severely damaged hepatocytes. By contrast, in carriers and patients with immune suppression, there may be large amounts of HBsAg in hepatocytes. A case was described of a Sardinian child with relapsing corticosteroid-dependent chronic hepatitis with viral particles in all hepatic cell nuclei, yet in very small numbers per nucleus (ALMEIDA *et al.*, 1973). Most of the studies on intrahepatic HBAg have been done in patients with acute hepatitis, or in carriers. KRAWCZYNSKI *et al.* (1972) have reported on the presence of HBsAg in liver, detected mainly by immunofluorescence, in cases of chronic aggressive hepatitis and cirrhosis, in which cytoplasmic particles of HBsAg were demonstrable in 54% and 31% of cases respectively. Notably, in these latter cases HBAg was not present in body fluids despite being present in the liver, although detailed studies on serum by sensitive techniques were not performed.

The most definitive study is that of GUDAT *et al.* (1975) in which four types of expression pattern of HBV in liver were described, ranging from few components (self limited hepatitis), abundant core, abundant surface antigen (chronic persistent disease) to spotty expression of both core and surface antigen particles (aggressive disease).

6. HBAg Outside the Liver—Immune Complexes

There are several references, cited by MACKAY and POPPER (1973), to HBsAg being associated with immune complex disease, the complexes being deposited particularly in vessel walls with all the features of vasculitis (GOCKE *et al.*, 1971) or polyarteritis nodosa (MARTINI *et al.*, 1972; BAKER *et al.*, 1972; GERBER *et al.*, 1972); deposits are associated with immunoglobulin and complement, and HBsAg was demonstrable in vessel walls by fluorescence microscopy. HBAg has been demonstrated in renal glomeruli (COMBES *et al.*, 1971) and in synovial fluid during the arthritis which can occur in the prodromal period of hepatitis (ONION *et al.*, 1971), and deposition of HBsAg in the synovium may be associated with a fall in serum complement (ALPERT *et al.*, 1971). In a series of 100 patients with viral hepatitis B, arthritis-arthralgia or rashes were recorded in 29 (KOHLER, 1973). The lesions of infantile papular acrodermatitis may be attributable to HBsAg (GIANOTTI, 1971). In a report from Poland (BRZOSKO *et al.*, 1974) it was stated that over 50% of 52 unselected cases of nephrotic syndrome in children were attributable to glomerular complexes containing HBsAg.

7. Non-Correlation between HBsAg in Serum and Presence and Type of Liver Disease

The presence of HBsAg in serum is in general associated with infectivity, but there is apparently no relationship between the amount demonstrable in serum or liver, and the incidence, severity and chronicity of liver disease, as judged by the following observations.

Serum HBsAg occurs in populations with a distinct geographical and, presumably, genetic background and with a strong male preponderance (SUTNICK *et al.*, 1971). The prevalence is low in developed Western communities e.g. for an Australian (Queensland) population of 52,893 blood donors, there were only 40 (0.07%) who were HBsAg positive; these included 32 males, and only 5 of the 40 had some abnormality in the medical history (MASON *et al.*, 1972). On the other hand, high prevalences have been reported from Mediterranean countries, and even higher from Pacific and African communities (BLUMBERG *et al.*, 1971a). The marked racial differences in prevalence of HBAg were well demonstrated amongst healthy racial groups in a common environment in Singapore, i.e., 7.5% in Chinese, 4.0% in Malays, 0.9% in Indians (YAP *et al.*, 1972), and such racial differences were demonstrable from 5—9 years of age.

The presence of HBsAg in serum is associated with a wide range of histological appearances of the liver (Fig. 7). There may be neither histological liver lesions (KLINGE *et al.*, 1970) nor biochemical changes (OKOCHI and MURAKAMI, 1968), or mild "non specific" histological alterations of the liver may be seen including steatosis (SINGLETON *et al.*, 1971; REINICKE *et al.*, 1972), or damage may be extensive. Thus serum HBsAg can be found in carriers with or without known preceding

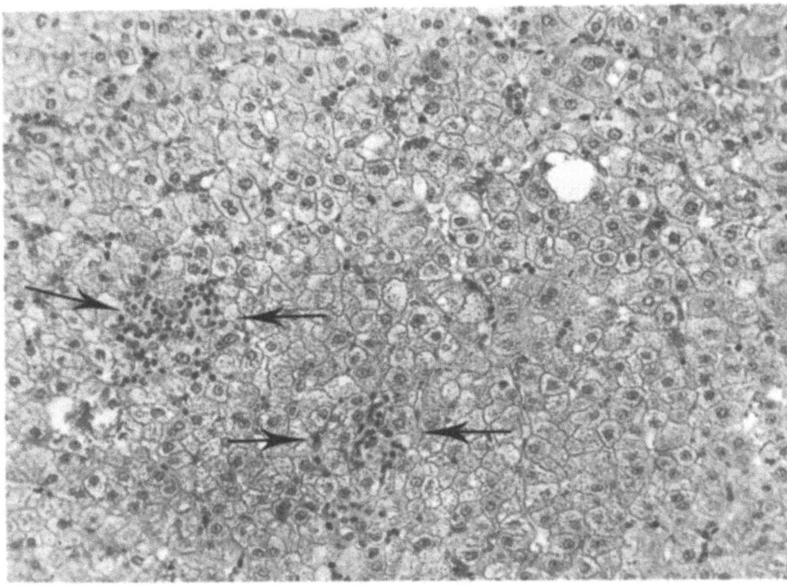

(a)

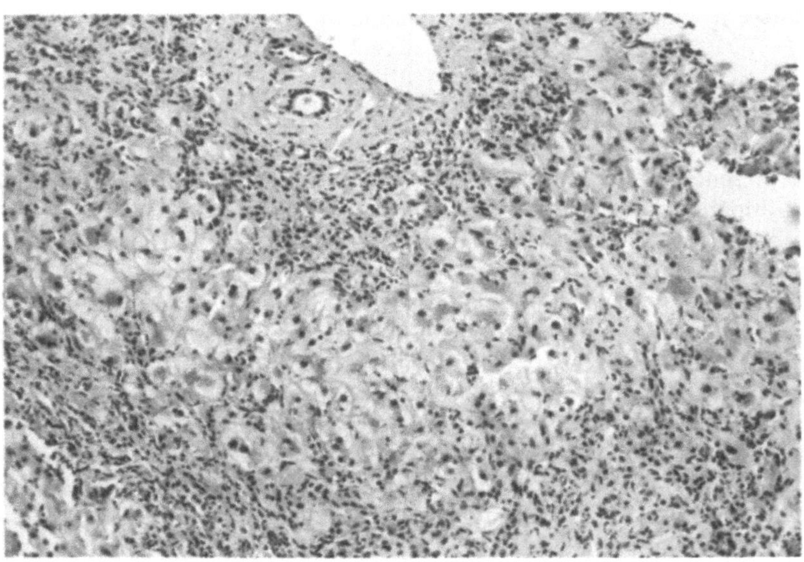

(b)

Fig. 7a and b. Range of histological changes in liver of chronic carriers of HBAg in serum. (a) Liver biopsy of 38 year old woman, persistent carrier of HBAg, three years after clinically diagnosed acute hepatitis: disarray of liver cell cords and foci of hepatocytolysis. HE ×100. (By courtesy of Dr. R.L. PETERS and University Park Press, Baltimore.) (b) Liver biopsy of 55 year old male mortuary attendant with HBAg associated chronic hepatitis following a clinically diagnosed acute hepatitis; the liver pattern is cirrhotic and changes of chronic active hepatitis are evident. (Case 2, MATHEWS and MACKAY, 1970.) (By courtesy of Editor of British Medical Journal) icteric or anicteric infection, in all forms of anicteric and icteric hepatitis, in massive hepatic necrosis, in which the antigen may disappear from the serum in the terminal stage (DUDLEY *et al.*, 1971), in diseases described as chronic active aggressive hepatitis (vide infra) and chronic persisting hepatitis (DUDLEY *et al.*, 1972), and in primary hepatic carcinomas with curious regional differences in prevalence (MACKAY and POPPER, 1973).

8. HBAg Associated Chronic Active Hepatitis

It is a matter of considerable importance (and controversy) as to whether HBsAg associated chronic active hepatitis can be identified as a specific clinical and pathogenetic entity and, in particular, distinguished from other types of chronic hepatitis. From observations in Melbourne (unpublished), the prototype patient would be of male sex, a migrant from abroad, perhaps but not necessarily having had an illness recognizable as acute viral hepatitis, continuously or recurrently elevated levels of serum transaminase, usually slight elevation of serum gamma globulin and absence of autoantibodies in serum. HBsAg would be regularly demonstrable in serum even by immunodiffusion, and in liver by electron microscopy. The histological picture would be variable: if there were changes specified as "aggressive", the condition would be called HB associated chronic active hepatitis and, if "hepatitic", chronic persisting hepatitis. A Ugandan study (ANTHONY *et al.*, 1973) showed HB associated chronic liver disease to be characterized by a particular type of cell damage, ballooning and dysplasia, and a macronodular more than a micronodular cirrhosis, but this is not invariable.

There are wide regional variations in the prevalence of HBsAg in cases of chronic hepatitis, this being quite low, less than 5% of all cases, in Australia (MATHEWS and MACKAY, 1970; COOKSLEY *et al.*, 1972) and in England (FOX *et al.*, 1969), corresponding to low carrier rates of HBsAg for the general population, and much higher, approximately 25%, in parts of the United States, Japan and parts of Europe, the relevant reports being cited by PRINCE (1971); the highest rate of 62% was cited by WEWALKA *et al.* (1970) for an Austrian series of cases with histological features of "chronic aggressive hepatitis". Although WEWALKA *et al.* (1970) stated that there was "no reason to assume that Au/SH antigen positive hepatitis is a special entity", detailed comparisons were not made with cases of "autoimmune type" chronic hepatitis.

In reports describing a relatively high incidence of HBsAg in chronic active hepatitis and cirrhosis (KRASSNITZKY *et al.*, 1970), there is the implication that the presence of this antigen is important in the development of chronic liver disease. However the frequency with which well-defined acute serum hepatitis (HBsAg positive) undergoes progressive transition under observation to chronic active hepatitis is uncertain. CREUTZFELDT *et al.* (1966) described an evolution of acute transfusion hepatitis to cirrhosis of the liver over nine months. NIELSEN *et al.* (1971) reported that chronic aggressive hepatitis supervened after acute sporadic hepatitis B in 8 of 112 patients, but did not provide individual case details. ARONOFF *et al.* (1973) described transition through acute hepatitis to chronic active hepatitis and "post-hepatitic cirrhosis" in 8 of 18 HBsAg positive cases in a transplantation unit. PETERS (1973) recorded in detail one fully documented example

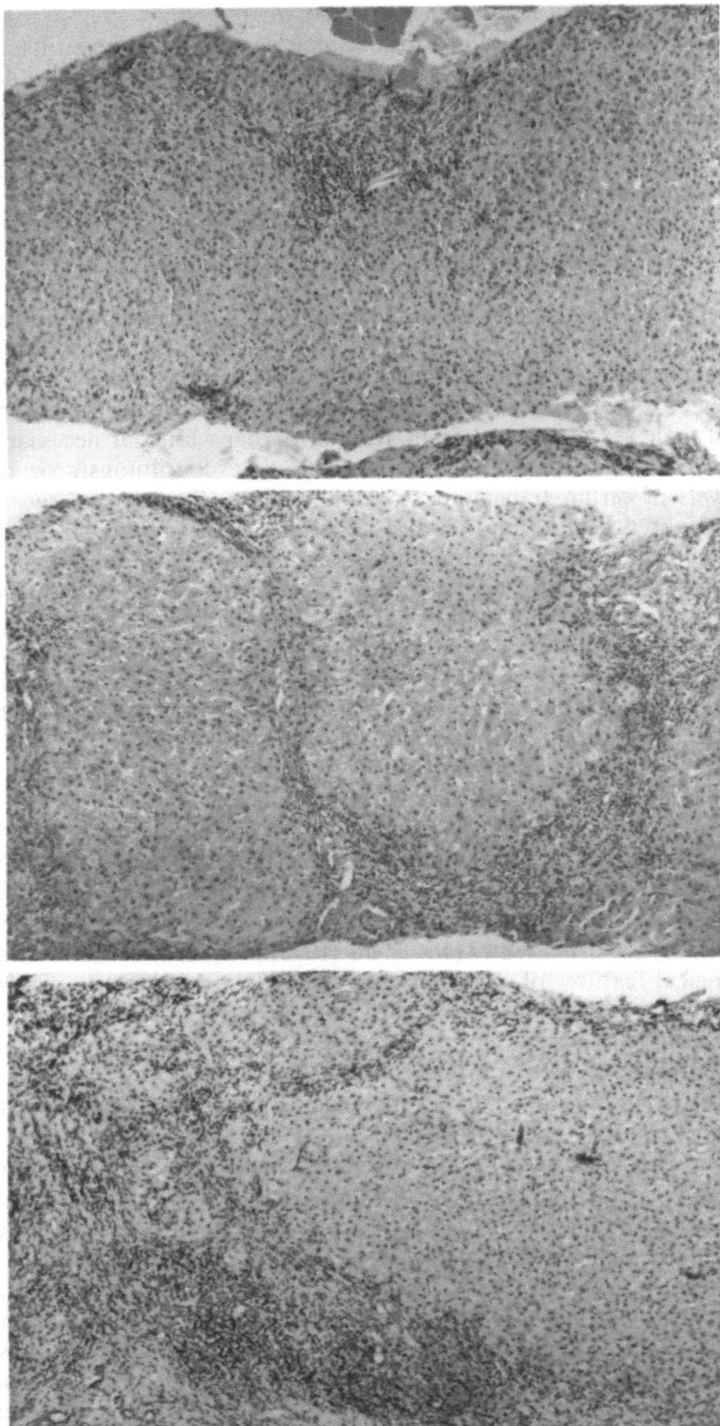

(a)

(b)

(c)

of a patient who certainly had acute hepatitis B and developed cirrhosis under observation, with persistence of antigenaemia. The conclusion is that there is such an entity as HBsAg positive chronic active hepatitis and cirrhosis, characterized by persistent carriage of HBsAg in serum and chronic "aggressive" changes in the liver histologically (Fig. 8a–c); the proportion of such cases among all cases of chronic active hepatitis will vary considerably according to locality.

9. Immune Responses to HBAg

a) Humoral Response to HBsAg. Antibody to the surface antigens of HBAg (anti HBs) is detected much less frequently in serum than is HBsAg with the usual techniques, but with sensitive techniques, haemagglutination or radioimmunoassay, anti HBs is more often demonstrable, e.g. after disappearance of the antigen in acute serum hepatitis (SHULMAN, 1970); whether or not the presence of anti HBs indicates infectivity is uncertain (PURCELL *et al.*, 1971). Antibody to HBsAg is demonstrable also in animals e.g. rabbits, deliberately immunized with HBAg (MELARTIN and BLUMBERG, 1966) and in naturally and deliberately infected chimpanzees (Section C.VI.2). LANDER *et al.* (1972) demonstrated in a population study an age related increase in frequency and geometric mean titre of anti HBs, the overall frequency being around 20%. However the incidence of anti HBs is as high as 82% in frequently transfused patients (LANDER *et al.*, 1971). BARKER *et al.* (1973a) found that 79.5% of persons developed serum antibody after exposure to serum hepatitis virus, and two patterns of antibody response were distinguished, a late low titre response designated as a "primary" response, and, in some persons resistant to infection, an early high titre response designated as a "secondary" anamnestic response.

Complexes of HBsAg and anti HBs in the blood are demonstrable by serological procedures (SHULMAN and BARKER, 1969; MILLMAN *et al.*, 1970), immunofluorescence (BRZOSKO *et al.*, 1971) and electron-microscopy (ALMEIDA and WATERSON, 1969). However it can be noted that liver injury does not result from deposition in the liver of complexes of HBsAg and anti HBs, in that no relationship could be shown between levels of immune complexes circulating in the serum and manifestations of chronic aggressive hepatitis (PRINCE and TREPO, 1971), nor between the extent of hepatitis and titre of HBsAg or third component of complement. Moreover, extracellular gamma globulin capable of binding complement is not demonstrable in the liver in acute hepatitis with massive necrosis, nor in chronic active hepatitis—conversely, even when there is demonstrable gamma globulin, presumably antibody, together with HBsAg, there may not be any tissue injury (GERBER *et al.*, 1972).

b) Cell Mediated Immunity and Hepatitis B. Specific cell-mediated immunity to components of HBsAg was reported by YEUNG LAIWAH (1971), using the *in*

◀ Fig. 8a–c. Progression of liver lesions associated with chronic hepatitis B infection. Biopsies at 2 year intervals from a 38 year old male Yugoslav showing evolution from (a) delayed resolution of acute hepatitis to (b) chronic active hepatitis with incipient cirrhosis, and to (c) established cirrhosis with continuing evidence of chronic hepatitis. HE ×70. HBAg particles were demonstrable in cytoplasm of liver cells, from third biopsy (Fig. 6b) *vitro* technique of lymphocyte transformation, with HBsAg positive serum as source of antigen, and by DUDLEY *et al.* (1972), using the leukocyte migration inhibition (LMI) procedure. There is confirmation of these claims in later reports. KNOLLE *et al.* (1973), using LMI, found a much higher frequency of positive tests in patients with hepatitis who cleared HBsAg than in those who failed to do so. YEUNG LAIWAH *et al.* (1973) used both HBsAg-rich serum and purified preparations of HBAg, and two *in vitro* methods, lymphocyte stimulation and leucocyte migration inhibition; positive results were demonstrable after recovery from acute hepatitis infection, but not in persistent carriers, indicative of anergy or tolerance to HBAg. DE GAST *et al.* (1973) using the lymphocyte transformation technique and purified heat-inactivated preparations of HBsAg likewise found responsiveness of lymphocytes after recovery from acute hepatitis B infection.

Integrity of cell-mediated immunity (CMI) to HBsAg was considered theoretically to be a major determinant of the outcome of the interaction of HB virus and the host, by analogy with other virus infections, and DUDLEY *et al.* (1972) analysed the possibilities as follows. With normal CMI (T lymphocytes) there would be elimination of HB virus and full recovery, but with defective CMI (vide infra), the virus will persist. In the latter case, the effects on the liver will range from nil, c.f. persisting tolerated infection with murine lymphocytic choriomeningitis virus, mild recurring damage as in "chronic persisting hepatitis", or severe destructive effects culminating in cirrhosis and liver failue. There are suggestions (GIUSTINO *et al.*, 1972) that the use of corticosteroid drugs in acute Type B hepatitis may predispose to persistent carriage of HBsAg, presumably by impairing the immune response to the HB virus. The involvement of the T-cell system in immune responses to HBsAg was established experimentally by ROBERTS *et al.* (1975), using conventional (Balb/c) and "nude" athymic mice; these were immunized with HBsAg in Freund's complete adjuvant. The conventional mice mounted typical delayed sensitivity reactions and produced good humoral immune responses whereas the athymic mice failed to do so.

The concept of immunodeficiency as a determinant of chronic infection would be strengthened if cell-mediated immune capacity could be shown to be depressed in carriers of HBsAg. Such depression may well operate in those diseases, including leprosy and chronic nephritis, in which an HBsAg carrier state may exist. However in apparently healthy carriers in Italy studied by SUTNICK *et al.* (1973b), lymphocyte function was normal as judged by transformation responses to PHA. In a study by NIELSEN *et al.* (1973b), comprehensive assessments of cell-mediated immunity (cutaneous responses to DNCB, haemocyanin and PPD, and mitogenic responses of lymphocytes to PHA) failed to show defective cell-mediated immunity, leading to the conclusion that general immunodeficiency was not a prerequisite for developing HB-antigenaemia. Cellular immunity, as judged by PHA response, was shown to be intact in HBsAg positive hepatitis, but there was a decline in the later phases of the disease (SODOMANN and HAVEMANN, 1973).

10. HBAg—A Unique Particle

It has long been recognized that there are curious inconsistencies between the presence and amount of HBsAg on the one hand and infectivity and disease on the other. BLUMBERG *et al.* (1971 b) considered the hepatitis B (Australia) antigen to have the combined properties of a peculiar infectious agent and a serum protein polymorphism, and hence they recommended a new term, "icron", to describe such a particle.

Some of the known inconsistencies can be restated. Some materials containing HBsAg transmit serum hepatitis in exquisitely small amounts, whereas transmission in other circumstances requires transfusion of large amounts of blood. Carriers of HBsAg, despite having large amounts of antigen in their serum and liver, do not readily transmit infection by contact (CHALMERS and ALTER, 1971), whereas contact infection from patients ill with serum hepatitis and who are HBAg positive is well established (SCHOLER *et al.*, 1970; HERSH *et al.*, 1971). Note may be made also of the noninfectivity of heat-treated albumin fractions of serum containing HBAg (HOLLAND *et al.*, 1971), the non-cytopathogenicity of HBAg in tissue culture (COYNE *et al.*, 1970), or organ culture (JENSON *et al.*, 1970; ZUCKERMAN and BAINES, 1972), and the absence in viral hepatitis of circulating interferon (HILL *et al.*, 1971) which is usually found in typical viral infections.

Reference may be made here to the remarkable report (unconfirmed in the subsequent two years) by BANATVALA and PAYNE (1973) that acute phase sera containing HBsAg induced necrotic changes in tobacco plants. The leaves of the plants were sprinkled with carborundum and then inoculated with 0.1 ml of test serum. After 7—9 days the leaves lost turgidity, became crinkled and by 14 days had become necrotic: only sera containing HBsAg induced these effects, and neutralization was demonstrable with convalescent sera. These observations raised the speculation that the hepatitis B agent was related to "viroids" (ZUCKERMAN, 1973), i.e., infectious plant pathogens with a structure like that of transfer RNA and having a single strand of RNA so folded that it has a partial double stranded structure; the prototype "viroid" is an agent causing potato spindle tuber disease (DIENER, 1972). However the cores of Dane particles contain circular DNA and DNA polymerase (ROBINSON, 1975), indicating that HBV is a DNA-virus.

11. Immune Aberrations and Persistence of Hepatitis B

The nature of the immune abèrration àllowing persistent carriage in serum and in liver cells of large amounts of a normally immunogenic particle, HBAg, is puzzling, and the following considerations could be relevant.

1. General immunodeficiency, particularly affecting cell-mediated immunity (DUDLEY *et al.*, 1972). Such deficiency could be associated with uraemia (note also the exposure to infection with HB virus during haemodialysis), various chronic immunodepressive disease states such as leukaemia and leprosy (BLUMBERG *et al.*, 1971 b; WELLS and FUDENBERG, 1972), possibly adverse socio-nutritional states (CHERUBIN *et al.*, 1972), or could be consequential to use of immunodepressive drugs including corticosteroids (vide C.V.9) and azathioprine.

2. Specific or limited immunodeficiency, unique to particular antigens of the HBAg particle. This may pertain with healthy carriers, particularly among certain racial groups who may have a genetically based incapacity for immune responsiveness to determinants of HBAg, and a relationship to histocompatibility antigens

is possible (MACKAY and POPPER, 1973). This may be the basis of the "genetic polymorphism" proposed for the carrier state by BLUMBERG *et al.* (1971 b).

3. Specific prenatally induced immune tolerance may operate in cases in which HBAg is transmitted from an infected mother either via the placenta (SCHWEITZER *et al.*, 1972) or neonatally (MERRILL *et al.*, 1972); or specific immune tolerance to the particle on the part of T cells may be acquired in the course of infection with hepatitis B virus.

4. The incorporation by the virus of host components into the coat material, with tolerogenesis, could represent an "adaptive" response to protect the virion from the immune response of the host.

VI. Infection of Animals with Hepatitis Viruses

Various animals are susceptible to hepatitis viruses, and these may be taken as models for human viral hepatitis. However most interest centres on infection of animals with human hepatitis viruses.

The human hepatitis viruses A and B have high specificity for the human species, the common laboratory animals being resistant; however certain primates are susceptible, particularly the marmoset in the case of virus A, and the chimpanzee in the case of virus B.

1. Viral Hepatitis in Animals

There are many viruses that produce hepatitis in animals and these infections provide good experimental models illustrating portals of entry, localization of virus particles in liver, patterns of liver injury, host response and immunity. Experimental viral hepatitis in animals was the subject of a monograph by PIAZZA (1969) and the more recent literature is discussed by SABESIN and KOFF (1974).

Among animals, mice are susceptible to hepatitis, and there is a group of contagious enteric viruses that cause mild disease. A carrier state may exist (cf. human hepatitis B) and latent disease can be reactivated by stress or by other infectious agents. Mice are susceptible also to ectromelia, a pox virus, which induces massive hepatic necrosis; replication of virus in lymphoid tissue including Kupffer cells may compromise host immune mechanisms.

The influence of genetic factors operating through immune pathways is illustrated by the differing susceptibility among mouse strains to mouse hepatitis virus type 3 (LE PREVOST *et al.*, 1975; DUPUY *et al.*, 1975). There was an innate high resistance to infection of strain A mice, whereas other strains were susceptible and died from liver necrosis. Resistance appeared to require both specific immunity (T cells) and non-specific immunity (macrophages). Thus, in the resistant strain, macrophages did not support infection, whereas in susceptible strains, and in the resistant strain after procedures interfering with T cell function, virus did proliferate in macrophages.

Dogs are susceptible to infection with a hepatotropic DNA-containing adenovirus with a range of disease manifestations including a chronic state. In the rat, virus hepatitis requires mitotic activity, so that induction in the adult requires partial hepatectomy; massive necrosis may occur with stromal collapse and nodular hyperplasia. Sheep and cattle are susceptible to Rift Valley fever virus which induces a range of lesions including massive necrosis.

2. Human Hepatitis A Infection of Marmosets

Considerable controversy has surrounded claims that primates can be infected with hepatitis A virus, and the literature is reviewed by DEINHARDT *et al.* (1972). The validity of the claims of DEINHARDT and colleagues on the infectivity of the marmoset is now accepted. This South American monkey was selected initially because its contact with humans was low, and so immunity to human viruses would be lacking. The definitive experimental studies were reported by DEINHARDT *et al.* in 1967 and yielded the following data. Sera from four patients with acute (presumably type A) hepatitis, and a known hepatitis inducing serum, and a control serum, were inoculated into small groups of marmosets and, although the monkeys did not become overtly ill, there was clear biochemical and morphological evidence of acute hepatitis. The biochemical evidence was based particularly on rises in serum of transaminase and dehydrogenase enzymes over 4—13 weeks after inoculation, and the morphological evidence on needle biopsy specimens of liver which showed changes quite similar to those of human infectious hepatitis (Fig. 9); these changes preceded the enzyme changes and persisted after them. Moreover transfer of acute-phase sera from marmoset to marmoset regularly reproduced hepatitis. In reviewing their experience, DEINHARDT'S group (1972) emphasized that 41 of 61 marmosets inoculated with hepatitis materials developed hepatitis as against none of 53 inoculated with control materials; moreover more than one hundred uninoculated control animals were subjected to prolonged observation and only one developed spontaneous hepatitis. DEINHARDT *et al.* (1972) therefore refuted earlier suggestions that their findings could be explained by activation of a latent

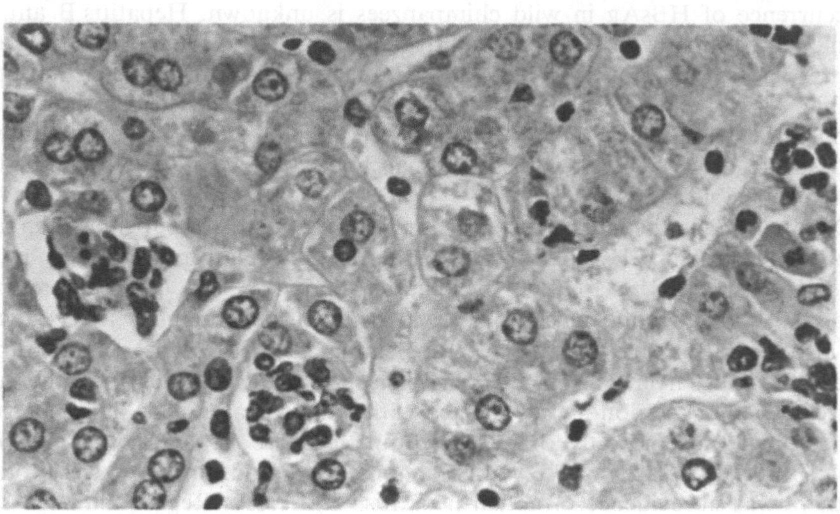

Fig. 9. Liver from marmoset infected with human infectious hepatitis virus (virus A) showing areas of focal hepatocellular necrosis. HE ×600. (By courtesy of Dr. F. DEINHARDT)

marmoset virus. Additional observations of importance included failure of infected marmosets to develop HBsAg, and non-susceptibility of marmosets to infection with HBsAg positive sera: these findings showed that the marmosets were susceptible specifically to hepatitis A virus. A further finding which is puzzling was that infected marmosets became resistant to a second infection with the same virus, but not necessarily resistant to a different isolate, indicative of strain variants of virus A.

Solid confirmation of Deinhardt's claims comes from a study in Costa Rica by MASCOLI *et al.* (1973) who intravenously inoculated 274 marmosets with blood from persons with hepatitis A or hepatitis B; only specimens from Type A hepatitis induced hepatitis. As final confirmation, HOLMES *et al.* (1973) showed that convalescent (presumably immune) sera from volunteers infected with Type A hepatitis (Krugman's MS-1 strain) were capable of neutralizing the infectious fractions of sera from subjects with Type A hepatitis; thus infectious sera with control material caused hepatitis in some 60–75% of inoculated marmosets whereas infectious sera mixed with convalescent serum caused hepatitis in only one of 20 inoculated marmosets, and in this monkey the incubation period was greatly prolonged.

3. Hepatitis B in Non-Human Primates

The WHO Scientific Group Report (1973) gives information on hepatitis B in primates. It notes that many attempts to transmit hepatitis B to primates initially yielded mostly negative results. However efforts were renewed when hepatitis B antigen and antibody were detected in serum of captive chimpanzees (6–12%), and also in orangoutangs and gibbons. Using sensitive radioimmunoassays, HBAg is said to be detectable in most captive chimpanzees, but these do not appear to develop a recognizable hepatitic illness, nor transmit hepatitis B to exposed humans, and the same holds for the orangoutang and gibbon. The frequency of occurrence of HBsAg in wild chimpanzees is unknown. Hepatitis B antibody is demonstrable in a wide variety of captive monkeys, the incidence in chimpanzees being 50%, and in other monkeys the frequency is about 10%. Although the possibility is not excluded that a different but related antigen elicits the anti HBs demonstrable in monkeys, the probability is very high that chimpanzees are infected, as a result of direct contact, with the human hepatitis B virus, and the *ad* subtype seems responsible.

Data relating to the infectivity of the human hepatitis B virus for the chimpanzee are presented in the WHO Report (1973), and in full detail in a study by BARKER and colleagues (1973b) (Fig. 10). Deliberately induced HBV infection resembles the disease in man quite closely. The biochemical abnormalities are equivalent. The histological changes in the liver are similar and HBAg is demonstrable in the cytoplasm of liver cells; acute phase plasmas are infectious for other chimpanzees, whether the donor was infected with human material or had a presumed natural infection. The only other susceptible primate is the rhesus monkey in which six serial passages of HBV was demonstrated, and antibody was produced, but there was no evidence of actual hepatitis. The WHO Report makes a strong point of the limitations imposed by the world shortage of non-human primates and the difficulties of using these for experiments relating to hepatitis B.

(a)

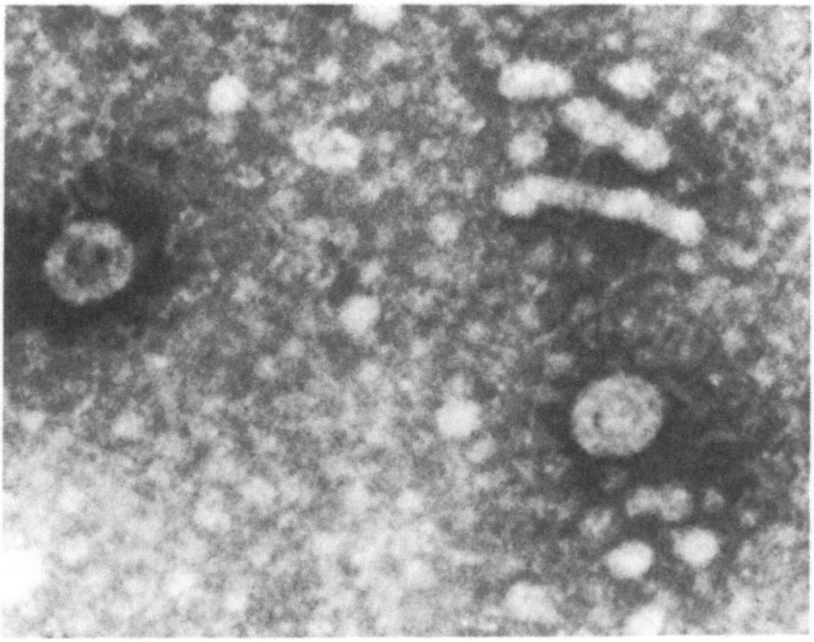

(b)

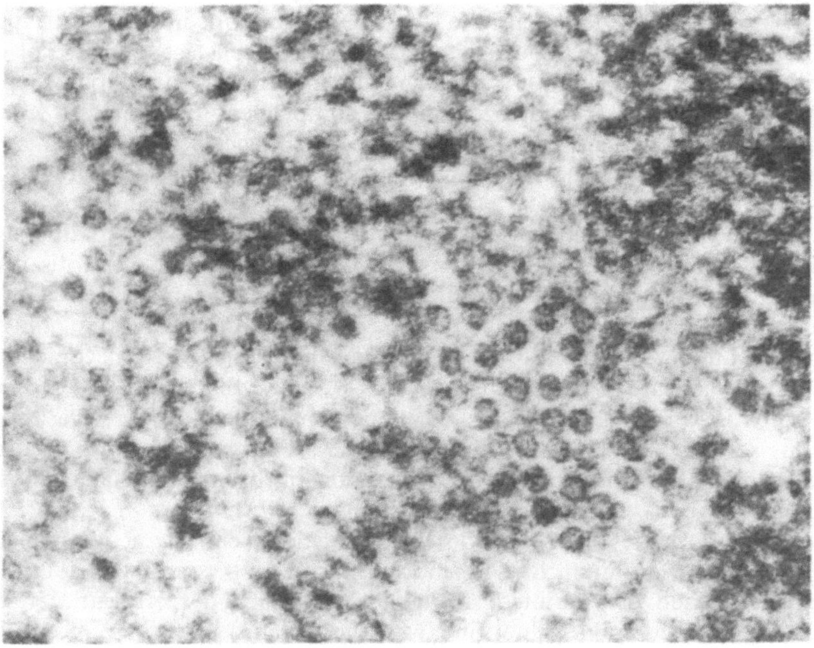

Fig. 10a and b. Electron micrograph preparations from chimpanzees infected with hepatitis virus B. (a) Serum showing HBAg as small particles, tubular structures and large double-shelled (Dane) particles (cf. Fig. 5). (b) Core particles in nucleoplasm of infected liver cell. × 125,000. (By courtesy of Dr. L.F. BARKER)

D. Liver Disease Associated with Autoimmune Reactions

I. History

The disease known today as chronic active hepatitis became recognized in the early nineteen fifties. Prior references exist (NEEFE, 1946), but such descriptions appear to have been protracted acute hepatitis. Increasing definition of the disease came after 1950 with the introduction to clinical practice of a number of new laboratory techniques, including electrophoresis, which disclosed the hypergammaglobulinaemia, liver biopsy, which showed the chronic inflammatory reaction in the liver, the LE cell test and other serological techniques, which indicated the underlying immune disturbance, and the transaminase test which as a "biochemical biopsy" allowed the activity of the disease to be assessed at will.

From 1950–1960 there were a number of clinical descriptions of chronic active hepatitis including those of WOOD *et al.* (1948) as "chronic virus hepatitis", WALDENSTROM (1950), KUNKEL and colleagues (1951) as an abstract, and later in 1956 as a detailed publication linking chronic hepatitis to collagen diseases (BEARN *et al.*, 1956), and SAINT and colleagues (1953) in a paper in which "active chronic hepatitis" was introduced in its present-day sense. The other major liver disease of immunological interest, primary biliary cirrhosis, was reviewed and designated as such by AHRENS *et al.* (1950) and this name replaced earlier ones including Hanot's cirrhosis, cholangiolitic cirrhosis, xanthomatous biliary cirrhosis and others. However this present name is still inappropriate in relation to the earlier non-cirrhotic stages of the disease, specified as "chronic non-suppurative destructive cholangitis" by RUBIN *et al.* (1965).

Immunological interest in chronic liver disease developed when JOSKE and KING (1955) observed a positive lupus erythematosus (LE) cell test in a case of chronic hepatitis, and MACKAY *et al.* (1956) introduced the concept of "lupoid hepatitis". GAJDUSEK and MACKAY recognized that a complement fixation test with tissue extracts served as an additional autoimmune serological marker, this becoming known as the autoimmune complement fixation (AICF) test (GAJDUSEK, 1958; MACKAY and GAJDUSEK, 1958; MACKAY and LARKIN, 1958), and positive results were obtained in systemic lupus erythematosus, chronic active hepatitis, and also in primary biliary cirrhosis (MACKAY, 1958). In 1961, lupoid hepatitis was cited as illustrating five "markers" of autoimmunity, and the concept was presented of "self-perpetuation" to explain the chronicity of certain diseases, including lupoid hepatitis (MACKAY, 1961). By 1963, immunofluorescence had become available as a clinical laboratory procedure, and this revealed that many cases of chronic active hepatitis in which LE cells were undemonstrable gave positive antinuclear reactions serologically (HOLBOROW *et al.*, 1963). Then it was shown by immunofluorescence that positive autoantibody reactions in primary biliary cirrhosis were due to an antibody reactive with mitochondria (WALKER *et al.*, 1965). Next, a further immunofluorescence reaction characteristic of chronic active hepatitis was discovered, that with an antigen in smooth muscle (JOHNSON *et al.*, 1966). Studies during this period also pointed strongly to a beneficial therapeutic effect from corticosteroid drugs and azathioprine (MACKAY, 1968a). The more recent developments in the history of chronic active hepatitis concern the recognition of subgroups, viz. that associated with hepatitis B antigen in serum, referred to in the previous Section (C.V.8), the prototype form associated with autoimmune features, and that associated with drug allergy, described in Section F; however it is still uncertain whether these subgroups represent different pathogenetic entities, either initially or in their later progression to chronicity (MACKAY and POPPER, 1973; MACKAY, 1974).

II. Autoimmune "Lupoid" Type of Chronic Hepatitis

1. Definition

This disease has been defined by the following criteria (MACKAY *et al.*, 1965).

a) Persistent activity for at least six months, usually with relapsing or continuing jaundice and/or elevated serum levels (200–1000 units) of transaminase enzymes.

b) Serum gamma globulin levels ranging from 2.0 to 10.0 g per 100 ml.

c) Histological features of perilobular "piecemeal" necrosis with disruption of the limiting plate of the lobule, hepatocellular regeneration, lymphoid-plasma cell infiltration, fibrosis and progression to cirrhosis.

d) Positive autoimmune type serological reactions, particularly to antigens of cell nuclei and smooth muscle.

e) Improvement with "anti-immune" drugs, including corticosteroids and azathioprine.

2. Clinical Features

The female: male disease incidence is about 4:1, and the age incidence is bimodal, with two peak incidences, in the 10–20 year decade and after age 60 (MACKAY, 1968b). The major symptoms are those of hepatitis (malaise, anorexia, jaundice, and bouts of right upper abdominal pain) (MACKAY and WOOD, 1962), but there may be few if any symptoms at all. Younger females show evidence of endocrine disturbance with amenorrhoea (sometimes the first symptom of the disease), striae and acne, attributable to impaired hepatic excretion of hormones. The liver is enlarged in the early stages but later becomes contracted and small. There may be many large spider naevi. Features of "multisystem disease" include arthralgia, and other autoimmune-type diseases may be present concurrently, or may supervene (*vide infra*). Splenomegaly in the early stages is attributable more to reticuloendothelial hyperplasia as part of the abnormal immune response than to portal hypertension, because the size of the spleen can fluctuate markedly according to the activity of the disease (MACKAY and WHITTINGHAM, 1967). The disease tends to progress to a cirrhotic stage with hepatic insufficiency and/or portal hypertension, but the tempo of this can be delayed or arrested by suppressive treatment (*vide infra*).

3. Biochemical and Haematological Features

The most characteristic biochemical feature is continuing or phasic elevations of blood levels of transaminase enzymes (O'BRIEN *et al.*, 1960), which presumably escape from damaged liver cells, and reflect the degree of hepatocellular necrosis. Transaminase levels are usually in the range of 200–1000 units during exacerbations (REYNOLDS *et al.*, 1964; MACKAY *et al.*, 1965). "Active" phases with hepatocellular necrosis are accompanied by other evidence of hepatic dysfunction including hyperbilirubinaemia, low serum albumin (< 3.0 g per 100 ml), increased retention of bromsulphalein (10–40% of injected dose in 45 min) and, as evidence of the abnormality in immune responses, gamma globulin levels up to 10.0 g per 100 ml. If necrosis stops and the transaminase level falls, as occurs after suppressive treatment, all of these indices revert synchronously towards normal (MACKAY, 1968a). The level of alkaline phosphatase may be mildly elevated, and the now obsolete flocculation tests of "liver function" give strongly positive results. Blood examination shows slight to moderate anaemia and leucopenia, and thrombocytopenia is seen particularly in patients with splenomegaly. Coagulation defects are late accompaniments attributable to impaired hepatic synthesis of clotting factors. An excess of plasma cells in the bone marrow in chronic liver disease was reported by JARROLD and VILTER (1949), and a "marked increase" in plasma cells in the marrow occurred in 15 of 17 patients with chronic active hepatitis, resembling multiple myeloma in two cases, according to HOENSCH and HARTWICH (1972).

4. Histopathological Features

No histological change can be specified as being characteristic of autoimmune chronic hepatitis, because of the long time-course and the gradual evolution from the acute to the chronic late stage of the disease. There is clustering of certain histopathological attributes in the early hepatitic or necrotic stage (GOLDSTEIN and MACKAY, 1967), i.e. perilobular necrosis, bridging necrosis, collapse, ballooned hepatocytes and infiltration of plasma cells, whereas the late cirrhotic stage is marked by fibrosis and nodulation, although some hepatitic changes will still be evident. The histological picture in the earliest stages may resemble that seen in slowly resolving acute infectious hepatitis, with hepatocellular necrosis, Councilman bodies as residues of necrosed liver cells, marked cellular infiltration in portal tracts and prominence of Kupffer cells together with numerous plasma cells.

Other histological features which are emphasized include hepatocellular damage, ballooning and necrosis in the periportal regions, called "piecemeal necrosis" (POPPER *et al.*, 1965), shown in Fig. 11, isolation of clumps of liver cells to form pseudoacinar structures, called "rosettes" (KLATSKIN, 1958; MISTILIS, 1968), dense lymphoid infiltrations including many plasma cells in portal areas, sometimes associated with lymph follicles with germinal centres (MACKAY, 1961), together with infiltration of plasma cells into the hepatic lobule around groups of liver cells, and hepatic cell "fallout" and "collapse", which may be of sufficient extent to involve the entire lobule (panlobular necrosis) or more than one lobule (submassive collapse) (MISTILIS, 1968). The areas of collapse tend to bridge portal areas, or portal areas and central veins, and fibrous strands, developing in association with these "collapse bridges" (BOYER and KLATSKIN, 1970), are the apparent precursors of the septa which determine architectural disorganization and nodular cirrhosis.

Cirrhosis tends to be established early in the disease. Thus in the series of 82 cases of chronic active hepatitis described by MISTILIS (1968), cirrhosis was present within one year in a third of the cases, the incidence rising to 90% of cases through the second to the eighth year of illness. It is a typical macronodular "post-necrotic" type cirrhosis, with broad fibrous bands enclosing large and small regenerative nodules (Fig. 12). The natural history, before present-day treatment

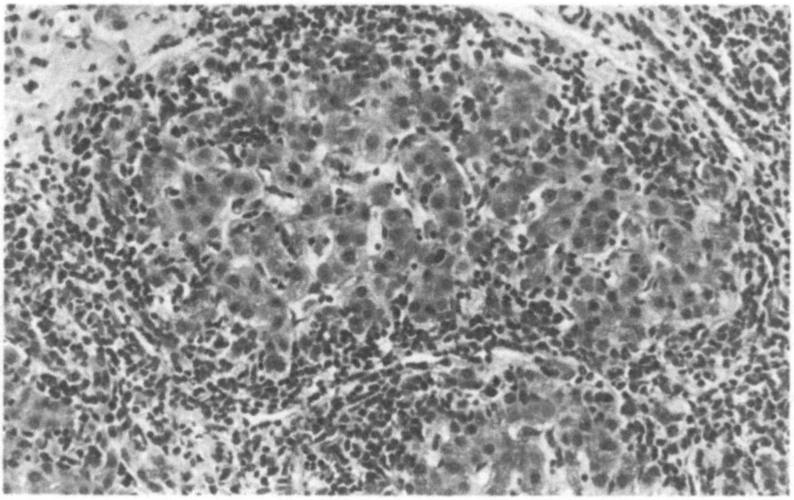

Fig. 11. Liver biopsy from woman aged 16 with typical autoimmune hepatitis: perilobular necrosis and dissection of lobule by invading immunocytes which are mostly plasma cells. HE ×300

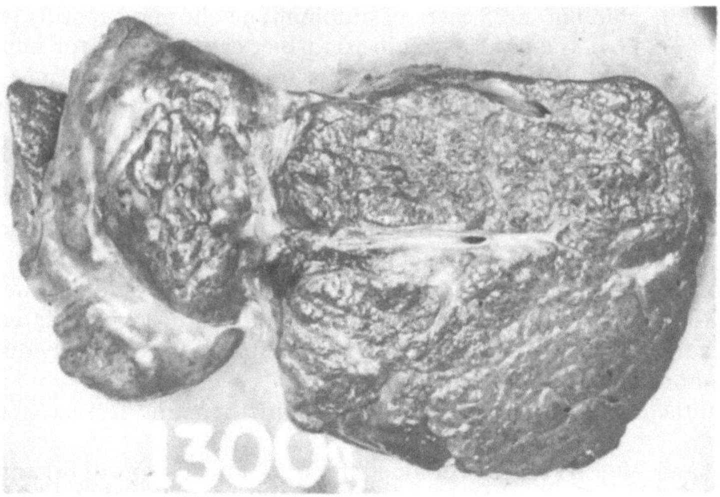

Fig. 12. Liver of woman aged 37 with autoimmune hepatitis showing coarse multilobular cirrhosis. (By courtesy of Editor of Postgraduate Medicine)

regimes, was for chronic active hepatitis usually to progress to liver failure (MACKAY, 1972b), but the disease occasionally became less active in time with spontaneous subsidence of necrosis and inflammatory reaction. With maintained suppressive treatment with corticosteroid drugs and azathioprine, there is recession of features of histological activity although full architectural restoration seldom occurs.

5. Hypergammaglobulinaemia and Humoral Autoantibodies

Hypergammaglobulinaemia and the serological demonstration of autoantibodies in the blood is a "hallmark" of autoimmune-type chronic active hepatitis; the major reactants are components of cell nuclei, smooth muscle and, less frequently, cell mitochondria (Fig. 13). The specificity of these autoantibodies for chronic liver disease is not fully defined because of (a) imperfect definition of the various chronic liver diseases (with the presence of autoantibody being used in itself as a diagnostic marker, as for mitochondrial antibody in primary biliary cirrhosis); (b) no standardisation of tissue substrates, reagents or methods for demonstration of autoantibodies (leading to wide variations in reported incidence of autoantibodies in various liver diseases); and (c) serological reactivity varying with phases of activity of the disease and response to treatment (*vide infra*). Also, there is no indication that the demonstrable autoantibodies are necessarily pathogenic and these may be no more than "markers" of immune aberration.

a) Hypergammaglobulinaemia. Raised levels of gamma globulin were the earliest recognized immunological anomaly in chronic hepatitis (KUNKEL *et al.*, 1951), with levels up to 10 g per 100 ml being reported (ZIMMERMAN *et al.*, 1951). Such increases are in contrast to levels in diffuse liver disease due to other causes, such as alcoholism. Studies in my clinic (MACKAY *et al.*, 1965; MACKAY, 1968b) on total gamma globulin in 25 cases of autoimmune chronic hepatitis gave a mean level of 3.3 (±S.D. 0.8) g per 100 ml; in 16 further cases studied for immunoglobulin classes, the serum levels per 100 ml were for IgG 3.57 g, for IgM 0.15 g and IgA 0.29 g, the latter two levels being only slightly elevated. Comparable data were reported by FEIZI (1968).

A further indication of immunoglobulin anomaly in chronic hepatitis is the occurrence of cryoglobulins and monoclonal proteins, the literature on which is discussed by ZLOTNICK *et al.* (1972) and ELIAKIM *et al.* (1972). These authors tabulated 19 cases of cryoglobulinaemia and, in most of the cases, the cryoprotein was of mixed type (IgG-IgM), representing an immune complex; the IgM component was more often monoclonal than polyclonal. A particular complication was the occurrence in several cases of glomerulonephritis, presumably due to deposition of immune complexes in the kidney.

The characteristic elevation of IgG in chronic hepatitis still lacks an accepted explanation.

TRIGER and WRIGHT (1973) examined this question in terms of (a) an abnormally reactive immune system, or (b) increased antigenic stimulation of a normal antibody-forming system. Under (a) would be included anomalies associated with autoimmunization, and the demonstrable autoantibodies would account, in part at least, for the hypergammaglobulinaemia. It cannot be said that the antibody-producing system is generally "hyperresponsive" in that deliberate antigenic challenge with test antigens of bacterial origin does not yield abnormally high antibody responses (CHERRICK *et al.*, 1959; LEE *et al.*, 1971). As an indication of increased stimulation of the immune system, there are in chronic hepatitis, increased titres of antibody (independent of known challenge) to dietary proteins (TRIGER *et al.*, 1972), gut associated bacteria (PROTELL *et al.*, 1971; BJORNEBOE, PRYTZ and ORSKOV, 1972), and measles and rubella viruses (TRIGER *et al.*, 1972). HENCE TRIGER and WRIGHT (1973) suggested that hyperglobulinaemia in liver disease is due to failure of the diseased liver to sequester antigens, either as a result of direct damage to Kupffer cells, or a bypassing of this cell system through a collateral circulation in the liver. But this seems quite unlikely as the sole explanation because the hyperglobulinaemia of chronic active hepatitis is most pronounced in earlier rather than later phases of the disease, and greatly exceeds that seen in conditions with equivalent hepatic disorganization, such as alcoholic cirrhosis. On the other hand, PRYTZ *et al.* (1973) showed that higher amounts of antibody to *E. coli* were demonstrable in alcoholic than in non-alcoholic cirrhosis.

A possibility not hitherto mentioned is that anti-idiotype antibody could account for the hyperglobulinaemia of chronic hepatitis. Immunoglobulin molecules themselves are known to expose new immunogenic determinants, antibodies to which are known as idiotypes. Thus once an immune response had been initiated in the liver the production of anti-antibody could result in a "cascade" reaction. Favouring this is the known occurrence in liver disease of antigamma-globulin reactivity (see under f. below).

b) Antibody to Cell Nuclei. This was first recognized in chronic hepatitis by the finding of positive tests for LE cells in two cases in Melbourne (JOSKE and KING, 1955), and the recognition of further cases gave rise to the term "lupoid hepatitis" (MACKAY *et al.*, 1956). However the LE cell reaction in chronic hepatitis, as contrasted with that in systemic lupus erythematosus (SLE), is likely to be "weaker" with fewer typical LE cells in the preparation, and more ephemeral, becoming negative with natural or therapeutically induced remissions (MACKAY *et al.*, 1965; SOLOWAY *et al.*, 1972a). The antinuclear reaction in chronic hepatitis was demonstrated in 1963 by immunofluorescence (HOLBOROW *et al.*, 1963), and this is now the conventional way of recognizing antinuclear autoantibodies in autoimmune chronic hepatitis.

In SLE there are different types of immunofluorescence reaction given by antinuclear antibodies including the "homogeneous" pattern given to antibody to nucleoprotein, the "shaggy" and "rim" patterns given by antibodies to DNA, and the "speckled" patterns given by antibodies to a soluble antigen referred to as SM (TAN, 1967); chronic hepatitis is associated with a narrower range of antinuclear antibodies in that only the "homogeneous" pattern is observed (Fig. 13). Also whereas in SLE reactivity to native double stranded DNA is characteristic, this in chronic hepatitis is most uncommon (HUGHES, 1973), the reactivity being only to single-stranded DNA (KOFFLER *et al.*, 1969). Finally there is a special nuclear specificity in chronic hepatitis, in that the antinuclear antibodies react to higher titre with the nuclei of polymorphonuclear leucocytes (PMNL) than with nuclei of lymphocytes or tissue cells (SMALLEY *et al.*, 1968), and there may be different reactivities with different tissue sources of nuclei (FABER and ELLING, 1967). Fluorescence tests using human blood smears are useful for demonstrating this differential nuclear reactivity in chronic hepatitis—and, as the titre of ANA against PMNL nuclei during activity may be extremely high, up to 10^8 and falls with remission, it is a useful marker of response (WHITTINGHAM, 1973). There are indications that the PMNL specific ANA can be responsible for development of LE cells in chronic hepatitis (SMALLEY *et al.*, 1968).

c) Antibody to Smooth Muscle (SMA). This is demonstrable by immunofluorescence, as described by JOHNSON *et al.* (1965), and has proved a most useful diagnostic marker, particularly as it is absent in SLE (WHITTINGHAM *et al.*, 1966). SMA is detectable using any mammalian source of smooth muscle, with rat stomach being suitable for routine diagnostic use (Fig. 13). SMA reacts also with smooth muscle in the wall of blood vessels, spleen, uterus, gut and elsewhere. SMA as demonstrated by immunofluorescence gives uniform staining of the entire cytoplasm; the antibody does not react by complement fixation or immunodiffusion, using smooth muscle extracts (WHITTINGHAM *et al.*, 1966).

The reactive antigen for SMA was recognized in tissues other than smooth muscle, e.g. the mesangium of the renal glomerulus, by WHITTINGHAM *et al.* (1966), and it now appears to be a very widely distributed tissue component. A filamentous immunofluorescence reaction was described between SMA and cells from fetal liver and lung grown as monolayers in culture (HOLBOROW, 1972), leading to the opinion that SMA reacts with an autoantigen resembling actinomyosin present as a contractile protein in the outer membrane of various cells. Also rabbit antisera raised to human platelets reacted with smooth muscle in a variety of sites (BECKER

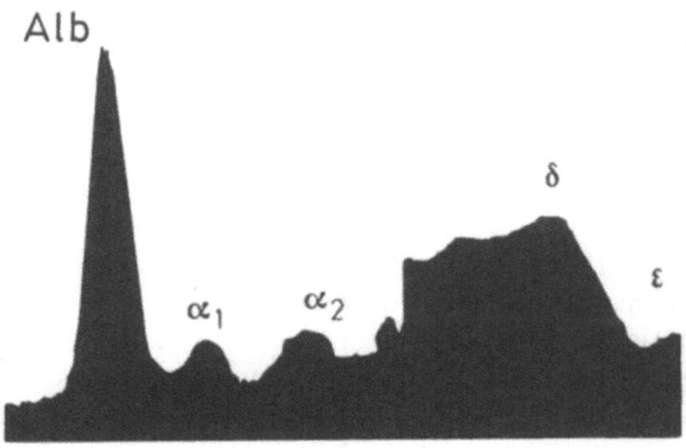

Fig. 13a

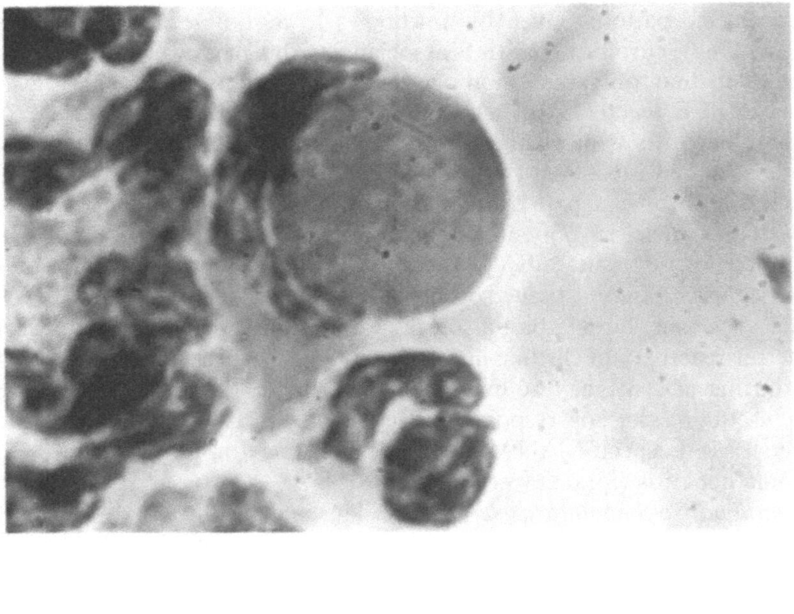

Fig. 13b

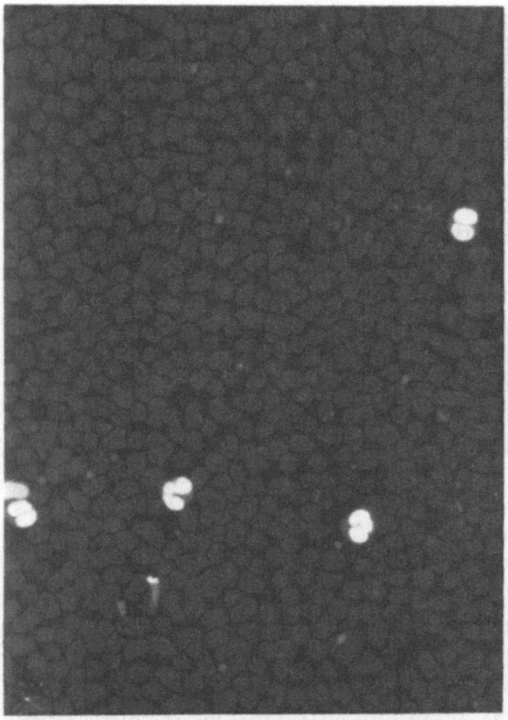

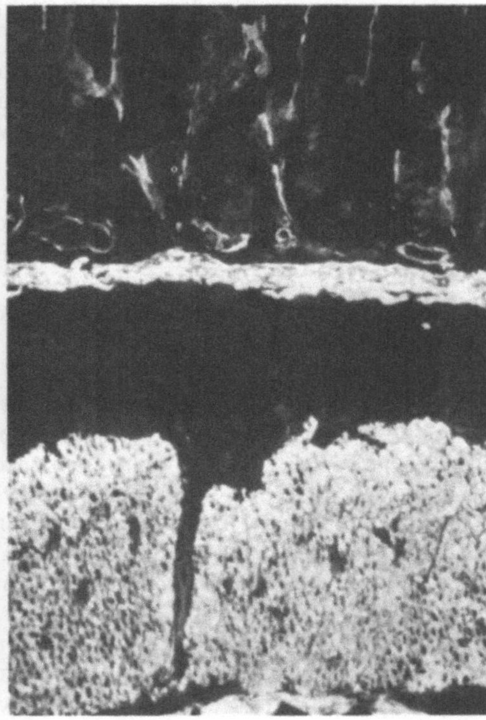

(d)

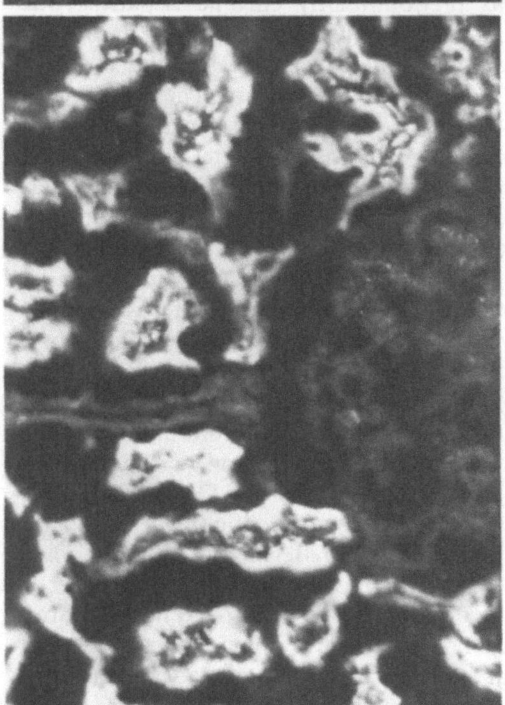

Fig. 13a—e. A montage illustrating the serological abnormalities of autoimmune hepatitis. (a) Moving boundary electrophoresis pattern from patient with "cirrhosis", redrawn from Stern and Reiner (1946). (b) Typical positive LE cell preparation from 55 year old woman with lupoid hepatitis. (c) Immunofluorescence reaction in chronic hepatitis for antinuclear antibody, using human blood film, illustrating granulocyte-specific antinuclear reaction. (d) Immunofluorescence reaction in chronic hepatitis illustrating reaction of serum with muscularis and muscularis mucosae of rat stomach. (e) Immunofluorescence reaction in primary biliary cirrhosis illustrating reaction of serum with mitochondria in proximal tubules of human kidney

and NACHMAN, 1973). Thus, although the mode of stimulation (immunogenesis) of SMA, and the reason for the specificity of SMA for hepatic disease, are uncertain, there are many possible sites of immunogenesis for SMA. These could include contractile proteins of hepatocyte membranes (*vide supra*), endothelial cells of liver sinusoids, or platelets, or possibly vessel walls or the smooth muscle present in the spleen.

According to GABBIANI *et al.* (1973), the reactivity of SMA can be absorbed out by lysed platelet extracts. The active component is a constituent of the contractile material of platelets, thrombosthenin, which contains actin. GABBIANI *et al.* (1973) claimed that SMA was in fact an antiactin antibody and that various "non-muscular" structures contained actin, notably platelets, hepatocytes, renal tubular cells, polymorphs, lymph node lymphocytes and fibroblasts. Thus the antigen of SMA is a very widely distributed tissue component.

d) Antibody to Mitochondria. This is more characteristic of cholangiolar than hepatic damage, and is described in the subsequent section on primary biliary cirrhosis (Fig. 13). The reported incidence in cases of chronic active hepatitis ranges from 11% (KLATSKIN and KANTOR, 1972) to 29% (DONIACH *et al.*, 1966), and it occurs especially in those cases of cirrhosis with "mixed" features of chronic hepatitis and primary biliary cirrhosis (DONIACH and WALKER, 1969).

e) Antibodies to Microsomes. In rare instances an antibody to microsomes demonstrable by immunofluorescence is present in chronic liver disease (RIZZETTO *et al.*, 1973). The tissues used to demonstrate the microsomal antibody included human and rat liver and kidney and certain other tissues. The underlying disease associated with microsomal antibody was predominantly chronic hepatitis, but of an unusual type in that males and females were equally represented and other of the characteristic serological markers of chronic hepatitis were lacking.

f) Complement-Fixing Antibodies to Cytoplasmic Components. These were recognized in liver disease in 1908 (NORUP, 1965) and were described by EATON *et al.* (1944) as occurring transiently in 30% of cases of acute hepatitis. The finding was made adventitiously by GAJDUSEK (1958) at the Hall Institute that a complement fixation reaction with fresh extracts of human liver and kidney was given by sera from patients with various chronic autoimmune diseases, notably SLE, lupoid hepatitis and primary biliary cirrhosis (see Section D.I). Subsequently, tissues from animals including rat (DONIACH *et al.*, 1966) and rhesus monkey (NORUP, 1965) were found to be equally reactive. The reactive cytoplasmic components included mitochondria, microsomes and a soluble cytoplasmic antigen (ASHERSON, 1959; DEICHER *et al.*, 1960). MACKAY and LARKIN (1958) reported an incidence of positive AICF reactions (titre >8) in cases of autoimmune chronic hepatitis of 27% (controls 3–4%), and comparable findings were reported by DONIACH *et al.* (1966) in London (30%) and NORUP (1967) in Denmark (30%). The AICF reaction in chronic hepatitis shows no tissue specificity, in particular for liver, but different reactive sera showed differing patterns of reactivity when tested against a panel of tissues (GAJDUSEK, 1958); however the pattern for a particular patient remained constant throughout the disease. Titres tended to drop in positivity after long remissions. The AICF reaction gave impetus to the concept of autoimmunity in chronic hepatitis but has now been superseded as a routine test by immunofluorescence, which is more convenient and discriminative.

It is uncertain whether the various anticytoplasmic autoantibodies demonstrable in liver disease are pathogenic, either directly or as components of antigen–antibody complexes; in fact, it was suggested that such antibodies could even be protective (WIEDERMANN and MIESCHER, 1965). A reaction analogous to AICF was demonstrated in rabbits after acute liver injury with carbon tetrachloride (WEIR, 1963), and within 12 weeks after experimental infection with pseudotuberculosis (THEWAINI and OAKLEY, 1967); in the latter study sera with high autoantibody titres were cytotoxic to cells in tissue culture. The possibility of cytotoxicity of sera containing autoantibodies relevant to human chronic hepatitis was examined by PARONETTO *et al.* (1973) using cell-lines derived from patients with liver diseases, particularly chronic active hepatitis. Although there was specific binding of serum to cells derived from liver, cytotoxic effects were not observed using a chromium release technique.

g) Antigammaglobulin Antibodies (Rheumatoid Factors). These were described in cirrhosis by HOWELL *et al.* (1960), and a high incidence of positive reactions with the latex test was reported by ATWATER and JACOX (1963); antigammaglobulin reactivity in liver disease is reported also by BONOMO *et al.* (1963) and BONOMO *et al.* (1966). We found that 14 of 28 patients with autoimmune chronic hepatitis reacted to a titre of 32 or greater in the sensitized sheep cell agglutination test (MACKAY *et al.*, 1965). It was shown in five of six cases of "post necrotic" cirrhosis, using fluorescein-labelled aggregated gammaglobulin, that lymphoid cells in the liver, including Kupffer cells, lymphocytes and plasma cells, were synthesizing rheumatoid factor (BONOMO *et al.*, 1966). Antiglobulins in serum in chronic liver disease were shown to exist as all three immunoglobulin classes, G, M and A (VISCHER and BÄNZIGER, 1972).

h) Coombs' Test. This was observed in 12% of cases of autoimmune chronic hepatitis (MACKAY *et al.*, 1965) with haemolysis occurring in some; however in this series no distinction was made between a "true" antiglobulin reaction and one due to complement adventitiously attached to the red cell surface. Coexistence of haemolytic anaemia and chronic hepatitis is cited in Section D.II.9.

i) Antibodies to Cardiolipin. These are responsible for the various serological tests for syphilis, and for the "false positive" tests for syphilis in diseases such as SLE. However these antibodies, rather surprisingly, are infrequently demonstrable in chronic hepatitis (MACLACHLAN *et al.*, 1965), despite the fact that the location of the reactive antigen in mitochondria is similar to that of the mitochondrial autoantibodies of primary biliary cirrhosis (DONIACH *et al.*, 1971).

j) Antibodies to "Thyrogastric" Antigens. These are autoantibodies to antigens of thyroid colloid, thyroid epithelial cell cytoplasm and gastric parietal cell cytoplasm; these autoantibodies "cluster" and "overlap" in autoimmune diseases of the thyroid gland and stomach (IRVINE *et al.*, 1962). The incidence in chronic active hepatitis of antibodies to thyroid cells was stated by DONIACH *et al.* (1966) to be significantly increased over that in matched controls, but not so in primary biliary cirrhosis and cryptogenic cirrhosis. However studies in my Unit (unpublished) have shown no increase in incidence over controls of organ specific thyroid or gastric antibodies in autoimmune liver disease.

k) Antibodies to Liver-Specific Antigens. Autoantibodies with specificity for liver cell components would have considerable theoretical significance for autoimmune concepts of pathogenesis of chronic hepatitis, if such were demonstrable. The presence has been shown in man and animals of liver specific antigens (SARGENT *et al.*, 1966; SCHUMACHER and SCHNEIDER, 1969; MEYER ZUM BÜSCHENFELDE and MIESCHER, 1972; ESPINOSA, 1973; SMITH and IVERSON, 1973), and there are claims that autoantibodies reactive with components of liver cell cytoplasm are demonstrable specifically in chronic hepatitis (SCHEIFFARTH *et al.*, 1965; SCHUMACHER, 1969); however it must be stated that organ-specific autoantibodies for liver are not readily demonstrable, at least by routine methods, as they are in immunopathic diseases involving other organ-systems. There are a few references to antibody in chronic hepatitis apparently reactive with bile canaliculi (JOHNSON *et al.*, 1966; DIEDERICHSEN, 1969; MACSWEEN *et al.*, 1973), as heteroantibody and as true autoantibody. Also, as possible evidence for the *in vivo* reactivity of autoantibody with liver antigen in chronic hepatitis, DAWKINS and JOSKE (1973) found that liver biopsy tissue of three patients gave reactivity with an anti-IgG fluorescein conjugate.

6. Serum Complement in Chronic Hepatitis

A reduced level of serum complement is an indicator of a given disease being due to an immunopathogenic process, and for a role of antigen-antibody complexes in tissue damage. For example, those types of glomerulonephritis due to deposition of immune complexes in glomeruli are associated with low levels of complement. No characteristic alterations have been found in levels of complement or complement-components in autoimmune chronic hepatitis, according to most reports. These include studies from my Clinic on total complement, cited by ASHERSON (1960) and MACKAY (1971), studies on beta 1C/1A in lupoid hepatitis by MUELLER-EBERHARD *et al.* (1970) and by FOX *et al.* (1971), although low levels were reported in cases of chronic active hepatitis by PAGALTSOS *et al.* (1972). Two groups, FINLAYSON *et al.* (1972), and POTTER *et al.* (1973), have reported detailed and definitive studies on levels of total complement and complement components in chronic active hepatitis. Thus chronic active hepatitis in the precirrhotic phase is not characteristically associated with marked lowering of complement components, and when such does occur it is more probably associated with poor synthetic function by the diseased liver rather than with the presence of autoantibodies.

7. Damage by Immune Complexes

The observations on levels of complement components, cited above, allow the conclusion that deposition of immune complexes in the liver would not be the usual cause of heptocellular damage in autoimmune-type chronic active hepatitis. However deposition of complexes of various autoantigens with antibody could account for extrahepatic manifestations of the disease, particularly the characteristic arthralgia. Also, deposits of gamma globulin have been identified in glomeruli by immunofluorescence in autoimmune chronic hepatitis (MACKAY, 1971) and such could account for associated renal lesions (SILVA *et al.*, 1965). Reference was made in Section D.II.5.a to cases of chronic hepatitis with mixed cryoglobulinaemia associated with IgG-IgM immune complexes; extensive lesions with purpura and neural damage were attributed to these complexes, together with glomerular deposits. It could be assumed that the IgM component of these complexes was an antibody to a determinant of IgG, possibly as an idiotypic response (see Section D.II.5.a).

8. Cell Mediated Immunity in Chronic Active Hepatitis

The earlier autoimmune serological studies in chronic hepatitis preceded the present era of interest in cell-mediated (T cell dependent) and humoral (B cell dependent) immune functions. For most autoimmune diseases, humoral autoantibodies could not be closely related to tissue damage, and this led to suppositions that tissue damage in such diseases would prove to be due to cell mediated activities, although proof of this has been difficult to obtain, and the mechanism(s) of autoimmune damage to solid tissues is still an open question.

a) Depressed General Cell-Mediated Immunity. Certain autoimmune diseases are characterized not only by autoantibodies to host antigens but also by depression of cellular reactivity to extrinsic antigens; primary biliary cirrhosis (see Section D.III.7) was the earliest disease to be studied in this context. In a comprehensive study on general cell-mediated immunity in autoimmune diseases (Toh *et al.*, 1973), there were included 24 cases of chronic active hepatitis. There was marked suppression of cell-mediated immune responses to a batch of five ubiquitous skin-test antigens, as compared with matched controls, and suppressive therapy could not be held entirely responsible for this finding. Correspondingly, patients with chronic hepatitis had depressed responsiveness of lymphocytes to the mitogen, phytohaemagglutinin (Toh *et al.*, 1973) although serum factors could be partly responsible for this (Newberry *et al.*, 1973). Toh *et al.* (1973) concluded that autoimmune-type hepatitis and other autoimmune conditions showed an immunological imbalance in the form of depressed cell-mediated immunity to extrinsic antigens and "hyperactive" humoral immune responses to self antigens and selected extrinsic antigens.

b) Augmented Specific Cell-Mediated Immunity. The methods available for testing of specific cell-mediated immunity (CMI) to autoantigens in man depend on demonstration of one or other effects of lymphokines, these being mediators released by activated T lymphocytes. There probably exist numerous lymphokines, each with a differing effect, although one particular lymphokine could have several different properties. Lymphokine effects are believed to determine (a) cutaneous delayed hypersensitivity reactions, (b) inhibition of migration of various indicator cells in capillary tubes, (c) lymphocyte-mediated cytotoxicity, (d) blastogenic transformation of cultured lymphocytes exposed to mitogen or antigen, and (e) slowing of macrophage migration in an electrophoretic field. The current status of these tests and their application to human disease are reviewed in a Progress Report (1973); few of the *in vitro* techniques have yet come into routine use in clinical immunology laboratories.

There are two reports (Tobias *et al.*, 1967; Warnatz, 1969) of transformation of peripheral blood lymphocytes on exposure to liver antigen in patients with chronic hepatitis and primary biliary cirrhosis, but these have not been further followed up.

The major findings of interest, as far as human autoimmune disease is concerned, have been obtained with the technique of SØBORG and BENDIXEN (1967), in which peripheral blood leucocytes are used as the source of both the reactive "sensitized" lymphocytes, and the migrating "indicator" cells, the latter including both granulocytes and monocytes. Applications of this test to various autoimmune diseases, of thyroid gland, adrenal gland, stomach and colon, are cited by BENDIXEN and NERUP (1971). Three groups have reported positive results in autoimmune liver disease. MEYER ZUM BÜSCHENFELDE *et al.* (1974), using liver-specific lipoprotein as antigen, obtained positive results in most of 34 cases of non-treated chronic active hepatitis, and in some cases of cirrhosis, but not in other types of liver disease, nor in treated chronic active hepatitis. MILLER *et al.* (1972), using liver specific lipoprotein as antigen, demonstrated leucocyte inhibitory activity in $^{11}/_{16}$ cases of chronic active hepatitis and $^{7}/_{12}$ cases of primary biliary cirrhosis, whilst BACON *et al.* (1972), using a whole liver cell extract as antigen, obtained positive results in 75% of 32 patients with either chronic hepatitis or primary biliary cirrhosis.

Cytotoxic activity of blood lymphocytes, as evidence of cellular immunity against autochthonous liver cells obtained by biopsy, was reported in two studies. PARONETTO and VERNACE (1975), assessing cytotoxicity visually, found this to be demonstrable in various types of chronic hepatitis, and in acute hepatitis, and there was no correlation with autoantibodies. WANDS and ISSELBACHER (1975), assessing cytotoxicity by chromium release, found that this could be demonstrable using as targets Chang liver cells and also autochthonous liver cells. In both studies, cytotoxicity was reduced by prednisolone treatment, and the authors felt that the findings indicated that liver cell destruction *in vivo* was caused by self-reactive lymphocytes.

9. Disease Associations in Chronic Active Hepatitis

The association or "clustering" of certain diseases has proven a useful pointer to autoimmunity as a systemically acting pathogenesis. Chronic hepatitis has been reported in coexistence with ulcerative colitis (GRAY *et al.*, 1958; HOLDSWORTH *et al.*, 1965), Hashimoto's thyroiditis (READ *et al.*, 1963), Graves' disease (THOMPSON and HART, 1973), haemolytic anemia (MACKAY *et al.*, 1965), fibrosing alveolitis of the lung (TURNER-WARWICK, 1968), Sjögren's disease (KROOK, 1961) and renal tubular acidosis, pulmonary diffusion defects and peripheral neuropathy (GOLDING and MASON, 1971; GOLDING *et al.*, 1973). Lupoid hepatitis was associated with a thymoma in one report (LINKE, 1965). Liver lesions are reported in rheumatoid arthritis (LANGNESS *et al.*, 1969) and Felty's syndrome (BLENDIS *et al.*, 1970), but these were more akin to non-specific reactive hepatitis. Autoimmune chronic hepatitis shares some features with SLE, but these diseases can be distinguished on several criteria, notably the absence in SLE of progressive hepatitis and smooth muscle antibody; there are, however, cases reported in which coexisting features of both diseases have made distinction impossible (BENNER *et al.*, 1968; FUNG *et al.*, 1969).

10. Genetic Aspects of Chronic Hepatitis

The relatively minor literature on presumed inherited and familial examples of cirrhosis and chronic hepatitis appears to discount any strong genetic component in autoimmune-type chronic hepatitis. The review of MADDREY and IBER (1964) cited previous literature and contributed eight cases of "familial cirrhosis" but autoimmune types of liver disease were not specifically considered. ELLING *et al.* (1966) examined 90 siblings of 38 cirrhotic probands, of whom 27 could have had autoimmune-type liver disease (post-hepatitic or cryptogenic cirrhosis); there were no instances of cirrhosis (on clinical criteria) in the relatives, although a higher than expected proportion had antinuclear factor (22%) and rheumatoid factor (17%), perhaps indicative of a familial tendency to autoimmune reactivity. A similar conclusion could be drawn from the occurrence of a greater mean level of gamma globulin in 31 maternal relatives of a proband with lupoid hepatitis (CAVELL and LEONHARDT, 1965), and from the excess occurrence of serological abnormalities in 28 relatives of 9 patients with lupoid hepatitis (MACLACHLAN *et al.*, 1965). Mixed autoimmune diseases have been described in kindreds, exemplified by lupoid hepatitis and myasthenia gravis (WHITTINGHAM *et al.*, 1970), and by a remarkable kindred in which five members had autoimmune-type hepatitis and cirrhosis and eight others had various abnormal autoimmune serological reactions (JOSKE and LAURENCE, 1970).

A possibly important clue was provided by the association of autoimmune-type hepatitis with histocompatibility antigens HL-A1 and 8 (MACKAY and MORRIS, 1972), later corroborated in two further studies (FREUDENBERG *et al.*, 1973; GALBRAITH *et al.*, 1974a; PAGE *et al.*, 1975); in the latter study there was an increased frequency of homozygosity for HLA-8. Histocompatibility antigens are known to be linked with immune responsiveness in animals, and are associated with certain immunopathogenic diseases in man. The coexistence of HL-A1 and 8, possibly as the haplotype 1, 8, was considered by MACKAY and MORRIS (1972) to predispose to the production of lymphocytes, presumably T lymphocytes, capable of being stimulated by self antigens, particularly if a minor somatic mutation (ineffective in other genotypes) had occurred. This genotype was assumed to be associated with high responsiveness to microbial and viral antigens, conferring "compensatory" survival advantages, and might account for raised levels of antibody to microbial antigens in chronic hepatitis (Section D.II.5.a), and could be linked with the occurrence of immunoglobulin abnormalities in relatives of patients with chronic hepatitis.

11. Anti-Immune Drugs in Treatment of Chronic Hepatitis

Certain drugs are known to influence the impact of cellular or humoral antibody on target tissues, and others to modify immune function by cellular suppression. These include "anti-inflammatory" drugs of which prototypes are aspirin and phenyl butazone, the corticosteroid drugs of which the prototype is prednisolone, and immunosuppressive drugs exemplified by azathioprine, cyclophosphamide and methotrexate. Such drugs, particularly prednisolone and azathioprine, have proved to be effective in suppressing disease activity in autoimmune chronic active hepatitis.

This has important implications—practical, in providing better treatment and improving the survival—and theoretical, in providing evidence for chronic hepatitis being due more to the response of the host than the activity of any extrinsic pathogenic agent. Historical aspects relating to the use of anti-immune drugs in chronic active hepatitis were summarized by MACKAY (1972a).

The effectiveness of corticosteroids in chronic hepatitis was controversial until publication of three well controlled trials (cited by MACKAY, 1972a) showing that corticosteroids not only suppressed biochemical evidence of disease activity (O'BRIEN *et al.*, 1960), but led to better survival. The mode of action of corticosteroid drugs in ameliorating immunopathic disease is still not clear, but possible actions in chronic active hepatitis were described by MACKAY and WOOD (1963) as follows. (a) They diminish the effectiveness of cell-bound antibody in damaging target cells, presumably by reducing the increase in permeability that would otherwise result. (b) They diminish the effectiveness of autoantigens in stimulating immunologically competent cells capable of producing γ-globulin. (c) As a result of (a), they diminish the amount of autoantigen available as a stimulus to antibody-producing cells. As a practical point, POWELL and AXELSEN (1972) showed that the conversion of prednisone to the biologically active form prednisolone is incomplete in severe liver disease, and hence prednisolone is the corticosteroid of choice.

Cytotoxic immunosuppressive drugs began to be used in clinical therapy around 1960 as awareness developed of immunopathogenic causes of disease, and their use increased as the effectiveness of azathioprine became apparent in rejection of organ transplants. Azathioprine came into increasing usage in chronic hepatitis in the early 1960's, and a comparative study by MACKAY (1968a) of groups of 15 patients treated with either prednisolone or azathioprine showed that both drugs were effective in maintaining remission over a three year period of treatment, with prednisolone being in some respects superior to azathioprine. The combination of prednisolone and azathioprine is at least as effective as either alone (SOLOWAY *et al.*, 1972b; MURRAY-LYON *et al.*, 1973), and lower doses of both drugs can be used. Observations on patients with chronic hepatitis treated for 3 year periods with anti-immune drugs indicate that their effect is more usually suppressive than curative in that relapse tends to occur after drugs are withdrawn (MACKAY, 1972b).

III. Autoimmune Cholangitis and Primary Biliary Cirrhosis (PBC)

1. Definition

Primary biliary cirrhosis can be defined as a chronic diffuse liver disease with persistent jaundice of obstructive type with patent extrahepatic bile ducts, obliterative damage to intrahepatic biliary ductules, and progression to a biliary-type cirrhosis.

2. Clinical Features

The disease spectrum of primary biliary cirrhosis ranges from an early stage, which can be designated as autoimmune cholangitis, to a terminal hepatic cirrhosis. The disease occurs predominantly in women of middle age (40—60 years), and the early features are determined by obstruction to the outflow of bile, bile salts and cholesterol, resulting in jaundice and itchiness of the skin. The later features are determined by (a) malabsorption and vitamin deficiencies, including osteomalacia due to vitamin D deficiency, (b) deposition of lipid in tissues including skin, producing xanthomas, and (c) progression over 5—7 years to cirrhosis with portal hypertension and hepatic failure.

3. Biochemical Features

These include persistently and highly raised levels in serum of alkaline phosphatase particularly, bilirubin and usually cholesterol. Levels in blood of hepatocellular enzymes (transaminases) are only moderately raised, to 100—200 units.

4. Histological Features

In the earlier stages the appearances are those of chronic cholangitis with lymphoid aggregates in portal areas, particularly surrounding damaged biliary ductules and sometimes showing lymph follicle formation (WILLIAMS, 1965), together with concentric periductular fibrosis and bile duct necrosis (Fig. 14); this precirrhotic stage was termed "chronic non-suppurative destructive cholangitis" by RUBIN *et al.* (1965), and could also be referred to as "autoimmune cholangitis". There is usually some degree of hepatocellular damage, usually periportal, but the prominent "piecemeal" necrosis seen in chronic active hepatitis is lacking, except in those infrequent cases in which features of both diseases coexist. In the later stages, bile ductules disappear, being replaced by pseudoductular structures, fibrosis becomes more prominent, and cirrhosis slowly develops. The exact mechanism of cirrhosis is not well defined, but, as in other chronic hepatitides, may be via formation of "collapse bridges" between portal tracts. Sarcoid-like granulomata may be a prominent feature in the early stages (GOUDIE *et al.*, 1966), and there is a report in which sarcoidosis appeared to coexist with primary biliary cirrhosis (STANLEY *et al.*, 1972).

5. Hypergammaglobulinaemia and Humoral Autoantibodies

a) Hypergammaglobulinaemia. There is a raised level of gamma globulin which, in contrast to chronic active hepatitis, is mostly of IgM class; the level of IgM is in the range of 200—600 mg per 100 ml (FEIZI, 1968).

b) Antibody to Mitochondria. This autoantibody was detected initially by complement fixation using whole tissue homogenates (MACKAY, 1958), and is specifically reactive with mitochondria by complement fixation (DONIACH and WALKER, 1972). The immunofluorescence procedure for mitochondrial (M) antibody was introduced by WALKER *et al.* (1965), and this is now the preferred technique, with fresh human kidney being a convenient source of antigen (Fig. 13). WALKER *et al.* (1965) emphasized the extremely high incidence (100% of 32 patients) and specificity for PBC of the immunofluorescence reaction for mitochondrial antibody, and particularly its absence in extrahepatic biliary obstruction, and the non-organ-specificity of the reaction. The incidence of mitochondrial antibody in PBC in

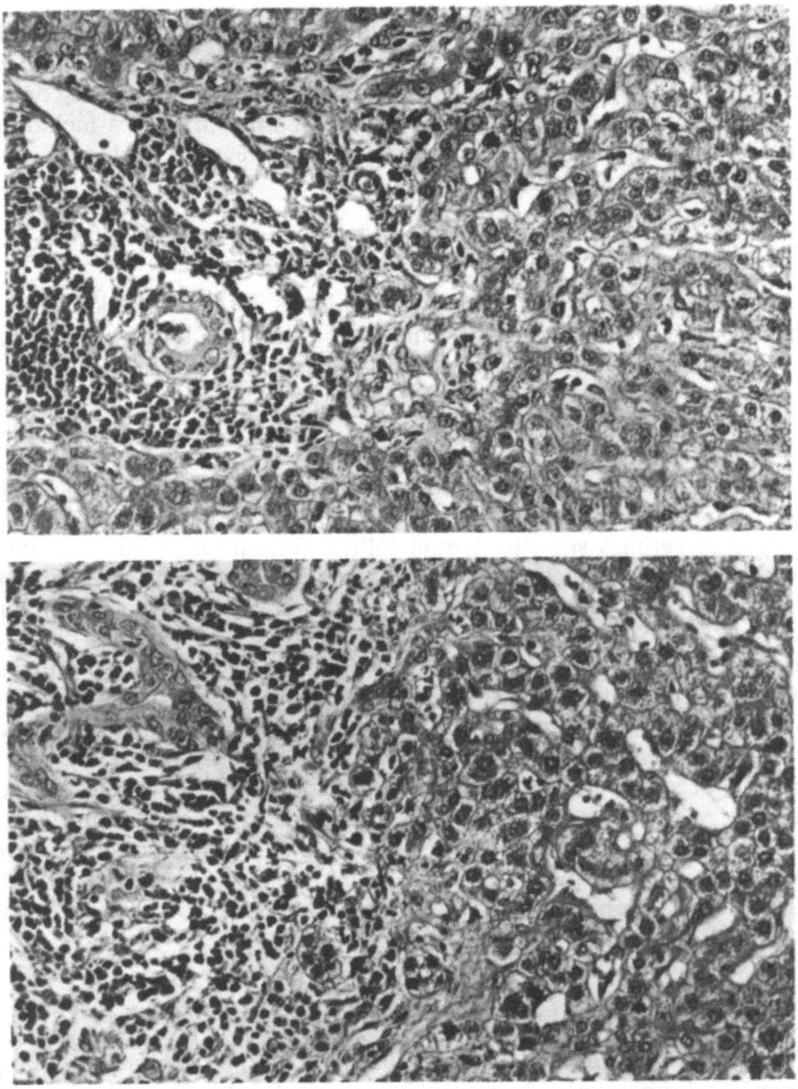

(a)

(b)

Fig. 14a and b. Lesions of primary biliary cirrhosis. (a) Early lesion showing enlarged portal tract with lymphoid cells surrounding a damaged bile duct. HE ×240. (b) Late lesion showing portal tract affected by chronic inflammation with absence of bile ducts and with formation of pseudoductules. HE ×240

other reports has ranged from 79% (PARONETTO *et al.*, 1967) to 87% (GOUDIE *et al.*, 1966); there appeared to be no apparent clinical or histological differences between the usual seropositive and the rare seronegative cases of primary biliary cirrhosis (GOUDIE *et al.*, 1966). In a recent comprehensive report on 188 patients with PBC by KLATSKIN and KANTOR (1972), the incidence of positive M antibody reactions in 188 patients was 84%.

The class of mitochondrial antibodies in primary biliary cirrhosis is IgM (PARONETTO *et al.*, 1967), consistent with the raised level of serum IgM.

Mitochondrial antibody has high but not absolute specificity for the disease PBC. Considering firstly liver diseases other than PBC, there is the practical question of diagnosis of intra versus extra hepatic biliary obstruction. Earlier studies (WALKER *et al.*, 1965) led to the belief that mitochondrial antibody did not occur in extrahepatic biliary obstruction. KLATSKIN and KANTOR (1972) reported a positive reaction in 4 (2%) of 180 cases of extrahepatic obstruction, resulting in all from biliary cancer. By contrast, LAM *et al.* (1972) claimed that positive immunofluorescence tests for mitochondrial antibody were obtainable in some three-fourths of 21 patients with chronic extrahepatic biliary obstruction of various types, in some cases to titres of 1:5000. Also KAPLOWITZ *et al.* (1973) cited seven patients in whom mitochondrial antibody was present with extrahepatic obstruction due to gall stones (4), ampullary strictures (2) and carcinoma (1), but in some of these cases the condition causing the obstruction may have developed after the onset of parenchymal liver diseases. However there is a problem in the interpretation of the two latter studies in that heterologous (rat) kidney was used and certain human sera contain a heteroantibody to rat tissues which simulates but is unrelated to the mitochondrial antibody reaction of primary biliary cirrhosis. Hence apparently positive fluorescence tests for mitochondrial antibody with rat tissue should be checked using a human tissue, e.g. human kidney (WHITTINGHAM, 1974).

The reported occurrence of mitochondrial antibody in chronic active hepatitis varies; cited incidences are 7% (GOUDIE *et al.*, 1966), 11% (KANTOR and KLATSKIN, 1972), and 5% (WHITTINGHAM, 1974), with the 28% incidence reported by DONIACH *et al.* (1966) being relatively high. In cryptogenic cirrhosis the reported incidence of M antibody has ranged from 6% (KLATSKIN and KANTOR, 1972) to 31% (DONIACH *et al.*, 1966). Claims that mitochondrial antibody is present in allergic liver injury (Section F.VI) require confirmation. KAPLOWITZ *et al.* (1973) reported on 45 positive tests for M antibody, and grouped these according to diagnoses of primary biliary cirrhosis (22 cases), extrahepatic biliary obstruction (7 cases, *vide supra*), and other liver diseases, mostly chronic active hepatitis and cryptogenic cirrhosis (16 cases). It is well recognized that some patients, usually elderly women, with "cryptogenic" cirrhosis give positive tests for M antibody, and these presumably represent a latent or terminal phase of PBC (DONIACH and WALKER, 1969, 1972).

"True" mitochondrial antibody occurs in some non-hepatic autoimmune diseases in low frequency (1–5%) according to DONIACH and WALKER (1972), such diseases including thyrogastric autoimmune disease, myasthenia gravis, autoimmune haemolytic anaemia and rheumatoid arthritis, and in somewhat higher frequency in SLE (5%) and Sjogren's disease (8%); a similarly high incidence of antimitochondrial antibody in Sjogren's syndrome (10 of 171 cases) was reported by WHALEY *et al.* (1973). Antimitochondrial antibodies associated with a "lupus-like" disease were demonstrated by complement fixation in 21 cases (20 men and one woman) by MAAS and SCHUBOTHE (1973), and in six cases by BERG *et al.* (1973); here again, it must be noted that rat kidney, which contains a heteroreactive antigen, was used to demonstrate this antibody.

The antigenic site for reactivity of M antibody was studied in detail by BERG *et al.* (1967), using subcellular fractions isolated by differential centrifugation and marker enzymes, and examination of mitochondria fragmented by various methods. The reactive antigen was associated with mitochondrial membranes, particularly the inner membranes, and antigenic activity was shown to depend upon an association of a protein component of the inner membrane with a phospholipid.

c) Antibody to Cell Nuclei. This antibody, demonstrable by immunofluorescence, occurred in 24% of 100 cases of PBC, and in 8% in titres above $^1/_{80}$ according to DONIACH and WALKER (1972). Moreover these authors stated that antinuclear-positive cases tended to be those in which the mitochondrial antibody is lacking; also, some half of the antinuclear reactions in PBC were of the speckled type.

d) Antibody to Smooth Muscle. This antibody was demonstrable by immunofluorescence in a high proportion, 49%, of 100 cases of PBC, and in high titre, above $^1/_{80}$, in 8%, according to DONIACH and WALKER (1972).

e) Antibody to Cell Cytoplasm. Mitochondria are one of the reactants in complement fixation tests using cell cytoplasm, this being the means by which mitochondrial antibody was first demonstrated (Section D.I); the incidence of reactivity in PBC is 83% (DONIACH and WALKER, 1972), similar to that using immunofluorescence.

f) Other Antibodies. PBC does not appear to be associated with any broad autoimmune serological disturbance, in that rheumatoid factors, anti-erythrocyte antibodies, and anti-platelet antibodies have received no comment in the literature. It is difficult to assess organ-specific thyroid and gastric antibody in PBC by immunofluorescence, as the mitochondrial reaction obscures other reactivities; the incidence of thyroid antibody was increased in PBC, but not significantly so (DONIACH *et al.*, 1966).

g) Bile-Duct Specific Antibodies. Specific reactivity of serum in PBC and other liver diseases with an antigen in newly regenerated biliary ducts has been claimed (PARONETTO *et al.*, 1964), but there have been no subsequent reports to confirm this.

6. Serum Complement

Increased mean values for total complement were reported by POTTER *et al.* (1973), and were attributed to an effect of biliary duct obstruction.

7. Cell-Mediated Immunity

a) Depressed General Cell-Mediated Immunity. Primary biliary cirrhosis is associated with general anergy to extrinsic antigens known to elicit cell-mediated immune reactions—indeed PBC was the first autoimmune disease shown to have this association. The initial findings of FOX *et al.* (1969) were that patients with PBC had depressed cutaneous reactivity to tuberculin and dinitrochlorobenzene (DNCB) and showed depressed lymphocyte responses to the mitogen PHA. FOX *et al.* (1973) reinvestigated this problem using haemocyanin to elicit delayed hypersensitivity skin reactions. Earlier findings with tuberculin and DNCB were corroborated, and five of nine patients failed to develop sensitivity to haemocyanin. The cause and significance of this impaired T cell function in PBC, and in other autoimmune disorders, is unknown.

b) Specific Cell-Mediated Immunity. To examine positive cell-mediated immunity to autoantigens in PBC, studies have been done with cell mitochondria which are the known reactant in tests for humoral autoantibody. Positive reactions were reported by BROSTOFF (1970), using the *in vitro* leucocyte migration inhibition (LMI) assay of SØBORG and BENDIXEN (1967) with liver mitochondria as antigen.

It was found by MILLER *et al.* (1972) and BACON *et al.* (1972) that leucocytes of patients with chronic active hepatitis and PBC were equally reactive in the LMI test when liver lipoprotein or whole liver extract was used as antigen; this is surprising as the two diseases are dissimilar, despite some overlap. However pronounced inhibition using liver mitochondria was likewise obtained in cases of autoimmune (Hashimoto) thyroiditis and thyrotoxicosis, and even after tissue damage (myocardial infarction), according to WARTENBERG *et al.* (1973). Thus the humoral immune reactivity with mitochondria, which is highly but not absolutely specific for PBC, appears not to have a correspondingly specific cellular immune counterpart.

A protein fraction of human bile was used as antigen in the LMI test in primary biliary cirrhosis; 8 of 10 cases of PBC gave a positive result (EDDLESTON *et al.*, 1973). The inference was that the autoimmunogen in PBC is present as a normal constituent of bile, with a possible origin from bile duct epithelial cells.

8. Disease Associations

The suggestion that primary biliary cirrhosis was a "multisystem" disease was made by MACKAY (1960) in reporting a case of PBC with associated diseases, interstitial nephritis and chronic gastritis. Although cases of PBC coexisting with other autoimmune disorders are infrequently reported, attention can be directed to the association between Sjögren's disease (sicca complex) and PBC. Examples were cited by GOLDING *et al.* (1970), and the association was further documented by ALARCÓN-SEGOVIA *et al.* (1973) and WHALEY *et al.* (1973). ALARCÓN-SEGOVIA and colleagues studied 14 cases of PBC using a range of tests capable of demonstrating salivary gland insufficiency; seven patients had ocular symptoms, seven showed histological abnormalities on labial biopsy, and three had antibodies to DNA. Other reported associations with PBC include scleroderma (MURRAY-LYON *et al.*, 1970; REYNOLDS *et al.*, 1971) and renal tubular acidosis (GOLDING and MASON, 1971).

9. Hepatitis B Antigen

The role of hepatitis B virus in primary biliary cirrhosis has evoked a considerable literature most of which is cited in a paper by MACSWEEN and associates (1973); surprisingly, however, there is omission of reference to the paper (KROHN *et al.*, 1970) making the strongest claims for a pathogenetic role of HBV in PBC. Consensus of opinion would be that of MADDREY *et al.* (1972) which is that when HBsAg is present in PBC, it is coincidental, and irrelevant to pathogenesis.

10. Genetic Determinant of PBC and Mitochondrial Antibody

Family studies in various autoimmune diseases have disclosed an increased incidence of both the relevant disease, and/or the relevant tissue antibodies, in close relatives of affected propositi. This holds particularly for thyrogastric autoimmune disease (DONIACH *et al.*, 1965) and to a lesser degree for systemic lupus erythematosus (LEONHARDT, 1961; LARSEN, 1972). There are two relevant reports, from the same source (FEIZI *et al.*, 1972; WALKER *et al.*, 1972) on familial occurrences of PBC and mitochondrial antibody. One report described a family with clustering of mitochondrial and other antibodies, together with liver disease diagnosed as PBC in five sisters. The other report described clinical and immunological studies on 126 close relatives of 27 patients with PBC. Mitochondrial antibodies were found in 7% of healthy relatives, and in none of the matched controls, and other autoantibodies (to smooth muscle, nuclei and other antigens) showed clustering in certain of the families. These observations imply strongly that there is a genetic factor in the pathogenesis of PBC but, as with other genetically determined immunopathies, the nature of this is obscure. Despite the sharing of "seroimmunologic abnormalities" among relatives of patients with chronic active hepatitis and PBC (GALBRAITH *et al.*, 1974b), the prevalence of histocompatibility antigen HL-A8 is not increased in PBC as it is in chronic active hepatitis.

E. Experimental Models of Chronic Hepatitis

I. Immune Induction of Chronic Liver Disease

The existence of an appropriate immunological model in an animal is usually taken as evidence for immunopathy as the cause of the analogous spontaneous disease in man. Experimental models of autoimmune disease are of two types, those induced by special immunizing procedures, e.g. thyroiditis in guinea pigs, rabbits and other animals by injection with thyroglobulin in Freund's complete adjuvant (FCA), and those which are naturally occurring in special strains of animals, e.g. autoimmune haemolytic anaemia and "lupus-like" disease of New Zealand mice.

1. Immunization with Liver in Freund's Complete Adjuvant

Despite many attempts in various species, a self sustaining experimental autoimmune hepatitis has proved difficult to induce by immunization with liver extract in FCA, even though species-specific and organ-specific hepatic antigens do exist (SARGENT *et al.*, 1966). BEHAR and TAL (1959) gave one injection of homologous liver in adjuvant into guinea pigs and hamsters and produced liver lesions mostly in the younger animals, but these were of necrotic character and unlike those of human chronic hepatitis, and serological studies were not done. JOHNSON *et al.* (1963) injected rat liver in FCA into rabbits and produced autoantibodies reactive with autologous liver *in vitro* by immunofluorescence, but these antibodies did not bind to the rabbit's liver *in vivo*, and liver lesions were not described. SOERGEL and FRIEDELL (1964) gave single and multiple injections of guinea pig liver in FCA into guinea pigs, but failed to induce liver lesions except for adjuvant granulomas, nor were produced autoantibodies specific for liver. DOBIAS and BALAZS (1967a) injected rabbits with homogenates of rat organs (liver, kidney, heart) in Freund's incomplete adjuvant, and obtained evidence of a hepatitic response, shown biochemically by transaminase elevations, histologically by necrosis and fibrosis, and serologically by production of autoantibodies; in a further study by DOBIAS and BALAZS (1967b), rats which were injected with a rabbit antiserum reactive with rat liver mitochondria developed changes in the liver similar to those in the actively immunized rabbits. Although DOBIAS and BALAZS (1967b) considered that immune reactions were responsible for some of the observed liver damage, the lesions which they illustrated in their papers did not appear to resemble those of chronic active hepatitis in man.

SCHEIFFARTH *et al.* (1967) induced a chronic hepatitis in mice by repetitive immunization with homologous mouse liver in FCA, and likened the disease to the classical diseases (of brain and thyroid) induced by this procedure. In a subsequent study (WARNATZ *et al.*, 1975), lymph node and spleen cells from liver-immunized mice showed specific cytotoxicity for syngeneic liver cells, and it was claimed that lymphocytes could be "educated" *in vitro* for acquisition of cytotoxicity.

Progress in this area has been made by Meyer zum Büschenfelde and colleagues (MEYER ZUM BÜSCHENFELDE *et al.*, 1972; MEYER ZUM BÜSCHENFELDE and MIESCHER, 1972). They have described the extraction and characterization, by differential centrifugation and gel filtration on Sephadex, of two proteins extractable from the cytoplasm of human liver cells, one a stable protein and the other an unstable membrane lipoprotein; both were immunogenic in rabbits, yielding reactive antisera. Immunization of rabbits with a preparation containing these proteins induced a chronic hepatitis which, as illustrated, resembled human autoimmune-type progressive chronic hepatitis which was claimed to persist even 3–5 months after the last immunization injection (Fig. 15). However, it should be noted (a) that a heterologous system was used (human liver into rabbit), and (b) that a very intense schedule of repetitive immunizations appeared necessary, extending over several months.

In continuing studies on this model (HOPF and MEYER ZUM BÜSCHENFELDE, 1974; MEYER ZUM BÜSCHENFELDE and HOPF, 1974), there was further documentation of chronic hepatitic lesions and a suggestion that lesions were mediated by antibody-dependent lymphocyte cytotoxicity.

2. Damage by Allogeneic Cells

Graft versus host (GVH) reactions in animals are held to represent models of human autoimmune disease (STASTNY *et al.*, 1965), in the sense that the lymphoid cell behaves as a pathogenic agent. There are reports of focal lesions in the liver occurring in GVH reactions (cited by MACKAY, 1971), but these are not a major feature, and could be attributed to infection. GVH disease as it affects the liver was rejected as a useful model of autoimmune hepatitis in man by NOUZA and BOHM (1966).

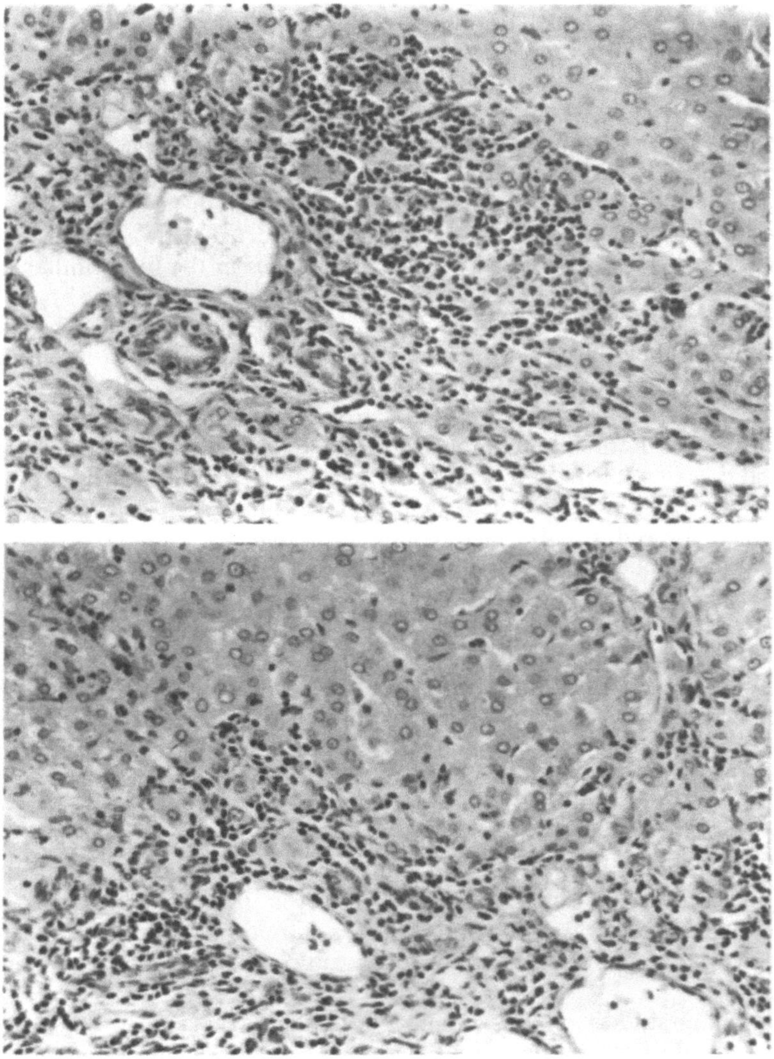

(a)

(b)

Fig. 15a and b. Experimental chronic hepatitis. Sections of liver from two rabbits given repetitive immunization of liver specific lipoprotein from human liver. Specimens obtained after five months of immunization. There is portal inflammation, periportal necrosis and incipient cirrhosis. HE ×400. (By courtesy of Dr. K.-H. MEYER ZUM BÜSCHENFELDE)

3. Damage by Antigen-Antibody Complexes

Acute liver damage was induced in rabbits by injection into the portal vein of soluble complexes of human serum albumin and homologous antibody (STEINER, 1961), and in rats by retrograde injection via the bile duct of antigen-antibody complexes, the antigens being whole horse serum and bovine serum albumin (PARONETTO *et al.*, 1962). In a different type of study, rats were sensitized by an antigen (heterologous serum albumin), and then challenged intravenously with it; in two studies (BLACKWELL, 1965a; FENNELL and SANTAMARIA, 1962), there was localization of the antigen in the liver and liver injury. One of these studies (BLACKWELL, 1965a) was of interest in that chronic liver damage was produced by repeated intravenous injections of albumin into sensitized rats, for periods from four to 37 weeks; the cirrhosis that developed in 70% of animals was attributed to recurring cycles of immunological tissue injury (BLACKWELL, 1965b). In another technique again, rats were given repetitive intraperitoneal injections of swine serum and horse serum; there was localization of immune complexes in vessels and connective tissue in the liver, and this was followed by cirrhosis (PARONETTO and POPPER, 1965). Also, the presence of antigen-antibody complexes in the liver could augment a pre-existing mild hepatic injury (PARONETTO and POPPER, 1966). All of the above studies show clearly that toxic antigen-antibody complexes are capable of producing hepatic lesions in animals, although the antigens concerned have been "extrinsic", and usually from heterologous species. They illustrate well that immunological reactions are capable of initiating and potentiating hepatocellular injury, but appear to have minor pathogenetic relevance to spontaneously developing autoimmune-type hepatitis in man.

II. Viral Induction of Chronic Liver Disease

1. Aleutian Mink

These develop a disease characterized by hypergammaglobulinaemia, fibrinoid necrosis of vessels and massive plasma cell infiltrations in various sites in the body, including the liver. The hepatic lesions are mainly related to biliary ducts and portal areas, and are not associated with ongoing destruction of liver cells or development of cirrhosis (LEADER *et al.*, 1963). Aleutian mink disease is due to a transmissible viral agent (EKLUND *et al.*, 1968) which induces a marked but apparently ineffectual immunoglobulin response, the immunogenic stimulus for which is uncertain. By analogy, an equivalent response to a hepatotropic virus, e.g. Type A or Type B hepatitis virus, could determine types of chronic active hepatitis in man.

2. Canine Hepatitis Virus

This provided another possible model in dogs for human chronic hepatitis (GOCKE *et al.*, 1967). These dogs, when rendered partially immune to canine hepatitis by passive immunization with hyperimmune serum, became predisposed to a protracted hepatitis with fibrosis, despite disappearance of virus from the liver; virus-antibody complexes possibly potentiated liver damage initiated by the virus itself.

3. Lymphocytic Choriomeningitis (LCM) Virus

Certain strains of mice are susceptible to chronic persisting infection with a tolerated virus. The prototype for this is lymphocytic choriomeningitis (LCM) virus infection of mice, the consideration of which lead to the original description of immune tolerance by BURNET and FENNER (1949). Mice infected neonatally with LCM virus develop a state of "persisting tolerated infection" in which most tissues contain LCM virus but show no lesions (HOTCHIN, 1971); however this state tends to fail in later life with various lesions ensuing, but liver damage is not prominent.

The complex pathology of LCM disease in the mouse was assessed in detail by LEHMANN-GRUBE (1972), some of whose observations can be summarized as follows. (a) From observations on cultured cells, the virus does not obviously harm the mouse cell in which it multiplies. (b) Virus-induced new antigens are demonstrable by transplantation experiments. (c) Infected mice tend to succumb at 1 year from a "late disease" akin to a "runting" syndrome. (d) Antibody to LCM virus is produced, and immune complexes of viral antigen with antibody can form, so that "tolerance" is not absolute. (e) Elimination of LCM virus depends entirely on cell-mediated immunity which is in some way abrogated in infected mice. (f) Operationally at least, pathological changes in LCM infected mice are of "autoimmune" nature, although it cannot be stated whether the "autoantigen" is mostly a resident virus, a virally modified host protein, or a host protein "demasked" by the virus, or a host hapten attached to the virus as a carrier.

4. Lactic Dehydrogenase (LDH) Virus

This can exist as a tolerated infection in mice, as does LCM virus. In LDH virus infection, there are elevated levels of plasma enzymes including transaminase, and hypergammaglobulinaemia, and pronounced lymphoid hyperplasia in the spleen, but liver lesions have not been described (NOTKINS *et al.*, 1966).

5. Reovirus 3

An interesting model disease was described by WALTERS *et al.* (1973) following neonatal infection of mice with reovirus 3. Of 11,532 mice inoculated, 147 (1.3%) showed a syndrome of jaundice and runting at 22 days. These authors cited their earlier work in which chronic reovirus infection was likened to human autoimmune processes, including chronic active hepatitis, and their study showed that there was development of smooth muscle antibody, and immune deposits in glomeruli in the mice with jaundice and runting.

6. Liver Disease in New Zealand Black (NZB) Mice

NZB mice, which are known to be subject to various autoimmune reactions, were reported to develop lesions in the liver suggestive of lupoid hepatitis (DUBOIS *et al.*, 1966). Liver lesions however have been inconspicuous in these mice studied in the Hall Institute, and such as do occur are attributable to infection.

As a concluding comment, the opinion here and that of other reviewers (PARONETTO and POPPER, 1968; VISCHER, 1971) is that as yet no convincing model in animals of human chronic hepatitis has yet been developed.

F. Liver Diseases Associated with Drug Reactions

I. Differentiations and Types of Drug-Associated Liver Injury

Writers on the subject of drug-induced hepatitis (SMETANA, 1963; ZIMMERMAN, 1963; KLATSKIN, 1968) have emphasized that drug-induced hepatic damage can be due either to a toxic effect of the drug on liver cells, or to an idiosyncratic response (presumably allergic) to the drug or a degradation product of it. True hepatotoxicity, which is relevant to this review only from the standpoint of its differentiation from hepatic damage due to hypersensitivity, may be direct or indirect. Direct hepatotoxicity is marked by the following criteria—the brevity of the interval between exposure and liver damage, the relationship of dose to damage, the occurrence of histologically distinct lesions in the liver and other organs, reproducibility in animals, a high incidence in exposed persons, and the drugs concerned being protoplasmic poisons. Indirect hepatotoxicity is associated with agents that interfere selectively with hepatic secretory or excretory pathways; most of the examples usually cited have little therapeutic relevance, except for the jaundice caused by C-17 alkyl substituted anabolic steroids.

Allergy (hypersensitivity) can be incriminated when liver damage occurs with minimal exposure to the drug, and occurs in a small proportion of exposed individuals, the features being the following (ZIMMERMAN, 1963): (a) a sensitization period of 1–4 weeks or previous exposure; (b) recurrences of liver damage on readministration of the drug; (c) desensitization with hepatic damage lessening on continued administration: (d) hepatic damage independent of the dose of the drug; (e) a low incidence of hepatic disease in exposed individuals; (f) a high incidence in affected persons of rash, fever and eosinophilia; (g) coincident occurrence of blood dyscrasias and other features of hypersensitivity; (h) histology consistent with hypersensitivity, or variable.

The three types of allergic liver injury are (a) cholestatic, with features of biliary obstruction, (b) hepatitic, with features of hepatocellular damage, and (c) granulomatous. Types (a) and (b) often co-exist as a mixed hepatitic-cholangitic lesion, and granulomata may coexist with either of the other types. Types (a) and (b) may be associated with acute or chronic liver injury, acute forms being the more usual. Guidelines for histological recognition of drug induced liver injury have been presented by an expert International Group (1974).

II. Allergic Cholangitis

1. Acute Allergic Cholangitis

The drugs known to, or believed to be capable of, inducing allergic cholangitis, according to ZIMMERMAN (1963) and SMETANA (1963), include particularly chlorpromazine and structurally related phenothiazines, e.g. prochlorperazine, mepazine and trifluoroperazine, promazine, chlordiazepoxide (librium), mepromabate, thiacetazone, alkylated testosterone derivatives including methyltestosterone and norethandrelone, and arsphenamine.

Acute allergic cholangitis mimics extra hepatic biliary obstruction. There is painless jaundice, often prolonged and deep, pruritus, and only slight hepatomegaly.

Biochemical tests on serum show raised levels of bilirubin and alkaline phosphatase with minimal or moderate alteration of transaminase. Histologically, there is pronounced canalicular bile stasis, particularly in centrilobular zones, a slight inflammatory reaction consisting of mononuclear cells and eosinophils in portal tracts, and in addition there is usually some degree of hepatocellular damage including necrosis (KLATSKIN, 1968), and fat (SMETANA, 1963); this hepatocellular damage may contribute to the cholestasis.

2. Chronic Allergic Cholangitis

This term can be applied when there is protraction of acute disease beyond a period of three months. ZIMMERMAN (1963), in reviewing 160 reported cases of allergic cholangitis due to chlorpromazine, found that some 30% had recovered by one month, and 65% by three months, with 35% pursuing a chronic course over one year; notably in 7% there was persistence over 12 months. The fact that chlorpromazine may be retained in the body for long periods may account for these protracted cases. There is little information as to whether chronic allergic cholangitis can undergo transition to a cirrhotic phase, i.e. be a precursor to a biliary-type cirrhosis. This was doubted by READ *et al.* (1961), but cases claimed to exemplify this were reported by WALKER and COMBES (1966).

III. Allergic Hepatitis

1. Acute Hepatitic Reactions

Many of the drugs known or believed to be capable of inducing allergic hepatitis, either as "pure" hepatitis or "mixed" hepatitis-cholangitis were cited by ZIMMERMAN (1963) according to their medical applications, and a list would include the following: psycho-active drugs, including chlorpromazine and congeners, and iproniazid; anticonvulsants, particularly diphenyl hydantoinate; thioureas; hypoglycaemic drugs; antibiotics, particularly erythromycin ester and possibly penicillin; antibacterial drugs including paraaminosalicylic acid, isoniazid, rifampicin, sulphonamides and sulfones; anticoagulants, particularly phenindione; the diuretic drug chlorthiazide, and the anaesthetic agent halothane. For most of the drugs cited above, the occurrence of allergic hepatitis is so uncommon that it does not contraindicate their use except in exceptional circumstances.

The clinical, biochemical and histological features of acute allergic hepatitis mimic those of acute infectious hepatitis (POPPER, 1973). However for some drugs at least, the disease is more severe and drawn-out, and mortality higher, e.g. 42% in those with halothane-related hepatitis (MOULT and SHERLOCK, 1975). The biochemical tests on serum show raised levels of hepatocellular enzymes, particularly transaminases. In many cases, the features are to some degree "mixed" with coexisting evidence of both hepatocellular damage and cholestasis. In addition, there may be systemic evidence of hypersensitivity including fever, arthralgia, rashes and urticaria, and eosinophilia in the blood. There is a close resemblance between hepatic lesions due to drug allergy and those of acute viral hepatitis, so much so that it could be suggested that similar immunological mechanisms determine damage in both viral and drug induced hepatitis (MACKAY and POPPER, 1973).

2. Chronic Hepatitic Reactions

The great majority of allergic hepatitic reactions resolve in the acute stage because the offending drug is readily recognized and withdrawn; this is indicative of the dependence of the reaction on the actual presence in the body of the drug. However certain drugs, by reason of being long retained in the body, or being taken intermittently or continuously, may induce a chronic drug-associated hepatitis. Particular examples of chronic hepatitis due to drugs to which exposure occurs over long periods include hepatitis associated with oxyphenisatin, alpha methyl dopa, isoniazid and in special circumstances halothane.

The clinical spectrum of drug associated chronic hepatitis ranges from a relapsing hepatitic illness resembling typical chronic active hepatitis to advanced cirrhosis of cryptogenic type as reported in a few long-time users of oxyphenisatin. A curious feature of some cases of drug-associated chronic hepatitis is the development of serological features usually associated with the autoimmune type of chronic hepatitis (lupoid hepatitis), i.e. positive tests for LE cells, antinuclear antibodies, and anti-smooth muscle antibodies, exemplified particularly by cases of hepatitis due to oxyphenisatin and alpha methyl dopa.

IV. Granulomatous Hepatic Reactions

A well recognized morphological expression in the liver of drug allergy is the occurrence of granulomas of the "tuberculoid" type, as seen in sarcoidosis and chronic infections. Examples cited in the literature include reactions to phenylbutazone (GOLDSTEIN, 1963; POPPER *et al.*, 1973) in which typical sarcoid like granulomata were demonstrable, sulphonylurea (BLOODWORTH, 1963) and chlorthiazide (HUSEBYE, 1964). In a case of hepatitis occurring rapidly after a second exposure to halothane, a liver biopsy on the third day post-exposure showed widespread parenchymal necrosis and also numerous tuberculoid granulomas with typical multinucleated giant cells, without necrosis or caseation (DORDAL *et al.*, 1970). Granulomatous hepatitic reactions have been reported also as an allergic response to sulphonamides by ESPIRITU *et al.* (1967), penicillin (WAUGH, 1952), hydrallazine (JORI and PESCHLE, 1973), and quinidine (CHAJEK *et al.*, 1975).

V. Specific Drugs

Reference will be made in this section to drugs which are more particularly prone to induce hepatitis, or about which controversy exists.

1. Iproniazid (Marsalid)

SHERLOCK (1968) cited a reported 0.2–0.4% of hepatitic reactions due to iproniazid, including an illustration of acute hepatic necrosis, this incidence leading to withdrawal of this drug from use.

2. Isoniazid

The substantial literature dealing with hepatitis associated with isoniazid was reviewed by MADDREY and BOITNOTT (1973). A number of well documented cases are described with fatal outcome (COHEN *et al.*, 1961), and in some a documented recurrence on rechallenge (MARTIN and ARTHAUD, 1970). Recently there has been very considerable interest in liver disease in patients with tuberculosis receiving this drug. BAILEY *et al.* (1973) cited previous reports and examined the question by monitoring hepatic function in 427 patients receiving isoniazid long-term, for 4–8 months. There were 37 (9%) in whom increases in transaminase occurred, and 13 had in addition other evidence of liver dysfunction, although isoniazid was not necessarily reponsible in all; in only five patients did the presumed isoniazid reaction compel withdrawal of the drug.

MADDREY and BOITNOTT (1973) reported 14 cases, mostly females, observed over a five year period; the illness was hepatitic in character, together with fever and eosinophilia in some, and there were three deaths from fulminant hepatic necrosis. In three cases there was a demonstrated exacerbation on rechallenge. Histologically, the features resembled viral hepatitis; notably, bridging necrosis was seen in five and eosinophils were prominent in the biopsy. In this study, associated autoimmune serological features, which coexist with some types of hypersensitivity hepatitis, were not reported. Further examples were cited by ROSSOUW and SAUNDERS (1975) in a study of hepatic reactions to antituberculous drugs; these authors reviewed the conflicting results of studies on *in vitro* demonstration of drug sensitization by the lymphocyte transformation test.

3. Phenazopyridine Hydrochloride (Pyridium)

This drug is widely used for dysuria. GOLDFINGER and MARX (1972) cited a reported case and described two further cases of hypersensitivitiy hepatitis due to this drug.

4. Diphenyl Hydantoin

A case of anicteric hepatitis associated with treatment with diphenyl hydantoin was reported by PEZZIMENTI and HAHN (1970), with review of nine previously reported cases; most of the 10 cases were associated with fever, rash and eosinophilia, two were fatal, and four were documented by rechallenge. A case with predominantly cholestatic features, together with eosinophilia and fever, was reported by MARTIN and RICKERS (1972).

5. Sulphonamides

Sulphonamides are usually cited as inducing allergic hepatitis (ZIMMERMAN, 1963) but well-documented examples are infrequent. KONTTINEN *et al.* (1972) reviewed earlier literature and noted only four cases in which there was documentation by challenge with a test dose. They added two further cases due to sulphamethoxypyridazine and sulphamethizole, both in older women. The clinical features were hepatitic, with high levels of hepatocellular enzymes in serum. SHAW and JACOBS (1970) cite a case of Stevens-Johnson syndrome with "toxic hepatitis" attributed to a long-acting sulphonamide.

6. Penicillin and Oxacillin

Penicillin-induced hepatitis appears remarkably rare considering the sensitizing properties of this drug. A case of acute hepatitis attributed to penicillin was reported by VALDIVIA-BARRIGA *et al.* (1963), a case described as "lupoid hepatitis" by GIRARD *et al.* (1967), and a granulomatous hepatitis by WAUGH (1952). Three examples of an hepatic hypersensitivity reaction to oxacillin were described by DISMUKES (1973).

7. Erythromycin Ester

Jaundice due to erythromycin estolate was recognized in 1961, and some 50 cases have been recorded, with recurring jaundice on rechallenge in 15 (OLIVER *et al.*, 1973). The hepatic reaction is of mixed cholestatic-hepatitic type, with upper abdominal pain as a prominent feature in some of the reported cases (OLIVER *et al.*, 1973). The biochemical changes included elevations of both transaminase and alkaline phosphatase levels, and the liver biopsy correspondingly showed features of hepatitis (periportal infiltrates) and cholestasis (bile plugging in canaliculi), together with eosinophilic infiltration in portal tracts. Abnormalities of liver function may last for some months, but permanent damage has not been reported. Although there are only some 50 recorded examples of hepato-cholangitis due to erythromycin ester in the literature, there have been no less than 113 examples of "hepatotoxicity" (presumably sensitivity reactions) reported from 1964–1973 to the Australian Drug Evaluation Committee; their opinion (1973) was that erythromycin estolate should be no longer be made available.

8. Halothane

Halothane hepatitis is of special interest by reason of the controversy over the existence of this entity. Hepatologists tend to take an affirmative view, with SHARPSTONE *et al.* (1971) reporting 11 cases and having little doubt that halothane was responsible for the hepatitis in the patients described, and with SHERLOCK (1971) concluding that halothane hepatitis has now been accepted, "at least in most quarters". Some anaesthesiologists take the negative view, with Simpson their major spokesman, claiming that the evidence for the existence of halothane hepatitis would not withstand careful scrutiny, and is sometimes even factually inaccurate (SIMPSON *et al.*, 1971, 1973).

The affirmative argument for "halothane hepatitis" as a clinical entity is based on two lines of evidence. Firstly, there is an apparently high frequency of cases in which hepatitis has occurred after halothane anaesthesia and particularly after second or multiple exposures to halothane, 92% in the series of MOULT and SHERLOCK (1975). Secondly there has been the occurrence of hepatitis in exposed persons other than patients undergoing anaesthesia; these including anaesthesiologists and an exposed factory worker (cited by SHERLOCK, 1971), an exposed laboratory technician (JOHNSTON and MENDELSOHN, 1971), and a prisoner who surreptitiously sniffed halothane (SCHATZKI *et al.*, 1973); the anaesthesiologist, whose case was reported by KLATSKIN and KIMBERG (1969), had recurrent attacks of hepatitis coinciding with his use of halothane. Other evidence includes the occurrence of fever with onset of hepatitis after halothane exposure, and the appearance of eosinophilia in the blood. Moreover, the chemically-related agent methoxyflurane is also reported to cause hepatitis with features of hypersensitivity (JOSHI and CONN, 1974). Simpson (vide supra) challenges all of the above evidence and exphasizes the difficulties in interpreting jaundice, rashes, fever and eosinophilia after surgery and anaesthesia. Indeed, there can be numerous causes of jaundice in the postoperative period, listed in the review by CARNEY and VAN DYKE (1972), these including hypoxia, sepsis, undernutrition and viral hepatitis.

Immunological studies have certainly not helped to resolve the question of the existence of halothane hepatitis as an immunologically-induced disease, mainly because drug sensitivity phenomena are difficult to validate by *in vitro* methods. RODRIGUEZ *et al.* (1969) claimed that mitochondrial antibody, characteristic of the immunopathic disease primary biliary cirrhosis, was demonstrable in halothane hepatitis, and DONIACH *et al.* (1966) also reported low-titre reactions. However findings from my laboratory (WHITTINGHAM, 1974) do not support this claim, and the problem of interpreting mitochondrial reactions using rat rather than the human sources of mitochondrial antigen (Section D.III.5) may be relevant here. OPOLON *et al.* (1969) described lymphoblastic transformation induced by drug antigens as an *in vitro* procedure for demonstrating sensitivity reactions. PARONETTO and POPPER (1970) reported that blood lymphocytes of 10 of 15 patients considered to have halothane hepatitis transformed when exposed *in vitro* to halothane. This latter study was criticized by WALTON *et al.* (1973) on several grounds and, moreover, neither WALTON *et al.* (1973) nor MOULT and SHERLOCK (1975) could demonstrate transformation of lymphocytes on exposure to halothane in any of the suspected halothane-sensitive subjects in their series, 15 and 12 cases respectively.

Majority opinion accepts the reality of halothane hepatitis as an example of allergic hepatitis but the evidence is circumstantial and indirect, and there is great need for the development of appropriate immunological methods to provide *in vitro* confirmation.

9. Oxphenisatin

The existence of chronic hepatitis associated with laxative abuse was described by REYNOLDS *et al.* (1971) and these authors drew attention to the association of autoimmune serological reactions to nuclear and smooth muscle antigens. Their cases were in middle-aged or older women who had been taking oxyphenisatin daily for 1–2 years. The clinical biochemical and histological features were those of "typical" chronic active hepatitis, except that the disease regressed when laxatives were ceased. However exacerbations occurred upon inadvertent re-exposure or deliberate challenge, pointing to the allergic basis of the disease.

Oxphenisatin induced hepatitis subsequently became recognized in other countries. In Australia, six cases were recognized in one city by WILLING and

HECKER (1971), and other reports, emphasizing the relative frequency and numerical contribution of oxyphenisatin hepatitis to chronic hepatitis cases, include those of COOKSLEY *et al.* (1973) and GOLDSTEIN *et al.* (1973), and the possibility that a "cryptogenic" cirrhosis could be accounted for by prolonged oxyphenisatin abuse was raised by SHANN (1971). The number of notified cases in Australia (21 as of 1972) led to oxphenisatin being withdrawn from the Australian market (Australian Drug Evaluation Committee, 1972). In Germany, oxphenisatin containing laxatives were associated with acute inflammatory episodes of liver disease in four patients known to have chronic progressive hepatitis (WILDHIRT, 1972).

10. Alpha Methyl Dopa ("Aldomet")

This drug is popular for the treatment of hypertension but is known to induce occasionally an autoimmune type of haemolytic anaemia (WORLLEDGE, 1973), and, quite rarely, lupus reactions (MACKAY *et al.*, 1968). A case was reported in detail by ELKINGTON *et al.* (1969), and these authors reviewed 17 previous reports relating to liver dysfunction in 52 patients receiving Aldomet. The causal role of Aldomet sensitivity could not be established in all of these cases, but in some exacerbation on rechallenge was established. ELKINGTON *et al.* (1969) stated that the onset of illness could be from one week to one year after starting the drug, the onset was usually acute, and the course benign; resolution occurred after withdrawal of the drug, and in a few cases despite its continued use. A case of Aldomet-hepatitis associated with the LE phenomenon was reported by ELIASTAM and HOLMES (1971), with full recovery after withdrawal of the drug, and further cases were included in the report of GOLDSTEIN *et al.* (1973). The topic of Aldomet-hepatitis was further reviewed, in the course of another case report, by TYSELL and KNAUER (1971), and the benign self-limiting nature of the hepatitis was emphasized. On the other hand, the potential seriousness of Aldomet-hepatitis is evidenced by cases progressing to fatal massive hepatic necrosis, illustrated by the reports of HOYUMPA and CONNELL (1973), REHMAN *et al.* (1973), TOGHILL *et al.* (1974), and MADDREY and BOITNOTT (1975).

11. Aspirin

Aspirin appeared to induce hepatitic liver injury in three patients with systemic lupus erythematosus, and in one chronic active hepatitis was suspected (SEAMAN *et al.*, 1974). In view of the widescale use of aspirin in the community, it seems important to establish whether aspirin-induced hepatitis is in fact a common occurrence.

12. Para-Aminosalicylic Acid (PAS)

In a large study of 7492 patients receiving antituberculous treatment, PAS was found to be the most common cause of drug hepatitis among 38 patients analysed (ROSSOUW and SAUNDERS, 1975). The interval between starting the drug and the onset of disease was mostly less than 90 days, the features were mostly hepatitic, rashes were frequent as were other markers of a hypersensitivity response.

VI. Immunological Basis of Allergic Liver Injury

1. Acute Reactions

A major problem in acute allergic liver injury is the nature and mode of action of the molecule which causes immunization, and the immunological process which elicits the damaging response. The sensitizing molecule could be the drug itself, the final metabolites, or the transitory intermediates in the metabolism of the drug. Halothane, for example, is broken down finally to bromide, chloride and an aliphatic compound, trifluoracetic acid, and the entire molecule, or any of the intermediates (see CARNEY and VAN DYKE, 1972) could be immunogenic by virtue of attachment of the drug as a hapten to a structural protein of the liver cell or biliary ductule. The same would hold for other drugs causing hepatitic reactions. The well-known model "sedormid purpura" (ACKROYD, 1949) could be taken as a possible analogue. In this classical situation, the drug attaches to platelets which provide the carrier molecule, and the antibody is reactive with the carrier-hapten complex; thrombocytopenia occurs only in the presence of the drug as hapten, platelet as carrier, and antibody. Neither *in vivo* nor *in vitro* systems for studying the possible humoral or cell-mediated immunological processes have been reliably developed for human drug-induced liver injury. In fact, the only direct evidence that an immunologic process is operating is that rechallenge, inadvertent or deliberate, with the suspected drug will rapidly evoke features of hepatic or cholangiolar damage.

2. Drug-Induced Hepatitis with Autoimmune Markers

This reaction is presumably analogous to other drug-induced autoimmune syndromes such as lupus erythematosus induced by hydrallazine (PERRY, 1973), procaine amide (WHITTINGHAM *et al.*, 1972), practolol (RAFFERTY and DENMAN, 1973) and autoimmune type haemolytic anaemia induced by alpha methyl dopa (WORLLEDGE, 1973). The drugs reported to induce an allergic-type hepatitis associated with a positive LE cell reaction include oxphenisatin and alpha methyl dopa (Sections F.V.9 and F.V.10) and also isoniazid (BICKERS *et al.*, 1961).

It is not certain in these drug-induced autoimmune syndromes whether (a) a particular attachment of the drug to a host protein provides an autoimmunogenic configuration, (b) the drug provides a special microenvironment in which immune induction can occur (WHITTINGHAM *et al.*, 1972), or (c) in the case of liver disease, whether autoimmune processes supervene upon initial allergic liver damage induced by the drug.

3. Experimental Models of Allergic Hepatitis

There has not been reported any animal model closely simulating drug-induced liver injury in man, so that progress in understanding these conditions has been retarded. TEN VEEN (1973) administered hydrallazine, isoniazid, procaine amide, and methyl dopa and chlorthalidone to three inbred strains of mice, these drugs being selected on the basis of their known effect in inducing autoimmune syndromes in man. Smooth muscle antibody (SMA), which is characteristic of human autoimmune-type hepatitis was induced by certain of these drugs, particularly alpha methyl dopa and chlorthalidone and rather inconspicuous liver infiltrates were demonstrable in some mice with positive reactions for SMA.

G. Conclusion: Immunology and the Liver

As a conclusion, emphasis will be placed on the importance of immunological function in relation to liver disease, from the standpoint of the role in liver disease of immune deficiency, hypersensitivity, persistent tolerated infection and autoimmunity, and the importance of immune mediated liver disease to the genesis of chronic hepatitis and cirrhosis of the liver.

I. Immune Deficiency

1. Phagocytic Function

The phagocytic function of the reticuloendothelial (Kupffer cell) system in the liver is depressed by the architectural disorganization of the liver associated with hepatic cirrhosis, and this facilitates the bacteraemia and systemic infections known to occur in patients with cirrhosis. The bypassing by intestinal microorganisms of the Kupffer cell system in cirrhosis, with resulting excessive antigenic stimulation in extrahepatic sites, was proposed as a partial explanation for the hypergammaglobulinaemia of cirrhosis (Section D.II.5).

2. Immunocyte Function

In so far as immune responsiveness is concerned with the riddance of microorganisms from the body, it is assumed that immune deficiency predisposes to the various parasitic, bacterial and viral diseases of the liver, described in Section B, and for persistence of hepatitis B virus. Although liver diseases due to infection are predisposed to by immune deficits associated with undernutrition, debilitation and ageing, such deficits may be subtle and not recognized by conventional testing in man of humoral and cell-mediated immune function. The complexities of host-parasite responses in parasitic infestations of man are discussed by OGILVIE and JONES (1973), with the impression being given that much remains to be learned.

II. "Hypersensitivity" Responses

"Hypersensitivity" responses may determine damage in infections of the liver, the most notable example being schistosomiasis in which the granulomatous reaction occurs as a manifestation of T cell mediated immunity. It is likely that other granulomatous reactions in liver in response to infection, e.g. brucellosis, tuberculosis and leprosy of the liver, have a similar basis.

III. Persistent Tolerated Infection: Hepatitis B Virus

The various disease manifestations associated with hepatitis B virus exemplify in man the state of "persistent tolerated infection", as seen in lymphocytic choriomeningitis virus infection in mice and Aleutian disease in mink. The mechanisms are unknown by which "slow", "latent" or "temperate" viruses of man and animals elude the immune defences of the host. In these infections, including chronic hepatitis B virus infection in man, the virus can exist in harmony with the host if full tolerance exists, but a partial ineffective immune response can set up a chronic or recurrent disease, either through a cell-mediated immune attack on tissues containing viral antigens, or by deposits in tissues of antigen-antibody complexes.

IV. Autoimmunity

The concept of autoimmunity as a disease mechanism has become well established for diseases such as thyroiditis, myasthenia gravis, systemic lupus erythematosus and others; the main items of evidence are the existence of autoantibodies reactive with disease-specific autoantigens and appropriate induced or spontaneous disease models in animals. The concept of autoimmunity as a cause of chronic hepatitis is based on more indirect evidence: hypergammaglobulinaemia; autoantibodies which have disease specificity but not liver specificity; lymphoid reactions in the liver; clustering of other immunopathological diseases with chronic active hepatitis; and an amelioration of chronic hepatitis with "anti-immune" drugs. But, notably, no intrinsic component of liver has been shown to readily induce an immunopathogenic type of hepatitis in animals, nor has a "target" antigen been demonstrable in the human disease. The presence of smooth muscle antibody in most cases has directed attention to actinomyosin of the membrane of liver cells as one potential "target", but this autoantibody is not demonstrable in all cases, and can be present in the absence of liver damage.

No single "basic" cause for autoimmunization has been identified, despite much experimentation and speculation. Proposed causal explanations range from the "deterministic", which involves an identifiable extrinsic immunogenic stimulus which "triggers" a response that overrides natural immune tolerance, to the "mutational" in which intrinsic somatic mutation gives rise to self-reactive thymus-derived lymphocytes.

The "deterministic" concept holds that various extrinsic stimuli can elicit autoimmune responses against self antigens. The simplest immunological explanation would be cross-reactivity depending on antigenic determinants shared by microorganisms and host-components: thus streptococcal cell wall proteins are claimed to provoke antibodies cross-reactive with heart muscle antigens; *E. coli* 012 to provoke antibodies cross-reactive with colon mucosal antigens; and mycoplasma to provoke antibodies reactive with the i antigen of erythrocytes. However viral infection may act in a more subtle manner. In the model proposed by BRETSCHER (1973) viral infection results in expression of new antigenic determinants on self-reactive but normally tolerant T lymphocytes; these new determinants on the T cell surface allow the T cell to receive a proliferative signal and so generate a "forbidden" self-reactive clone. Previous evidence of raised antibody titres to viral antigens in chronic active hepatitis (Section D.II.5) was recently supplemented by a further report on associations between chronic active hepatitis and high titres of antibody to measles and rubella (LAITINEN and VAHERI, 1974).

The "mutational" approach to the genesis of autoimmunity holds that mutability and change of pattern of receptors is an intrinsic property of immunocytes, and that extrinsic influences (infection, trauma) do no more than provide an appropriate microenvironment for proliferation of self-reactive T immunocytes arising by a process of intrinsic mutagenesis.

A germ-line genetic component must be considered for autoimmune chronic active hepatitis by reason of the demonstrated association of this disease with histocompatibility antigens 1 and 8 (MACKAY and MORRIS, 1972). This phenotype could be associated with immune-response genes which code for antigen receptors closely related to autoantigens so that minor somatic mutations in T cells would result in the generation of immunocytes with self-reactive properties.

V. The Chronic Hepatitis-Cirrhosis Problem

1. Extent of Problem

The magnitude of chronic hepatitis and cirrhosis as a health problem can be illustrated by the estimate of MARTINI (1973) that there are some 310,000 deaths annually from cirrhosis of the liver throughout the world. Considering European countries, SCHEUER (1973) cited World Health Organization figures for 1969 showing that deaths from cirrhosis per 100,000 population ranged from 3.2 in England to 35.3 in France, the latter reflecting a higher incidence of alcoholic cirrhosis. MARTINI (1973) referred to some 30 possible types of cirrhosis but many of these would be extremely rare and some might not even exist as entities. Many authorities see only three major types of cirrhosis—alcoholic, post-hepatitic, and cryptogenic (of unknown cause)—and some minor types, namely those associated with haemochromatosis, Wilson's disease, certain rare metabolic disorders, and cardiac disease.

Alcoholic cirrhosis accounts for 50% or more of all cases of cirrhosis, particularly in Western countries; cryptogenic cirrhosis for some 20—30% of cases in Western countries, and apparently for most of the cases in the Far East and parts of South America and Africa; and "post-hepatitic cirrhosis" for most of the remainder. "Post-hepatitic" has the connotation of a cirrhosis occurring as a direct consequence of, and sequel to, infectious (viral) hepatitis, but this is established only for hepatitis B infection; hence "post-hepatitic" would better used in the more general sense of cirrhosis occurring after any type of acute or chronic hepatitis, including the various types of chronic active hepatitis.

2. Subtypes of Chronic Hepatitis?

The broadest interpretation of chronic hepatitis would be to consider all diffuse parenchymal diseases of the liver in terms of three temporal phases, acute, chronic active and cirrhotic (MACKAY, 1972), with progression from acute to chronic liver injury requiring either continued exposure to the initiating agent, or the supervention of a new pathogenetic process such as an aberrant immune response (immunoaggression).

The pathogeneses which are concerned in chronic active hepatitis and post-hepatitic cirrhosis include the following.

Viral infection, with serum hepatitis virus (HB virus) persisting in serum and in liver cells as hepatitis B antigen (HBAg), and causing progressive liver disease (Section C.V.5).

Autoimmune reactions, which could either occur *de novo*, or supervene on other types of liver damage to cause perpetuation and progression to cirrhosis.

Drug allergies, which include acute reversible hepatitic and cholangitic reactions, and chronic hepatitic reactions which occasionally may progress to cirrhosis.

Cryptogenic liver disease is based on the term "cryptogenic cirrhosis" introduced by DIBLE (1951); this is now used with the connotations of (a) liver disease with no clue as to pathogeneses, and (b) histologically "inactive" cirrhosis (BHATHAL *et al.*, 1973). However in cases of "inactive" cirrhosis associated with positive tests for HBsAg or autoantibodies, which point to an antecedent pathogenesis, the term "cryptogenic" would be inappropriate.

"Chronic active hepatitis" and "post-hepatitic cirrhosis" have been discussed extensively over the past two decades, but two fundamental questions remain unresolved. The first is whether various types of chronic active hepatitis can be distinguished, on the basis of autoimmune markers, HBsAg in serum or drug induction, or whether they should be considered in a general category of "chronic active liver disease" (SOLOWAY and SUMMERSKILL, 1973). The second is whether there are recognizable morphological appearances which characterize transition of chronic hepatitis to cirrhosis.

The features of the autoimmune (lupoid) type of chronic active hepatitis and cirrhosis (Section D.II) include female sex, "multisystem" disease, responsiveness of disease to corticosteroid drugs and azathioprine, biopsy features which include lymphoid-plasma ell reactions in the liver with marked "piecemeal" periportal necrosis, hypergammaglobulinaemia, autoimmune serological reactions (to cell nuclei and smooth muscle) and a high frequency of histocompatibility antigens 1 and 8; however the relative weighting of these various attributes in the definition of autoimmune chronic hepatitis is still uncertain.

The features of the hepatitis B associated type of chronic active hepatitis, described in Section C.V.8, include male sex, extrahepatic disease manifested as arthritis and arteritis, variable responsiveness to immunosuppressive drugs, biopsy features of chronic aggressive hepatitis but with a less pronounced plasma cell response, and persistence of HBsAg in serum and liver cells. Most hepatologists find that cases of chronic active hepatitis segregate according to tests for HBsAg and autoantibodies in serum, in that positivity for HBsAg is associated with negativity for autoantibodies.

This is the reported experience from (a) American sources, including WRIGHT *et al.* (1969) from New Haven, BULKLEY *et al.* (1970) from Boston, FINLAYSON *et al.* (1972) from New York, and PETERS (1973) from Los Angeles, (b) English sources, including FOX *et al.* (1969), VISCHER (1970), and DUDLEY *et al.* (1973), and (c) from Australia, by COOKSLEY *et al.* (1972). On the other hand, coexisting positivity of tests for HBAg and autoantibodies in chronic hepatitis was reported from the Mayo Clinic by SOLOWAY *et al.* (1972), from Italy by BIANCHI *et al.* (1972), and from England by REED *et al.* (1973).

The allergic type of chronic active hepatitis, described in Section F.III, is considered to be infrequent but may account for a substantial proportion of cases of chronic hepatitis in older females. The main feature is that a known potentially "sensitizing" drug has been taken over a long period, improvement occurs when the drug is withdrawn, and there is relapse on rechallenge; the coexistence in some cases of the autoantibody reactions associated with autoimmune type hepatitis is unexplained.

In a study of 39 HBsAg negative cases of chronic active hepatitis, a high proportion (62%) was found to give positive reactions in the leucocyte migration assay for cell-mediated immunity to HBsAg (LEE *et al.*, 1975). This indication that HBV infection may initiate the autoimmune type of chronic active hepatitis is in line with hypotheses of POPPER and MACKAY (1972) and EDDLESTON and WILLIAMS (1975), but further evidence is needed.

Finally there are cases of chronic active hepatitis (and cirrhosis) which cannot be attributed to any of the above categories, there being negative tests for autoantibodies and HBsAg, and no known exposure to drugs or toxins. It is elected to call these cryptogenic chronic active hepatitis and cirrhosis (BHATHAL *et al.*, 1973; PETERS, 1973), and this group probably comprises various pathogenetic entities yet to be identified. Such cases constitute a relatively small proportion of all cases of chronic active hepatitis and cirrhosis in Caucasian communities (COOKSLEY *et al.*, 1972), but appear to constitute the major proportion in Asian communities (LEE, 1973; WHITTINGHAM *et al.*, 1973).

3. Morphological Correlates of Transition of Hepatitis to Cirrhosis?

The histological characteristics of "classical" chronic active hepatitis were described and referenced in Section D.II.4. An attempt was made by an International Group (1971) to obtain a consensus of opinion on histological features characteristic of chronic hepatitis, and the Group distinguished two entities. These were *chronic persisting hepatitis* with hepatitic features but no indications of architectural disorganization or likelihood of progression, and *chronic aggressive hepatitis* (a morphological counterpart of clinically designated chronic active hepatitis), with histological features that might specify inevitable transition through chronic hepatitis to cirrhosis, these being portal tract enlargement with irregularity of portal tract borders, extensive periportal necrosis, a high density of infiltrating mononuclear and plasma cells, and inflammatory septa extending into hepatic lobules. In cases described by BOYER and KLATSKIN (1970), key histological features specifying transition of acute hepatitis to chronic hepatitis and post-necrotic cirrhosis were bridging lesions of necrosis and collapse between portal tracts and central veins (subacute hepatic necrosis). These lesions can be identified also in the autoimmune types of chronic hepatitis (lupoid hepatitis) and in transition of alcoholic liver injury to alcoholic cirrhosis (GERBER and POPPER, 1972), and may well be an important determinant of disordered regeneration and architectural loss after recurring episodes of damage to the liver of any type.

The important point is seen to be that, despite controversy on what does constitute "aggressive" hepatitis, there is a polarization in appearances constituting "persistent" and "aggressive" hepatitis with relatively few cases showing intermediate features. This, taken with the frequency of autoimmune markers in cases in the "aggressive" category and absence of such markers in cases in the "persistent" category speaks for specificity in the association between autoimmune reactions and the "aggressive" lesion.

4. Immunopathogenesis of Chronic Hepatitis—Neoantigen or Autoantigen

Whilst it is still not resolved whether the HBsAg associated, autoimmune and drug associated (allergic) types of chronic hepatitis are in fact separable as subgroups of chronic active hepatitis, each type may undergo transition to cirrhosis through a common immune-mediated pathogenetic pathway, specified as an "immunoaggressive" reaction. This could be associated with (a) a response to an immunogenic neoantigen in the liver, or (b) a response to a natural autoantigen of liver.

One type of immunogenic neoantigen would be hepatitis B virus within liver cells. By analogy with persisting tolerated infection in mice with lymphocytic choriomeningitis (LCM) virus, host cells would be damaged by reactions of varying intensity directed either against the passenger virus itself, or against liver cell proteins associated with the virus particle (Section E.II.3). Another type of immunogenic neoantigen would be a drug, or a breakdown product of it, attached to a liver cell protein as carrier; ongoing damage appears to require continued administration of the drug, and the meachanism would be analogous to the classical "sedormid purpura" model of thrombocytopenia (Section F.VI.1). The immunogenic autoantigen, as mentioned above, has not been identified, but actinomyosin components of the cell membrane might be concerned.

5. Effector Mechanisms in Immune-Mediated Liver Disease

Effector mechanisms of Immune tissue injury are usually specified in terms of the Types I—IV reactions as described by COOMBS and GELL (1968), these being Type I—anaphylactic or reaginic antibody (IgE), Type II—cytotoxic antibody, Type III—immune complexes, and Type IV—cytotoxic T lymphocytes; to these are now added a Type V reaction, represented by antibody reactive with cell membranes or receptors with functionally important effects (CARNEGIE and MACKAY, 1975) and Type VI, in which specifically reactive humoral antibody facilitates the attachment to the target cell of a non-specifically reactive cell (K cell) which has an Fc receptor and, once attached, can effect target cell lysis (NELSON, 1974).

Which mechanism(s) is operative in presumed immune-mediated liver diseases is uncertain. As evidence for Type II reactions (cytotoxic antibody), there is autoantibody to actinomyosin, a component of liver cell membrane, in serum but no cytotoxic liver-specific autoantibody is demonstrable in chronic hepatitis. There is some evidence for Type III reactions, i.e. deposition of immune complexes, in HBsAg associated chronic hepatitis. Type IV reactions are usually held to operate in most putative autoimmune disorders, but this is mainly by reason of failure to implicate other mechanisms; in fact it has been difficult to demonstrate specific cell-mediated immunity in most human autoimmune diseases, although the findings with the leucocyte migration inhibition technique (Section D.II.8) are a hopeful development. Finally, as discussed by HOPF and MEYER ZUM BÜSCHENFELDE (1974) and EDDLESTON and WILLIAMS (1974), cytotoxicity by specific antibody acting in association with non-specifically reactive lymphocytes (Type VI) is a possible but unproven mechanism.

Dysfunction of the immune system is clearly of major importance in the genesis of post-hepatitic and cryptogenic types of cirrhosis: these constitute some 50% of all cases of chronic diffuse parenchymal liver disease in many countries. The origin of the immune dysfunction and mediation of damage to the target tissue in chronic liver disease remains uncertain and no single mechanism could cover all cases. However this holds for autoimmunity in general, and other types of immunopathy, in man, and also in experimental animals in which critical dissection of immunological events should be most easily accomplished. Meanwhile the present understanding of immune-mediated liver disease has made great contributions to hepatology in the areas of diagnosis and treatment.

Abbreviations

AICF	autoimmune complement fixation
ANA	antinuclear antibody
Au antigen	Australia antigen, synonymous with hepatitis B antigen
B cell	lymphocyte maturing in bone marrow
CMI	cell-mediated immunity
FCA	Freund's complete adjuvant
GOT	glutamic oxaloacetic transaminase
GVH	graft versus host
HBsAg	hepatitis B surface antigen
LCM (virus)	lymphocytic choriomeningitis (virus)
LDH (virus)	lactic dehydrogenase (virus)
LMI	leucocyte migration inhibition
M antibody (MA)	antimitochondrial antibody
nm	nanometre
NZB (mice)	New Zealand black (mice)
PBC	primary biliary cirrhosis
PMNL	polymorphonuclear leucocytes
SLE	systemic lupus erythematosus
SMA	smooth muscle antibody
T cell	lymphocyte maturing in thymus
WHO	World Health Organization

References

ACKROYD, J.F.: The pathogenesis of thrombocytopenic purpura due to hypersensitivity to sedormid. Clin. Sci. **7**, 249 (1949).

AHRENS, E.H., PAYNE, M.A., KUNKEL, H.G., EISENMENGER, W.J., BLONDHEIM, S.H.: Primary biliary cirrhosis. Medicine (Baltimore), **29**, 299 (1950).

AJDUKIEWICZ, A.B., DUDLEY, F.J., FOX, R.A., DONIACH, D., SHERLOCK, S.: Immunological studies in an epidemic of infective, short-incubation hepatitis. Lancet **1972 II**, 803.

ALARCÓN-SEGOVIA, D., DIAZ-JOUANEN, E., FISHBEIN, E.: Features of Sjogren's syndrome in primary biliary cirrhosis. Ann. intern. Med. **79**, 31 (1973).

ALKAN, W.J., EVENCHIK, Z., ESCHAR, J.: Q fever and infectious hepatitis. Amer. J. Med. **38**, 54 (1965).

ALLEN, U.R., BASS, B.H.: Fatal hepatic necrosis in glandular fever. J. clin. Path. **16**, 337 (1963).
ALMEIDA, J.D., GIOANNINI, P., SCALISE, G., HARRISON, C.V.: Electron microscope study of a case of Australia antigen-positive chronic hepatitis. J. clin. Path. **26**, 113 (1973).
ALMEIDA, J.D., RUBENSTEIN, D., SCOTT, E.J.: New antigen-antibody system in Australia antigen positive hepatitis. Lancet **1971 II**, 1225.
ALMEIDA, J.D., WATERSON, A.P.: Immune complexes in hepatitis. Lancet **1969 II**, 983.
ALPERT, E., ISSELBACHER, K.J., SCHUR, P.H.: The pathogenesis of arthritis associated with viral hepatitis. New Engl. J. Med. **285**, 185 (1971).
ALTER, H.J., BARKER, L.F., HOLLAND, P.V.: Hepatitis B immune globulin evaluation of clinical trials and rationale for usage. New Engl. J. Med. **293**, 1093 (1975).
ALTER, H.J., BLUMBERG, B.S.: Further studies on a "new" human isoprecipitin system (Australia antigen). Blood **27**, 297 (1966).
ALTER, H.J., HOLLAND, P.V., PURCELL, R.H., LANDER, J.J., FEINSTONE, S.M., MORROW, A.G., SCHMIDT, P.J.: Posttransfusion hepatitis after exclusion of commercial and hepatitis-B antigen-positive donors. Ann. intern. Med. **77**, 691 (1972).
ANDRADE, Z.A.: Hepatic schistosomiasis: morphological aspects, chap. 16 in: Progress in Liver Disease, vol. 2 (POPPER, H. and SCHAFFNER, F., eds.). London: Heinemann 1965.
ANSTEY, L.: Granulomatous ascaris hepatitis. S. Afr. med. J. **40**, 13 (1960).
ANTHONY, P.P., VOGEL, C.L., SADIKALI, F., BARKER, L.F., PETERSON, M.R.: Hepatitis-associated antigen and antibody in Uganda: Correlation of serological testing with histopathology. Brit. med. J. **1**, 403 (1973).
AREAN, V.M.: The pathologic anatomy and pathogenesis of fatal human leptospirosis (Weil's disease). Amer. J. Path. **40**, 393 (1962).
ARONOFF, A., GAULT, M.H., HUANG, S.N., LAL, S., WU, K.T., MOINUDDIN, M.D., SPENCE, L., MACLEAN, L.D.: Hepatitis with Australia antigenemia following renal transplantation. Canad. med. Ass. J. **108**, 43 (1973).
ASHERSON, G.L.: Antibodies against nuclear and cytoplasmic cell constituents in systemic lupus erythematosus and other diseases. Brit. J. exp. Path. **40**, 209 (1959).
ASHERSON, G.L.: Serum complement levels in systemic lupus erythematosus and other diseases. Aust. Ann. Med. **9**, 57 (1960).
ATWATER, E.C., JACOX, R.F.: The latex-fixation test in patients with liver disease. Ann. intern. Med. **58**, 419 (1963).
Australian Drug Evaluation Committee: Withdrawal of oxyphenisatin acetate, diacetoxydiphenolisatin and triacetyldiphenolisatin from the Australian market. Med. J. Aust. **1**, 1051 (1972).
Australian Drug Evaluation Committee: The erythromycins. Med. J. Aust. **2**, 192 (1973).
AYHAN, A., GOKOZ, A., KARACADAG, S., TELAFAR, H.: The liver in typhoid fever. Amer. J. Gastroent. **59**, 141 (1973).
BACON, P.A., BERRY, H., BOWN, R.: Cell-mediated immune reactivity in liver disease. Gut **13**, 427 (1972).
BAILEY, W.C., TAYLOR, S.L., DASCOMB, H.E., GREENBERG, H.B., ZISKIND, M.M.: Disturbed hepatic function during isoniazid chemoprophylaxis. Amer. Rev. resp. Dis. **107**, 523 (1973).
BAKER, A.L., KAPLAN, M.M., BENZ, W.C., SIDEL, J.S., WOLFE, H.J.: Polyarteritis associated with Australia antigen positive hepatitis. Gastroenterology **62**, 105 (1972).
BANATVALA, J.E., PAYNE, C.: Effects on plants of sera from patients with HBAg-associated hepatitis. Lancet **1973 I**, 1359.
BANCROFT, W.H., MUNDON, F.K., RUSSELL, P.K.: Detection of additional antigen determinants of hepatitis B antigen. J. Immunol. **109**, 842 (1972).
BARKER, L.F., CHISARI, F.V., MCGRATH, P.P., DALGARD, D.W., KIRSCHSTEIN, R.L., ALMEIDA, J.D., EDGINGTON, T.S., SHARP, D.G., PETERSON, M.R.: Transmission of type B viral hepatitis to chimpanzees. J. infect. Dis. **127**, 648 (1973b).
BARKER, L.F., PETERSON, M.R.: Detection of hepatitis-associated antigen and antibody—Comparison of methods and their application. Canad. med. Ass. J. **106**, 486 (1972).
BARKER, L.F., PETERSON, M.R., SHULMAN, N.R., MURRAY, R.: Antibody responses in viral hepatitis, Type B. J. Amer. med. Ass. **223**, 1005 (1973a).
BARKER, L.F., STEVENS, D.P., HILLIS, W.D.: Identification of reovirus type 2 in cell cultures inoculated with hepatitis sera. Proc. Soc. exp. Biol. (N.Y.) **131**, 262 (1969).
BATEMAN, N.T., EYKYN, S.J., PHILLIPS, I.: Pyogenic liver abscess caused by *Streptococcus milleri*. Lancet **1975 I**, 657.
BAYER, M.E., BLUMBERG, B.S., WERNER, B.: Particles associated with Australia antigen in the sera of patients with leukemia, Down's syndrome and hepatitis. Nature (Lond.) **218**, 1057 (1968).
BEARN, A.G., KUNKEL, H.G., SLATER, R.J.: The problem of chronic liver disease in young women. Amer. J. Med. **21**, 3 (1956).
BECHTELSHEIMER, H., KORB, G., GEDIGK, P.: The morphology and pathogenesis of "Marburg virus" hepatitis. Human Path. **3**, 255 (1972).

BECKER, C.G., NACHMAN, R.L.: Contractile proteins of endothelial cells, platelets and smooth muscle. Amer. J. Path. **71**, 1 (1973).
BECKER, M.D., SCHEUER, P.J., BAPTISTA, A., SHERLOCK, S.: Prognosis of chronic persistent hepatitis. Lancet **1970 I**, 53.
BEHAR, A.J., TAL, C.: Experimental liver necrosis produced by the injection of homologous whole liver with adjuvant. J. Path. Bact. **77**, 591 (1959).
BENDIXEN, G., NERUP, J.: Cellular (delayed) hypersensitivity to tissue antigens, Immunopathology. VIth International Symposium, Grindelwald, p. 323–332, ed. by P.A. MIESCHER. Basel: Schwabe 1971.
BENNER, E.J., GOURLEY, R.T., COOPER, R.A., BENSON, J.A.: Chronic active hepatitis with lupus nephritis. Ann. intern. Med. **68**, 405 (1968).
BENNETT, H.D., FRANKEL, J.J., BEDINGER, P., BAKER, L.S.: Infectious mononucleosis with hepatitis. Arch. intern. Med. **86**, 391 (1950).
BERG, P.A., DONIACH, D., ROITT, I.M.: Mitochondrial antibodies in primary biliary cirrhosis: I. Localization of the antigen to mitochondrial membranes. J. exp. Med. **126**, 277 (1967).
BERG, P.A., TRAUNECKER, U., MARKER, A.: Mitochondriale Antikörper bei nicht hepatischen Krankheiten. Häufigkeit, Signifikanz und differential-diagnostische Bedeutung. Dtsch. med. Wschr. **98**, 1186 (1973).
BERQUIST, K.R., MAYNARD, J.E., SHELLER, M., SCHABLE, C.A.: Comparative studies of hepatitis "candidate" agents and parvovirus in Detroit-6 cell cultures. J. infect. Dis. **126**, 203 (1972).
BHATHAL, P.S., DWYER, J.M., MACKAY, I.R., MATHEWS, J.D., ROBSON, G., STRICKLAND, R.G., WHITTINGHAM, S.: The spectrum of liver disease in an Australian teaching hospital: a prospective study of 205 patients. Med. J. Aust. **2**, 1085 (1973).
BIANCHI, P., PORRO, C.B., COLTORTI, M., DARDANONI, L., BLANCO, C.D.V., FAGIOLO, U., FARINI, R., MENOZZI, I., NACCARATO, R., PAGLIARO, L., SPANO, C., VERME, G.: Occurrence of Australia antigen in chronic hepatitis in Italy. Gastroenterology **63**, 482 (1972).
BICKERS, J.N., BUECHNER, H.A., HOOD, B.J., ALVAREZ-CHIESA, G.: Hypersensitivity reaction to antituberculous drugs with hepatitis, lupus phenomenon and myocardial infarction. New Engl. J. Med. **265**, 131 (1961).
BJORNEBOE, M., PRYTZ, H., ORSKOV, F.: Antibodies to intestinal microbes in serum of patients with cirrhosis of the liver. Lancet **1972 I**, 58.
BLACKWELL, J.B.: The effects on the liver of sensitised rats of intravenous injection of antigen. J. Path. Bact. **90**, 259 (1965a).
BLACKWELL, J.B.: Cirrhosis resulting from repeated injections of antigen. J. Path. Bact. **90**, 245 (1965b).
BLENDIS, L.M., ANSELL, I.D., JONES, K.L., HAMILTON, E., WILLIAMS, R.: Liver in Felty's syndrome. Brit. med. J. **1**, 131 (1970).
BLOODWORTH, J.M.B. JR.: Morphologic changes associated with sulfonylurea therapy. Metabolism **12**, 287 (1963).
BLUMBERG, B.S., ALTER, H.J., VISNICK, S.: A "new" antigen in leukemia sera. J. Amer. med. Ass. **191**, 541 (1965).
BLUMBERG, B.S., GERSTLEY, D.A., HUNGERFORD, D.A., LONDON, W.T., SUTNICK, A.I.: A serum antigen (Australia antigen) in Down's syndrome leukemia and hepatitis. Ann. intern. Med. **66**, 924 (1967).
BLUMBERG, B.S., MELARTIN, L., GUINTO, R.A., WERNER, B.: Family studies of a human serum isoantigen system (Australia antigen). Amer. J. hum. Genet. **18**, 594 (1966).
BLUMBERG, B.S., MILLMAN, I., SUTNICK, A.I., LONDON, W.T.: The nature of Australia antigen and its relation to antigen-antibody complex formation. J. exp. Med. **134**, 320 (1971b).
BLUMBERG, B.S., SUTNICK, A.I., LONDON, W.T., MILLMAN, I.: Australia antigen and hepatitis. New Engl. J. Med. **283**, 349 (1970).
BLUMBERG, B.S., SUTNICK, A.I., LONDON, W.T., MILLMAN, I.: The discovery of Australia antigen and its relation to viral hepatitis. Perspect. Virology **7**, 223 (1971a).
BODURTHA, A., KIM, Y.H., LAUCIUS, J.F., DONATO, R.A., MASTRANGELO, M.J.: Hepatic granulomas and other hepatic lesions associated with BCG immunotherapy for cancer. Amer. J. clin. Path. **61**, 747 (1974).
BOGGS, J.D., MELNICK, J.L., CONRAD, M.E., FELSHER, B.F.: Viral hepatitis. Clinical and tissue culture studies. J. Amer. med. Ass. **214**, 1041 (1970).
BONOMO, L., LOSPALLUTO, J., ZIFF, M.: Anti-gamma globulin factors in liver disease. Arthr. and Rheum. **6**, 104 (1963).
BONOMO, L., TURSI, A., MINERVA, V.: Immunofluorescence study of rheumatoid factor in liver tissue of patients with rheumatoid arthritis and hepatic diseases. J. Path. Bact. **92**, 423 (1966).
BOROS, D.L., WARREN, K.S.: Delayed hypersensitivity-type granuloma formation and dermal reaction induced and elicited by a soluble factor isolated from *Schistosoma mansoni* eggs. J. exp. Med. **132**, 488 (1970).
BOTHWELL, P.W., MACARA, A.W., MARTIN D., SKONE, J.F., WOFINDEN, R.C.: Infectious hepatitis in Bristol, 1959–1962. Brit. med. J. **2**, 1613 (1963).

BOYER, J.L., KLATSKIN, G.: Pattern of necrosis in acute viral hepatitis: Prognostic value of bridging (subacute hepatic necrosis). New Engl. J. Med. **283**, 1063 (1970).

BRETSCHER, P.: Hypothesis: a model for generalised autoimmunity. Cell. Immunol. **6**, 1 (1973).

BROSTOFF, J.: Migration inhibition studies in human disease. Proc. roy. Soc. Med. **63**, 905 (1970).

BROTMAN, B., PRINCE, A.M., GODFREY, H.R.: Role of arthropods in transmission of hepatitis-B virus in the tropics. Lancet **1973, I**, 1305.

BRZOSKO, W.J., KRAWCZYNSKI, K., NAZAREWICZ, T., MORZYCKA, M., NOWOSLAWSKI, A.: Glomerulonephritis associated with hepatitis-B surface antigen immune complexes in children. Lancet **1974 II**, 477.

BRZOSKO, W.J., MADALINSKI, K., KRAWCZYNSKI, K., SKWARSKA, H., NOWOSLAWSKI, A.: Australian-antigen immune complexes in patients with different forms of hepatitis. J. infect. Dis. **123**, 251 (1971).

BUCHANAN, R.D., FINE D.P., COLLEY, D.G.: *Schistosoma mansoni* infection in mice depleted of thymus dependent lymphocytes. II. Pathology and altered pathogenesis. Amer. J. Path. **71**, 207 (1973).

BULKLEY, B.H., HEIZER, W.D., GOLDFINGER, S.E., ISSELBACHER, K.J., SHULMAN, N.R.: Distinctions in chronic active hepatitis based on circulating hepatitis-associated antigen. Lancet **1970 II**, 1323.

BURCH, G.E., TSUI, C.Y., HARB, J.M.: Hepatitis in mice infected with Coxsackie Virus B1. Brit. J. exp. Path. **54**, 249 (1973).

BURNET, F.M., FENNER, F.: The Production of Antibodies, 2nd ed. Melbourne: Macmillan 1949.

BURRELL, C.J., PROUDFOOT, E., KEEN, G.A., MARMION, B.P.: Carbohydrates in hepatitis B antigen. Nature (Lond.) **243**, 260 (1973).

CALLAHAN, W.P., JR., RUSSELL, W.O., SMITH, M.G.: Human toxoplasmosis. A clinicopathologic study with presentation of five cases and review of the literature. Medicine (Baltimore) **25**, 343 (1946).

CARNEGIE, P.R., MACKAY, I.R.: Vulnerability of cell surface receptors to autoimmune reactions. Lancet **1975 II**, 684.

CARNEY, F.M.T., VAN DYKE, R.A.: Halothane hepatitis: A critical review. Anaesth. and Analgesia **51**, 135 (1972).

CAVELL, B., LEONHARDT, T.: Hereditary hypergammaglobulinemia and lupoid hepatitis. Acta med. scand. **177**, 751 (1965).

CHAJEK, T., LEHRER, B., GELTNER, D., LEVIJ, I.S.: Quinidine-induced granulomatous hepatitis. Ann. intern. Med. **81**, 774 (1974).

CHALMERS, T.C., ALTER, H.J.: Management of the asymptomatic carriers of the hepatitis associated (Australia) antigen. New Engl. J. Med. **285**, 613 (1971).

CHERRICK, G.R., POTHIER, L., DEFOUR, J-J., SHERLOCK, S.: Immunologic response to tetanus toxoid inoculation in patients with hepatic cirrhosis. New Engl. J. Med. **261**, 340 (1959).

CHERUBIN, C.E., HARGRAVE, R.L., PRINCE, A.M.: The serum hepatitis related antigen (SH) in illicit drug users. Amer. J. Epidem. **91**, 510 (1970).

CHERUBIN, C.E., PURCELL, R.H., LANDER, J.J., MCGINN, T.G., CONE, L.A.: Acquisition of antibody to hepatitis B antigen in three socioeconomically different medical populations. Lancet **1972 II**, 149.

CHUNG, W.K., MOON, S.K., GERSHON, R.K., PRINCE, A.M., POPPER, H.: Anicteric hepatitis in Korea. Arch. intern. Med. **113**, 535 (1964).

CHUTTANI, H.K., SIDHU, A.S., WIG, K.L., GUPTA, D,N., RAMALINGASWAMI, V.: Follow-up study of cases from the Delhi epidemic of infectious hepatitis, 1955–1956. Brit. med. J. **2**, 676 (1966).

COHEN, R., KALSER, M.H., THOMSON, R.V.: Fatal hepatic necrosis secondary to isoniazid therapy. J. Amer. med. Ass. **176**, 877 (1961).

COLE, R.A.: Viral agents from patients with infective hepatitis. Aust. J. exp. Biol. med. Sci. **43**, 497 (1965).

COMBES, B., STASTNY, P., SHOREY, J., EIGENBRODT, E.H., BARRERA, A., HULL, A.R., CARTER, N.W.: Glomerulonephritis with deposition of Australia antigen-antibody complexes in glomerular basement membrane. Lancet **1971 II**, 234.

CONRAD, M.E.: Endemic viral hepatitis in U.S. soldiers: causative factors and the effect of prophylactic gamma globulin. Canad. med Ass. J. **106**, 456 (1972).

COOKSLEY, W.G.E., COWEN, A.E., POWELL, L.W.: The incidence of oxyphenisatin ingestion in active chronic hepatitis: a retrospective controlled study of 29 patients. Aust. N.Z. J. Med. **3**, 124 (1973).

COOKSLEY, W.G., POWELL, L.W., MISTILIS, S.P., OLSEN, G., MATHEWS, J.D., MACKAY, I.R.: Australia antigen in active chronic hepatitis in Australia: results in 130 patients from three centres. Aust. N.Z. J. Med. **2**, 261 (1972).

COOMBS, R.R.A., GELL P.G.H.: Classification of allergic reactions responsible for clinical hypersensitivity and disease. In: Clinical Aspects of Immunology, 2nd ed. (GELL, P.G.H., and COOMBS, R.R.A., eds.), pp. 575–596. Oxford: Blackwell 1968.

COOPER, W.C., GERSHON, R.K., SUN, S.C., FRESH, J.W.: Anicteric viral hepatitis: A clinicopathological follow-up study in Taiwan. New Engl. J. Med. **274**, 585 (1966).

Co-operative Study. Prophylactic gamma globulin for prevention of epidemic hepatitis. Arch. intern. Med. **128**, 723 (1971).

COPE, V.Z.: Human Actinomycosis. London: Heinemann 1952.
CORCORAN, I.E., HEGSTROM, G.J., ZOECKLER, S.J., KEIL, P.G.: Liver structure in nonfatal malaria. Gastroenterology **24**, 53 (1953).
COYNE, V.E., MILLMAN, I., CERDA, J., GERSTLEY, B.J.S., LONDON, T., SUTNICK, A., BLUMBERG, B.S.: The localization of Australia antigen by immunofluorescence. J. exp. Med. **131**, 307 (1970).
CREUTZFELDT, W., SEVERIDT, H.J., SCHMITT, A., GALLASCH, E., ARNDT, H.J., BRACHMANN, H., SCHMIDT, G., TSCHAEPE, J.: Untersuchungen über Häufigkeit und Verlauf der ikterischen und anikterischen Transfusionshepatitis. Dtsch. med. Wschr. **91**, 1813 (1966).
CULLINAN, E.R., KING, R.C., RIVERS, J.S.: The prognosis of infective hepatitis: A preliminary account of a long-term follow-up. Brit. med. J. **1**, 1315 (1968).
DANE, D.S., CAMERON, C.H., BRIGGS, M.: Virus-like particles in serum of patients with Australia antigen-associated hepatitis. Lancet **1970I**, 695.
DAWKINS, R.L., JOSKE, R.A.: Immunoglobulin deposition in liver of patients with active chronic hepatitis and antibody against smooth muscle. Brit. med. J. **2**, 643 (1973).
DEFRONZO, R.A., MURRAY, G.F., MADDREY, W.C.: Aeromonas septicemia from hepatobiliary disease. Amer. J. dig. Dis. **18**, 323 (1973).
DE GAST, G.C., HOUWEN, B., NIEWEG, H.O.: Specific lymphocyte stimulation by purified head-inactivated hepatitis-B antigen. Brit. med. J. **4**, 707 (1973).
DE GROOTE, J., DESMET, V.J., GEDIGK, P., KORB, G., POPPER, H., POULSEN, H., SCHEUER, P.J., SCHMID, M., THALER, H., UEHLINGER, E., WEPLER, W.: A classification of chronic hepatitis. Lancet **1968II**, 626.
DEICHER, H.R.G., HOLMAN, H.R., KUNKE, H.G.: Anti-cytoplasmic factors in the sera of patients with systemic lupus erythematosus and certain other diseases. Arthr. and Rheum. **3**, 1 (1960).
DEINHARDT, F., HOLMES, A.W., CAPPS, R.B., POPPER, H.: Studies on the transmission of human viral hepatitis to marmoset monkeys. I. Transmission of disease, serial passages and descritpion of liver lesions. J. exp. Med. **125**, 673 (1967).
DEINHARDT, F., WOLFE, L., JUNGE, U., HOLMES, A.W.: Viral hepatitis in non-human primates. Canad. med. Ass. J. **106**, 468 (1972).
DEL PRETE, S., CONSTANTINO, M., DOGLIA, M., FABIANI, M.P., BORIN, R.: Epidemic hepatitis associated antigen. Cand. med. Ass. J. **106**, 493 (1972).
DEW, H.: Hydatid disease. Sydney: Australian Medical Publishing Co. Ltd. 1928.
DIBLE, J.H.: Degeneration, necrosis, and fibrosis in the liver. Brit. med. J. **1**, 833 (1951).
DIEDERICHSEN, H.: Hetero-antibody against bile canaliculi in patients with chronic, clinically active hepatitis. Acta med. scand. **186**, 299 (1969).
DIENER, T.O.: Is the scrapie agent a viroid? Nature (Lond.) New Biol. **235**, 218 (1972).
DISMUKES, W.E.: Oxacillin-induced hepatic dysfunction. J. Amer. med. Ass. **226**, 861 (1973).
DOBIAS, G., BALAZS, M.: Studies of the pathogenetic role of humoral antibodies reacting with subcellular organ antigens: I. Active immunization of rabbits with rat-organ antigens. Immunology **12**, 373 (1967a).
DOBIAS, G., BALAZS, M.: Studies of the pathogenetic role of humoral antibodies reacting with subcellular organ antigens: II. Passive immunization of rats with anti-rat rabbit immune sera. Immunology **12**, 389 (1967b).
DONIACH, D., LINDQVIST, H.L., BERG, P.A.: Non-organ specific cytoplasmic antibodies detected by immunofluorescence. Int. Arch. Allergy **41**, 501 (1971).
DONIACH, D., ROITT, I.M., TAYLOR, K.B.: Autoimmunity in pernicious anaemia and thyroiditis. A family study. Ann. N.Y. Acad. Sci. **124**, 605 (1965).
DONIACH, D., ROITT, I.M., WALKER, J.G., SHERLOCK, S.: Tissue antibodies in primary biliary cirrhosis, active chronic (lupoid) hepatitis, cryptogenic cirrhosis and other liver diseases and their clinical implications. Clin. exp. Immunol. **1**, 237 (1966).
DONIACH, D., WALKER, J.G.: A unified concept of autoimmune hepatitis. Lancet **1969I**, 813.
DONIACH, D., WALKER, J.G.: Immunopathology of liver disease. Progr. Liver Dis. **4**, 381 (1972).
DORDAL, E., GLAGOV, S., ORLANDO, R.A., PLATZ, C.: Fatal halothane hepatitis with transient granulomas. New Engl. J. Med. **283**, 357 (1970).
DOUGHERTY, W.J., ALTMAN, R.: Viral hepatitis in New Jersey, 1960–1961. Amer. J. Med. **32**, 704 (1962).
DRURY, R.A.B.: Larval granulomata in the liver. Gut **3**, 289 (1962).
DUBOIS, E.L., HOROWITZ, R.E., DEMOPOULOS, H.B., TEPLITZ, R.: NZB/NZW mice as a model of systemic lupus erythematosus. J. Amer. med. Ass. **195**, 285 (1966).
DUDLEY, F.J., FOX, R.A., SHERLOCK, S.: Relationship of hepatitis-associated antigen (HAA) to acute and chronic liver injury. Lancet **1971II**, 1.
DUDLEY, F.J., FOX, R.H., SHERLOCK, S.: Cellular immunity and hepatitis associated Australia antigen liver disease. Lancet **1972I**, 723.
DUDLEY, F.J., GIUSTINO, V., SHERLOCK, S.: Cell mediated immunity in patients positive for hepatitis-associated antigen. Brit. med. J. **4**, 754 (1972).
DUDLEY, F.J., O'SHEA, M.J., AJDUKIEWICZ, A., SHERLOCK, S.: Serum autoantibodies and immunoglobulins in hepatitis-associated antigen (HAA)-positive and -negative liver disease. Gut **14**, 360 (1973).

DUDLEY, F.J., SCHEUER, P.J., SHERLOCK, S.: Natural history of hepatitis-associated antigen-positive chronic liver disease. Lancet **1972II**, 1388.
DUPONT, H.L., HORNICK, R.B., LEVIN, H.S., RAPAPORT, M.I., WOODWARD, T.E.: Q fever hepatitis. Ann. intern. Med. **74**, 198 (1971).
DUPUY, J.M., LEVEY-LEBLOND, E., LE PREVOST, C.: Immunopathology of mouse hepatitis virus type 3 infection. II. Effect of immunosuppression in resistant mice. J. Immunol. **114**, 226 (1975).
EATON, M.D., MURPHY, W.D., HANFORD, V.L.: Heterogenetic antibodies in acute hepatitis. J. exp. Med. **79**, 539 (1944).
EDDLESTON, A.L.W.F., MCFARLANE, I.G., MITCHELL, C.G., REED, W.D., WILLIAMS, R.: Cell-mediated immune response in primary biliary cirrhosis to a protein fraction from human bile. Brit. med. J. **4**, 274 (1973).
EDDLESTON, A.L.W.F., WILLIAMS, R.: Inadequate antibody response to HBAg or suppressor T-cell defect in development of active chronic hepatitis. Lancet **1974II**, 1543.
EDGINGTON, T.S., RITT, D.J.: Infected cells specify different membrane glycoproteins. Proc. nat. Acad. Sci. (Wash.) **65**, 865 (1970).
EDGINTON, T.W., RITT, D.J.: Intrahepatic expression of serum hepatitis virus associated antigens. J. exp. Med. **134**, 871 (1971).
Editorial Comment: Subtypes of Australia antigen. Brit. med. J. **1**, 127 (1973).
Editorial Comment,: Herpes hepatitis in adults. Brit. med. J. **1**, 248 (1973).
EKLUND, C.M., HADLOW, W.J., KENNEDY, R.C., BOYLE, G.C.: Aleutian disease of mink: Properties of the etiologic agent and the host responses. J. infect. Dis. **118**, 510 (1968).
ELIAKIM, M., ZLOTNICK, A., SLAVIN, S.: Gammopathy in liver disease. Progr. Liver Dis. **4**, 403 (1972).
ELIASTAM, M., HOLMES, A.W.: Hepatitis, arthritis and lupus cell phenomena caused by methyldopa. Am. J. dig. Dis. **16**, 1014 (1971).
ELKINGTON, S.G., SCHREIBER, W.M, CONN, H.O.: Hepatic injury caused by L-alpha-methyl dopa. Circulation **40**, 589 (1969).
ELLING, P., RANLØV, P., BILDSØE, P.: A genetic approach to the pathogenesis of hepatic cirrhosis. Acta med. scand. **179**, 527 (1966).
EPPINGER, H.: Die Pathogenie des Icterus. Ergebn. inn. Med. Kinderheilk. **1**, 107 (1908).
ESCHAR, J., REIF, L., WARON, M., ALKAN, W.J.: Hepatic lesion in chickenpox. Gastroenterology **64**, 462 (1973).
ESPINOSA, E.: Circulating tissue antigens. II. Studies on an organ specific antigen of human liver. Lab. Invest. **29**, 556 (1973).
ESPIRITU, C.R., KIM, T.S., LEVINE, R.A.: Granulomatous hepatitis associated with sulfadimethoxine hypersensitivity. J. Amer. med. Ass. **202**, 985 (1967).
ESTERLY, J.R., SLUSSER, R.J., RUEBNER, B.H.: Hepatic lesions in the congenital rubella syndrome. J. Pediat. **71**, 676 (1967).
FABER, V., ELLING, P.: Anti-nuclear factors in hepatic cirrhosis, with special reference to the different nuclear antigenicity of various tissues. Acta. path. microbiol. scand. **69**, 11 (1967).
FACEY, R.V., MARSDEN, P.D.: Fascioliasis in man: an outbreak in Hampshire. Brit. med. J. **2**, 619 (1960).
FARROW, L.J., HOLBOROW, E.J., JOHNSON, G.D., LAMB, S.G., STEWART, J.S., TAYLOR, P.E., ZUCKERMAN, A.J.: Autoantibodies and the hepatitis-associated antigen in acute infective hepatitis. Brit. med. J. **2**, 693 (1970).
FEHER, J., SOMOGYI, T., TIMMER, M., JOZSA, L.: Early syphilitic hepatitis. Lancet **1975II**, 896.
FEIGIN, R.E., ANDERSON, D.C.: Human leptospirosis, CRC Crit. Rev. Clin. Lab. Sci. **5**, 413 (1975).
FEINSTONE, S.M., KAPIKIAN, A.Z., PURCELL, R.H.: Hepatitis A: detection by immune electron microscopy of a virus-like agent associated with acute illness. Science **182**, 1026 (1973).
FEINSTONE, S.M., KAPIKIAN, A.Z., PURCELL, R.H., ALTER, H.J., HOLLAND, P.V.: Transfusion-associated hepatitis not due to viral hepatitis type A or B. New Engl. J. Med. **292**, 767 (1975).
FEIZI, T.: Immunoglobulins in chronic liver disease. Gut **9**, 193 (1968).
FEIZI, T., NACCARATO, R., SHERLOCK, S., DONIACH, D.: Mitochondrial and other tissue antibodies in relatives of patients with primary biliary cirrhosis. Clin. exp. Immunol. **10**, 609 (1972).
FENNELL, R.H., SANTAMARIA, A.: Anaphylaxis in the rat: Immunohistochemical and histochemical studies of the liver. Amer. J. Path. **41**, 521 (1962).
FERRIS, A.A.: Antigens in infectious hepatitis. Brit. med. Bull. **28**, 131 (1972).
FERRIS, A.A., COLE, R.A.: Detroit 6 cells and infective hepatitis. Med. J. Austr. **2**, 1213 (1966).
FINLAYSON, N.D.C., KROHN, K., ANDERSON, K.E., JOKELAINEN, P.T., PRINCE, A.M.: Interrelations of hepatitis B antigen and autoantibodies in chronic idiopathic liver disease. Gastroenterology **63**, 646 (1972).
FINLAYSON, N.D.C., KROHN, K., FAUCONNET, M.H., ANDERSON, K.E.: Significance of serum complement levels in chronic liver disease. Gastroenterology, **63**, 653 (1972).
FLEGEL, H.: Über die Leberveränderungen bei der Lues congenita. Zbl. allg. Path. path. Anat. **87**, 302 (1951).

FOX, R.A., DUDLEY, F.J., SHERLOCK, S.: The serum concentration of the third component of complement $\beta 1C/\beta 1A$ in liver disease. Gut **12**, 574 (1971).

FOX, R.A., DUDLEY, F.J., SHERLOCK, S.: The primary immune response to hemocyanin in patients with primary biliary cirrhosis. Clin. exp. Immunol. **14**, 473 (1973).

FOX, R.A., JAMES, D.G., SCHEUER, P.J., SHARMA, O., SHERLOCK, S.: Impaired delayed hypersensitivity in primary biliary cirrhosis. Lancet **1969I**, 959.

FOX, R.A., NIAZI, S.P., SHERLOCK, S.: Hepatitis-associated antigen in chronic liver disease. Lancet **1969II**, 609.

FRANKEN, F.H., AMELUNG, D., GARKE, P., POHLE, D., LIEBERMEISTER, H., DEUPMANN, F.J.: Zur Frage der posthepatitischen Lebercirrhose. Dtsch. med. Wschr. **94**, 1309 (1969).

FREUDENBERG, J., ERDMANN, K., MEYER ZUM BÜSCHENFELDE, K.H., FÖRSTER, E. BERGER, J.: HL-A bei Lebererkrankungen. Klin. Wschr. **51**, 1075 (1973).

FUNG, W.P., CHEW, B.K., TAN K.K.: Active chronic hepatitis with positive L.E. cell test and lupus nephritis. Aust. Ann. Med. **18**, 288 (1969).

FUTCH, C., ZIKRIA, B.A., NEU, H.C.: Bacteroides liver abscess. Surgery **73**, 59 (1973).

GABBIANI, G., RYAN, G.B., LAMELIN, J-P., VASSALLI, P., MAJNO, G., BOUVIER, C.A., CRUCHAUD, A., LUSCHER, E.F.: Human smooth muscle autoantibody—its identification as antiactin antibody and a study of its binding to "nonmuscular" cells. Amer. J. Path. **72**, 473 (1973).

GAJDUSEK, D.C.: An "autoimmune" reaction against human tissue antigens in certain acute and chronic diseases: I. Serological investigations. Arch. intern. Med. **101**, 9 (1958).

GALBRAITH, R.M., EDDLESTON, A.L.W.F., SMITH, M.G.M., WILLIAMS, R., MACSWEEN, R.N.M., WATKINSON, G., DICK, H., KENNEDY, L.A., BATCHELOR, J.R.: Histocompatibility antigens in active chronic hepatitis and primary biliary cirrhosis. Brit. med. J. **3**, 604 (1974b).

GALBRAITH, R.M., SMITH, M., MACKENZIE, R.M., TEE, D.E., DONIACH, D., WILLIAMS, R.: High prevalence of sero-immunologic abnormalities in relatives of patients with active chronic hepatitis or primary biliary cirrhosis. New Engl. J. Med. **290**, 63 (1974a).

GALLAGHER, N.D., GOULSTON, S.J.M.: Persistent acute viral hepatitis. Brit. med. J. **1**, 906 (1962).

GARIBALDI, R.A., HATCH, F.E., BISNO, A.L., HATCH, M.H., GREGG, M.B.: Nonparenteral serum hepatitis. Report on an outbreak. J. Amer. med. Ass. **220**, 963 (1972).

GERBER, M.A., BRODIN, A., STEINBERG, D., VERNACE, S., YANG, C., PARONETTO, F.: Periarteritis nodosa, Australia antigen and lymphatic leukemia. New Engl. J. Med. **286**, 14 (1972).

GERBER, P., GOLDSTEIN, G.: Relationship of Epstein-Barr virus-induced membrane antigens in lymphoid cells to viral envelop antigens. J. Immunol. **105**, 793 (1970).

GERBER, M.A., POPPER, H.: Relation between central canals and portal tracts in alcoholic hepatitis. A contribution to the pathogenesis of cirrhosis in alcoholics. Human Path. **3**, 199 (1972).

GERBER, M.A., SCHAFFNER, F., PARONETTO, F.: Immunoelectron microscopy of hepatitis B antigen in liver. Proc. Soc. exp. Biol. (N.Y.) **140**, 13 (1972).

GERIN, J.L., SHIH, J.W.-K., KAPLAN, P.M.: Biophysical and biochemical characterization of hepatitis B antigen. Amer. J. med. Sci. **270**, 115 (1975).

GIANOTTI, F.: The Australia antigen in infantile papular acrodermatitis. Gut **12**, 763 (1971).

GILES, J.P., KRUGMAN, S.: Viral hepatitis. Immunoglobulin response during the course of the disease. J. Amer. med. Ass. **208**, 497 (1969).

GILES, J.P., MCCOLLUM, R.W., BERNDTSON, L.W., KRUGMAN, S.: Viral hepatitis: relation of Australia/SH antigen to the Willowbrook MS-2 strain. New Engl. J. Med. **281**, 119 (1969).

GILLE, G., RINGERZ, O., ZETTERBERG, B.: Serum hepatitis among Swedish track finders. II. A clinical study. Acta med. scand. **182**, 129 (1967).

GIRARD, J.P., HAENNI, B., BERGOZ, R., KAPANCI, Y., CRUCHAUD, A.: Lupoid hepatitis following administration of penicillin. Helv. med. Acta **34**, 23 (1967).

GIUSTINO, V., DUDLEY, F.J., SHERLOCK, S.: Thymus dependent lymphocyte function in patients with hepatitis associated antigen. Lancet **1972II**, 850.

GOCKE, D.J., HSU, K., MORGAN, C., BOMBARDIERI, S., LOCKSHIN, M., CHRISTIAN, C.L.: Vasculitis in association with Australia antigen. J. exp. Med. **134**, 330s (1971).

GOCKE, D.J., KAVEY, N.B.: Hepatitis antigen. Lancet **1969I**, 1055.

GOCKE, D.J., PREISIG, R., MORRIS, T.Z., MCKAY, D.G., BRADLEY, S.E.: Esperimental viral hepatitis in the dog: Production of persistent disease in partially immune animals. J. clin. Invest. **46**, 1506 (1967).

GOLDFINGER, S.E., MARX, S.: Hypersensitivity hepatitis due to phenazopyridine hydrochloride. New Engl. J. Med. **286**, 1090 (1972).

GOLDING, P.L., BOWN, R., MASON, A.M.S., TAYLOR, E.: "Sicca complex" in liver disease. Brit. med. J. **4**, 340 (1970).

GOLDING, P.L., MASON, A.M.S.: Renal tubular acidosis and autoimmune liver disease. Gut **12**, 153 (1971).

GOLDING, P.L., SMITH, M., WILLIAMS, R.: Multisystem involvement in chronic liver disease. Studies on the incidence and pathogenesis. Amer. J. Med. **55**, 772 (1973).

GOLDSTEIN, A.G.: Sarcoid reaction associated with phenylbutazone hypersensitivity. Ann. Intern. Med. **59**, 97 (1963).

GOLDSTEIN, G., MACKAY, I.R.: Lupoid hepatitis: Computer analysis defining "hepatitis" and "cirrhosis" phases and relationships between hepatocellular damage and immune reactions in the liver. Aust. Ann. Med. **16**, 62 (1967).
GOLDSTEIN, G.B., LAM, K.C., MISTILIS, S.P.: Drug-induced active chronic hepatitis. Amer. J. dig. Dis. **18**, 177 (1973).
GORDON, I., BERBERIAN, M., STEVENSON, D., REDECKER, A.G.: Distribution of hepatitis B antigenic determinants in different forms of viral hepatitis. J. infect. Dis. **126**, 569 (1972).
GOUDIE, R.B., MACSWEEN, R.N.M., GOLDBERG, D.M.: Serological and histological diagnosis of primary biliary cirrhosis. J. clin. Path. **19**, 527 (1966).
GRADY, G.F.: Australia antigen and viral hepatitis. Viewpoints on digest. Dis. **2**, No. 2 (1970).
GRAY, N., MACKAY, I.R., TAFT, L.I., WEIDEN S., WOOD, I.J.: Hepatitis, colitis and lupus manifestations. Amer. J. dig. Dis. **3**, 481 (1958).
GUDAT, F., BIANCHI, L., SONNABEND, W., THIEL, G., AENISHAENSLIN, W., STALDER, G.A.: Pattern of core and surface expression in liver tissue reflects state of specific immune response in hepatitis B. Lab. Invest. **32**, 1 (1975).
HADZIYANNIS, S., GERBER, M.A., VISSOULIS, C., POPPER, H.: Cytoplasmic hepatitis B antigen in "ground-glass" hepatocytes of carriers. Arch. Path. **96**, 327 (1973).
HADZIYANNIS. S., MOUSSOUROS, A., VISSOULIS, C., AFROUDAKIS, A.: Cytoplasmic localization of Australia antigen in the liver. Lancet **1972I**, 976.
HAEX, A.J.CH., VAN BEEK, C.: Tuberculosis and aspiration liver biopsy; its clinical significance. In: Diagnosis and Therapy. Haarlem: DEERVEN, F., BOHN, N.V. 1955.
HAHN, R.D.: Syphilis of the liver. Amer. J. Syph. **27**, 529 (1943).
HANSHAW, J.B., BETTS, R.F., SIMON, G., BOYNTON, R.C.: Acquired cytomegalvirus infection. New Engl. J. Med. **272**, 602 (1965).
HAUG, H.: Die "persistierende Hepatitis" im Vergleich mit den anderen chronischen Verlaufsformen nach epidemischer Virushepatitis. Klin. Wschr. **46**, 221 (1968).
HAVENS, P.: Viral hepatitis. Clinical patterns and diagnosis. Amer. J. Med. **32**, 665 (1962).
HEATHCOTE, J., SHERLOCK, S.: Spread of acute hepatitis B in London. Lancet **1973I**, 1468.
HELSKE, T., NEVANLINNA, H.R.: Familial accumulation of carriers of Au antigen. J. med. Genet. **10**, 270 (1973).
HERSEY, D.F., SHAW, E.D.: Viral agents in hepatitis. A review, Lab. Invest. **19**, 558 (1968).
HERSH, T., MELNICK, J.L., GOYAL, R.F., GOLLINGER, F.B.: Nonparenteral transmission of viral hepatitis type B (Australia antigen-associated serum hepatitis). New Engl. J. Med. **285**, 1363 (1971).
HILL, P.A., WALSHE, J.H., PURCELL, R.M.: Failure to demonstrate circulating interferon during incubation period and acute stage of transfusion-associated hepatitis. Proc. Soc. exp. Biol. (N.Y.) **136**, 853 (1971).
HIRSCHMAN, R.J., SHULMAN, N.R., BARKER, L.F., SMITH, K.O.: Virus-like particles in sera of patients with infectious and serum hepatitis. J. Amer. med. Ass. **208**, 1667 (1969).
HOENSCH, H., HARTWICH, C.: Panzytopenien und Knochenmarksveränderungen bei chronisch-aggressiver Hepatitis. Dtsch. med. Wschr. **97**, 1491 (1972).
HOFSTAD, M.S., MCGEHEE, E.H., BENNETT, P.C.: Avian infectious hepatitis. Avian Dis. **2**, 358 (1958).
HOLBOROW, E.J.: Immunological aspects of viral hepatitis. Brit. med. Bull. **28**, 142 (1972).
HOLBOROW, E.J., ASHERSON, G.L., JOHNSON, G.D., BARNES, R.D.S., CARMICHAEL, D.S.: Antinuclear factor and other antibodies in blood and liver diseases. Brit. med. J. **1**, 656 (1963).
HOLBOROW, E.J., HEMSTED, E.H., MEAD, S.V.: Smooth muscle auto-antibodies in infectious mononucleosis. Brit. med. J. **3**, 323 (1973).
HOLDSWORTH, C.D., HALL, E.W., DAWSON, A.M., SHERLOCK, S.: Ulcerative colitis in chronic liver disease. Quart. J. Med. **34**, 211 (1965).
HOLLAND, J.J., KIEHN, E.D.: Influenza virus effects on cell membrane proteins. Science **167**, 202 (1970).
HOLLAND, P.V., ALTER, H.J., PURCELL, R.H., SCOURIS, J.T.: Hepatitis-associated antigen and antibody in cold ethanol fractionates of human blood. Vox Sang. (Basel) **20**, 464 (1971).
HOLLAND, P.V., PURCELL, R.H., SMITH, H., ALTER, H.J.: Subtyping of hepatitis-associated antigen (HBAg); simplified technique with counter-electrophoresis. Immunology **109**, 420 (1972).
HOLMES, A.W., DEINHARDT, F., WOLFE, L., FROESNER, G., PETERSON, D., CASTO, B.: Specific neutralization of human hepatitis type A in marmoset monkeys. Nature (Lond.) **243**, 419 (1973).
HOOFNAGLE, J.H., GERETY, R.J., BARKER, L.F.: Antibody to hepatitis-B-virus core in man. Lancet **1973II**, 869.
HOOFNAGLE, J.H., GERETY, R.J., NI, L.Y., BARKER, L.F.: Antibody to hepatitis B core antigen. A sensitive indicator of hepatitis B virus replication. New Engl. J. Med. **290**, 1336 (1974).
HOPF, U., MEYER ZUM BÜSCHENFELDE, K.H.: Studies on the pathogenesis of experimental chronic active hepatitis in rabbits. II. Demonstration of immunoglobulin on isolated hepatocytes. Brit. J. exp. Path. **55**, 509 (1974).
HOTCHIN, J.: A concept of persistent virus infection. In: Viruses Affecting Man and Animals (SANDERS, M. and SCHAEFFER, M., eds.), p. 213. St. Louis, Missouri: Warren Green 1971.

HOU, P.C., PANG, I.S.C.: Chlonorchis sinensis infestation in man in Hong Kong. J. Path. Bact. **87**, 245 (1964).

HOWELL, D.S., MALCOLM, J.M., PIKE, R.: The F11 agglutinating factor in serums of patients. Amer. J. Med. **29**, 662 (1960).

HOYUMPA, A.M., CONNELL, A.M.: Methyldopa hepatitis. Amer. J. dig. Dis. **18**, 213 (1973).

HUGHES, G.R.V.: The diagnosis of systemic lupus erythematosus. Brit. J. Haemat. **25**, 409 (1973).

HUNT, J.S., SILVERSTEIN, M.J., SPARKS, F.C., HASKELL, C.M., PILCH, Y.H., MORTON, D.L.: Granulomatous hepatitis: a complication of BCG immunotherapy. Lancet **1973II**, 820.

HUSEBYE, K.O.: Jaundice with persisting pericholangiolitic inflammation in a patient treated with chlorthiazide. Amer. J. dig. Dis. **9**, 439 (1964).

HUTT, M.S.P.: Some aspects of liver disease in Ugandan Africans. Trans. trop. Med. Hyg. **54**, 273 (1971).

International Group: Morphological criteria in viral hepatitis. Lancet **1971I**, 333.

International Group: Guideline for diagnosis of therapeutic drug-induced liver injury in liver biopsies. Lancet **1974I**, 854.

IRVINE, W.J., DAVIES, S.H., DELAMORE, I.W., WILLIAMS, A.W.: Immunological relationship between pernicious anaemia and thyroid disease. Brit. med. J. **2**, 454 (1962).

ISRAEL, H.I., GOLDSTEIN, R.A.: Hepatic granulomatosis and sarcoidosis, Ann. intern. Med. **79**, 669 (1973).

IVERSEN, P., ROHOLM, K.: An aspirative biopsy of the liver with remarks on its diagnostic significance. Acta med. scand. **102**, 1 (1939).

IWARSON, S., LUNDIN, P., HERMODSSON, S.: Liver morphology in acute viral hepatitis related to the hepatitis B antigen. J. clin. Path. **25**, 850 (1972).

IWARSON, S., MAGNIUS, L., LINDHOLM, A., LUNDIN, P.: Subtypes of hepatitis B antigen in blood donors and post-transfusion hepatitis: clinical and epidemiological aspects. Brit. med. J. **1**, 84 (1973).

JARROLD, R., VILTER, R.W.: Hematologic observations in patients with chronic hepatic insufficiency. J. clin. Invest. **28**, 286 (1949).

JEFFRIES, D.J., JAMES, W.H., JEFFERISS, F.J.G., MACLEOD, K.G., WILLCOX, R.R.: Australia (hepatitis-associated) antigen in patients attending a veneral disease clinic. Brit. med. J. **2**, 455 (1973).

JENSON, A.B., MCCOMBES, R.M., SAKURADA, M., MELNICK, J.L.: Organ cultures inoculated with serum from hepatitis patient with Au antigenemia. Exp. molec. Path. **13**, 217 (1970).

JOHNSON, G.D., ASHERSON, G.L., KAKLAMANIS, E., DUMONDE, D.C.: Demonstration by immunofluorescence of auto-antibody in the serum of rabbits given injections of rat tissue. J. Path. Bact. **86**, 521 (1963).

JOHNSON, G.D., HOLBOROW, E.J., GLYNN, L.E.: Antibody to smooth muscle in patients with liver disease. Lancet **1965II**, 878.

JOHNSON, G.D., HOLBOROW, E.J., GLYNN, L.E.: Antibody to liver in lupoid hepatitis. Lancet **1966II**, 416.

JOHNSTON, G.I., MENDELSOHN, F.: Halothane hepatitis in a laboratory technician. Aust. N.Z.J. Med. **2**, 171 (1971).

JORDAN, W.S., JR., ALBRIGHT, R.W.: Liver function tests in infectious mononucleosis. J. Lab. clin. Med. **35**, 688 (1950).

JORI, G.P., PESCHLE, C.: Hydralazine disease associated with transient granulomas in the liver. Gastroenterology **64**, 1163 (1973).

JOSEPH, T.J., VOGT, P.J.: Disseminated herpes with hepatoadrenal necrosis in an adult. Amer. J. Med. **56**, 735 (1974).

JOSHI, P.H., CONN, H.O.: The syndrome of methoxyflurane-associated hepatitis. Ann. intern. Med. **80**, 395 (1974).

JOSKE, R.A., FINCKH, E.S.: Hepatic changes in human brucellosis. Med. J. Aust. **1**, 266 (1955).

JOSKE, R.A., KEALL, D.D., LEAK, P.J., STANLEY, N.F., WALTERS, M.N.I.: Hepatitis-encephalitis in humans with reovirus infection. Arch. intern. Med. **113**, 811 (1964).

JOSKE, R.A., KING, W.E.: The L.E. cell phenomenon in active chronic viral hepatitis. Lancet **1955II**, 477.

JOSKE, R.A., LAURENCE, B.H.: Familial cirrhosis with autoimmune features and raised immunoglobulin levels, Gastroenterology **59**, 546 (1970).

KAPLAN, P.M., GREENMAN, R.L., GERIN, J.L., PURCELL, R.H., ROBINS, W.S.: DNA polymerase associated with human hepatitis B antigen. J. Virol. **12**, 995 (1973).

KAPLOWITZ, N., FINLAYSON, N.D.C., WALMSLEY, P., THURNHERR, N., JAVITT, N.B.: Hepatobiliary diseases associated with serum antimitochondrial antibody (AMA). Amer. J. Med. **54**, 725 (1973).

KARAT, A.B.A., JOB, C.K., RAO, F.S.S.: Liver in leprosy: histological and biochemical findings. Brit. med. J. **1**, 307 (1971).

KATZ, R., RODRIGUEZ, J., WARD, R.: Post-transfusion hepatitis-effect of modified gamma globulin added to blood *in vitro*. New Engl. J. Med. **285**, 925 (1971).

KIM, C.Y.: Hepatitis associated antigen. Its biologic properties and nucleic acid. Vox Sang. (Basel) **20**, 461 (1971).
KIM, C.Y., BISSELL, D.M.: Stability of the lipid protein of hepatitis-associated (Australia) antigen. J. infect. Dis. **123**, 470 (1971).
KLATSKIN, G.: Subacute hepatic necrosis and postnecrotic cirrhosis due to anicteric infections with the hepatitis virus. Amer. J. Med. **25**, 333 (1958).
KLATSKIN, G.: Mechanisms of toxic and drug induced hepatic injury, chap. 14, Toxicity of Anaesthetics. New York: Williams and Wilkins 1968.
KLATSKIN, G.: Hepatitis associated with systemic infections, chap. 21 in: Diseases of the Liver, 4th ed., ed. by SCHIFF, L. Philadelphia: Lippincott 1975.
KLATSKIN, G., KANTOR, F.S.: Mitochondrial antibody in primary biliary cirrhous and other diseases. Ann. intern. Med. **77**, 533 (1972).
KLATSKIN, G., KIMBERG, D.V.: Recurrent hepatitis attributable to halothane, sensitization in an anesthetist. New Engl. J. Med. **280**, 515 (1969).
KLINGE, O., KABOTH, U., ARNOLD, R.: Histologische Leberuntersuchungen bei gesunden Australia (SH)-Antigen-und-Antikörper-Trägern. Dtsch. med. Wschr. **95**, 2583 (1970).
KNOLLE, J., MEYER ZUM BÜSCHENFELDE, K.H., BOLTE, J.P., BERGER, J.: Cellular immune response to hepatitis associated antigen and homologous liver specific protein in acute HAA positive hepatitis. Klin. Wschr. **51**, 1172 (1973).
KOFF, R.S., GRADY, G.F., CHALMERS, T.C., MOSLEY, J.W., SWARTZ, B.L.: Viral hepatitis in a group of Boston hospitals. III. Importance of exposure to shellfish in a non-epidemic period. New Engl. J. Med. **276**, 703 (1967).
KOFF, R.S., ISSELBACHER, K.J.: Changing concepts in the epidemiology of viral hepatitis. New Engl. J. Med. **278**, 1371 (1968).
KOFFLER, D., CARR, R.J., AGNELLO, V., FEIZI, T., KUNKEL, H.G.: Antibodies to polynucleotides. Distribution in human serums. Science **166**, 1648 (1969).
KOHLER, P.: Clinical immune complex disease. Manifestations in systemic lupus erythematosus and hepatitis B virus infection. Medicine (Baltimore) **52**, 419 (1973).
KONTTINEN, A., PERÄSALO, J.O.S., EISALO, A.: Sulfonamide hepatitis. Acta med. scand. **191**, 389 (1972).
KORN, R.J., KELLOW, W.F., HELLER, P., CHOMET, B., ZIMMERMAN, H.J.: Hepatic involvement in extrapulmonary tuberculosis; histologic and functional characteristics. Amer. J. Med. **27**, 60 (1959).
KRASSNITSKY, O., PESENDORFER, F., WEWALKA, F.: Australia-SH-Antigen und Lebererkrankungen. Dtsch. med. Wschr. **95**, 249 (1970).
KRAWCZYNSKY, K., NAZAREWICZ, T., BRZOSKO, W.J., NOWOSLAWSKI, A.: Cellular localization of hepatitis-associated antigen in livers of patients with different forms of hepatitis. J. infect. Dis. **126**, 372 (1972).
KROHN, K., FINLAYSON, N.D.C., JOKELAINEN, P.T., ANDERSON, K.E., PRINCE, A.M.: Electron microscopical and immunological observations of the serum-hepatitis (S.H.) antigen in primary biliary cirrhosis. Lancet **1970II**, 379.
KROOK, H.: Liver cirrhosis in patients with a lupus erythematosus-like syndrome. Acta med. scand. **169**, 713 (1961).
KRUGMAN, S., FRIEDMAN, H., LATTIMER, C.: Viral hepatitis, type A: Identification by specific complement fixation and immune adherence tests. New Engl. J. Med. **292**, 1141 (1975).
KRUGMAN, S., GILES, J.P.: Viral hepatitis. New light on an old disease. J. Amer. med. Ass. **212**, 1019 (1970).
KRUGMAN, S., GILES J.P.: Viral hepatitis, Type B (MS-2 strain). Further observations on natural history and prevention. New Engl. J. Med. **238**, 755 (1973).
KRUGMAN, S., GILES, J.P., HAMMOND, J.: Infectious hepatitis. Evidence for two distinctive clinical epidemological and immunological types of infection. J. Amer. med. Ass. **200**, 365 (1967).
KRUGMAN, S., GILES, J.P., HAMMOND J.: Viral hepatitis, Type B MS-2 strain. Prevention with specific hepatitis B immune serum globulin. J. Amer. med. Ass. **218**, 1665 (1971).
KRUGMAN, S., WARD, R., GILES, J.P.: The natural history of infectious hepatitis. Amer. J. Med. **32**, 717 (1962).
KUNKEL, H.G., AHRENS, E.H., EISENMENGER, W.J., BONGIOVANNI, A.M., SLATER, R.J.: E treme hypergammaglobulinemia in young women with liver disease. J. clin. Invest. **30**, 654 (1951).
LAITINEN, O., VAHERI, A.: Very high measles and rubella virus antibody titres associated with hepatitis, systemic lupus erythematosus and infectious mononucleosis. Lancet **1974I**, 194.
LAM, K.C., MISTILIS, S.P., PERROTT, N.: Positive tissue antibody tests in patients with prolonged extrahepatic biliary obstruction. New Engl. J. Med. **286**, 1400 (1972).
LAMB, S.G., STERN, H.: Cytomegalovirus mononucleosis with jaundice. Lancet **1966II**, 1003.
Lancet Editorial: What about Type A hepatitis. Lancet **1973II**, 1007.
Lancet Editorial: e and anti-e. Lancet **1975II**, 1191.
LANDER, J.L., ALTER, H.J., PURCELL, R.H.: Frequency of antibody to hepatitis-associated antigen as measured by a new radioimmunoassay technique. J. Immunol. **106**, 1166 (1971).

LANDER, J.J., HOLLAND, P.V., ALTER, H.J., CHANOCK, R.M., PURCELL, R.H.: Antibody to hepatitis-associated antigen. Frequency and pattern of response as detected by radioimmunoprecipitation. J. Amer. med. Ass. **220**, 1079 (1972).

LANGNESS, U., SELMAIR, H., OPITZ, K.: Rheumatoid hepatitis? Münch. med. Wschr. **111**, 2486 (1969).

LARSEN, R.A.: Family studies in systemic lupus erythematosus, Suppl. 543 to Acta med. scand. (1972).

LAZARCHICK, J., DE SOUZA, E., SILVA, N.A., NICHOLS, D.R., WASHINGTON, J.A.: Pyogenic liver abscess. Mayo Clin. Proc. **48**, 349 (1973).

LEADER, R.W., WAGNER, B.M., HENSON, J.B., GORHAM, J.R.: Structural and histochemical observations of liver and kidney in Aleutian disease of mink. Amer. J. Path. **43**, 33 (1963).

LEBOUVIER, G.L.: The heterogeneity of Australia antigen. J. infect. Dis. **123**, 671 (1972).

LEBOUVIER, G.L.: Subtypes of hepatitis-B antigen: Clinical relevance. Ann. intern. Med. **79**, 894 (1973).

LEBOUVIER, G.L., MCCOLLUM, R.W., HIERHOLZER, W.J., JR., IRWIN, G.R., KRUGMAN, S., GILES, J.P.: Subtypes of Australia antigen and hepatitis-B virus. J. Amer. med. Ass. **222**, 928 (1972).

LEE, A.K.Y.: Auto-antibodies in cirrhosis and hepatocellular carcinoma. Aust. N.Z. J. Med. **3**, 268 (1973).

LEE, A.K.Y., MACKAY, I.R., ROWLEY, M.J., YAP, C.Y.: Measurement of antibody-producing capacity to flagellin in man. IV. Studies in autoimmune disease, allergy, and after azathioprine treatment. Clin. exp. Immunol. **9**, 507 (1971).

LEE, W.M., REED, W.D., MITCHELL, C.G., GALBRAITH, R.M., EDDLESTON, A.L.W.F., ZUCKERMAN, A.J., WILLIAMS, R.: Cellular and humoral immunity to hepatitis-B surface antigen in active chronic hepatitis. Brit. med. J. **1**, 705 (1975).

LEHMANN-GRUBE, F.: Persistent infection of the mouse with the virus of lymphocytic choriomeningitis. J. clin. Path. **25**, 8 (1972).

LEONHARDT, T.: Family studies in systemic lupus erythematosus. Acta med. scand. Suppl. 416 to vol. **176** (1964).

LEPREVOST, C., LEVEY-LEBLOND, E., VIRELIZIER, J.L., DUPUY, J.M.: Immunopathology of mouse hepatitis virus type 3 infection. I. Role of humoral and cell-mediated immunity in resistance mechanisms. J. Immunol. **114**, 221 (1975).

LINKE, A.: Thymustumor mit lupoider Hepatitis. Schweiz. med. Wschr. **95**, 1492 (1965).

LURMAN, A.: Eine Icterusepidemie. Berl. klin. Wschr. **22**, 20 (1885).

LYFORD, J., III, JOHNSON, R.W., JR., BLACKMAN, S., SCOTT, R.B.: Pathologic findings in a fatal case of disseminated granuloma inguinale with miliary bone and joint involvement. Bull. Johns Hopk. Hosp. **79**, 349 (1946).

MAAS, D., SCHUBOTHE, M.: Lupus-erythematodes – ähnliches Syndrom. Dtsch. med. Wschr. **98**, 131 (1973).

MAASS, G., HAAS, R., OEHLERT, W.: Experimental infections of monkeys with the causative agent of the Frankfurt-Marburg syndrome (FMS). Lab. Anim. Handb. **4**, 155 (1970).

MACCALLUM, F.O.: Historical perspectives (viral hepatitis). Canad. med. Ass. J. **26**, 423 (1972).

MACKAY, I.R.: Primary biliary cirrhosis showing a higher titer of autoantibody. New Engl. J. Med. **258**, 185 (1958).

MACKAY I.R.: Primary biliary cirrhosis: A case with systemic lesions and circulating anti-tissue antibody. Lancet **1960II**, 521.

MACKAY, I.R.: The problem of persisting destructive disease of the liver. Gastroenterology **40**, 617 (1961).

MACKAY, I.R.: Chronic hepatitis: Effect of prolonged suppressive treatment and comparison of azathioprine with prednisolone. Quart. J. Med. **37**, 379 (1968a).

MACKAY, I.R.: Lupoid hepatitis and primary biliary cirrhosis: Autoimmune diseases of the liver? Bull. rheum. Dis. **18**, 487 (1968b).

MACKAY, I.R.: Cirrhosis and other diseases of the liver. In: Immunological Diseases, 2nd ed., ed. by SAMTER, M., TALMAGE, D.W., ROSE, B., SHERMAN, W.B., and VAUGHAN, J.H., vol. II., part V, sect. IV, 1323. Boston:Little, Brown and Co., 1971.

MACKAY, I.R.: Immunosuppressive drugs and chronic hepatitis. Med. J. Aust. **1**, 1207 (1972a).

MACKAY, I.R.: Chronic hepatitis. Canad. med. Ass. J. **106**, 519 (1972b).

MACKAY, I.R.: Etiology of chronic hepatitis. In: The Liver and its Diseases, ed. by SCHAFFNER, F., SHERLOCK, S., LEEVY, C., chap. 20. New York: Intercontinental Medical Book Corporation 1974.

MACKAY, I.R., COWLING, D.C., HURLEY, T.H.: Drug-induced autoimmune disease. Haemolytic anaemia and lupus cells after treatment with methyl dopa. Med. J. Aust. **2**, 1047 (1968).

MACKAY, I.R., GAJDUSEK, D.C.: An "autoimmune" reaction against human tissue antigens in certain acute and chronic diseases: II. Clinical correlations. Arch. intern. Med. **101**, 30 (1958).

MACKAY, I.R., LARKIN, L.: The significance of the presence in human serum of complement-fixing antibodies to human tissue antigens. Aust. Ann. Med. **7**, 251 (1958).

MACKAY, I.R., MORRIS, P.J.: Association of autoimmune active chronic hepatitis with HL-A1, 8. Lancet **1972II**, 793.

MACKAY, I.R., POPPER, H.: Immunopathogenesis of chronic hepatitis: A review. Aust. N.Z.J. Med. **1**, 79 (1973).

MACKAY, I.R., TAFT, L.I., COWLING, D.C.: Lupoid hepatitis. Lancet **1956II**, 1323.

MACKAY, I.R., WEIDEN, S., HASKER, J.: Autoimmune hepatitis. Ann. N.Y. Acad. Sci. **124**, 767 (1965).

MACKAY, I.R., WHITTINGHAM, S.: "Auto-immune" chronic hepatitis. Postgrad. Med. **41**, 72 (1967).

MACKAY, I.R., WOOD, I.J.: Lupoid hepatitis: A comparison of 22 cases with other types of chronic liver disease. Quart. J. Med. **31**, 485 (1962).

MACKAY, I.R., WOOD, I.J.: The course and treatment of lupoid hepatitis. Gastroenterology **45**, 4 (1963).

MACLACHLAN, M.J., RODNAN, G.P., COOPER, W.M., FENNELL, R.H.: Chronic active ("lupoid") hepatitis: A clinical, serological and pathological study of 20 patients. Ann. intern. Med. **62**, 425 (1965).

MACSWEEN, R.N.M.: Australia antigen and primary biliary cirrhosis. J. clin. Path. **26**, 335 (1973).

MACSWEEN, R.N.M., ARMSTRONG, E.M., GRAY, K.G., MASON, M.: Bile canalicular antibody in primary biliary cirrhosis and in other liver diseases. Lancet **1973I**, 1419.

MADDREY, W.C., BOITNOTT, J.K.: Isoniazid hepatitis. Ann. intern. Med. **79**, 1 (1973).

MADDREY, W.C., BOITNOTT, J.K.: Severe hepatitis from methyldopa. Gastroenterology **68**, 351 (1975).

MADDREY, W.C., IBER, F.L.: Familial cirrhosis—a clinical and pathological study. Ann. intern. Med. **61**, 667 (1964).

MADDREY, W.C., JOHNS, C.J., BOITNOTT, J.K., IBER, F.L.: Sarcoidosis and chronic hepatic disease: a clinical and pathologic study of 20 patients. Medicine (Baltimore) **49**, 375 (1970).

MADDREY, W.C., SAITO, S., SHULMAN, N.R., KLATSKIN, G.: Coincidental Australia antigenemia in primary biliary cirrhosis. Ann. intern. Med. **76**, 705 (1972).

MAGNIUS, L.O., ESPMARK, A.: New specificities in Australia antigen positive sera distinct from the LeBouvier determinants. J. Immunol. **109**, 1017 (1972).

MANGOS, P., MENZIES, S.: Human fascioliasis in Australia. Med. J. Aust. **1**, 295 (1973).

MARCIAL-ROJAS, R.A.: Parasitic diseases of the liver. In: The Liver (GALL, E.A., and MOSTOFI, F.K., eds.), p. 431. Baltimore: Williams and Wilkins Company, 1973.

MARTIN, C.E., ARTHAUD, J.B.: Hepatitis after isoniazid administration. New Engl. J. Med. **282**, 433 (1970).

MARTIN, D.S., SMITH, D.T.: Blastomycosis (American blastomycosis, Gilchrist's disease); report of 13 new cases. Am. Rev. Tuberc. **39**, 488 (1939).

MARTIN, W., RICKERS, J.: Cholestätische Hepatose nach Diphenyl-hydantoin. Wien. klin. Wschr. **84**, 41 (1972).

MARTINI, G.A.: Cirrhosis in Europe. In: Liver—Proceedings of an International Liver Conference (SAUNDERS, S.J., and TERBLANCHE, J., eds.), p. 255. London: Pitman Medical 1973.

MARTINI, G.A., STROHMEYER, G., SODOMANN, C.P.: Die Panarteritis Nodosa bei chronischer Hepatitis mit Australia Antigen Nachweis. Dtsch. med. Wschr. **97**, 642 (1972).

MASCOLI, C.C., ITTENSOHN, O.I., VILLAREJOS, V.M., ARQUEDAS, J.A., PROVOST, P.J., HILLEMAN, M.R.: Recovery of hepatitis agents in the marmoset from human cases occurring in Costa Rica. Proc. Soc. exp. Biol. (N.Y.) **142**, 276 (1973).

MASON, E.C., SHAW, A.E., HARDING, M.J., WITNEY, K.J.: High voltage immunoelectro-osmophoresis in Australia antigen screening of blood donors. Med. J. Aust. **1**, 1020 (1972).

MATHER, G., DAWSON, J., HOYLE, C.: Liver biopsy in sarcoidosis. Quart. J. Med. **24**, 331 (1955).

MATHEWS, J.D., MACKAY, I.R.: Australia antigen in chronic hepatitis in Australia. Brit. med. J. **1**, 259 (1970).

MCBRIDE, R.A., CORSON, J.M., DAMMIN, G.J.: Mucormycosis, two cases of disseminated disease with cultural identification of Rhizopus: review of literature. Am. J. Med. **28**, 832 (1960).

MCCOLLUM, R.W., BECH, V., ISACSON, P., RIORDAN, J.T.: A survey for hemagglutinins in viral hepatitis. Amer. J. Med. **27**, 703 (1959).

MCCOLLUM, R.W.: Serum antigens in viral hepatitis. Report of a conference. J. Infect. Dis. **120**, 641 (1969).

MCCULLOUGH, N.B., EISELE, C.W.: Brucella hepatitis leading to cirrhosis of the liver. Arch. intern. Med. **88**, 793 (1951).

MCDONALD, S.: Acute yellow atrophy. Edinb. med. J. **15**, 208 (1908).

MEDEARIS, D.N., JR.: Observations concerning human cytomegalovirus infection and disease. Bull. Johns Hopk. Hosp. **114**, 181 (1964).

MELARTIN, L., BLUMBERG, B.S.: Production of antibody against Australia antigen in rabbits. Nature (Lond.) **210**, 1340 (1966).

MELNICK, J.L., BOGGS, J.D.: Human volunteer and tissue culture studies of viral hepatitis. Canad. med. Ass. J. **106**, 461 (1972).

MERRILL, D.A., DUBOIS, R.S., KOHLER, P.F.: Neonatal onset of the hepatitis-associated antigen carrier state. New Engl. J. Med. 1280 (1972).

MEYER ZUM BÜSCHENFELDE, K.H., HOPF, W.: Studies on the pathogenesis of experimental chronic active hepatitis in rabbits. I. Induction of the disease and protective effect of allogeneic liver specific proteins. Brit. J. exp. Path. **55**, 498 (1974).

MEYER ZUM BÜSCHENFELDE, K.H., KNOLLE, J., BERGER, J.: Celluläre Immunreaktionen gegenüber homologen leberspezifischen Antigenen (HLP) bei chronischen Leberentzündungen. Klin. Wschr. **52**, 246 (1974).

MEYER ZUM BÜSCHENFELDE, K.H., KOSSLING, F.K., MIESCHER, P.A.: Experimental chronic active hepatitis in rabbits following immunization with human liver proteins. Clin. exp. Immunol. **11**, 99 (1972).
MEYER ZUM BÜSCHENFELDE, K.H., MIESCHER, P.A.: Liver specific antigens. Pqrification and characterization. Clin. exp. Immunol. **10**, 89 (1972).
MILLER, J., SMITH, M.G.M., MITCHELL, C.G., REED, W.D., EDDLESTON, A.L.W.F., WILLIAMS, R.: Cell-mediated immunity to a human liver-specific antigen in patients with active chronic hepatitis and primary biliary cirrhosis. Lancet **1972II**, 296.
MILLER, W.J., PROVOST, P.J., MCALEER, W.J., ITTENSOHN, O.L., VILLAREJOS, V.M., HILLEMAN, M.R.: Specific immune adherence assay for human hepatitis A antibody. Application to diagnostic and epidemiologic investigations. Proc. Soc. exp. Biol. (N.Y.) **149**, 254 (1975).
MILLMAN, I., LOEB, L.A., BAYER, M.E., BLUMBERG, B.S.: Australia antigen (a hepatitis-associated antigen). Purification and physical properties. J. exp. Med. **131**, 1190 (1970).
MISTILIS, S.P.: Pericholangitis and ulcerative colitis. I. Pathology, aetiology and pathogenesis. Ann. intern. Med. **63**, 1 (1965).
MISTILIS, S.P.: Natural history of active chronic hepatitis: II. Pathology, pathogenesis, and clinicopathological correlation. Aust. Ann. Med. **17**, 277 (1968).
MORROW, R.H., JR., SAI, F.T., BARKER, L.F.: Australia antigen and hepatitis in Accra, Ghana. Brit. med. J. **4**, 389 (1971).
MOSLEY, J.W.: Viral hepatitis: a group of epidemiologic entities. Canad. med. Ass. J. **106**, 427 (1972).
MOULT, P.J.A., SHERLOCK, S.: Halothane-related hepatitis: A clincal study of twenty-six cases. Quart. J. Med. **44**, 99 (1975).
MUELLER-EBERHARD, C., KRETZSCHMER, G., KUHN, H.A.: Untersuchungen zur Bedeutung des β1C/1A-Gehaltes im Serum von Patienten mit sog. "Lupoider" Hepatitis. Klin. Wschr. **48**, 491 (1970).
MURPHY, F.A., SIMPSON, D.I.H., WHITFIELD, S.G., ZLOTNIK, I., CARTER, G.B.: Marburg virus infection in monkeys. Ultrastructural studies. Lab. Invest. **24**, 279 (1971).
MURRAY-LYON, I.M., STERN, R.B., WILLIAMS, R.: Controlled trial of prednisolone and azathioprine in active chronic hepatitis. Lancet **1973I**, 735.
MURRAY-LYON, I.M., THOMPSON, R.P.H., ANSELL, I.D., WILLIAMS, R.: Scleroderma and primary biliary cirrhosis. Brit. med. J. **3**, 258 (1970).
NEEFE, J.M.: Recent advances in knowledge of "virus hepatitis". Med. Clin. N. Amer. **39**, 1407 (1946).
NELSON, D.W.: Immunity to infection, allograft immunity and tumour immunity: parallels and contrasts. Transplant. Rev. **19**, 226 (1974).
NEWBERRY, W.M., SHOREY, J.W., SANFORD, J.P., COMBES, B.: Depression of lymphocyte reactivity to phytohemagglutinin by serum patients with liver disease. Cell. Immunol. **6**, 87 (1973).
NIEDERMAN, J.C., MCCOLLUM, R.W., HENLE, G., HENLE, W.: Infectious mononucleosis: clinical manifestations in relation to EB virus antibodies. J. Amer. med. Ass. **208**, 205 (1968).
NIELSEN, J.O., DIETRICHSON, O., ELLING, P., CHRISTOFFERSEN, P.: Incidence and meaning of persistence of Australia antigen in patients with acute viral hepatitis: development of chronic hepatitis. New Engl. J. Med. **285**, 1157 (1971).
NIELSEN, J.O., DIETRICHSON, O., JUHL, E.: Incidence and meaning of the "e" determinant among hepatitis-B-antigen positive patients with acute and chronic liver diseases. Lancet **1974II**, 913.
NIELSEN, J.O., LEBOUVIER, G.L., the Copenhagen Hepatitis Acute Program: Subtypes of Australia Antigen among patients and healthy carriers in Copenhagen. New Engl. J. Med. **288**, 1257 (1973a).
NIELSEN, J.O., NIELSEN, M.H., ELLING, P.: Differential distribution of Australia-antigen-associated particles in patients with liver diseases and normal carriers. New Engl. J. Med. **288**, 484 (1973).
NIELSEN, J.O., REINICKE, V., DIETRICHSON, O., ANDERSEN, V., THOMSEN, M., ANDERSEN, E.: Immunological studies of Australia antigen carriers with and without liver diseases. Clin. exp. Immunol. **15**, 9 (1973b).
NORUP, G.: Complement-fixing liver antibodies: I. Occurrence in a material of normal blood donors. Acta path. microbiol. scand **65**, 405 (1965).
NORUP, G.: Complement-fixing liver antibodies: II. Occurrence in a material of patients with chronic hepatitis. Acta path. microbiol. scand. **69**, 404 (1967).
NOTKINS, A.L., MERGENHAGEN, S.E., RIZZO, A.A., SCHEELE, C., WALDMANN, T.Z.: Elevated γ-globulin and increased antibody production in mice infected with lactic dehydrogenase virus. J. exp. Med. **123**, 347 (1966).
NOUZA, K., BOHM, F.: The changes in the liver of F1 hybrids following administration of parental lymphoid cells: A model of the autoimmune reaction against the liver tissue? Folia biol. (Praha) **12**, 355 (1966).
O'BRIEN, E.N., PATERSON, B., RALSTON, M., MACKAY, I.R.: Plasma transaminase in liver disease. Aust. Ann. Med. **9**, 295 (1960).
OGILVIE, B.M., JONES, V.E.: Immunity in the parasitic relationship between helminths and hosts. Progr. Allergy **17**, 94 (1973).
OGRA, P.L.: Immunologic aspects of hepatitis-associated antigen and antibody in human body fluids. J. Immunol. **110**, 1197 (1973).

OHBAYASHI, A., OKOCHI, K., MAYUMI, M.: Familial clustering of asymptomatic carriers of Australia antigen and patients with chronic liver disease or primary liver cancer. Gastroenterology **62**, 618 (1972).

OKOCHI, K., MURAKAMI, S.: Observations on Australia antigen in Japanese. Vox Sang. (Basel) **15**, 374 (1968).

OKUDAIRA, M., STRAUB, M., SCHWARZ, I.: The etiology of discrete splenic and hepatic calcifications in an endemic area of histoplasmosis. Amer. J. Path. **39**, 599 (1961).

OLIVER, L.E., ISER, J.H., STENING, G.F., SMALLWOOD, R.A.: "Biliary colic" and ilosone. Med. J. Aust. **1**, 1148 (1973).

ONION, D.K., CRUMPAKER, C.S., GILLILAND, B.C.: Arthritis of hepatitis associated with Australia antigen. Ann. intern. Med. **75**, 29 (1971).

OPOLON, P., CARTRON, J., CHICOT, D., CAROLI, J.: Application du test de transformation lymphoblastique (TTL) au diagnosis de certaines hepatites médicamenteuses. Presse méd. **77**, 204 (1969).

O'SHAUGHNESSEY, W.J., BÜCHNER, H.A.: Hepatitis associated with a coxsackie B5 virus infection during late pregnancy. J. Amer. med. Ass. **179**, 71 (1962).

PAGALTSOS, A.P., SMITH, M.G.M., EDDLESTON, A.L.W.F., WILLIAMS, R.: Total haemolytic complement after liver transplantation and in liver disease. Transplantation **14**, 41 (1972).

PAGE, A.R., SHARP, H.L., GREENBERG, L.J., YUNIS, E.J.: Genetic analysis of patients with chronic active hepatitis. J. clin. Invest. **56**, 530 (1975).

PARONETTO, F., GERBER, M., VERNACE, S.J.: Immunological studies in patients with chronic active hepatitis and primary biliary cirrhosis I. Cytotoxic activity and binding of sera to human liver cells grown in tissue culture. Proc. Soc. exp. Biol. (N.Y.) **143**, 756 (1973).

PARONETTO, F., POPPER, H.: Aggravation of hepatic lesions in mice by *in vivo* localization of immune complexes (Auer hepatitis). Amer. J. Path. **47**, 549 (1965).

PARONETTO, F., POPPER, H.: Chronic liver injury induced by immunologic reactions. Amer. J. Path. **49**, 1087 (1966).

PARONETTO, F., POPPER, H.: Hetero, iso- and autoimmune phenomena in the liver, p. 563, in: Text-book of Immunopathology, ed. by MIESCHER, P., and MÜLLER-EBERHARD, H., New York: Grune and Stratton 1968.

PARONETTO, F., POPPER, H.: Lymphocyte stimulation induced by halothane in patients with hepatitis following exposure to halothane. New Engl. J. Med. **283**, 277 (1970).

PARONETTO, F., SCHAFFNER, F., POPPER, H.: Immunocytochemical and serologic observations in primary biliary cirrhosis. New Engl. J. Med. **271**, 1123 (1964).

PARONETTO, F., SCHAFFNER, F., POPPER, H.: Antibodies to cytoplasmic antigens in primary biliary cirrhosis and chronic active hepatitis. J. Lab. clin. Med. **69**, 979 (1967).

PARONETTO, F., VERNACE, S.: Immunologic studies in patients with chronic active hepatitis. Cytotoxic activity of lymphocytes to autochthonous liver cells grown in tissue culture. Clin. exp. Immunol. **19**, 99 (1975).

PARONETTO, F., WOOLF, N., KOFFLER, D., POPPER, H.: Response of the liver to soluble antigen-antibody complexes. Gastroenterology **43**, 539 (1962).

PERRY, H.M.: Late toxicity to hydralazine resembling systemic lupus erythematosus or rheumatoid arthritis. Amer. J. Med. **54**, 58 (1973).

PETERS, R.L.: Hepatitis B antigen and chronic hepatic conditions. In: Australia Antigen (PRIER, J.E. and FRIEDMAN, H., eds.), chap. 10. Baltimore: Park Press 1973.

PEZZIMENTI, J.F., HAHN, A.L.: Anicteric hepatitis induced by diphenylhydantoin. Arch. intern. Med. **125**, 118 (1970).

PIAZZA, M.: Experimental Viral Hepatitis. Thomas, Springfield, Illinois, 1969.

PONS-ROMERO, F., HEATHCOTE, J., SHERLOCK, S.: The epidemiological importance of 'ay' and 'ad' subtypes of HB-Ag. Gut **15**, 733 (1974).

POPPER, H.: Drug-induced liver injury. In: The Liver (GALL, E.A. and MOSTOFI, F.K., eds.), p. 182. Baltimore: The Williams and Wilqins Company 1973.

POPPER, H., GERBER, M., VERNACE, S.: Immunologic factors in liver disease. Israel J. med. Sci. **9**, 103 (1973).

POPPER, H., MACKAY, I.R.: Relation between Australia antigen and autoimmune hepatitis. Lancet **1972I**, 1161.

POPPER, H., PARONETTO, F., SCHAFFNER, F.: Immune processes in the pathogenesis of liver disease. Ann. N.Y. Acad. Sci. **124**, 781 (1965).

POTTER, B.J., TRUEMAN, A.M., JONES, E.A.: Serum complement in chronic liver disease. Gut **14**, 451 (1973).

POWELL, L.W., AXELSEN, E.: Corticosteroids in liver disease: studies on the biological conversion of prednisone to prednisolone and plasma protein binding. Gut **13**, 690 (1972).

POWELL, O.W.: Liver involvement in "Q" fever. Aust. Ann. Med. **10**, 52 (1961).

POWELL, S.J.: Amoebic liver disease. Ghana med. J. **8**, 100 (1969).

PRINCE, A.M.: An antigen detected in the blood during the incubation period of serum hepatitis. Proc. nat. Acad. Sci. (Wash.) **60**, 814 (1968).

PRINCE, A.M.: Role of serum hepatitis virus in chronic liver disease. Gastroenterology **60**, 913 (1971).
PRINCE, A.M., HARGROVE, R.L., SZUMESS, W., CHERUBIN, C.E., FONTANA, V.J., JEFFRIES, G.H.: Immunologic distinction between infectious and serum hepatitis. New Engl. J. Med. **282**, 987 (1970).
PRINCE, A.M., METSELAAR, D., KAFUKO, G.W., MUKWAYA, L.G., LING, C.M., OVERBY, L.R.: Hepatitis B antigen in wild-caught mosquitoes in Africa. Lancet **1972II**, 247.
PRINCE, A.M., TREPO, C.: Role of immune complexes involving SH antigen in pathogenesis of chronic active hepatitis and polyarteritis nodosa. Lancet **1971I**, 1309.
Progress Report: In vitro methods in cell-mediated immunity. Cell. Immunol. **6**, 331 (1973).
PROTELL, R.L., SOLOWAY, R.D., MARTIN, W.J., SCHOENFELD, L.J., SUMMERSKILL, W.H.J.: Anti-salmonella agglutinins in chronic active liver disease. Lancet **1971I**, 330.
PROVOST, P.J., ITTENSOHN, O.L., VILLAREJOS, V.M., HILLEMAN, M.R.: A specific complement-fixation test for human hepatitis A employing CR326 virus antigen. Diagnosis and epidemiology. Proc. Soc. exp. Biol. (N.Y.) **148**, 962 (1975).
PRYTZ, H., BJORNEBOE, M., ORSKOV, F., HILDEN, M.: Antibodies to escherichia coli in alcoholic and non-alcoholic patients with cirrhosis of the liver or fatty liver. Scand. J. Gastroent. **4**, 433 (1973).
PURCELL, R.H., DEINSTAG, J.L., FEINSTONE, S.M., KAPIKIAN, A.Z.: Relationship of hepatitis A antigen to viral hepatitis. Amer. J. med. Sci. **270**, 61 (1975).
PURCELL, R.H., WALSHE, J.H., HOLLAND, P.V., MORROW, A.G., WOOD, S., CHANOCK, R.M.: Serial epidemiological studies of transfusion-associated hepatitis. J. infect. Dis. **123**, 406 (1971).
RAFFERTY, E.B., DENMAN, A.M.: Systemic lupus erythematosus syndrome induced by practolol. Brit. med. J. **2**, 452 (1973).
RAMACHANDRAN, S., DE SARAM, R., RAJAPAKSE, C.N.A., SIVALINGAM, S.: Hepatic manifestations during amoebic dysentery. Postgrad. med. J. **49**, 261 (1973).
READ, A.E., HARRISON, C.V., SHERLOCK, S.: Chronic chlorpromazine jaundice with particular reference to its relationship to primary biliary cirrhosis. Amer. J. Med. **31**, 249 (1961).
READ, A.E., SHERLOCK, S. HARRISON, C.V.: Active 'juvenile' cirrhosis as part of a systemic disease and the effect of corticosteroid therapy. Gut **4**, 378 (1963).
REDEKER, A.G.: Viral hepatitis: Current concepts. Postgrad. Med. **53**, 77 (1973).
REED, W.D., EDDLESTON, A.L.W.F., STERN, R.B., WILLIAMS, R., ZUCKERMAN, A.J., BOWES, A., EARL, P.M.: Detection of hepatitis-B antigen by radioimmunoassay in chronic liver disease and hepatocellular carcinoma in Great Britain. Lwncet **1973II**, 690.
REHMAN, O.U., KEITH, T.A., GALL, E.A.: Methyldopa-induced submassive hepatic necrosis. J. Amer. med. Ass. **224**, 1390 (1973).
REINICKE, V., DYBKJAER, E., POULSEN, H., BANKE, O., LYLLOFF, K., NORDENFELT, E.: A study of Australia-antigen-positive blood donors and their recipients, with special reference to liver histology. New Engl. J. Med. **286**, 867 (1972).
RELLER, L.B.: Granulomatous hepatitis associated with acute cytomegalovirus infection. Lancet **1973I**, 20.
REYNOLDS, T.B., DENISON, E.K., FRANKL, H.D., LIEBERMAN, F.L., PETERS, R.L.: Primary biliary cirrhosis with scleroderma, Raynaud's phenomenon and telangioctasia. Amer. J. Med. **50**, 302 (1971).
REYNOLDS, T.B., EDMONDSON, H.A., PETERS, R.L., REDEKER, A.: Lupoid hepatitis. Ann. intern. Med. **61**, 650 (1964).
REYNOLDS, T.B., PETERS, R.L., YAMADA, S.: Chronic active and lupoid hepatitis caused by a laxative oxyphenisatin. New Engl. J. Med. **280**, 813 (1971).
RIGHTSEL, W.A., KELTSCH, R.A., TEKUSHAN, F.M., MCLEAN, I.W.: Tissue culture cultivation of cytopathogenic agents from patients with clinical hepatitis. Science **124**, 226 (1956).
RINGERZ, O., ZETTERBERG, B.: Serum hepatitis among Swedish trackfinders. An epidemiologic study. New Engl. J. Med. **276**, 540 (1967).
RIZZETTO, M., SWANA, G., DONIACH, D.: Microsomal antibodies in active chronic hepatitis and other disorders. Clin. exp. Immunol. **15**, 331 (1973).
ROBERTS, I.M., BERNARD, C.C., VYAS, G.N., MACKAY, I.R.: T-cell dependence of immune response to hepatitis B antigen in mice. Nature (Lond.) **254**, 606 (1975).
ROBINSON, W.S.: DNA and DNA polymerase in the core of the Dane particle of hepatitis B. Amer. J. med. Sci. **270**, 151 (1975).
ROBSON, G.S., MACKAY, I.R.: Generalized cytomegalovirus infection in a patient with lupoid hepatitis. Aust. Ann. Med. **18**, 147 (1969).
RODRIGUEZ, M., PARONETTO, F., SCHAFFNER, F., POPPER, H.: Antimitochondrial antibodies in jaundice following drug administration. J. Amer. med. Ass. **208**, 148 (1969).
ROHOLM, K., IVERSEN, P.: Leberveränderungen bei akuter epidemischer Hepatitis. Verh. dtsch. Ges. inn. Med. **51**, 359 (1939).
ROSSOUW, J.E., SAUNDERS, S.J.: Hepatic complications of antituberculous therapy. Quart. J. Med. **44**, 1 (1975).
ROTT, R., DRZENIEK, R., SABER, M.S., REICHERT, E.: Blood groups substances, Forssman, and mononucleosis antigens in lipid containing RNA viruses. Arch. ges. Virusforsch. **19**, 273 (1966).

ROWE, W.P., HARTLEY, J.W., CRAMBLETT, H.G., MASTROTA, F.M.: Detection of human salivary gland virus in the mouth and urine of children. Am. J. Hyg. **67**, 57 (1958).
ROWLAND, A.J., SKONE, J.F.: Epidemiology of infectious hepatitis. Brit. med. Bull. **28**, 149 (1972).
ROZEN, P., KORN, R.J., ZIMMERMAN, H.J.: Computer analysis of liver function tests and their interrelationships in 347 cases of viral hepatitis. Israel J. med. Sci. **6**, 67 (1970).
RUBIN, E., SCHAFFNER, F., POPPER, H.: Primary biliary cirrhosis: Chronic non-suppurative destructive cholangitis. Amer. J. Path. **46**, 387 (1965).
SABESIN, S.M., FALLON, H.J., ANDRIOLE, V.T.: Hepatic failure as a manifestation of cryptococcosis. Arch. intern. Med. **111**, 661 (1963).
SABESIN, S.M., and KOFF, R.S.: Pathogenesis of experimental viral hepatitis, Part I and Part II. New Engl. J. Med. **290**, 944 and 996 (1974).
SAINT, E.G., KING, W.E., JOSKE, R.A., FINCKH, E.S.: The course of infection hepatitis with special reference to prognosis and the chronic stage. Aust. Ann. Med. **2**, 113 (1953).
SARGENT, A.U., MYERS, J., ROSE, B., RICHTER, M.: Organ and species specificity of rat hepato-cellular antigens. Immunology **10**, 199 (1966).
SCHAFFNER, F., POPPER, H.: Nonspecific reactive hepatitis in aged and infirm people. Amer. J. dig. Dis. **4**, 389 (1959).
SCHATZKI, P.F., KAY, S., MCGAVIE, J.D.: Ultrastructural pathology of a case of halothane hepatitis. Amer. J. dig. Dis. **18**, 905 (1973).
SCHEIFFARTH, F., WARNATZ, H., ESSING, H.G.: Serological studies of autoantibodies in acute and chronic liver disease. Int. Arch. Allergy **28**, 240 (1965).
SCHEIFFART, F., WARNATZ, H., SCHMIDT, H.J.: Immunological studies on the development of experimental hepatitis in thymectomized mice. Int. Arch. Allergy **32**, 308 (1967).
SCHEUER, P.: Liver biopsy interpretation. London: Balliere 1968.
SCHEUER, P.J.: Chronic liver disease: size and scope of the problem. J. roy. Coll. Phycns. Lond. **8**, 17 (1973).
SCHOLER, A., THOMSSEN, R., KABOTH, V., WIERCH, R.: Nachweis in parental Infektionen im Rahmen eines Ausbruchs von übertragbarer Gelbsucht mit positiven Australia (SH) Antigen Befund. Dtsch. med. Wschr. **95**, 2852 (1970).
SCHUMACHER, K.: Untersuchungen zur Spezifität anticytoplasmatischer Antikörper bei chronisch progressiver Hepatitis. Klin. Wschr. **47**, 965 (1969).
SCHUMACHER, K., SCHNEIDER, W.: Differenzierung und Isolierung löslicher Organantigene aus Human-Leber. Klin. Wschr. **47**, 806 (1969).
SCHWARTZ, J., MUTH, J.: Coccidioidomycosis: a review. Amer. J. med. Sci. **221**, 89 (1951).
SCHWEITZER, I.L., WING, A., MCPEAK, C., SPEARS, R.L.: Hepatitis and hepatitis-associated antigen in 56 mother-infant pairs. J. Amer. med. Ass. **220**, 1092 (1972).
SEAMAN, W.E., ISHAK, K.G., PLOTZ, P.H.: Aspirin induced hepatotoxicity in patients with systemic lupus erythematosus. Ann. intern. Med. **80**, 1 (1974).
SELMAIR, H., VIDO, I., KABOTH, U., SCHOBER, A.: Australia (SH)-Antigen-Befunde bei floriden und ausgeheilten chronisch-persistierenden Hepatitiden. Dtsch. med. Wschr. **96**, 1908 (1971).
SHANN, F.: Jaundice associated with oxyphenisatin. Lancet **1971II**, 44.
SHARPSTONE, P., MEDLEY, D.R.K., WILLIAMS, R.: Halothane hepatitis—A preventable disease? Brit. med. J. **1**, 448 (1971).
SHAW, D.J., JACOBS, R.P.: Simultaneous occurrence of toxic hepatitis and Stevens-Johnson syndrome following therapy with sulfisoxazole and sulfamethoxazole. Bull. Johns Hopk. Hosp. **126**, 130 (1970).
SHERLOCK, S.: Diseases of the liver and biliary system, 4 th ed. Oxford: Blackwell 1968.
SHERLOCK, S.: Halothane hepatitis. Gut **12**, 324 (1971).
SHERLOCK, S.: Chronic hepatitis B antigen disease. J. roy. Coll. Phycns. Lond. **8**, 24 (1973).
SHULMAN, N.R.: Hepatitis-associated antigen. Amer. J. Med. **49**, 669 (1970).
SHULMAN, N.R., BARKER, L.F.: Virus-like antigen, antibody and antigen-antibody complexes in hepatitis measured by complement fixation. Science **165**, 304 (1969).
SILVA, H., HALL, E., HILL, K.R., SHALDON, S., SHERLOCK, S.: Renal involvement in active 'juvenile' cirrhosis. J. clin. Path. **18**, 157 (1965).
SIMON, H.B., WOLFF, S.W.: Granulomatous hepatitis and prolonged fever of unknown origin: a study of 13 patients. Medicine (Baltimore) **52**, 1 (1973).
SIMPSON, B.R., STRUMIN, L., WALTON, B.: The halothane dilemma; a case for the defence. Brit. med. J. **4**, 96 (1971).
SIMPSON, B.R., STRUMIN, L., WALTON, B.: Halothane hepatitis—fact or fallacy. Proc. roy. Soc. Med. **66**, 56 (1973).
SINGLETON, J.W., MERRILL, D.A., RUSSELL, A.F., KOHLER, P.F., FETTBERG, W.A.H.: Liver disease in Australia-antigen-positive blood donors. Lancet **1971II**, 1.
SMALLEY, M.J., MACKAY, I.R., WHITTINGHAM, S.: Antinuclear factors and human leucocytes: Reaction with granulocytes and lymphocytes. Aust. Ann. Med. **17**, 28 (1968).

SMETANA, H.F.: The histologic diagnosis of viral hepatitis by needle biopsy. Gastroenterology **26**, 612 (1954).
SMETANA, H.F.: The histopathology of drug-induced liver disease. Ann. N.Y. Acad. Sci. **104**, 821 (1963).
SMITH, J.B., IVERSON, G.M.: Occurrence of liver-specific antigen in adult human serum. Clin. exp. Immunol. **13**, 209 (1973).
SMITH, V.A., FRANCIS, T.I., DAVID-WEST, T.S.: Autoantibodies in acute viral hepatitis, yellow fever and hepatocellular carcinomas: clinical and experimental findings. J. Path. Bact. **109**, 83 (1973).
SOBEL, H.J., WOLF, E.H.: Liver involvement in early syphilis. Arch. Path. **93**, 565 (1972).
SØBORG, M., BENDIXEN, G.: Human leucocyte migration as a parameter of hypersensitivity. Acta med. scand. **181**, 247 (1967).
SODOMANN, C.-P., HAVEMANN, K.: Die Bedeutung cellulärer Immunreaktionen bei der Hepatitis. Internist (Berl.) **14**, 583 (1973).
SOERGEL, K.H., FRIEDELL, G.H.: Non-specific effects of liver extract-adjuvant injection in guinea pigs. A morphologic and immunologic study. J. Lab. clin. Med. **64**, 51 (1964).
SOLOWAY, R.D., SUMMERSKILL, W.H.J.: Chronic active liver disease: classification and treatment. Postgrad. Med. **53**, 88 (1973).
SOLOWAY, R.D., SUMMERSKILL, W.H.J., BAGGENSTOSS, A.H., SCHOENFELD, L.J.: Lupoid hepatitis, a non-entity in the spectrum of chronic active liver disease. Gastroenterology **63**, 458 (1972a).
SOLOWAY, R.D., SUMMERSKILL, W.H.J., BAGGENSTOSS, A.H., GEALL, M.G., GITNICK, G.L., ELVEBACK, L.R., SCHOENFELD, L.J.: Clinical, biochemical and histological remission of severe chronic active liver disease: a controlled study of treatment and early prognosis. Gastroenterology **63**, 820 (1972b).
SPINK, W.W., HOFFBAUER, F.W., WALKER, W.W., GREEN, R.A.: Histopathology of the liver in human brucellosis. J. Lab. clin. Med. **34**, 40 (1949).
STANLEY, N.N., FOX, R.A., WHIMSTER, W.F., SHERLOCK, S., JAMES, D.G.: Primary biliary cirrhosis or sarcoidosis—or both. New Engl. J. Med. **287**, 1282 (1972).
STASTNY, P., STEMBRIDGE, V.A., VISCHER, T., ZIFF, M.: Homologous disease in the adult rat, a model for autoimmune disease: II. Findings in the joints, heart and other tissues. J. exp. Med. **122**, 681 (1965).
STEIN, O., FAINARU, M., STEIN, Y.: Visualization of virus-like particles in endoplasmic reticulum of hepatocytes of Australia antigen carriers. Lab. Invest. **26**, 262 (1972).
STEINER, J.: Investigations of allergic liver injury. I. Light, fluorescent and electron microscopic study of the effects of soluble immune aggregates. Amer. J. Path. **38**, 411 (1961).
STERN, H.: Isolation of cytomegalovirus and clinical manifestations of infection at different ages. Brit. med. J. **1**, 665 (1968).
STEVENS, C.E., PALMER BEASLEY, R., TSUI, J., LEE, W.-C.: Vertical transmission of hepatitis B antigen in Taiwan. New Engl. J. Med. **292**, 771 (1975).
STEVENS, D.P., BARKERR, L.F., KETCHAM, A.S., MEYER, H.M., JR.: Asymptomatic cytomegalovirus infection following blood transfusion in tumor surgery. J. Amer. med. Ass. **211**, 1341 (1970).
SUTNICK, A.I., BUGBEE, S.J., LONDON, W.T., LOEB, L.A., PEYRETTI, F., LITWIN, S., BLUMBERG, B.S.: Lymphocyte function in normal people with persistent Australia antigen. J. Lab. clin. Med. **32**, 79 (1973b).
SUTNICK, A.I., LONDON, W.T., LEVINE, P.H., BLUMBERG, B.B.: Frequency of Australia antigen in patients with leukemia in different countries. Lancet **1971I**, 1200.
SUTNICK, A.I., SENIOR, J.R., GOESER, E., MILLMAN, I.: Similarity of hepatitis following transfusion of Australia-antigen positive and negative blood. Lancet **1973aII**, 461.
TAN, E.M.: Relationship of nuclear staining patterns with precipitating antibodies in systemic lupus erythematosus. J. Lab. clin. Med. **70**, 800 (1967).
TAYLOR, A.R., RIGHTSEL, W.A., BOGGS, J.D., MCLEAN, I.W.: Tissue culture of hepatitis virus. Amer. J. Med. **32**, 679 (1962).
TAYLOR, P.E.: Laboratory tests for Australia (hepatitis associated) antigen and antibody. Brit. med. Bull. **28**, 138 (1972).
TEN VEEN, J.H.: Studies on drug-induced lupus erythematosus in mice. II. Drug induced smooth muscle and skeletal muscle antibodies. Clin. exp. Immunol. **15**, 375 (1973).
TERRY, R.B., GUNNAR, R.M.: Primary miliary tuberculosis of the liver. J. Amer. med. Ass. **164**, 150 (1957).
THEWAINI ALI, A.J., OAKLEY, C.L.: Auto-antibodies in experimental chronic infective disease. J. Path. Bact. **93**, 413 (1967).
THOMPSON, W.G., HART, I.R.: Chronic active hepatitis and Graves' disease. Amer. J. dig. Dis. **18**, 111 (1973).
TOBIAS, H., SAFRAN, A.P., SCHAFFNER, F.: Lymphocyte stimulation and chronic liver disease. Lancet **1967I**, 193.
TOGHILL, P.J., BAILEY, M.E., WILLIAMS, R., ZEEGEN, R., BOWN, R.: Cytomegalovirus hepatitis in the adult. Lancet **1967I**, 1351.

TOGHILL, P.J., SMITH, P.G., BENTON, P., BROWN, R.C., MATTHEWS, H.L.: Methyldopa liver damage. Brit. med. J. **3**, 545 (1974).
TOH, B.H., ROBERTS-THOMSON, I.C., MATHEWS, J.D., WHITTINGHAM, S., MACKAY, I.R.: Depression of cell-mediated immunity in old age and the immunopathic diseases, lupus erythematosus, chronic hepatitis and rheumatoid arthritis. Clin. exp. Immunol. **14**, 193 (1973).
TONGE, J.I., DERRICK, E.H.: A fatal case of "Q" fever associated with hepatic necrosis. Med. J. Aust. **1**, 594 (1959).
TRIGER, D.R., ALP, M.H., WRIGHT, R.: Bacterial and dietary antibodies in liver disease. Lancet **1972I**, 60.
TRIGER, D.R., MURTZ, J.B., MACCALLUM, F.O., WRIGHT, R.: Raised antibody titers to measles and rubella viruses in chronic active hepatitis. Lancet **1972I**, 665.
TRIGER, D.R., WRIGHT, R.: Hyperglobulinaemia in liver disease. Lancet **1973I**, 1494.
TUCKER, E.S., III, SCOFIELD, G.F.: Hepatoadrenal necrosis: fatal systemic herpes simplex infection; review of literature and report of two cases. Arch. Path. **71**, 538 (1961).
TURNER, L.H.: Leptospirosis. Brit. med. J. **1**, 537 (1973).
TURNER-WARWICK, M.: Fibrosing alveolitis and chronic liver disease. Quart. J. Med. **37**, 133 (1968).
TYSELL, J.E., JR., KNAUER, C.M.: Hepatitis induced by methyldopa (Aldomet): report of a case and review of the literature. Amer. J. dig. Dis. **16**, 849 (1971).
VALDIVIA-BARRIGA, V., FELDMAN, A., ORELLANA, J.: Generalized hypersensitivity with hepatitis and jaundice after the use of penicillin and streptomycin. Gastroenterology **45**, 114 (1963).
VICKERS, F.N., MALONEY, P.J.: Gonococcal perihepatitis; report of three cases with comments on diagnosis and treatment. Arch. intern. Med. **114**, 120 (1964).
VIRCHOW, R.: Über das Vorkommen und den Nachweis des hepatogenen, insbesondere des katarrhalischen Icterus. Virchows Arch. path. Anat. **32**, 117 (1865).
VISCHER, T.L.: Australia antigen and autoantibodies in chronic hepatitis. Brit. med. J. **2**, 695 (1970).
VISCHER, T.L.: Immunologic aspects of chronic hepatitis. Progr. Allergy **15**, 268 (1971).
VISCHER, T.L., BÄNZIGER, A.E.: Quantitative determination of antiglobulins of the IgG, IgA and IgM class in sera of patients with rheumatoid arthritis or chronic liver disease and of healthy persons. Rev. Europ. Études clin. Biol. **15**, 422 (1972).
VISCHER, T.L., BERNHEIM, C., ENGELBRECHT, E.: Two cases of hepatitis due to toxoplasma gondii. Lancet **1937II**, 919.
VOEGT, H.: Zur Aetiologie der Hepatitis epidemica. Münch. med. Wschr. **89**, 76 (1942).
VON LICHTENBERG, F., ERIKSON, D.G., SADUN, E.H.: Comparative histopathology of schistosome granulomas in the hamster. Amer. J. Path. **72**, 149 (1973).
WALDENSTROM, J.: Leber: Blutproteine und Nahrungseiweiß Stoffwechsel. Krh., Sonderband: XV. Tagung, Bad Kissingen, p. 8., 1950.
WALKER, C.O., COMBES, B.: Biliary cirrhosis induced by chlorpromazine. Gastroenterology **51**, 631 (1966).
WALKER, J.G., BATES, D., DONIACH, D., BALL, P.A.J., SHERLOCK, S.: Chronic liver disease and mitochondrial antibodies: A family study. Brit. med. J. **1**, 146 (1972).
WALKER, J.G., DONIACH, D., ROITT, I.M., SHERLOCK, S.: Serological tests in diagnosis of primary biliary cirrhosis. Lancet **1965I**, 827.
WALTERS, M.L., STANLEY, N.F., DAWKINS, R.L., ALPERS, M.P.: Immunological assessment of mice with chronic jaundice and runting induced by reovirus 3. Brit. J. exp. Path. **54**, 329 (1973).
WALTON, B., DUMONDE, D.C., WILLIAMS, C., JONES, D., STRUNIN, J.M., LAYTON, J.M., STRUNIN, L., SIMPSON, R.: Lymphocyte transformation. Absence of increased responses in alleged halothane jaundice. J. Amer. med. Ass. **225**, 494 (1973).
WANDS, J.R., ISSELBACHER, K.J.: Lymphocyte cytotoxicity to autologous liver cells in chronic active hepatitis. Proc. nat. Acad. Sci. (Wash.) **72**, 1301 (1975).
WARNATZ, H.: DAS Phänomen der Lymphocyten-Transformation in der Pathogenese und Diagnostik von Autoimmunerkrankungen. Z. ges. exp. Med. **149**, 64 (1969).
WARNATZ, H., SCHEIFFARTH, F., SCHMEISSNER, R.: Studies on the cytotoxic effect of *in vivo* and *in vitro* immunized lymphocytes on liver target cells. Clin. exp. Immunol. **21**, 250 (1975).
WARREN, K.S., DOMINGO, E.O., COWAN, R.B.T.: Granuloma formation around schistosome eggs as a manifestation of delayed hypersensitivity. Amer. J. Path. **51**, 735 (1967).
WARTENBERG, J., DONIACH, D., BROSTOFF, J., ROITT, I.M.: Leucocyte migration inhibition with mitochondria in human autoimmune thyroid disorders. Clin. exp. Immunol. **14**, 203 (1973).
WAUGH, D.: Myocarditis, arteritis, and focal hepatic, splenic and renal granulomas apparently due to penicillin sensitivitiy. Amer. J. Path. **28**, 437 (1952).
WEIR, D.M.: Liver autoantibodies in the rat. Immunology **6**, 581 (1963).
WELLER, T.H., HANSHAW, J.B.: Virologic and clinical observations in cytomegalic inclusion disease. New Engl. J. Med. **256**, 1284 (1962).
WELLS, J.V., FUDENBERG, H.H.: Australia antigen (hepatitis-associated antigen). Aust. N.Z.J. Med. **3**, 278 (1972).

WEWALKA, F., GNAN, F., KRASSNITZKY, O., PESENDORFER, F.: Au/SH antigen in liver disease. Vox Sang. (Basel) **19**, 311 (1970).
WHALEY, K., WEBB, J., MCAVOY, B.A., HUGHES, G.R.V., LEE, P., MACSWEEN, R.N.M., BUCHANAN, W.W.: Sjegren's syndrome. 2. Clinical associations and immunological phenomena. Quart. J. Med. **42**, 513 (1973).
WHENHAM, G.R., CARLSON, H.C., AKSEL, A.: Avian vibrionic hepatitis in Alberta. Canad. vet. J. **2**, 3 (1961).
WHITTINGHAM, S.: Serological methods in autoimmune disease in man. In: Vol. 1 of: Research in Immunochemistry and Immunobiology, ed. by J.B.G. KWAPINSKI, p. 121–176. Baltimore: University Park Press 1973.
WHITTINGHAM, S.: Immunofluorescence reactions in patients with prolonged extrahepatic biliary obstruction. Gastroenterology **66**, 169 (1974).
WHITTINGHAM, S., IRWIN, J., MACKAY, I.R., SMALLEY, M.: Smooth muscle autoantibody (SMA) in "autoimmune" hepatitis. Gastroenterology **51**, 499 (1966).
WHITTINGHAM, S., MACKAY, I.R., IRWIN, J.: Autoimmune hepatitis: Immunofluorescence reactions with cytoplasm of smooth muscle and renal glomerular cells. Lancet **1966I**, 1333.
WHITTINGHAM, S., MACKAY, I.R., KISS, Z.S.: An interplay of genetic and environmental factors in familial hepatitis and myasthenia gravis. Gut **11**, 811 (1970).
WHITTINGHAM, S., MACKAY, I.R., THANABALASUNDRUM, R.S., CHUTTANI, H.K., MANJURAN, R., SEAH, C.S., YU, M., VIRANUVATTI, V.: Chronic liver disease: Differences in autoimmune serological reactions between Australians and Asians. Brit. med. J. **4**, 517 (1973).
WHITTINGHAM, S., MACKAY, I.R., WHITWORTH, J.A., SLOMAN, J.G.: Antinuclear antibody response to procainamide in man and laboratory animals. Amer. Heart J. **84**, 228 (1972).
W.H.O. Scientific Group: Viral hepatitis. Wld Hlth Org. techn. Rep. Ser. No. 412 (1973).
W.H.O. Scientific Group: Viral hepatitis. Wld Hlth Org. techn. Rep. Ser. No. 570 (1975).
WIEDERMANN, G., MIESCHER, P.A.: Cytoplasmic antibodies in patients with systemic lupus erythematosus. Ann. N.Y. Acad. Sci. **124**, 807 (1965).
WILDHIRT, E.: Leberschädigung durch Abführmittel. Dtsch. med. Wschr. **97**, 1131 (1972).
WILLIAMS, A., JACK, I.: Hepatic necrosis in neonatal herpes simplex infection. Med. J. Aust. **1**, 392 (1965).
WILLIAMS, G.E.G.: Pericholangiolitic biliary cirrhosis. J. Path. Bact. **89**, 23 (1965).
WILLING, R.L., HECKER, R.: Oxyphenisatin and liver damage. Med. J. Aust. **1**, 1179 (1971).
WOLLHEIM, F.A.: Immunoglobulins in the course of viral hepatitis and in cholestatic and obstructive jaundice. Acta med. scand. **183**, 473 (1968).
WOOD, I.J., KING, W.E., PARSONS, P.J., PERRY, J.W., FREEMAN, M., LIMBRICK, L.: Non-suppurative hepatitis: A study of acute and chronic forms with special reference to biochemical and histological changes. Med. J. Aust. **1**, 249 (1948).
WORLLEDGE, S.: Immune drug-induced hemolytic anemias. Semin. Hemat. **10**, 327 (1973).
YAP, E.H., ONG, Y.W., SIMONS, M.J., OKOCHI, K., KAYUMI, M., NISHIOKA, K.: Australia antigen in Singapore. II. Differential frequency in Chinese, Malays and Indians. Vox Sang. (Basel) **22**, 371 (1972).
YEUNG LAIWAH, A.A.C.: Lymphocyte transformation by Australia antigen. Lancet **1971II**, 470.
YEUNG LAIWAH, A.A.C., CHAUDHURI, A.K.R., ANDERSON, J.R.: Lymphocyte transformation and leucocyte migration-inhibition by Australia antigen. Clin. exp. Immunol. **15**, 27 (1973).
YOW, E.M., BRENNAN, J.C., PRESTON, J., LEVY, S.: The pathology of psittacosis: a report of 2 cases with hepatitis. Amer. J. Med. **27**, 739 (1959).
ZIMMERMAN, H.J.: Clinical and laboratory manifestations of hepatotoxicity. Ann. N.Y. Acad. Sci. **104**, 954 (1963).
ZIMMERMAN, H.J., HELLER, P., HILL, R.P.: Extreme hyperglobulinemia in subacute hepatic necrosis. New Engl. J. Med. **244**, 245 (1951).
ZLOTNICK, A., SLAVIN, S., ELIAKIM, M.: Mixed cryoglobulinemia with a monoclonal IgM component, associated with chronic liver disease. Israel J. med. Sci. **8**, 1968 (1972).
ZUCKERMAN, A.J.: Virus diseases of the liver. London: Butterworth 1970.
ZUCKERMAN, A.J.: Hepatitis associated antigen and viruses. Amsterdam: North Holland 1972.
ZUCKERMAN, A.J.: Is hepatitis caused by viroids. Lancet **1973I**, 1486.
ZUCKERMAN, A.J., BAINES, P.M.: Australia antigen as a marker of propagation of the serum hepatitis virus in liver cultures. Nature (Lond.) **236**, 78 (1972).

Radiation-Induced Injury of the Liver *

RAINER LESCH

With 32 Figures

A. Introduction

Because of its primary role in body metabolism, the liver is exposed to numerous chemical and physical noxae. While, for example, toxic-nutritive damages (alcohol) or damages due to poison or drugs often cause dysfunction and thus the symptoms of disease at an early stage, changes and dysfunction due to irradiation often are seen only after a long asymptomatic interval or they remain latent. This situation led to the controversy—still alive today—about the radiosensitivity of the liver and to the opinion that the liver is a relatively radioresistant organ (FRIEDMAN, 1942; ZOLLINGER, 1960).

Because human and animal tissues exhibit different sensitivities to X-rays, so-called sensitivity scales were set up on the basis of animal experiments and clinical trials (WETTERER, 1922; HOLTHUSEN, 1931, 1947; MUTH, 1961; HELLRIEGEL, 1965). In radiology, they are particularly important for the assessment of reactions to radiation of deep-seated organs and tissues because direct observation is not possible. Although according to the fundamental rules of radiation biology, one should expect a high sensitivity to irradiation due to its high metabolic activity, the liver was graded among the less sensitive organs and tissues. This assessment was made despite its central metabolic functions, its excretory tasks, and its role in the intestinal circulatory system which includes drainage of the total blood supply from the portal vein. According to the classification of WARREN (1936) into radiosensitive organs (2,500 R or less kills or seriously injures many cells) and radioresistant organs (over 5,000 R are necessary to kill or injure many cells), the liver must be included among the radioresistant organs. While the liver is still designated as being "moderately radiosensitive" by ELLINGER (1945, 1957) and by BERDJIS (1971), this concept has, during the last 15 years, undergone a fundamental change. Today it is held that liver tissue is a radiosensitive tissue (SCHERER, 1963). Only the quickly proliferating tissues such as the mucosae of the gastointestinal tract, bone marrow, and lymphatic tissue (BIRZLE, 1965; OGATA *et al.*, 1963; OEHLERT, 1973) are more radiosensitive. The clinical experience that irradiation of the upper abdominal region, which includes parts of the liver, is

* Die Untersuchungen des eigenen Arbeitskreises wurden dankenswerterweise von der Deutschen Forschungsgemeinschaft, Bonn-Bad Godesberg (Forschergruppe Leber) und von der Schutzkommission beim Bundesministerium des Inneren gefördert.

poorly tolerated by the patients, also points to a high radiosensitivity (BIRZLE, 1965). The false view of the radioresistancy of the liver was, according to GRAUL and SCHERER (1958) due to the lack of appropriate test reactions for evidence of liver damage. The fact that the effect of local irradiation of an organ was deduced from the effects observed in the same organ following whole-body irradiation rendered the information inadmissable (BLOOM, 1948; RAJEWSKY, 1956).

Because information on therapeutic irradiation of the liver was scarce (BIRZLE, 1965) and because radiodiagnosis has be carried out in a routine fashion only for a few years (STIRRET, 1954), there was no great stimulus for experimental clinical radiology of the liver. The situation changed in the last few years, particularly because work at Stanford University School of Medicine led to a clarification of the clinical picture of human radiation hepatitis (INGOLD *et al.*, 1965; KAPLAN and BAGSHAW, 1968; LEWIN and MILLIS, 1973) and because, following the atomic bomb explosions after the 2nd World War at the Bikini atoll, severe liver damage due to radioactive fallout (TSUZUKI, 1955) was observed.

B. Preliminary Remarks

I. Preliminary Remarks on Physical Facts

1. Radiation Spectrum

High-frequency rays with waves of 10^{-5} to 10^{-12} cm cause changes in tissues and organs and constitute the largest part of the radiation spectrum. These include the so-called corpuscular rays (DUNLAP, 1961; GLASSER *et al.*, 1949) that send out alpha and beta particles, neutrons, protons, and other heavy particles and the electromagnetic rays, i.e., X-rays and gamma rays. All are characterized by their ionizing effect when they hit matter (Report, 1962), whereby, their high speed is powerfully reduced. Only neutrons are not able to ionize matter directly.

2. Radiation Units

The roentgen unit "R" is used as a measure for X-rays and gamma rays. It is directly measured in air with the help of an ionization chamber. Because this system is not applicable to neutron rays. DACQUISTO and HARTGERING (1959) called the energy absorption unit for neutrons "rad". This term is used by many workers for all kinds of irradiation. It stands for the absorption of 100 ergs/g of irradiated material. In comparison, 1 R leads to the absorption of 87 erg/g.

3. Radiation Sources

An organism can be exposed to radiation from external sources such as X-rays, radioactive fallout, and nuclear reactions or to internally accumulated radioactive substances. The internal radiation sources consist predominantly of alpha- and beta-particles. All radioactive substances which get into the organism accumulate in certain organs and are not proportionately distributed.

II. Radiosensitivity

1. Definition

The assessment of reactions to radiation, particularly, identification of radiation damage that is just developing, is of special importance for radiotherapy. It is, however, difficult to define the radiosensitivity of an organ, because it is difficult to compare radiosensitivities. In one case, only functional tissue changes can be established, in another, early changes can be observed only microscopically, and in a third case, there are damages that can be ascertained only macroscopically. Often one cannot decide whether the damage is a direct or an indirect consequence of irradiation (BIRZLE, 1965). The *threshold dose* and the *tolerance* or *critical dose* are important for radiotherapy. The threshold dose is that radiation dose that causes a slight functional or morphological change in tissue. The tolerance dose or critical dose, however, is that radiation dose which is just tolerated without causing irreversible damage. In the sense of radiation protection, the tolerance dose also represents that dose under which no traceable changes occur (MELCHING, 1962). In radiotherapy, however, the tolerance dose characterizes the critical level above which an irreversible damage may occur (HOLTHUSEN, 1947; FRIEDMAN, 1954; BRICK, 1955). The threshold dose and the tolerance dose are two quantities that are characteristic for each tissue. They delimit the "range of sensitivity" that is so important for radiotherapy and that determines the radiotherapeutically useful sphere of action.

2. General Remarks on Radiosensitivity

The establishment of just-developing radiation damages is thus of particular importance for radiotherapy. It is especially desirable for deep seated organs and tissues because the role of skin reactions as a biological control has been superseded by technical progress in the field of radiotherapy. Reaction diagnostics are the most advanced in radiohematology (HEILMEYER, 1961; FLIEDNER and STODTMEISTER, 1962). Observations of radiation reactions of nervous tissue (ARNOLD *et al.*, 1954; BIBIKOVA, 1961; BREIT, 1962; CROMPTON and LAYTON, 1961; DIHLMANN, 1961; GUARINO and PERONI, 1961; LEBEDINSKY and NAKHILNITSKAYA, 1963; LIKHACHEV and NEMIROVSKAYA, 1963; MASCIDCCHI and CAZZOLA, 1962; PALLIS *et al.*, 1961; PECH *et al.*, 1961; RÜBER, 1962; SCHINZ, 1964; SCHÜMMELFEDER, 1962; ZEMAN, 1961) and of bone tissue (BARNHARD and GEYER, 1962; BIRKNER *et al.*, 1956; BROOKS and HILLSTROM, 1933; FLACHI and PIEROTTI, 1963; FRITZ, 1959; HORVATH *et al.*, 1962; HULTH and WESTERBORN, 1960, 1962; KOLAR and BABICKY, 1959, 1962, 1963; KOSCHITZ-KOSIC, 1961; LEABHART and BONFIGLIO, 1961; MACH, 1962; PAPPAS and COHEN, 1963; PFEIFFER and BUTTENBERG, 1959; SARRAZIN *et al.*, 1961; WÄCHTLER, 1961; ZUPPINGER, 1962; GRABIGER, 1964; HELD, 1925) brought about a change in the views on the radiosensitivities of these tissues.

Non-observance of the sensitivity of normal tissue can result in grave therapeutic accidents (O'MALLEY *et al.*, 1963; WARTHIN, 1967; WILLIS and BACHEM, 1927; DOMAGK, 1927).

In estimating the tissue reactions that one should expect after irradiation, factors such as regeneration ability, changes in blood circulation and metabolism (EVANS and NAYLOR, 1963; UMEGAKI and MATSUZAWA, 1963; PALMIERI and MICELLI, 1959; TSUCHIYA *et al.*, 1963), age (TUDWAY, 1962), and deviations due to the time of day (PIZZARELLO *et al.*, 1963; RUGH, 1963) must also be considered. Furthermore, the fact that the regenerative ability of a tissue is also influenced by a change in the metabolic activity of cells and tissue (LAMARQUE, 1954) must be taken into account.

3. Remarks on the Radiosensitivity of the Liver

Since, in general, damage of the liver produces a disturbance in essential body functions, the liver must be categorized as a "critical organ" (BERDJIS, 1971). Three factors play an important role: 1. radiosensitivity, 2. the degree of exposure to radiation, 3. the significance for the body function (Report, 1962). One can say that the liver is highly radiosensitive only if one defines sensitivity in terms of a just perceptible, slight, transient functional or morphological damage. A slight or a marked radioresistancy is then present when sensitivity signifies irreversible damage. Therefore the question is not that of the high or low radiosensitivity of the liver but that of determining from which radiation dose onward a reaction becomes perceptible and from which radiation dose onward irreversible damage can be expected.

III. Process of Radiation Damage

1. General

In human organs as well as in other cell systems, the process of radiation damage starts, at the cellular level, with ionization (Fig. 1). After a latent period

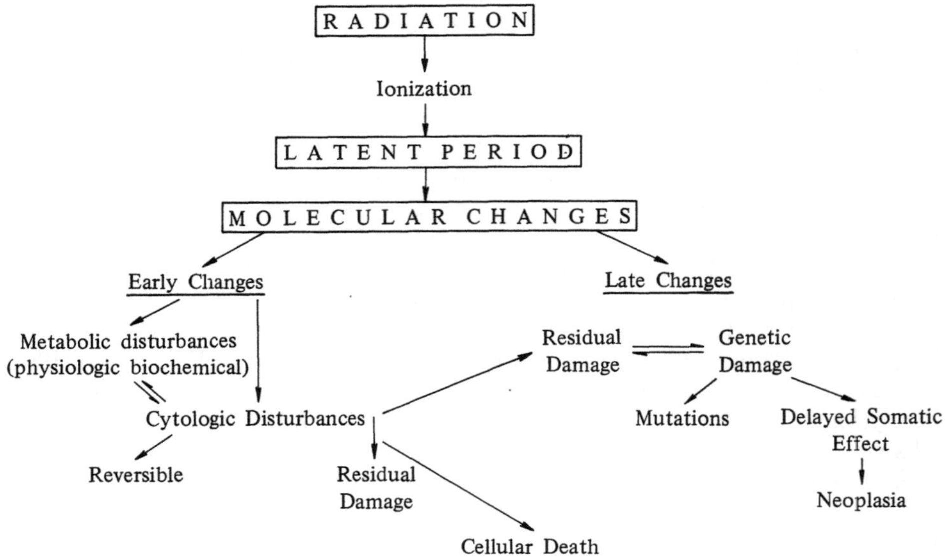

Fig. 1. Radiation injury in the cell. Schematic description of biological and histological effects of irradiation at cellular level

that cannot be accurately defined molecular changes take place which can be differentiated into early and late changes. Depending on the specific radiosensitivity and on the degree of ionization, these changes may be lethal or sublethal (RUGH, 1968). In the sublethal condition, cells can survive, increase in number, and develop anomalies as well as tumors. The latent period can last for minutes or for decades, again depending on the degree of radiation damage (RUGH, 1968).

2. Liver

a) *Morphological Characteristics*

The progression of radiation damage is marked by the morphological characteristics of the liver. These are determined from a structural and functional compartmentalization of the liver tissue into different kinds of cells and tissues. The mass of hepatocytes in which the metabolic processes essential for the organism take place, e.g., syntheses of glycogen, albumin, and fibrinogen or the conjugation of bile salts, make up the liver parenchyma. It constitutes approximately 90% of the total liver weight. The remaining 10% consists of the reticulohistiocytary system with the sinus endothelia as well as Kupffer cells, and the vessels, connective tissue, and the bile ducts of the portal tracts.

b) *Process of Radiation Damage*

Results of experimental trials and a series of clinical observations revealed that in the liver tissue, one must distinguish between acute and chronic changes, and that these changes show a marked dose dependence (INGOLD *et al.*, 1965; TEFFT, 1970).

α) Acute Radiation Reactions

Acute radiation reactions can be shown by light microscopic examination of the parenchyma (Table 1). Edemas of cell and nucleus, fatty degeneration, pyknoses, and necroses are most clearly seen, but one can also note a remarkable capacity for repair and regeneration (BUCHER, 1963). These acute radiation damages, however, are not characteristic or even pathognomonic of the influence of ionizing rays.

Table 1. Acute and chronic changes of the liver tissue in radiation hepatitis

Time after radiation in weeks	Parenchyma	Capillaries	Vessels	Structure
2–4	Necroses Atrophy	Hyperemia	Dilatation Alterations of the wall	Fibrosis
6–14	Necroses Atrophy	Hyperemia	Stenosis Obliteration	Fibrosis
20–50	Necroses Hyperplasia	—	Stenosis Obliteration	Fibrosis Cirrhosis

They are similar to those observed, in animal experiments, in the parenchyma under oxygen deficiency (MORGENROTH and THEMANN, 1964).

β) Late Radiation Changes

In contrast, radiation reactions can be seen in changes of the vascular apparatus, of the bile ducts, and the reticulohistiocytary system (Table 1). They are characterized by proliferative processes that produce a disturbance in the hepatic architecture or even cirrhotic alterations. Particularly important are the obliterative vascular changes that cause severe disturbance of blood circulation in the liver. The changes which occur in chronic liver damage are not pathognomonic of ionizing rays. They are observed in man, for example, as Budd-Chiari syndrome (REED and COX, 1966; OGATA *et al.*, 1963; INGOLD *et al.*, 1965).

c) Interrelations with Neighboring Organs

When finally assessing radiation damages of the liver, one must take into account that the morphological and biochemical changes are also influenced by neighboring organ systems. This relationship applies not only in the case of exposure of the whole body to irradiation but also in the case of irradiation of the liver alone or of irradiation when the liver is protected from the rays. So far, the assumption that the different organ systems mutually influence the reaction pattern holds, whether the pattern is organ specific or not, i.e., present in all organs.

For instance, the intensity of oxidative demethylation of aminopyrine by the liver is reduced in male rats for at least 4–5 days after whole-body X-irradiation (850 rads) but not in female rats (KNOTT and WILLS, 1974). The isolated irradiation of the testes exhibits the same effect. The injection of testosterone following the irradiation normalizes the process nearly completely.

C. Radiation-Induced Changes of the Human Liver

For a long time, clinical radiologists paid little attention to radiation-induced changes in the liver. Only a few primary liver diseases such as the rare hemangiomas of children and of adults and the rare primary carcinomas of the liver (BIRZLE, 1965) require radiotherapy. Thus, during irradiation of the gastrointestinal tract, only seldom was the liver protected. From the viewpoint of the clinical physician, interest was confined to those cases in which, on external irradiation of the liver region, overdose caused deficiencies, and in which long-living radioactive substances used as contrast media in radiodiagnostics and stored in the reticulohistiocytary system, especially in the liver, exhibited carcinogenic effects.

I. Irradiation by External Radiation Sources

Primary functional changes following therapeutic irradiation of the liver region led to the definition of the syndrome of "radiation sickness" or Roentgenkater. In addition to objectively perceptible changes, i.e. disturbances of specific metabolic

Table 2. Clinical findings in radiation hepatitis (increase in %)

Time after radiation in months	Alkaline phosphatase	Total bilirubine	LDH	SGOT	SGPT	BSP
1	100%	increased	normal	100%	100%	600%
2	100%	normal	normal	100%	normal	increased
4–5	normal	normal	normal	normal	normal	increased
10	normal	normal	normal	normal	normal	increased
24	normal	normal	normal	normal	normal	increased

functions of the liver, these terms also include subjective complaints, e.g., nausea, vomiting, etc. The term "radiation hepatitis" was coined (INGOLD, 1965; KAPLAN and BAGSHAW, 1968; SAMUELS *et al.*, 1971), to include different complications following irradiation of the human liver with large doses (1,300–5,100 rads) (Table 2). The demonstration of hepatomegaly, ascites, jaundice, a prolongation of bromsulphthalein excretion, and of other dysfunctions that are transient or can cause death in liver coma, led to the coining of this term (LACASSAGNE, 1971; OEHLERT, 1973). The term however, was not well chosen, because the changes of the human liver after irradiation have no resemblance to the inflammatory-degenerative and destructive changes of a true hepatitis (OEHLERT, 1973; KAPLAN and BAGSHAW, 1968; WARREN and FRIEDMAN, 1942). One is more justified in speaking of a veno-occlusive disease with subsequent Budd-Chiari syndrome than of "radiation hepatitis" (REED and COX, 1966; OGATA *et al.*, 1963; INGOLD, 1965).

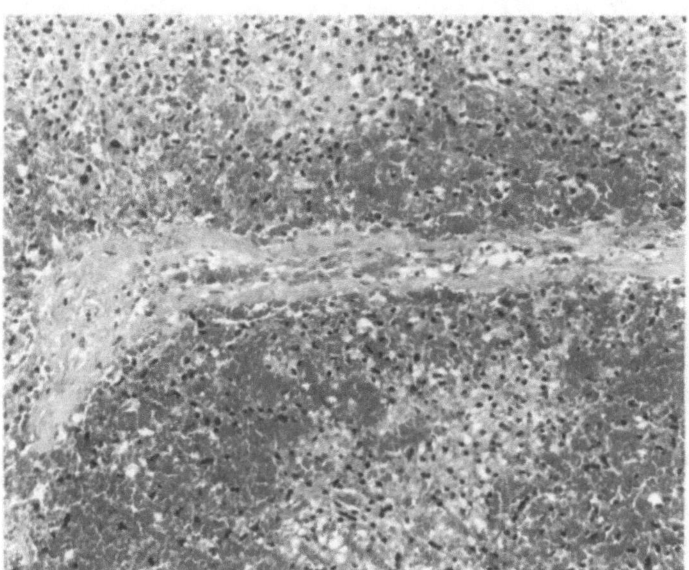

Fig. 2. Acute radiation hepatitis showing marked centrilobular congestion. Note sclerosis of central vein and intense surrounding congestion (HE: ×30). (Figs. 2–10 from LEWIN and MILLIS, 1973)

(a)

(b)

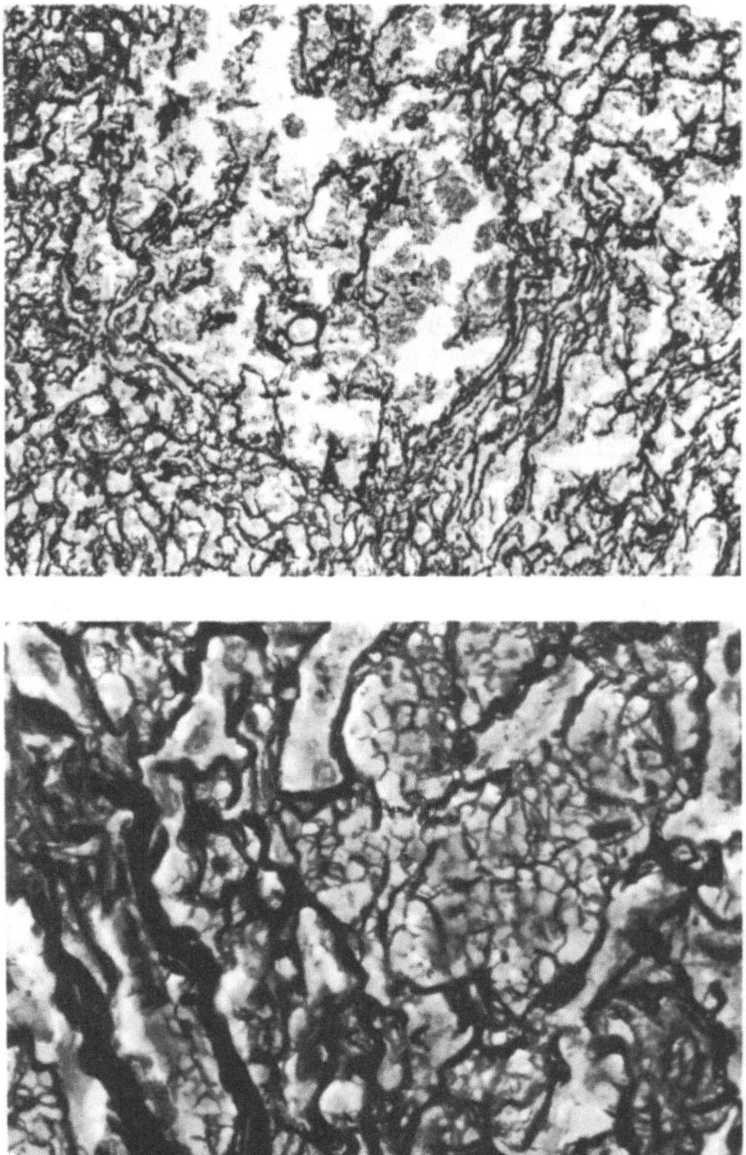

Fig. 3. (a) Acute radiation hepatitis showing distension and disruption of sinusoidal reticulin network (Gordon and Sweets: ×100). (b) Acute radiation hepatitis showing marked sinusoidal proliferation of reticulin (Gordon and Sweet: ×600)

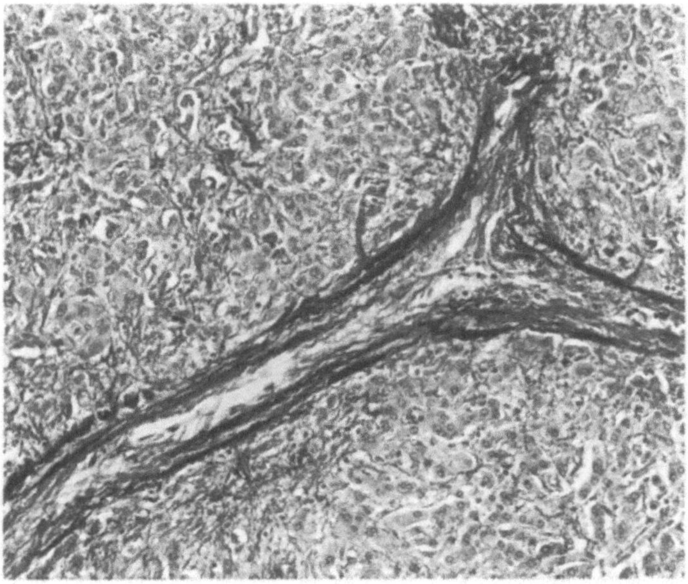

Fig. 4. Centrilobular venous sclerosis in radiation hepatitis. Note proliferation of reticulin fibers both within and around the vein (Gordon and Sweet: × 120)

1. Acute Radiation Changes

In the acute phase of hepatic radiation disease, degenerative changes in the parenchyma, observed in experimental animals can also be seen in man (Figs. 2—4). These changes, which cannot be compensated by the enormous regenerative power of the liver, can result in severe hyperemia with dilatation of the sinusoids and even centrolobular hemorrhages and liver cell atrophy (INGOLD, 1965; OGATA *et al.*, 1963; REED and COX, 1966). The severity of the clinical picture need not correlate with the degree of morphological changes in the liver. Thus abnormal liver function tests and evidence of hepatic injury obtained by needle biopsy could be demonstrated, while clinically the picture was asymptomatic (INGOLD, 1965). LEWIN and MILLIS (1973), at the time of death, observed severe liver dysfunctions in patients with acute radiation hepatitis, but not in those patients with chronic radiation hepatitis. The course of acute radiation hepatitis is variable. A few patients die, the majority survive, and 100 days after irradiation, demonstrate a restitution of the histological changes (OGATA *et al.*, 1963; INGOLD, 1965; REED and COX, 1966; WARREN and FRIEDMAN, 1947).

2. Effects of Chronic Irradiation

The continuing process of radiation damage is determined not by changes of the parenchyma but by changes of the mesenchymal structures which, in most

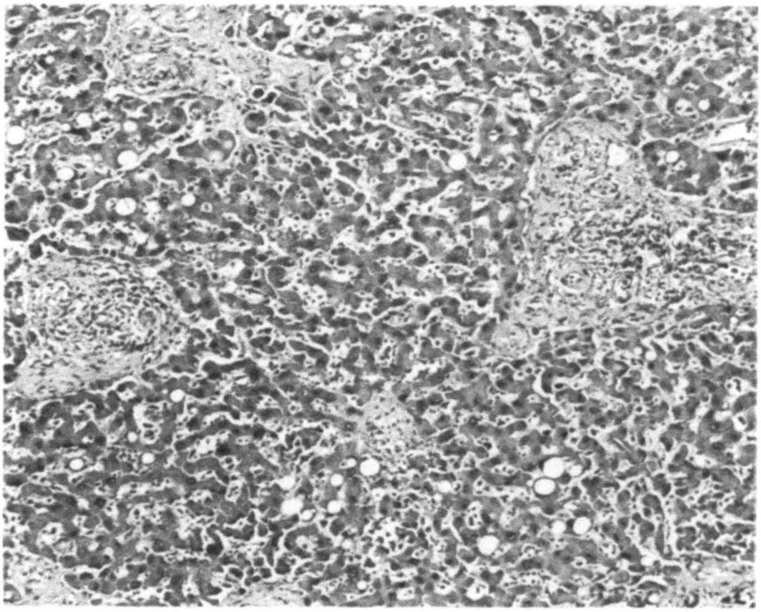

Fig. 5. Chronic radiation hepatitis showing portal fibrosis and distortion of lobular architecture (HE: ×65)

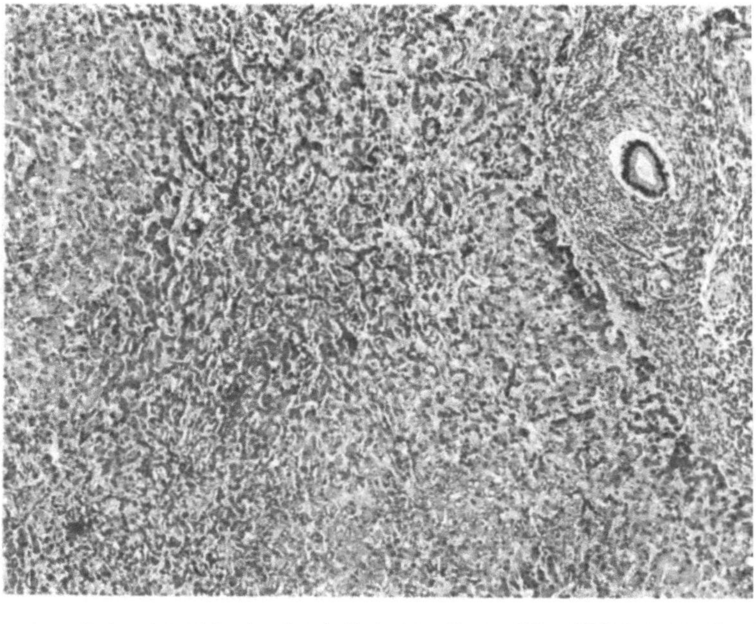

Fig. 6. Chronic radiation hepatitis showing indistinct outlines of liver lobules, atrophy of liver cell plates, and interstitial fibrosis. Note also sclerosis of central vein (HE: ×120)

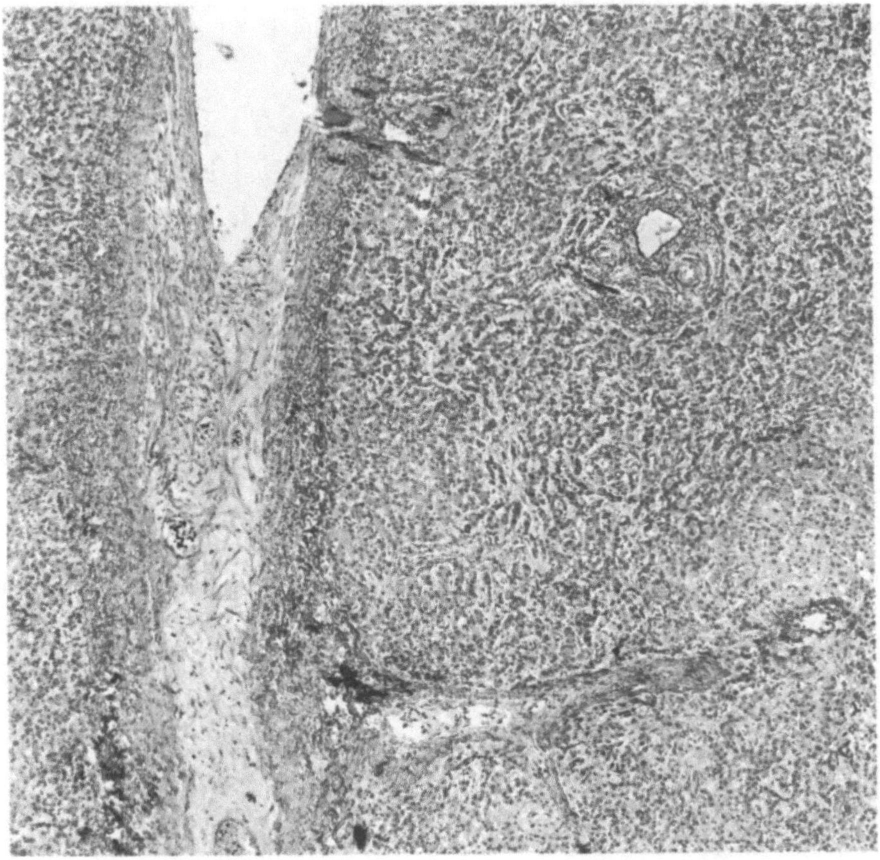

Fig. 7. Chronic radiation hepatitis showing marked intimal sclerosis of sublobular hepatic vein (HE: ×120)

cases, develop slowly. After irradiation of the entire liver with 3,000—6,000 rads, within a few weeks fibrotic obliterations of the small branches of the liver veins can occur, as well as increasing collagenization in the area of the portal tracts and the central lobule sections with a lobular collapse (Figs. 5—10). These vascular changes begin with a loss of endothelium, followed by an increase of argyrophilic fibers and vascular occlusion by granulation tissue. These massive changes, beginning in the area of the portal tracts and including interstitial fibrosis and capillarization of the liver parenchyma, soon developing into complete vascular occlusion, produce such extensive circulatory changes together with malnutrition of liver tissue, that the clinical picture of a portal stasis results (OGATA *et al.*, 1963; REED and COX, 1966; LEWIN and MILLIS, 1973). The terminal stage presents the same unspecific picture of a veno-occlusive disease that may also appear in chronic intoxication with Senecio- and Crotalaria alkaloids in man and in experimental animals (BRAS *et al.*, 1954; BRAS and MCLEAN, 1963; MCLEAN, 1970; GRASES and BECKER, 1972). The liver changes associated with the Budd-Chiari syndrome

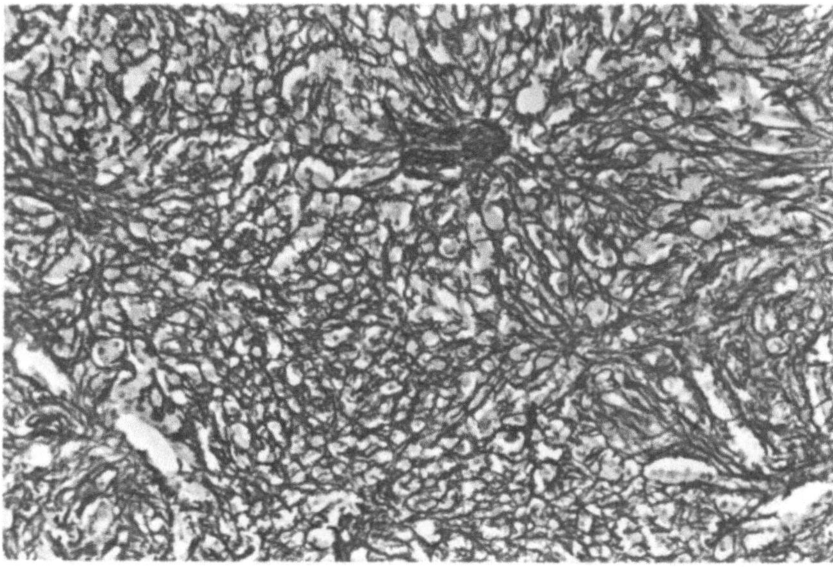

Fig. 8. Chronic radiation hepatitis showing marked increase in reticulin network and indistinct outline of liver lobules (Gordon and Sweet: ×100)

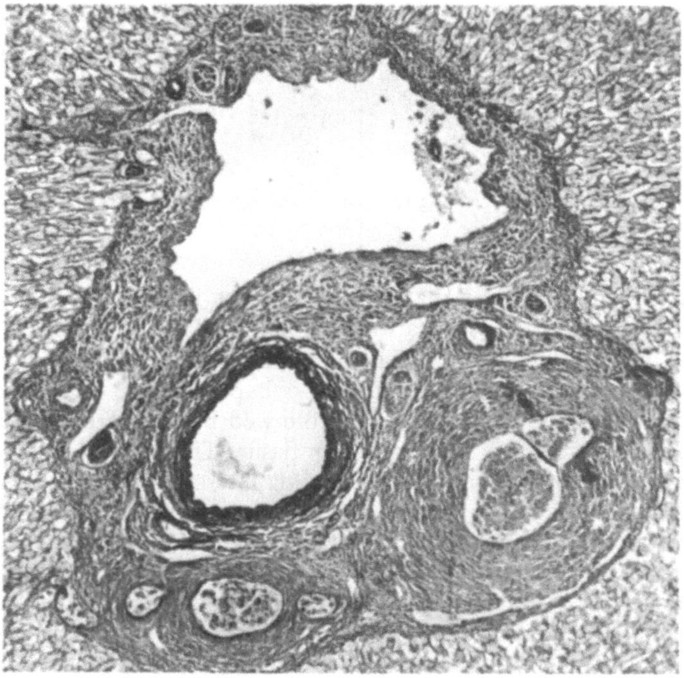

Fig. 9. Chronic radiation hepatitis showing portal tract fibrosis. Note concentric deposition of fibrous tissue around bile ducts (elastic van Gieson: ×100)

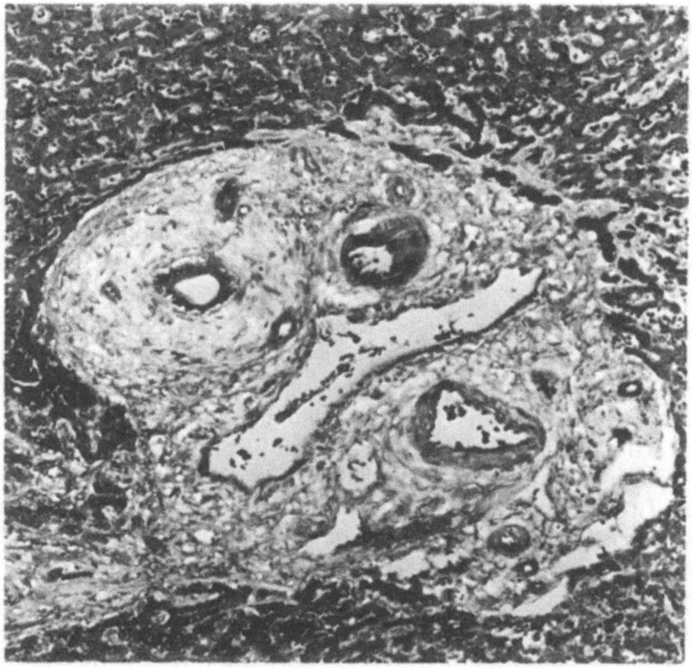

Fig. 10. Chronic radiation hepatitis showing characteristic edema of portal tracts (elastic van Gieson: ×100)

possibly cannot be differentiated from those occurring in radiation hepatitis, whilst the liver does not show the centrolobular changes and the lobular collapse with portal fibrosis present in a vitium cordis (REED and COX, 1966). ROBACK *et al.* (1971) described the case of a $6^1/_2$-years-old child who, $2^1/_2$ years after gamma-irradiation of a nephroblastoma, developed a veno-occlusive disease of the liver with portal hypertension and ascites.

CASE and WARTHIN (1924) following a histological examination of 3 livers after autopsy, described degenerative changes of the bile duct epithelium, particularly in the smaller bile ducts. In cases of irradiations that dated back only a few months, also atypical regenerated tissue could be demonstrated. Other authors observed heavily dilated sinusoids in the region of the sclerosed central veins as well as extramedullary blood formation (FELLOWS *et al.*, 1968). Sclerosing changes in the area of the central vein were also observed after irradiation of the whole body with cobalt 60 (DELCLOS *et al.*, 1963; LANSING *et al.*, 1968; WHARTON *et al.*, 1973). These findings could not be confirmed by other authors (LEWIN and MILLIS, 1973).

All patients in whom these findings could be ascertained had been treated with large radiation doses of over 7,200 rads. They survived radiotherapy only for some weeks, maximally for 2 years (FRYDL, 1962). The clinically observed terminal states and their deleterious result are attributed exclusively to the vascular changes.

In particular, the observations of INGOLD *et al.* (1965) and of BRICK (1955) permit the statement that a chronic liver disease due to irradiation has to be reckoned with if a dose of 4,000 rads is exceeded in the liver tissue. If the patient survives the severe obliterating changes for more than 4 months, then effective blood circulation of the liver can be rebuilt (REED and COX, 1966). Two years after irradiation, FRYDL (1962) observed regenerated parenchymal nodes in the irradiated atrophic and heavily fibrosed liver lobes. Angiectasis with hyalinization of the hepatic veins, including endothelial vacuolization and hemosiderin deposits and thrombosis of the bile ducts were present. Even though acute changes, e.g., damage of the liver parenchyma, are also observed when smaller doses are given, it can be assumed that doses of 3,000–3,500 rads are less dangerous when administered fractionally to the entire liver over a period of 3–4 weeks (INGOLD *et al.*, 1965; KAPLAN and BAGSHAW, 1968). In the case of acute changes, it is usually difficult to distinguish between symptoms which represent parenchymal damage due directly to irradiation and those that are conditioned by a secondary parenchymal damage resulting from the release of toxic catabolic products of disintegrating tumor masses. In general, these acute changes recede without any consequences. Changes characteristic of chronic radiation disease such as vascular obliterations and cirrhotic transformation do not develop.

These findings revive the old discussion that in the liver as well as in other organs the primary radiopathologic effect becomes manifest in the vascular and connective tissue while acute changes of the liver parenchyma are only representative of an indirect secondary effect (OGATA *et al.*, 1963; REED and COX, 1966).

In atomic bomb survivors at Hiroshima and Nagasaki delayed radiation effects on the liver such as cirrhosis and cancer (SCHREIBER *et al.*, 1971; MORIYAMA *et al.*, 1973) or veno-occlusive disease (STEER, 1974) could not be evaluated with respect to the radiation dose. This may also be due to the high incidence of liver cirrhosis and hepatoma following viral hepatitis and parasitosis in western Japan. MOORE and FERRANTE (1974) observed the development of a metastasizing hepatoma in a 32-year-old woman 20 years after X-irradiation of a liver hemangioma.

3. Detection of Lesions by Radioactive Hepatography

Vascular and parenchymal deficiencies occurring in chronic disease can be demonstrated scintigraphically after application of ^{131}I-labeled rose bengal and ^{198}Au (TAPLIN *et al.*, 1955; JOHNSON *et al.*, 1967; CONCANNON *et al.*, 1967; USSELMAN, 1966; KAPLAN and BAGSHAW, 1968; FELLOWS *et al.*, 1968). Using those compounds, JOHNSON *et al.* (1967) observed by scintillation scanning the reversibility of the changes. The phagocytic capacity of the Kupffer cells could be controlled using ^{198}Au. Six weeks after application of 3,900–5,500 R, JOHNSON *et al.* (1967) observed a suppression of the function of the reticulohistiocytary system, but could not trace other clinical signs of liver damage. Normal function was restored within 84–106 days after the last irradiation. Experiments with this method by KUROHARA *et al.* (1967) also indicated that there are no changes when doses under 300 rads are applied. Changes following irradiation with 4,000–5,000 rads are also to a large extent reversible if the whole liver was not exposed. The tests furthermore demonstrate that reticular cells are more radiosensitive than hepatocytes.

II. Irradiation by Internal Radiation Sources

To improve angiocardiography of the organs, a number of metal colloids were introduced into radiodiagnosis and examined in experimental animals in 1928 (BLÜHBAUM *et al.*, 1928). Thorium oxide proved to be the most useful. OKA (1929) injected rabbits and dogs intravenously with thorium dioxide and got an accumulation of the radio-opaque material in the reticulohistiocytary system, thereby rendering the liver and spleen visible. This procedure was also applied to hepatolienography of humans (RADT, 1929, 1930) and yielded excellent results. Under the name of thorotrast, thorium dioxide quickly became widely used as a contrast medium (KADRNKA, 1932).

Like other radioactive elements, e.g., the relatively short-lived polonium thorotrast is stored in the reticulo-histiocytary system, predominantly in liver, spleen, and lymph nodes (MUTH *et al.*, 1971). POPPER and KLEIN (1931) were the first to observe storage even 7 months after injection. Finally it was realized that it is not eliminated, but remains permanently in the reticulohistiocytary system.

Thorium, like polonium, emits predominantly alpha particles; in contrast to Po, however, it has an extremely long half-life of several million years (BAUER, 1949; DIEM and LEUTNER, 1968). In addition to alpha particles, beta particles are emitted with a ten times smaller energy. The equally emitted gamma rays are negligible (WACHSMUTH, 1948). The range of alpha particles in the tissue amounts to a maximum of 80 μ (WEGENER *et al.*, 1973). Due to the irreversible retention of the substance, the surrounding area is permanently exposed to radiation (BASERGA *et al.*, 1960). According to the radiation protection rules, this permanent radioactive irradiation exceeds the admissible dose by a factor of 10. The amount of secondary radiation is 6 times that of the primary radiation. In a diagnostic X-ray examination, the dose increase may reach 300—500 R. In a fractionated irradiation, focal doses up to 50,000 R may occur (JAKOB and WACHSMUTH, 1948). A large part of the injected material is stored in the liver (TAFT, 1937; ADACHI, 1940; RÖSSLE, 1949). Determination of the mid-concentration of the ^{232}thorium content showed that after the spleen and lymph nodes, the liver ranks 3rd as a storage organ (WEGENER *et al.*, 1973). The occurrence of the first radiation damages, hepatic and extrahepatic damages (NICAUD and HAMBURGER, 1937; MATTHES, 1954; BAUER, 1937) and OBERLING'S and GUERIN'S demonstration (1933) that in experiments in the rat, thorotrast has a radiocarcinogenic effect, caused the council of pharmacy and chemistry (1932) and other institutions to oppose thorotrast as contrast medium in radiology. Even guinea pigs, which are otherwise very tumor-resistant, developed carcinomas and sarcomas after thorotrast application (WARREN and GATES, 1941; LAVEDAN and COURTIAL 1949). BAUER (1943, 1948) warned against further administration because of the carcinogenic effect. On the basis of theoretical considerations, he hypothesized that cancer would appear after 12—18 years (BAUER, 1949). The inducibility of liver damages, particularly that of tumors, by thorotrast in animal experiments was repeatedly confirmed during the following years (TRIPOLI and HAAM, 1932; IRWIN, 1932; POHLE and RITCHIE, 1934; ROUSSY *et al.*, 1934; FOULDS, 1939; GUIMARES *et al.*, 1955). In 1947, the first case of liver sarcoma that had occurred was published in a woman 18 years after injection of thorotrast (MCMAHON *et al.*, 1947). From then until today, many deleterious cases were observed in which tumors occurred in the area of thorotrast deposits. There is also a good correlation with the mid-latent period of 15–20 years for radiocancer in humans (LACASSAGNE, 1971). SCHEIBE (1937) has reported on the formation of metastases of a cholangiary carcinoma in the liver induced by thorotrast. These tumors must be considered a consequence of the fact that, despite urgent warnings, radiologists and particularly surgeons continued to use thorotrast as contrast medium until about 1945; thus they can be termed as a true "iatrogenic disease" (BATZENSCHLAGER *et al.*, 1963; DALGREN, 1961; FRÜHLING *et al.*, 1956; GUIMARES *et al.*, 1955; HORTA DA SILVA *et al.*, 1961; LOONEY, 1960; MORI *et al.*, 1967; NIELSEN and KRACHT, 1958; TESLUK and NORDIN, 1955; THOMAS *et al.*, 1951).

GRASES (1966) compiled a great number of cases in which arteriograms and hepatolienograms had been made before the changes in liver and spleen were observed. In addition to local sarcomas of the soft tissue in the neighborhood of the injection site, osteosarcomas and leukemias (MCLEAN and BUDY, 1964; SABIN *et al.*, 1932) changes of the liver, liver fibroses and liver cirrhoses, liver carcinomas (MATTHES, 1954, 1956; BATZENSCHLAGER and WILHELM, 1957; FEDERLIN and SCIOR, 1957; OKINAKA *et al.*, 1957; MORGAN *et al.*, 1958; WERTHEMANN, 1959; KOHOUTEK and NOVAK, 1960; DAHLGREN, 1961; SUCKOW *et al.*, 1961; MÖBIUS and LEMBCKE, 1963; FREEZE and KEMNITZ, 1964; GROSSIORD *et al.*, 1956; SCHEIBE, 1973), and especially hemangioendotheliomata are most frequently observed (MACMAHON *et al.*, 1947; LÜDIN, 1953; SILVA-HORTA, 1953; 1956; TESLUK and NORDIN, 1955; CAROLI *et al.*, 1956; GRAMPA and TOMMASINI DEGNA, 1958; HIERONYMI, 1958; ROSENBAUM, 1959; GROS *et al.*, 1960; NETTLESHIP and FING, 1961; SCHREINER, 1961; MÖBIUS and LEMBCKE, 1963; FREEZE and KEMNITZ, 1964; GRASES, 1966; TRÜBESTEIN and CITOLER, 1973; FRÜHLING *et al.*, 1955). Many hepatic tumors developed in individuals in whom thorotrast had been used for bronchography, mammography, salpingography, dacryocystography, and for demonstration of the maxillary sinus (ZOLLINGER, 1949; FREEZE and KEMNITZ, 1964; VÖGTLIN and MINDER, 1952; ROTHE, 1957; AUSTONI, 1950; BRODY, and CULLEN, 1957; RUDOLPHI, 1950; HOFER, 1952; GROS *et al.*, 1955; HOHENSTATT, 1965; VELLENGA, 1965; SCHWANZER and FEDERLIN, 1957).

The frequent occurrence of late damages in the liver is quite striking. In comparison, late damages are observed only seldom in spleen and lymph nodes, even though general radiographs show that thorotrast is stored to the same if not a higher extent and that it is deposited more densely (Fig. 11). In a very dense agglomeration of thorotrast particles, such as can be observed in lymph nodes and spleen, a high percentage of radiation energy is destroyed by alpha-self-absorption. This phenomenon should not be expected in the liver, since the deposits of contrast medium are more finely dispersed (ROTBLAT and WARD, 1953, 1956; WEGENER and ZAHNERT, 1970; WEGENER *et al.*, 1971; KAUL and HEYDER, 1971; MUTH *et al.*, 1971). The deposits of foreign material in the liver can be clearly demonstrated macroscopically and microscopically (Figs. 12, 13). In the autoradiograph, the emission of alpha particles can be shown by the occurrence of tracks in the photo emulsion (LESCH and OEHLERT, 1968; OEHLERT and LESCH, 1966)

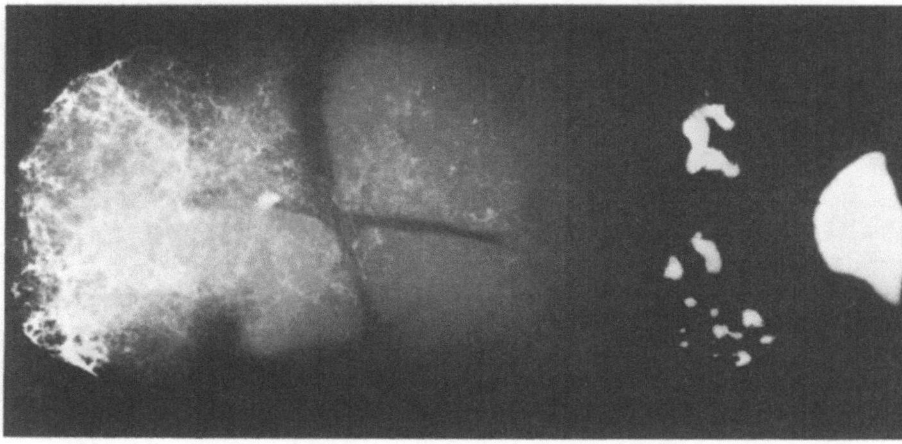

Fig. 11. Postmortem X-ray. Liver and superior mesenteric lymph nodes showing heavy deposits of roentgen-opaque thorotrast. (From GRASES, 1966)

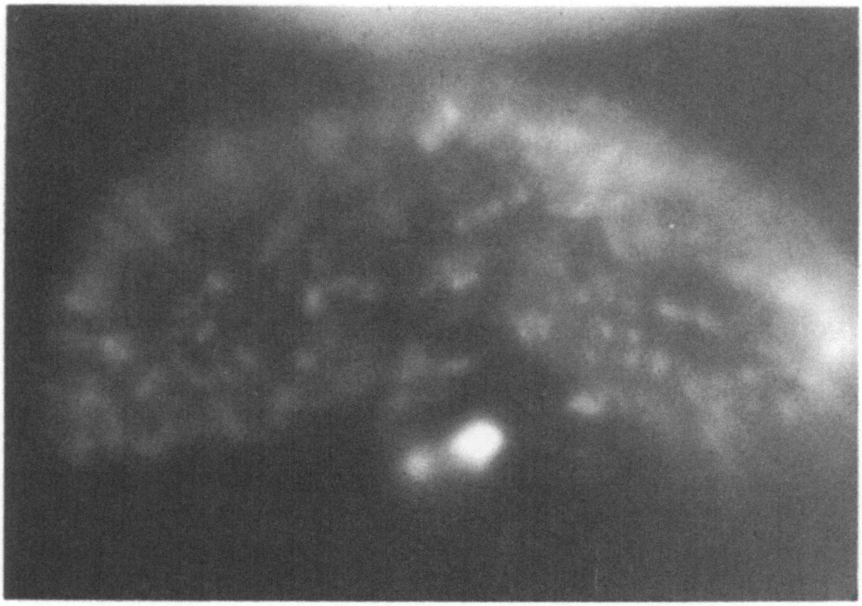

Fig. 12. X-ray film autoradiograph of formalin-fixed liver slice containing deposits of thorotrast after 4 weeks, exposure. Alpha-tracks induce blackening (in picture white spots) of film

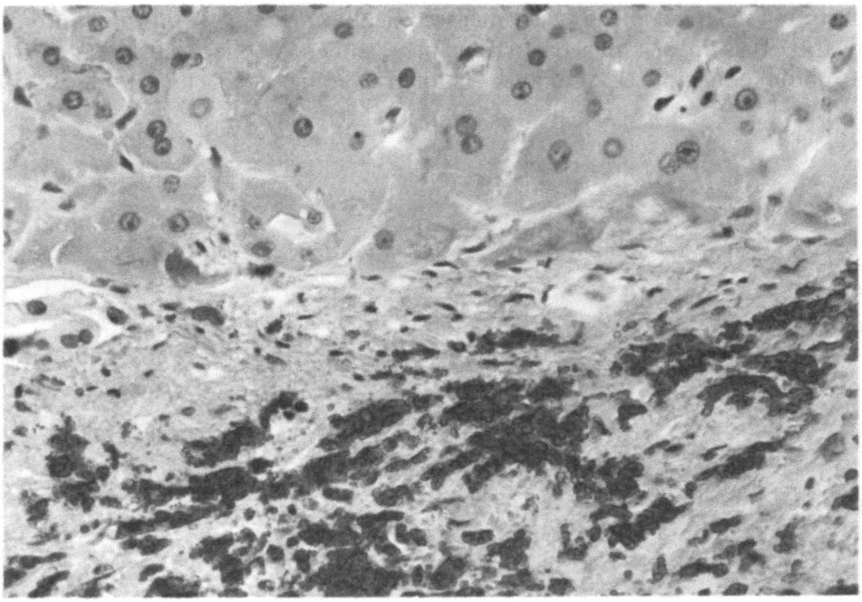

Fig. 13. Human liver cirrhosis after thorotrast application for radiograph of bile ducts. Development of large scar formation with heavy deposits of thorotrast particles (van Gieson: ×900)

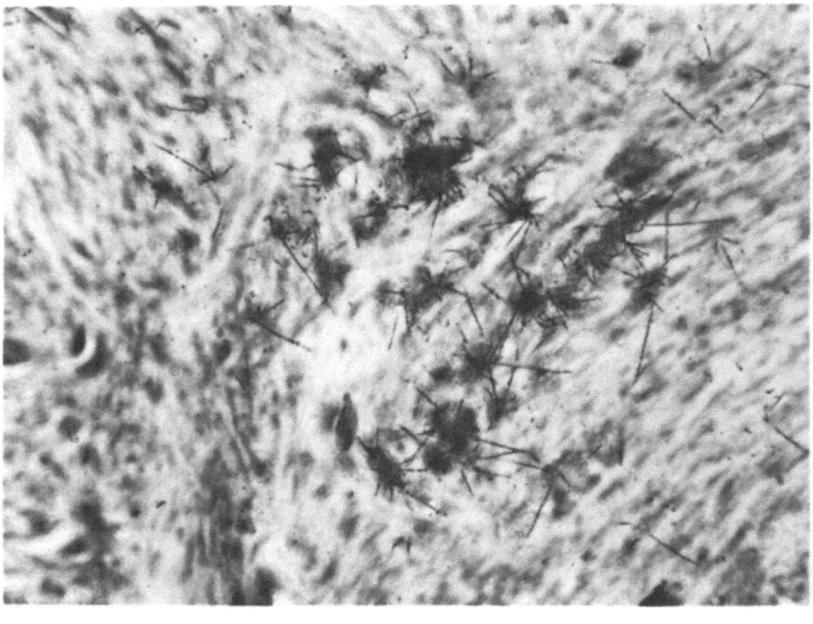

Fig. 14. Autoradiograph of thorotrast-containing liver. Note Alpha-tracks emitted by thorotrast particles (HE: ×900)

(Fig. 14). Using X-ray diffraction, the element thorium can be unequivocally identified in the foreign material deposits (GRASES, 1966). Neutron activation analysis permits determination of the concentration of thorotrast in the different tissues (EDDINGTON, 1967; SCHEER *et al.*, 1967; KAMPMANN *et al.*, 1968, 1969; LOONEY, 1960; UNNEWEHR *et al.*, 1964).

1. Morphological Findings in the Liver

Histological examinations of liver damages following thorotrast application permit the differentiation of two phases of late damages. Phase 1 is characterized by the development of liver fibrosis and cirrhosis. In phase 2, tumors develop in those cells that were within the radiation range of thorotrast deposits. Phase 1 thus represents an unspecific late damage, and phase 2 represents a specific late damage (WEGENER *et al.*, 1973; LACASSAGNE, 1971). If a tumor has already developed, both types of late changes are observed together. The development of tumors in the cirrhotic liver is equivalent to the formation of radiation cancer in other organs (ZOLLINGER, 1960) and to the chemical carcinogenesis of the liver in animal experiments (BANNASCH and REISS, 1971). The latency period of the changes is distinctly dose-dependent (ROUSSY and GUERIN, 1941).

Because of its widespread distribution in the liver, the alpha radiation of thorotrast only covers and necroses small cell groups. This process is followed by continuous regeneration of the liver parenchyma and a gradual development of liver cirrhosis. When this occurs one can no longer determine whether the subsequent tumor developed as a result of the cirrhosis, of direct radiation damage by thorotrast, or as a consequence of carcinogenesis and radiation (WEGENER *et al.*, 1973).

a) Radiocirrhosis of the Liver

Investigations by RIGLER *et al.* (1935), JACOBSON and ROSENBAUM (1938), and GILBERT (1942) demonstrated the progression of liver damages following injection of thorotrast. After one month, no changes are observed in the liver epithelium and stroma; after 6 months, there is only passive congestion. Changes of the cells adjacent to the thorotrast-loaden Kupffer cells or a fibrosis have not developed after 8–9 months. After 5 years, scar formation can be observed, and after 8 years, cirrhosis due to scar formation (Fig. 13). Even when the development of a tumor is preceded by a long latent period the formation of fibrosis and cirrhosis contraindicates the application of thorotrast (THOMAS *et al.*, 1951). In addition to the scars and diffuse interstitial sclerosis, older hemorrhages with hemosiderin deposits, regeneration, and formation of adenomas of the parenchyma, as well as bile duct proliferation can be observed. On the whole, however, changes of the vascular and connective tissue predominate—just as in the case of the late changes following external irradiation.

b) Radiocancers of the Liver

Thorotrast-induced hepatic tumors are usually sarcomas and are only occasionally cholangiar or hepatocellular carcinomas. These findings are in contrast to the fact that most primary hepatic tumors—aside from the consideration of etiology—are carcinomas. LACASSAGNE (1971) found in 50 cases described in the literature, 33 sarcomas and 17 carcinomas, GRASES (1966), in 33 cases, 14 sarcomas and 19 carcinomas. Sarcomas induced by thorotrast are predominantly hemangioendotheliomata which otherwise occur only rarely. The latency period for formation of sarcomas is 13 years, while that for carcinomas, is longer, i.e., 18 years (LACASSAGNE, 1971). Age does not influence the latency period. LACASSAGNE (1971) mentions the case of a man who at the age of 12 years had been injected with thorotrast and who died of cancer of the liver at the age of 30. There are no sexual distinctions either. While spontaneously forming hepatic tumors occur more often in men, tumors due to thorotrast occur with equal frequency in men and women. The same relationship has been observed with the formation of skin carcinoma following therapeutic application of X-rays or radium rays (LACASSAGNE, 1945).

2. Effects of Other Radioactive Elements

Some publications have reported the cirrhogenic and carcinogenic effects of other radioactive elements. A small platinum tube containing 2 mg of radium was accidently lost in the thorax, during an implantation because of a mamma carcinoma. At autopsy, it was found in the diaphragm over the liver; in addition to a local necrosis, it caused the development of a hemangioendothelioma in the liver (ROSS, 1932). Acute intoxication with different radio elements was observed in 23 Japanese sailors who happened to get into the fallout of the atomic bomb explosion of Bikini on March 1st, 1954. All of them exhibited skin and blood changes. After the 3rd month, 17 of them developed liver symptoms. A 40-year-old sailor died on the 207th day. At autopsy, liver atrophy with massive sclerosis and bile duct proliferation was found (TSUZUKI, 1955).

JUSTIN-BESANCON *et al.* (1958) reported an accidental polonium exposure. The autopsy of the 28-year-old engineer revealed multiple liver carcinomas without fibrosis or cirrhosis. Physical proof of gamma or alpha emission in the liver tissue, however, could not be furnished.

The application of monomeric and polymeric ^{239}Plutonium to rats of different ages (ranging from 0 to 140 days) leads to a different distribution pattern. As shown by means of autoradiography and radioanalysis of the various tissues the polymeric plutonium is stored mainly in the liver and the spleen, while monomeric plutonium is predominantly found in the skeleton (MAHLUM *et al.*, 1973).

D. Experimental Investigations of the Radiation Effect

In 1904, BERGONIE and TRIBONDEAU (1904) laid down the first radiation principle: the radiosensitivity of cells is directly proportional to the mitotic activity and indirectly proportional to the degree of differentiation. Since, according to BERTALANFFY and LAU (1962), cell regeneration is directly correlated with the mitotic activity of a tissue, i.e., many mitoses in the tissue are indicative or per-

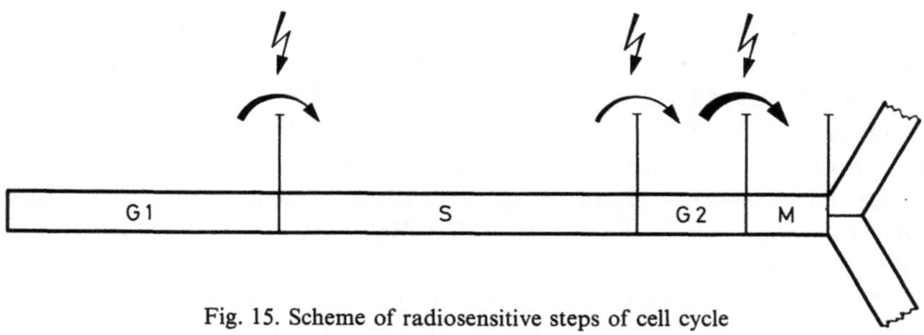

Fig. 15. Scheme of radiosensitive steps of cell cycle

manent cell regeneration and the existence of only a few suggests little or no cell regeneration, the observations of SCHOLTZ (1904) and SELDING (1904) could be easily explained. After application of radium rays and X-rays to the hepatic region, no morphological changes could be demonstrated in the resting liver, while the skin, which was rich in mitoses, showed extensive ulceration. The early findings that chromosome aberrations occur in growing, proliferating tissues also pointed to the close correlation between irradiation and cell division (BARDEEN, 1907; HERTWIG, 1911, 1920; KAUFMANN, 1954). Aberrations can be preserved for many cell generations (BARDEEN, 1907) and can develop when mitoses are arrested in the early prophase (CARLSON, 1940; KAUFMANN, 1954). They can have an essential influence on cell division and on cell survival (WOLFF, 1968). From studies on chromosome aberrations, MOORE (1965) and WOLFF (1968) drew conclusions concerning the radiosensitivity of the various phases of the cell cycle (Fig. 15). The variable sensitivities of the different phases of the cell cycle once more indicated that the radiation response of the various tissues is dependent on their proliferative activity and on the degree of differentiation (FABRIKANT, 1971). However, the existence of a general relation between cell proliferation and degree of differentiation on the one hand and radiosensitivity on the other hand is not necessarily inevitable (LEBLOND and WALKER, 1956; PRICE, 1958; STOLMAN, 1959; LAMERTON and FRY, 1963; LEBLOND, 1964; CLEAVER, 1967; PATT and QUASTLER, 1963).

I. Preliminary Remarks

To make radiation effects on the liver understandable, some preliminary remarks on the normal process of cell proliferation should be made. Based upon their proliferative state, four cell types can be distinguished: increasing populations, decreasing populations, stationary systems, and renewal populations (LEBLOND and WALKER, 1956; LEBLOND, 1964; CLEAVER, 1967; MESSIER and LEBLOND, 1960). The non-stationary cell systems, in plants as well as in animals, *in vitro* and *in vivo*, exhibit four phases in the cell cycle (Fig. 15): the mitotic phase (M), the pre-DNA-synthetic phase (G_1), the DNA-synthetic phase (S), and the post-DNA-synthetic phase (G_2). In most mammalian cells, the length of phase M is about 1 hr, that of S, 4—10 hrs, and that of G_2, 2—3 hrs, while the length of G_1 can range from minutes to months (PATT and QUASTLER, 1963).

The parenchyma of the adult liver is a stationary cell system with normally few proliferation cells. Thus according to the ideas and findings presented, radiation effects can only be traced with great difficulty, even after extremely large radiation doses. It represents a cell population of completely differentiated cells potentially capable of proliferation (G_0-population) that can be triggered into the cell cycle, e.g., during compensatory repair or regeneration (LESCH *et al.*, 1970; BUCHER, 1963; OEHLERT *et al.*, 1963; GRISHAM, 1962; BASERGA, 1968; STÖCKER and ALTMANN, 1964; FABRIKANT, 1968a, b). A G_0 population is one which can either again go through a proliferative phase or can die without so doing.

The fact that the G_0 population can, by partial hepatectomy, be stimulated again to go through the cell cycle, makes the liver an interesting system in which to examine the influence of radiation on the individual phases of cell proliferation and the process of DNA synthesis. In this context, it is particularly important that the partially hepatectomized liver represent a largely synchronized cell population, i.e., a majority of cells should be in the same phase of the cell cycle. Consideration of the effects of radiation on cell proliferation was for a long time in the limelight because of the proliferation-inhibiting effect of the ionizing rays, which is essential for clinical tumor radiology.

In contrast to the effects of radiation on DNA synthesis and mitosis, the influence on numerous other metabolic activities such as protein or lipid synthesis, oxidation or carbohydrate metabolism, and other activities cannot be precisely adjoined to the different phases of the cell cycle. They do not occur exclusively in certain phases but can be demonstrated during all phases of the cell cycle. Consideration of the influence of radiation on these metabolic events is of special importance, because they are associated with the metabolism of other body organs, and because many other metabolic reactions with which radiation may interfere take place in the liver (FRIEDMAN, 1942; GERBER and ALTMANN, 1970).

Finally, investigations during the last few years have shown (LESCH *et al.*, 1972; OEHLERT, 1973) that the combination of ionizing rays with other chemical noxae produces an influence on the reaction pattern of the liver in experimental animals.

From this fact and from historical considerations, the data acquired by experimental irradiation of the animal liver can be divided into four types: 1. early and late radiation changes morphologically demonstrable, 2. influence on DNA synthesis and morphological findings in the partially hepatectomized liver exposed to irradiation, 3. effects on metabolic activities other than DNA synthesis, 4. effects of combined radiation and drug application on liver function.

II. Early and Late Morphological Radiation Changes

The literature about experimental trials of radiation effects on the liver is full of contradictory findings, which primarily must be attributed to differing experimental procedures. Thus in the beginning, predominantly short-term experiments were carried out with a great variety of animal species. Under the light microscope, these experiments always produced negative results. Thus SCHOLTZ (1904) and SELDING (1904) were not able to produce morphological changes in the liver by external application of radium and X-rays, while the skin above the irradiation zones showed extensive ulcerations, and the sperma epithelium of the testis, irradiated at the same time, demonstrated striking lesions. With 6–12 fractionized irradiations of half of the liver of young rabbits—the other half of the liver was shielded by lead—after one month, no histological changes could be observed, as compared to the non-irradiated halves. Only after 2.5 months and 20 irradiations, was there a small narrowing of the trabeculae and of the volume of the irradiated lobules (HUDELLET, 1906, 1907). Extensive necrotic changes were observed in kittens exposed to fractionized irradiation for 20 days, starting on the 3rd day after birth, and killed 3 weeks later (TRIBONDEAU and HUDELLET, 1907). The authors assumed that in this experiment the radiosensitivity of the liver was a consequence of growth.

In 1928, in experiments with frog livers, TSCHASSOWRIKOW (1928) for the first time drew attention to early changes in the hepatocytic nucleus. POHLE and BUNTING (1932) observed slight, transitory radiation changes from the 1st–30th day after application of 600–2,500 R. Never did necrosis occur. Slight edema and fatty degeneration with a maximum on the 2nd day after irradiation were present; on the 30th day, however, they had disappeared. On application of up to 5,250 R on exteriorized dog livers, some of the animals died shortly afterwards of hemorrhage, peritonitis, or pneumonia. Others that survived up to 507 days died between the 15th and 16th months of liver failure with jaundice and ascites. The livers demonstrated extensive fibroses that had developed as early as 6 weeks after irradiation (BOLLIGER and INGLIS, 1933). By additional starving between 1 and 3 days before application of a single dose of 5,000–12,000 R X-rays in mice, a reduction in liver weight and a decrease in the size of those hepatocytes in which the nucleus-cytoplasm ratio had increased could be produced (WILSON and STOWELL, 1953). Three days after irradiation of mouse livers with 5,000 R, SUSSMAN (1956) observed an increase of about 15–18% in the size of the hepatocyte nuclei. On a single irradiation of rats with 800 R, significant nuclear growth could only be observed in the 3rd month after irradiation, which is within the time of the chronic radiation damage (SCHNEIKERT, 1973; WENIG, 1974). These differing findings led to the distinction between early and late histological radiation changes. The time between 8 and 20 days (BRENDLEIN and OEHLERT, 1974), or 50 days (KOVACS, 1974) after irradiation is supposed to be the early phase. Changes occurring later are regarded as late radiation-induced liver damages.

1. Early Radiation Changes of the Liver

a) Findings by Light Microscopy

The histological picture of the early radiation-induced changes following single (2,000–3,500 R) and fractionized irradiation with X-rays is characterized by an interstitial edema in periportal lobular areas (BRENDLEIN and OEHLERT, 1974; KOVACS, 1971; ARGAWAL and MEHROTRA, 1964; ARIEL, 1951; BOLLIGER and INGLIS, 1933; ELLINGER, 1957; WILSON and STOWELL, 1953). In addition, a slight decrease in the glycogen content of the hepatocytes (BRENDLEIN and OEHLERT, 1974; KOVACS, 1971) and moderate fatty degeneration in the centers of the lobules are present

(BRENDLEIN and OEHLERT, 1974; BACQ and ALEXANDER, 1966; BARONCHELLI, 1957; SZCZUREK, 1967; WILSON and STOWELL, 1953). In contrast, UNGER (1968) observed a decrease in the lipid content. These contrasting findings may be explained by the observation that the lipid content of the liver can change cyclically after irradiation (ELLINGER, 1957). BIRZLE (1965) made morphological investigations in rabbit livers exposed to X-rays of different doses. With small doses, applied just once (2,000—5,000 R), only slight reversible histological changes could be found within 12 and 54 days.

Short-term nuclear changes (BRENDLEIN and OEHLERT, 1974) with an increase in size of about 15—18% (SUSSMAN, 1956) as well as a slight increase in mitotic activity 8 days after the beginning of the investigation can be interpreted as a manifestation of increased metabolic activity and short-term regeneration of the parenchymal damages caused by irradiation. From this time to about the 31st day after irradiation, an essential intensification of mitotic activity could not be demonstrated (BRENDLEIN and OEHLERT, 1974). In accordance with this fact, liver cell damages as seen in the number of individual cell necroses were slight. Correspondingly, the indices of necrosis in irradiated and non-irradiated liver sections were about the same (KADOWAKY, 1956). Other authors (KOVACS, 1971; MIRONESCU and DRAGOMIR, 1967; SCHERER and STENDER, 1963; SUSSMAN, 1956) interpreted these nuclear changes as well as the edema which develops in the periportal liver sections as radiation-induced changes of the parenchymal blood circulation.

b) Electronmicroscopic Features

Changes of the liver observed under the electron microscope directly after irradiation are more impressive. They represent radiation effects, but they are not characteristic of radiation injury (FASSKE and THEMANN, 1963). Comparable alterations are to be found following acute hypoxemia (MÖLBERT and GUERRITORE, 1957) and temporary ischemia (HÜBNER and BERNHARD, 1961). They could first be shown in the organelles of the cytoplasm (GLAUSER, 1956; BRAUN, 1963; MORGENROTH and THEMANN, 1964) (Figs. 16—18). After 24 hrs, the structures of the nucleus and of the nucleolus were still intact, while the endoplasmic reticulum and the mitochondria demonstrated moderate vacuolization. The mitochondria showed a shortening of the cristae mitochondriales and even a complete loss of internal structures. JORDAN *et al.* (1972) pointed out that mitochondrial changes in mouse liver irradiated with less than 200,000 rads are difficult to distinguish from preparative artifacts, whereas doses higher than 600,000 rads produce swelling of the mitochondria followed by an ablatio of the cristae and the appearance of homogeneous turbidities of the structures. The structure of the double lamellae of the endoplasmatic reticulum was completely irregular. Using methods of ultrastructural morphometry, CHRISTOV and coworkers (1974) could demonstrate that even 24 hrs after X-irradiation of 300 rads, the numerical and volume density of peroxisomes and, in addition, of surface density of the rough endoplasmic reticulum were increased. At the same time, the number of mitochondria was reduced. The number of lipid particles in the cytoplasm and lysosomes was increased. After a single irradiation of the whole body with 1,000 R and local irradiation with doses of up to 5,000 R the nuclei demonstrated, also electronmicroscopically, shifts into higher nuclei classes (BRAUN, 1963). SCHERER (1956), SUSSMAN (1956), and WILSON and STOWELL (1953) made the same observations. Structural changes in the nucleus following X-ray irradiation with cobalt 60 can be seen

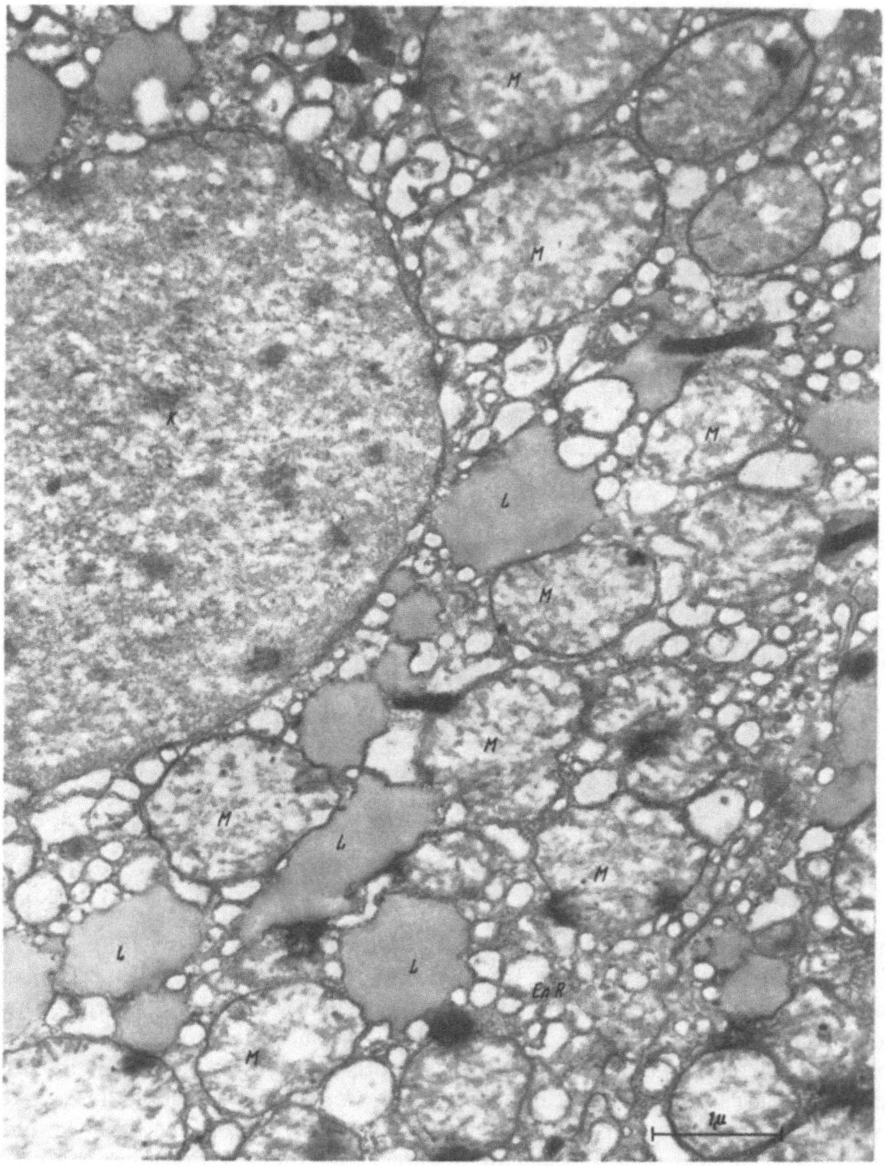

Fig. 16. Mouse hepatocyte 24 hrs after total body X-irradiation with 3,000 R. Note vacuolation of endoplasmic reticulum, enlargement of mitochondria, and lipid droplets (× 17,100). (*K* nucleus, *L* lipid droplets, *m* mitochondria.) (Figs. 16—18 from MORGENROTH and THEMANN, 1964)

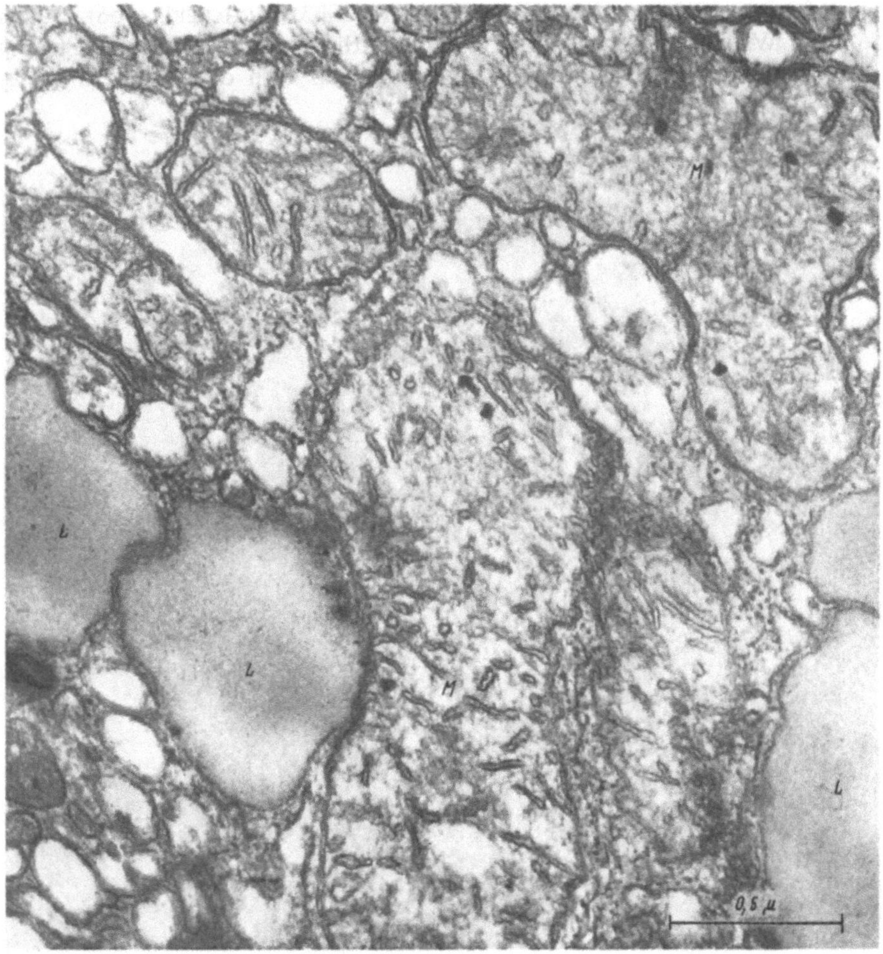

Fig. 17. Detail from Fig. 16. Enlargement of mitochondria with shortening of cristae mitochondriales (×45,500)

under the light microscope. These changes include nuclear swelling, formation of giant cells, nuclear vacuoles, nuclear pyknoses, pleated nuclear membranes, karyolysis, and karyorrhexis and can be further specified under the electron microscope (FASSKE and THEMANN, 1963) (Table 3). Vacuolization of the intermembranous space, caused by a partial lifting of the outer lamella of the nuclear membrane, can occur as early as the 1st hr after irradiation (BRAUN, 1960). These are the juxtanuclear vacuoles that can be seen with the light microscope after irradiation. Finally, the nuclear membrane can disintegrate. When consolidated and made more dense, the chromosomal material can often be observed near the inner lamella of the nuclear membrane. A loss of the chromatin can also occasionally be seen (FASSKE and THEMANN, 1963).

In contrast to the findings in bone marrow, lymph nodes, spleen, and thymus, which exhibit a continuous, intensive cell turnover, radiation-induced changes in the DNA of liver nuclei usually cannot be demonstrated in rabbits after incorpo-

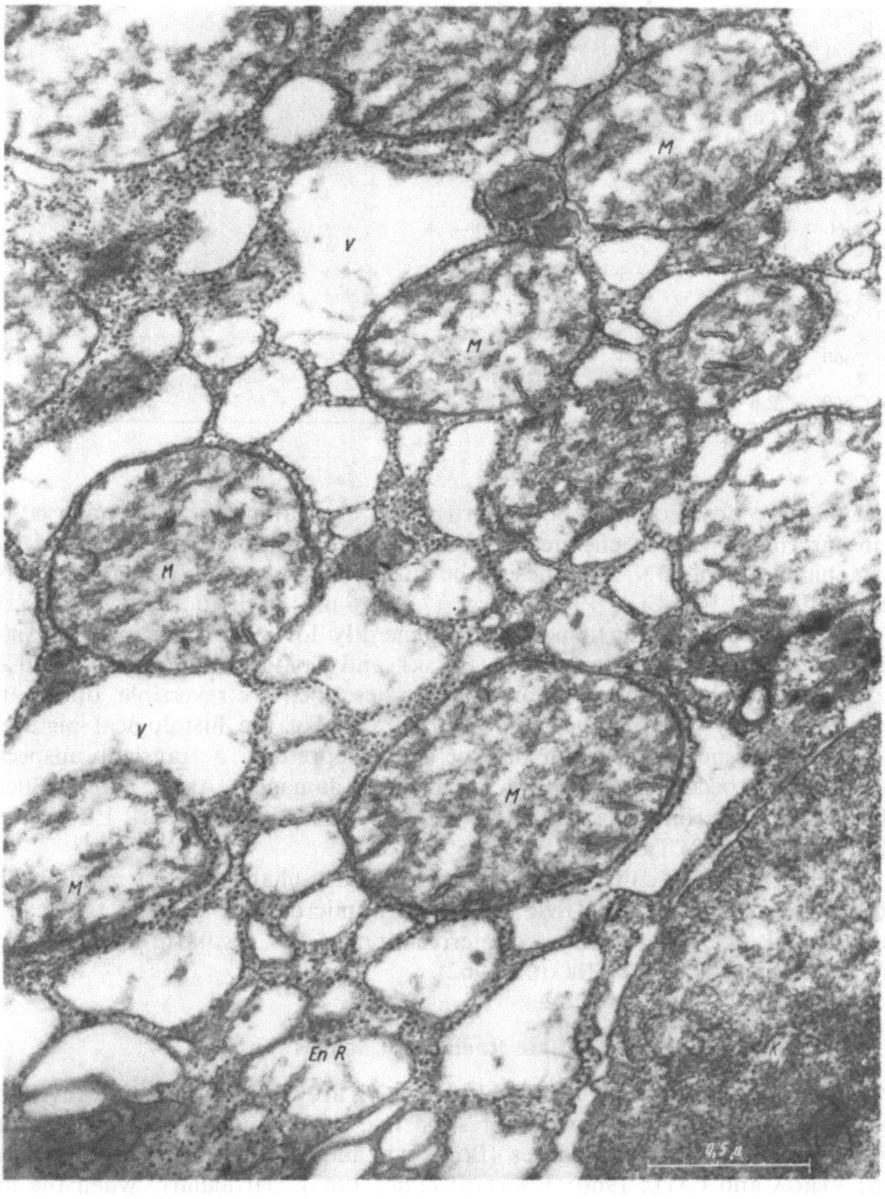

Fig. 18. Mouse hepatocyte 72 hrs after total body X-irradiation with 9,000 R. Heavy vacuolation (V) of endoplasmic reticulum and loss of mitochondrial structure (×41,500)

Table 3. Nuclear changes in mouse liver after X- and cobalt 60-irradiation in correlation to the dose or radiation and time course. (From FASSKE and THEMANN, 1963)

Dosage	Interval	Nuclear swelling	Giant cells	Nuclear vacuoles	Pyk-noses	Pleating nuclear membranes	Karyo-lysis	Karyo-rhexis
250 R	3 days	++	−	+	+	+	−	−
300 R	24 h	++	+	++	+	+	+	−
300 Co60	24 h	++	+	+++	+	+	+	−
300 R	3 days	+	+	++	++	++	+	+
300 R	7 days	+	−	+	++	++	++	+
300 R	14 days	−	−	+	++	+	+	−
300 R	24 days	−	−	−	+	+	−	−
800 R	3 days	++	+	+++	++	++	++	+
9,000 R	immediately	+	−	+	+	−	−	−
9,000 R	2 h	+++	−	+++	+	+	+	+
9,000 Co60	2 h	+++	−	+++	++	+	+	+
9,000 R	17 h	+++	+	+++	+++	+++	++	+
9,000 Co60	17 h	+++	+	+++	+++	+++	+++	+
9,000 R	24 h	++	+	+++	+++	+++	+++	++
9,000 Co60	24 h	++	+	+++	+++	+++	+++	++
9,000 R	48 h	++	+	++	+++	+++	+++	++
9,000 Co60	48 h	++	+	++	+++	+++	+++	+
9,000 R	72 h	+	+	+	++	+++	+++	++
9,000 Co60	72 h	+	+	++	+++	+++	+++	+++

ration of large doses of radiophosphorus. The electronmicroscopic observations are in agreement with biochemical examinations of the same animals. In organs with a high rate of DNA synthesis, the differences between ^{32}P-labeled DNA after small (7 × 0.16 mCi, ^{32}P) and large (7 × 5.66 mCi, ^{32}P) doses of the isotope are very marked. In liver tissue with a generally low incorporation rate, such a difference cannot be demonstrated (FASSKE and THEMANN, 1963). Since all the histological and electronmicroscopic changes described are reversible, one cannot say with certainty whether the later normalization of the histological picture is the result of tissue regeneration or whether it represents a transient unspecific reaction which occurs if the entire organism is damaged (ARIEL, 1951; BIRZLE and FLIEGEL, 1965; BARONCHELLI, 1957; MACCARDLE and CONGDON, 1955; RUBIN and CASARETT, 1968; TRASINO *et al.*, 1959).

Therefore it is difficult to say whether the early changes are a manifestation of the radiosensitivity of the liver. The electronmicroscopic changes that can be demonstrated at a time when a counterreaction of the organism is improbable, seem to advocate this view (BRAUN, 1962).

2. Late Radiation Changes

The early radiation changes of the liver, which are without exception reversible, contrast sharply with the more impressive late radiation changes that are only produced by large radiation doses (BOLLIGER and INGLIS, 1933; INGOLD *et al.*, 1965; VERGA and CALL, 1960; WESELOH *et al.*, 1967), particularly when the liver is examined after irradiation of the whole body. After hemi-irradiation of the liver with a dose of 4,000 R from observations made up to 555 days, LACASSAGNE and co-workers (1963, 1965) showed that the irradiated part of the liver exhibited a progressive atrophy corresponding to the suppressed mitotic activity. The loss of weight of the irradiated liver sections was compensated by a parallel hypertrophy of the covered lobules in which mitotic activity was sharply increased (Fig. 19).

In these experiments at $2^1/_2$ months after irradiation even though microscopic changes in the hepatocytes could not be demonstrated in either the irradiated or non-irradiated liver sections, broadening of the portal tracts and fibrosis of the vascular tissue were evident. The atrophic liver parenchyma was successively replaced by connective tissue (Fig. 19).

Five months later, increased proliferation of bile duct epithelium was observed in the non-irradiated lobules. These changes of the biliary tree were also seen after irradiation of the total organ with doses of 2,000—3,500 R (BRENDLEIN and OEHLERT, 1974). As early as 8—20 days after irradiation, cell damage and cell necroses which later produce a noticeable increase in the proliferative activity of the biliary epithelium are developing within the region of the bile ducts.

Distinct mitotic alterations which include formation of atypical giant nuclei and polynuclear epithelial giant cells can also be demonstrated. The increasing proliferative activity which reaches beyond the portal tracts causes the extensive proliferation of bile duct epithelium, which contributes to a change of the architecture of the liver tissue, i.e., to a liver cirrhosis (Figs. 20 and 21). Such changes could also be observed in long-term experiments with rabbits which received frac-

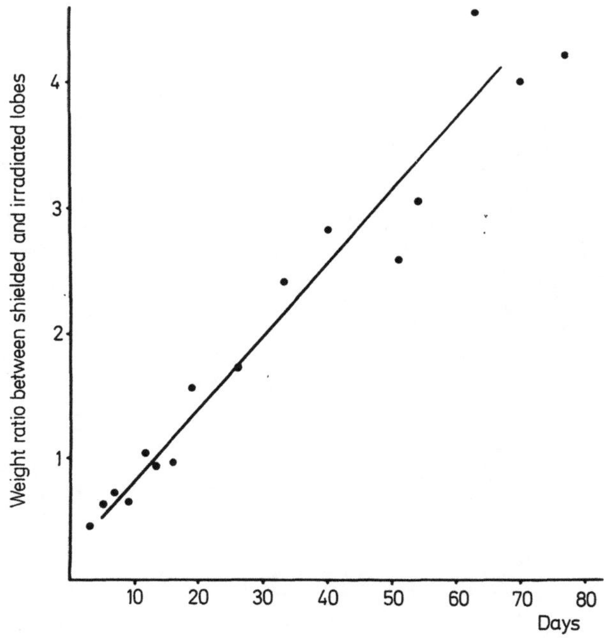

Fig. 19. Weight ratio between shielded and irradiated lobes. Shielded lobes represent initially 32% of total weight of liver. Weight ratio with lobes to be irradiated is thus 0.47. Graph shows development of compensative hypertrophy during first 3 months following irradiation. (From LACASSAGNE, 1971)

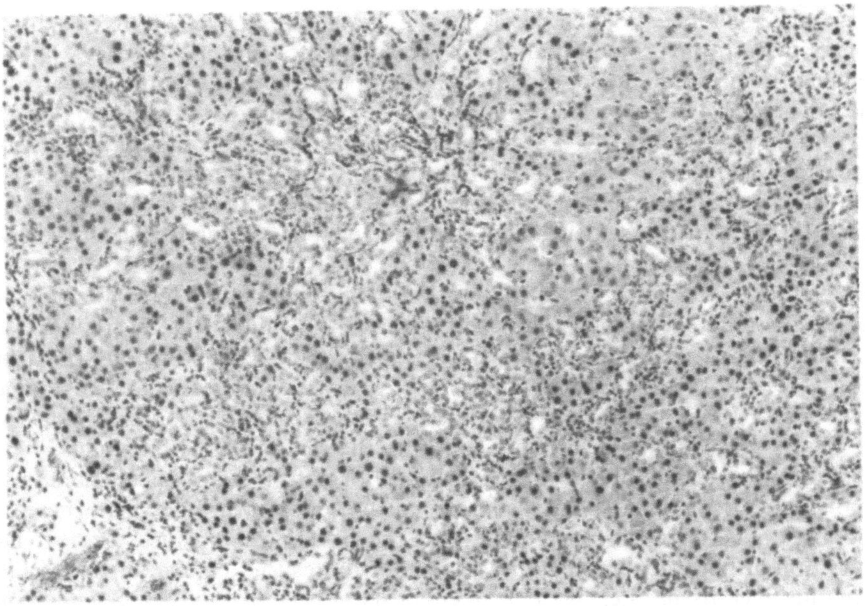

Fig. 20. Rat liver after X-irradiation of 2,000 R after 100 days. Striking proliferation of bile ducts throughout the liver with marked destruction of liver architecture toward liver cirrhosis (HE: ×65)

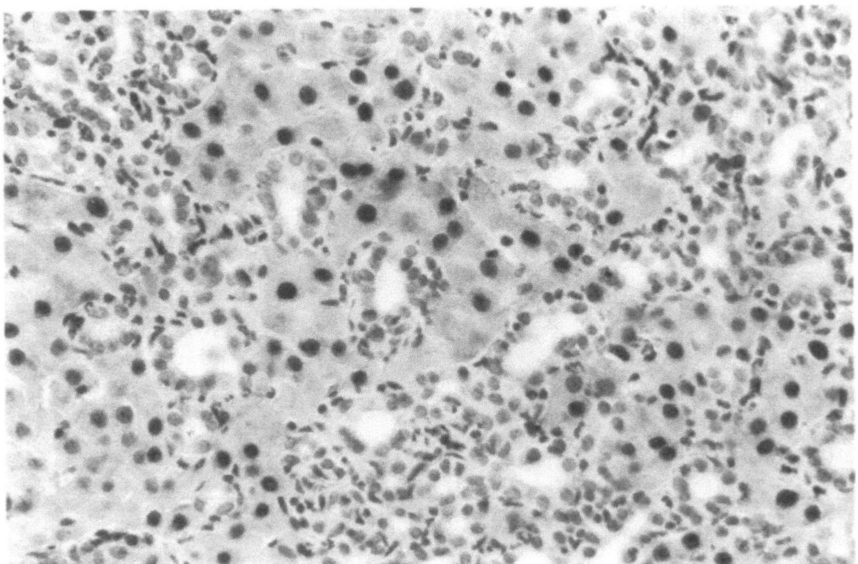

Fig. 21. Higher magnification of Fig. 20 (HE: ×600)

tionized doses of irradiation ranging from 10,000–20,000 R (BIRZLE, 1965). Between 12 and 27 days after irradiation, massive atypical biliary regeneration, as well as heavy damage of the liver parenchyma with marked portal fibrosis and transition into fibroses, were noted. Rats chronically intoxicated with the amino sugar galactosamine in the region of the biliary tree exhibited the identical symptoms (LESCH *et al.*, 1970; LESCH *et al.*, 1973). Thus it may be that this peculiar proliferative activity of the bile duct epithelium, which includes formation of conglomerates of biliary sprouts, does not represent a specific radiation damage but rather a characteristic reaction of the rat liver to intoxication.

At the same time, following single as well as fractionized irradiation, severe nuclear and cytoplasmic anomalies of the parenchyma can be demonstrated in rat and rabbit livers, e.g., formation of giant nuclei, double nuclei in the hepatocytes, atypical mitotic figures, giant nucleoli, and cytoplasmatic vacuolizations (BRENDLEIN and OEHLERT, 1974). If one supposes that the nuclear polymorphy is also a result of mitotic disturbances, the degree of nuclear polymorphy in the liver tissue must be dependent on the number of cell cycles that occurred in the meantime. If we assume that the mean lifetime of the liver epithelia of adult rats amounts to 150 days, then within a period of 31 days about $^1/_5$ of all liver epithelia would have gone through mitotic divisions which, in the case of pertinent mitotic disturbances, resulted in nuclear polymorphy. If one considers, however, the fact that immediately after a single irradiation of the liver an obvious increase in cell regeneration occurred, the increased mitotic activity of which could still be demonstrated on the 8th day after irradiation then $^1/_3$ or even half of all liver epithelia have already gone through a mitosis. This situation could then result in massive nuclear polymorphy. Nuclear polymorphy which occurs late after irradiation is in good correlation with the results of extensive nuclear measurements after a single irradiation with 800 R which caused a significant increase in nuclear growth only in the 3rd month after irradiation. Additional increase of polymorphy between the 40th and 100th day after irradiation can probably be attributed to the fact that during this period, the number of single cell necroses increases considerably and the rate of mitotic activity thereby continues to rise (BRENDLEIN and OEHLERT, 1974). Although nuclear polymorphy presents an impressive picture under the light microscope, its importance to the function of the liver is minimal. Despite the development of atypical mitoses, which may account for 80% of all mitoses, parenchymal regeneration is guaranteed, though it occurs very slowly. Moreover, liver parenchyma function is not disturbed (see later paragraph). On the other hand WILEY and co-workers (1973) reported that in addition to occurrence of atypical mitoses, X-irradiated mouse liver tissue reacts against proliferative stimuli with an enhanced rate of hepatomas.

The glycogen content of the hepatocytes increased in animals which were exposed to fractionized irradiation. In the late phase after irradiation, glycogen distribution was, however, varied. The changes in activity of acid phosphatase and of oxidative enzymes observed in the early phase remain unchanged up to the 150th day (KOVACS, 1971).

As in the human liver, experiments with animals have confirmed the importance of late radiation changes in the mesenchymal structures of the liver, specifically in the vascular system. The medium-sized and large branches of the portal vein are also especially affected. In rat livers exposed to a single dose of 2,000—3,500 R the first change observed by BRENDLEIN and OEHLERT (1974), as early as 20 days later, was severe perivascular edema of the medium-sized and large branches of the portal vein; after 30 days, they observed extensive thrombosis of the vessels, some of which were completely occluded. At the same time, the branches of the arteria hepatica showed hyalinization and thickening of the walls (Fig. 22a and b). The intrahepatic occlusions explain the ascites which were observed in the animals at the same time. The insular reconstitution, which is only discretely marked up to the 62nd day, cannot be supposed to be the cause of ascites. Thus the changes in the branches of the portal vein, including thrombosis comparable to that observed in the Budd-Chiari syndrome, must be regarded as the direct cause of the congestion in the portal veins of the formation of ascites and of the considerable growth of the spleen. The late focal and spotty necroses in the liver parenchyma are also due to these vascular occlusions. Later in the experiment, they again stimulate liver regeneration. The severe disturbances in blood circulation in the liver tissue must be regarded as a primary cause of insular reconstruction of the liver parenchyma and the development of cirrhosis. Bile duct proliferation described previously may be also due to the disturbances in blood circulation caused by necroses of bile duct epithelia. Also, internal radiation with colloidal ^{198}Au in various doses up to 67,000 rads in dogs causes severe alterations of the vascular system of the liver with occlusion of the vessels and cirrhotic fibrous proliferation followed by ascites formation and parenchymal degeneration (HAHN *et al.*, 1951).

The destruction of parenchymal cells and the proliferation of portal and intralobular bile duct cells are accompanied by intense activity of the Kupffer cells, beginning with hypertrophy, when the irradiation dose exceeds 3,300 R (VERGA and CALL, 1960). At the same time, enzymatic activity of acid phosphatase and of oxidative enzymes increases considerably in the Kupffer cells and in the mesenchymal cells of the portal fields (KOVACS, 1971). The reticulin fibers of the liver parenchyma which are fragmented in centrolobular regions early in the experiment (KOVACS, 1971), later on, particularly after irradiation doses of 7,400 R, become swollen and thickened, but retain their stainability for silver (VERGA and CALL, 1960).

3. Radiation Effect on Fetal Liver Tissue

DUPLAN and IZADIAN (1959) investigated the effect of X-rays applied on the 13th and 18th day after conception on the fetal liver. They applied X-rays doses of 200—1,000 R and killed the animals at different times between 24 and 120 hrs. About 30% of the fetuses which were irradiated before the 16th day of intrauterine life with 800 R died within 72 hrs. When the pregnancy continued, depending upon the applied radiation dose and the time of irradiation, the weight of the liver could barely be measured. The weight reduction was too great to be explained only by the destruction of fetal blood-forming tissue. The findings suggest that the actively proliferating liver parenchyma of the fetus is much more radiosensitive than that of the adult liver. On the 13th day of fetal life of a mouse, the hepatocytes and the cells of the hematopoietic systems were equally radiosensitive (DUPLAN, 1963). Using far smaller doses of 10 to 80 R/day during the periods of blastogenesis,

(a)

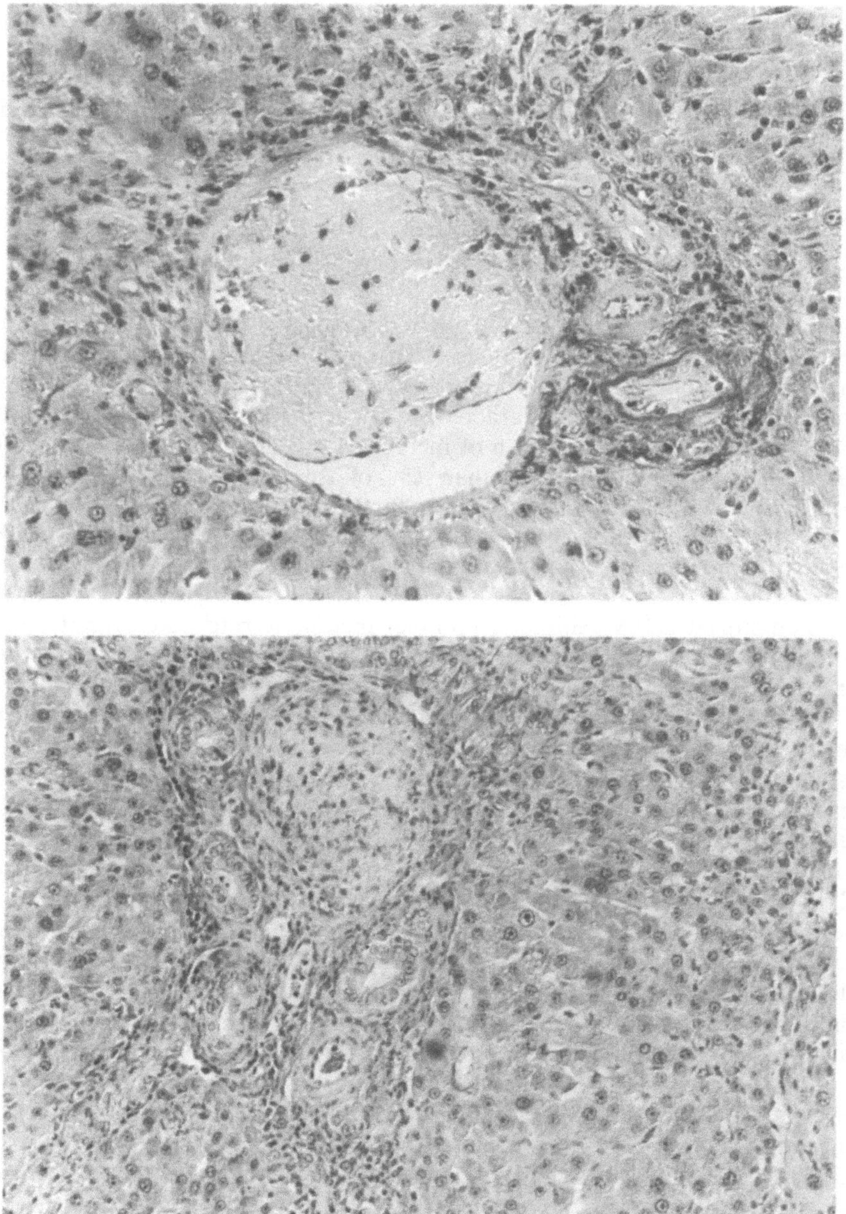

(b)

Fig. 22. (a) Rat liver 100 days after X-irradiation with 2,000 R. Thrombosis of portal vein with beginning organization (HE: ×370). (b) Same series as Fig. 22a. Complete obliteration of portal vein with granulation tissue. Thickening of wall of arteria hepatica (HE: ×370) organogenesis, fetogenesis, early and late embryogenesis respectively, KONERMANN (1975) demonstrated an enhanced growth activity within all experimental groups. This inducibility decreases with growing age. In these experiments, the mass ratio of hepatic and hemopoietic cells is not altered, compared with non-irradiated controls with respect to the postnatal disappearance of the hemopoietic cells.

III. Radiation Effect on Liver Regeneration with Special Regard to the Influence of Nucleic Acid Synthesis

With increasing age, the normal rat liver shows a rapidly decreasing rate of cell proliferation and of DNA synthesis (STÖCKER, 1973). The rate of proliferation in the liver of adult rats is low; more than 99% of all hepatocytes are in the G_0 phase, which is, however, characterized by active protein and RNA synthesis. Thus the low rate of incorporation of metabolic precursors into the nuclear DNA corresponds to the fact that less than 1% of the hepatocytes are in the DNA synthesis phase (FAUSTO and VAN LANCKER, 1965; NYGAARD and POTTER, 1959). The moderate rate of DNA synthesis indicates that the cytoplasmic enzymes involved in pyrimidine metabolism are only minimally active (SMITH and LOW-BEER, 1957).

Mitochondrial DNA exhibits a minimal metabolic rate that cannot be traced autoradiographically, but which has been demonstrated biochemically (CHANG and LOONEY, 1967; GERBER *et al.*, 1960; GERBER and REMY-DEFRAIGNE, 1946). So far there have been only a few statements in the literature on the radiosensitivity of this process, and it is assumed that the biosynthesis of mitochondrial DNA is less radiosensitive than that of the nuclei (CHANG and LOONEY, 1967). An alteration in the metabolic rate of mitochondrial DNA, however, obviously does not have any effect on radiation-induced liver damage.

Investigation of intermitotic cell systems, such as the epithelia of the gastrointestinal tract (OEHLERT, 1971), showed that proliferating cells are particularly radiosensitive during the periods of transition from one generation cycle to another. In contrast, the G_1 or G_0 phases, i.e., those phases that in general determine the lifetime of the cell, seem to be relatively insensitive. This assumption, however, is valid only as long as the cell remains in the G_1 or in the G_0 phase. If a population of reversible postmitotic cells, e.g. hepatocytes, is forced to proliferate late after a single irradiation and thus to pass from the G_0 phase into the S phase, mitotic disturbances, including chromosomal aberrations, cytological alterations, and even cell death (OEHLERT, 1971; WEINBREN *et al.*, 1960; WENIG, 1974), and a delay of DNA synthesis (LADDAGA and ROMAGNOLI, 1961) can be observed. Comparable observations of a transient cessation of mitosis and the production of atypical mitoses in fertile tissues were described previously by LACASSAGNE and MONOD (1927) in tumors, by ALBERTI and POLITZER (1923) in the corneal epithelium of urodele-larvae, and by STRANGEWAYS and OAKLEY (1923) in chorioid cultures of chick embryos.

The damage produced in a reversible postmitotic cell population remains latent and invisible in the histological or cytological picture, as long as the cells remain in the G_0 phase. It is only at the moment when a mitosis is being prepared or carried out, that the radiation-induced damage is unmasked by different forms of mitotic dysfunction.

1. DNA Synthesis and Liver Proliferation after Partial Hepatectomy

KELLY and PAYLE (1953) investigated the effect of total irradiation of mice on DNA synthesis during the period of regeneration after administration of CCl_4. The liver after partial hepatectomy, however, turned out to be the best experimental model for the study of radiation effects on DNA synthesis and cell proliferation. Liver proliferation after partial hepatectomy and the metabolic activities needed for this, particularly those which occur in the prereplicative phase of regeneration, have been described by many authors (for surveys see BUCHER, 1963; BASERGA, 1968; BUCHER and MALT, 1971; FABRIKANT, 1968a, b, c). About 18 hrs after partial hepatectomy, DNA synthesis begins in the remaining part of the liver and reaches a maximum between 24 and 30 hrs (BUCHER, 1963). Autoradiographic experiments confirmed the time course of regenerative proliferation determined biochemically. It turned out that up to the time of the most intensive incorporation of radioactive metabolic precursors, the highest labeling intensity could be demonstrated for hepatocytes. The maximal rates of proliferation for bile duct epithelia and Kupffer cells are reached later (OEHLERT *et al.*, 1963; BUCHER, 1963; GRISHAM, 1962; FABRIKANT, 1968a; RABES *et al.*, 1973). Characteristically, the parenchymal proliferation begins in the peripheral sections of the lobules and shifts to centrolobular areas, the longer after partial hepatectomy it is. Within 2—3 weeks, the remaining liver segment regains its former cell number and weight by compensatory hyperplasia (BUCHER, 1963; BUCHER and MALT, 1971), in the course of which 90% of the parenchymal cells divide within 24—28 hrs after operation. Investigation of radiation effects on DNA, RNA, and protein synthesis in the partially hepatectomized liver can be carried out as follows (VAN LANCKER, 1966):

1. The liver is irradiated at different times after partial hepatectomy (Section a)
2. The animals are partially hepatectomized at different times after irradiation (Section b)
3. Irradiation is carried out in animals which were not partially hepatectomized (Section c)

a) Irradiation of the Liver after Partial Hepatectomy: Metabolic Processes

The biochemical reactions in the different phases of regeneration which are influenced by exposure to radiation are summarized in Table 4 (for rev. see BUCHER, 1963; GAUTIER, 1961, 1967; VAN LANCKER, 1966, 1969). In the following, the effects of irradiation on different metabolic processes necessary for proliferation will be considered:

1. Delay of liver regeneration by irradiation (α)
2. Influence of irradiation on RNA synthesis (β)
3. Influence of irradiation on enzyme protein synthesis (γ)
4. Influence of irradiation on DNA synthesis in DNA-replicating cells (δ)

Table 4. Biochemical processes in regenerating liver and their alteration by irradiation at different times after partial hepatectomy. (From GERBER and ALTMAN, 1970)

Experimental conditions	0–6 hrs	6–12 hrs	12–18 hrs	18–24 hrs	24 hrs and later
Normal pattern of regeneration	Latency period: no significant biochemical change	Increased activity of RNA polymerase and synthesis of nuclear RNA; synthesis of cytoplasmic RNA enhanced later.	Synthesis of enzymes needed for DNA synthesis (dTR and dTMP phosphotransferases, dCMP aminohydrolase, DNA polymerase)	DNA synthesis (S phase)	Mitosis, eventually followed by another cell cycle
Pattern of regeneration when irradiated at some time during the period indicated	Low doses (200 R) delay all regeneration-related reactions	Low to intermediate doses delay enzyme formation and DNA synthesis and depress synthesis of nuclear RNA and later of cytoplasmic RNA	Intermediate doses delay enzyme and DNA synthesis; no effect on enzymes already formed	High doses (1000 R) immediately depress DNA synthesis and delay mitosis; no immediate effect on enzymes or primer activity	Intermediate doses delay mitosis and affect subsequent cell cycle

α) Irradiation of the whole body or irradiation of the liver at the time of partial hepatectomy suppresses the incorporation of different metabolic precursors into DNA during a period of 18–24 hrs after partial hepatectomy. Thus, irradiation with doses of between 150 and 3,000 R at different times after partial hepatectomy only delays the incorporation of ^{32}P, ^{14}C-orotate, ^{3}H-thymidine, and of labeled monophosphates, which are incorporated into DNA in smaller concentrations (CATER *et al.*, 1956; JAFFE *et al.*, 1959; HOLMES and MEE, 1955; HOLMES, 1956; BELTZ *et al.*, 1957; ALBERT and BUCHER, 1960; LEHNERT and OKADA, 1962, 1964; GERBER and REMY-DEFRAIGNE, 1966; VAN LANCKER, 1960). Following exposure to a dose as small as 450 R, the first DNA wave and the normally subsequent mitotic wave fail to appear, as measured by the rate of incorporation of ^{32}P into DNA (CATER *et al.*, 1956) (Fig. 23) and after application of ^{3}H-thymidine (BARBASON, 1974) when the liver is irradiated during the first 12 hrs after partial hepatectomy. Even when irradiation is applied 21 days after partial hepatectomy, DNA synthesis is reduced. If the liver is irradiated 17 or 24 hrs after partial hepatectomy, an immediate injection of ^{3}H-thymidine indicates replication of the hepatocytes within about 5 hrs (LOONEY *et al.*, 1960) which means that no inhibition can be observed (BARBASON, 1974). With doses of less than 2,000 R the regenerative ability is delayed but not abolished (HOLMES and MEE, 1955). The suppression of DNA synthesis and of the development of mitoses cannot be explained by an impairment of DNA synthesis alone (CATER *et al.*, 1956).

It is possibly the result of interference with phosphorylation (LOONEY *et al.*, 1965; KELLY, 1957). Following larger radiation doses, the time interval between maximal DNA synthesis and maximal mitotic activity increases, i.e., a delay in mitotic activity occurs in the G_2 phase (HOLMES, 1956). Irradiation during the

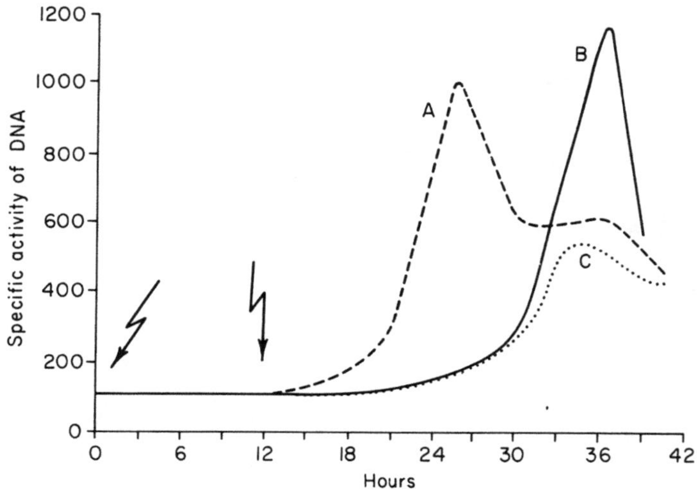

Fig. 23. Rate of DNA synthesis in regenerating rat liver after total body X-irradiation. *A*, nonirradiated control *B*, irradiated 12 hrs after partial hepatectomy; *C*, irradiated shortly before partial hepatectomy; arrows, time of X-irradiation (450 R). Specific activity of DNA: cpm/0.1 mg DNA. Abscissa: Hrs after hepatectomy. (From HOLMES, 1956)

S-phase (28 hrs after partial hepatectomy) with 450 R also leads to an inhibition of the suceeding mitotic wave (BARBASON, 1974). Local irradiation of the regenerating liver 1 hr, after application of ^{3}H-thymidine does not produce a loss of labeled DNA after 3,000–6,000 R. Only on irradiation with 12,000 R can a moderate degradation of DNA be observed. Excessive degradation of DNA observed in *Escherichia coli* is not observed in mammalian cells either *in vivo* or *in vitro*. Therefore, one can exclude degradation as the cause of the significant depression in the rate of DNA synthesis (LOONEY and CHANG, 1969). The effects of X-rays and electron rays applied in doses of 450 R were each compared by RUDNICKI (1963). The degree of DNA synthesis and of delayed formation of mitoses was about the same.

β) The formation of messenger RNA precedes the de novo synthesis of protein. One of the first indications of regeneration is the increase of acid-soluble ribonucleotides and the increased activity of RNA polymerase (BUCHER, 1963; BUCHER and MALT, 1971). The rate of incorporation of metabolic precursors into nuclear RNA increases accordingly and is followed by the synthesis of those enzymes necessary for DNA synthesis (FAUSTO and VAN LANCKER, 1965; GIUDICE and NOVELLI, 1963; TSUKADA and LIEBERMAN, 1964). In earlier studies, the effect of irradiation on the incorporation of ^{32}P into the total RNA could neither be observed in regenerating livers nor in normal livers. However, the studies in which ^{14}C-orotate was used as precursor showed that nuclear RNA synthesis is stimulated within 6–12 hrs after partial hepatectomy (BERG and GOUTIER, 1967; UCHIYAMA *et al.*, 1965) (Fig. 24). The stimulation of nuclear RNA synthesis is delayed if the liver was irradiated shortly before or after operation (BERG and GOUTIER, 1966; UCHIYAMA *et al.*, 1966).

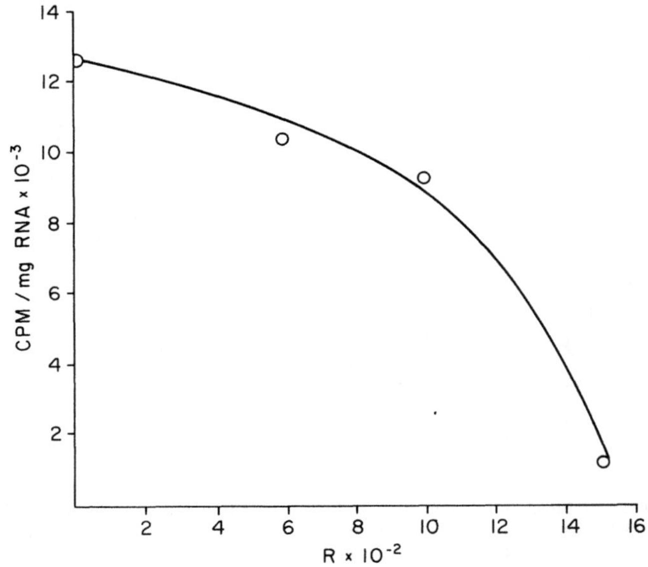

Fig. 24. Incorporation of orotate-^{14}C into rapidly labeled, nuclear RNA as function of radiation dose. Radiation dose in roentgens is plotted against specific activity of RNA. Rats were hepatectomized 24 hrs and X-irradiated (total body) 6 hrs before sacrifice. Each point on curve represents average value obtained with three pooled livers. (From UCHIYAMA *et al.*, 1965)

In the early phase of regeneration, the synthesis of cytoplasmatic RNA is influenced only to a small extent, while from 5 hrs after the operation on, the specific activity decreases markedly in contrast to that of nuclear RNA, which increases (Fig. 25) (BERG and GOUTIER, 1966, 1967). This effect may be the result of a delayed transfer of RNA from the nucleus into the cytoplasm; it may, however, depend also on the rate of turnover of the pCpCA terminal end of cytoplasmic RNA.

With respect to the various size classes of RNA, the high molecular weight RNA shows the greatest stimulation during regeneration after partial hepatectomy. This same RNA fraction is the one whose synthesis is most sharply decreased after irradiation, as shown by velocity sedimentation analysis in sucrose gradients. Measurements of the ultraviolet absorption showed that the relative content of the different nuclear RNA fractions is, however, not altered (BERG and GOUTIER, 1966; UCHIYAMA *et al.*, 1966). The labeling of cytoplasmic RNA with orotate after irradiation is decreased to the same degree in all fractions of cytoplasmic RNA.

The reduced incorporation of metabolic precursors into RNA may be the result of a changed precursor pool which in turn is due to a dilution with catabolic products from organs which contain radiosensitive RNA. Furthermore, there may be a reduction in the rate of formation of nucleotide-triphosphates, the activity of RNA-polymerase may be reduced, and finally, there may be structural changes of the chromosomes in which RNA is formed. So far, only results for the influence of irradiation on RNA polymerase have been obtained. Its formation is clearly

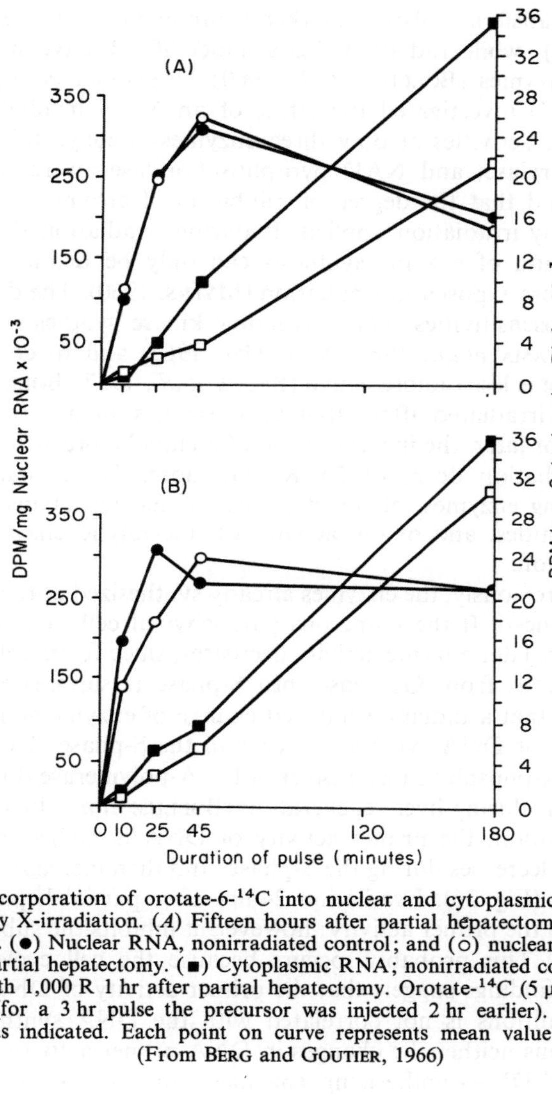

Fig. 25A and B. Incorporation of orotate-6-^{14}C into nuclear and cytoplasmic RNA of regenerating liver after total body X-irradiation. (*A*) Fifteen hours after partial hepatectomy, and (*B*) 12 hrs after partial hepatectomy. (●) Nuclear RNA, nonirradiated control; and (○) nuclear RNA; irradiated with 1,000 R 1 hr after partial hepatectomy. (■) Cytoplasmic RNA; nonirradiated control. (□) Cytoplasmic RNA, irradiated with 1,000 R 1 hr after partial hepatectomy. Orotate-^{14}C (5 μCi) was injected 12 hrs after hepatectomy (for a 3 hr pulse the precursor was injected 2 hr earlier). Rats were killed after injection at times as indicated. Each point on curve represents mean value obtained with 3 rats. (From BERG and GOUTIER, 1966)

delayed (BERG and GOUTIER, 1966, 1967; KLOUWEN, 1960; UCHIYAMA *et al.*, 1965; VANDERGOTEN and GOUTIER, 1966; WELLING and COHEN, 1960).

γ) The activity of the cytoplasmic enzymes necessary for DNA synthesis and for the formation of its metabolic precursors increases shortly before the onset of DNA synthesis. Liver irradiation 15 hrs before or 15 hrs after partial hepatectomy delays de novo synthesis of enzymes, but it does not have any effect on those enzymes that are already present in the liver. Thus, radiation doses of up to 1,500 R applied 6–7 hrs after partial hepatectomy inhibit thymidine kinase synthesis by as much as 99% (BELTZ, 1962; BELTZ and APPLEGATE, 1959; BOLLUM *et al.*, 1960). With these irradiation doses, the synthesis of thymidine kinase and

DNA-nucleotidyl-transferase also is markedly inhibited (UCHIYAMA *et al.*, 1965; Bollum *et al.*, 1960), while radiation doses under 700 R have no effect on the neoformation of enzymes (BOLLUM *et al.*, 1960; UCHIYAMA *et al.*, 1965). MYERS and DEWOLFE (1962) investigated the effect of an X-ray irradiation of 1,500 R on 24 enzymes. The activities of only three enzymes—deoxycytidilate deaminase, thymidine phosphorylase, and NAD pyrophosphorylase—were reduced. On the whole, it can be said that the degree of inhibition of enzyme synthesis depends on the dose of X-ray irradiation applied. If during irradiation the liver is partly covered, an inhibition of enzyme synthesis can only be demonstrated in those liver sections that were exposed to irradiation (MYERS, 1960). The different enzymes have different radiosensitivities. Thus thymidine kinase synthesis is extremely radiosensitive (UCHIYAMA *et al.*, 1965; WEN-MEI, 1963) and in contrast, synthesis of DNA polymerase is less radiosensitive (BELTZ *et al.*, 1957; BOLLUM *et al.*, 1960).

δ) If the liver is irradiated after DNA synthesis has already begun, i.e., 18 hrs after the operation or later, the incorporation of metabolic precursors is immediately inhibited by radiation doses of 500 R and more. Thus, changes of activity in DNA-synthesizing enzymes, of the structure of nucleoproteins, of the content of deoxyribonucleotides, and of the activity of nucleolytic enzymes may be the cause of his inhibition.

As mentioned previously, the enzymes already synthesized at the time of irradiation, are not influenced. If the numerous parenchymal cells are irradiated in the S-phase, some hours later enzyme activity decreases, since fewer cells enter mitosis, and transition of cells from G_1-phase into S-phase is suppressed. Therefore, it cannot be assumed that a radiation-induced change of enzyme activities represents the limiting factor for DNA synthesis in cells in the S-phase. Thus, for example, the activities of dTR-phosphotransferase or of DNA-polymerase do not run parallel with DNA synthesis during liver regeneration (BOLLUM *et al.*, 1960).

During regeneration, the primer activity of DNA is highest before the onset of DNA synthesis, decreases during the S-phase, and then increases again (LEHNERT and OKADA, 1964) (Fig. 26). Irradiation 24 hrs after partial hepatectomy has no immediate effect on the primer activity; however, it inhibits the subsequent increase of DNA synthesis. This probably, occurs because the cell cycle is blocked by irradiation. These findings suggest that the primer activity of DNA as determined under *in vitro* conditions is not correlated with the DNA synthesis rate *in vivo* (STACEY, 1961). Thus neither the changes in DNA-primer activity nor the changes in the activities of DNA-synthesizing enzymes can provide an explanation for the immediate effect of irradiation on DNA synthesis.

Furthermore, DNA synthesis can be influenced by nucleoproteins. As yet, however, only little is known about the mechanism. Most authors report that irradiation has no effect on nucleoprotein synthesis, either *in vitro*, or *in vivo* (BUTLER *et al.*, 1957; GERBAULET *et al.*, 1963; RICHMOND *et al.*, 1957). LOGAN (1959) and LOGAN *et al.* (1959) point out that there are distinct differences in the incorporation of radioactive amino acids into the irradiated nuclei. Histone synthesis is not disturbed if the hepatocytes are irradiated during the S-phase (LEHNERT and ODAKA, 1963, 1964). After irradiation, the acid-insoluble nucleoproteins, however, demonstrate a reduced incorporation of ^{14}C-lysine (LEHNERT and OKADA, 1966). Since, during the decrease of DNA synthesis after irradiation, nucleoprotein-synthe-

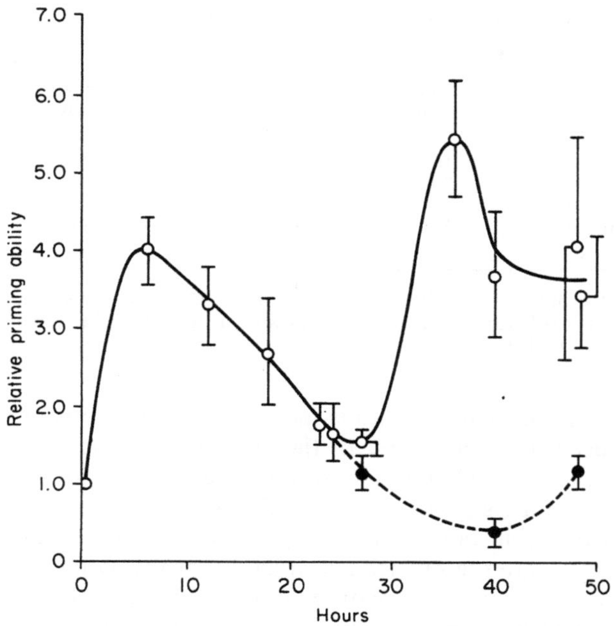

Fig. 26. Altered priming ability of isolated rat liver nuclei after partial hepatectomy and later total body X-irradiation. (○) Nuclei of nonirradiated, regenerating liver; and (●) nuclei of regenerating livers after 800 R total body X-irradiation administered 24 hrs after partial hepatectomy. (From LEHNERT and OKADA, 1964)

sis is maintained, a greater protein content can be shown as compared to DNA in irradiated nuclei than in normal ones.

After irradiation with 1,000 R a transitory decrease of the concentrations of histones and nucleoglobulins can be observed 10—24 hrs later in the nuclei of normal livers (ERNST, 1962, 1963b; HAGEN, 1960). This loss of nucleoproteins is irreversible in lymphoid organs and precedes cell death in the interphase. In the liver, however, normal concentrations are attained after 2—3 days. The solubility of nucleoproteins in salt solutions increases in lymphoid tissues, but not in the regenerating liver (GOUTIER, 1967).

In the regenerating liver, the content of deoxyribonucleotides increases shortly before the onset of DNA synthesis (SCHNEIDER and BROWNELL, 1957). This increase fails to appear if the liver is irradiated at the time of partial hepatectomy (JAFFE *et al.*, 1959). Possibly, the enzymes necessary for the synthesis of deoxyribonucleotides are not formed after irradiation. Earlier in the experiment, about 6—12 hrs after exposure to irradiation, the deoxyribonucleotides accumulate in the normal liver and to an even greater degree in the regenerating liver (SOŠKA *et al.*, 1962) (Table 5). This increase is in good agreement with the increased excretion of dCR in the urine (DIENSTBIER, 1965). These observations show that the liver, specifically the segment which remains after partial hepatectomy, is not able to metabolize the deoxycytidine that is released as a consequence of DNA catabolism in radiosensitive organs.

Table 5. Effects of X-irradiation on nucleoside content in regenerating liver. (From GERBER and ALTMAN, 1970)[a]

Group	Deoxy-cytidine	Methylde-oxycytidine	Deoxy-uridine	Thymidine
Control[b]	18	1.1	2.0	2.8
Irradiated[b]	26	0.5	0.17	0.4
Partially hepatectomized	24	1.9	0.76	4.6
Partially hepatectomized and irradiated	31	0.4	1.30	2.3

[a] Nucleoside content expressed as millimicromoles per gram of tissue. Rats were exposed to 600 R x-rays (total body) 24 hrs before partial hepatectomy and killed 24 hrs after surgery.
[b] Nonregenerating, normal liver.

The activity of lysosomal enzymes is increased in numerous organs as a result of radiation-induced tissue necroses. In the regenerating liver, DNase II in lysosomes and DNase I in mitochondria show an increased activity some hours before the onset of DNA synthesis (GOUTIER, 1967; GOUTIER-PIROTTE and GOUTIER, 1962). This increased activity is not modified by irradiation. One part of DNase II, however, passes over into the supernatant fraction, probably because the lysosomes become more fragile through irradiation (GOUTIER-PIROTTE and GOUTIER, 1962). A comparable increase in the activity of DNase II in the supernatant fraction can also be observed in normal irradiated livers and can be correlated with simultaneously occurring changes of the pH (GOUTIER, 1961). In the normal mouse liver, DNase I activity is changed only slightly by an irradiation of the whole body with 500—780 R (FELLAS *et al.*, 1954; KURNICK *et al.*, 1959). The total activity of ribonuclease of the rat liver increases 2—3 days after irradiation of the whole body with 600 R and decreases during the post-irradiation period (ROTH *et al.*, 1953). Whether changes in the concentration of an inhibitor are the cause for this effect is discussed by HILL *et al.* (1956).

The particular radiosensitivity of the proliferating liver can also be seen in rat fetuses after irradiation of pregnant animals between the 16th and 20th day of pregnancy with 500 R of cobalt 60. In the fetal liver, an inhibition of DNA synthesis occurs which lasts about one cell generation. RNA and protein synthesis are reduced but are going on during the inhibition of DNA synthesis. The effects of fractionized irradiation with 100 R each day from the 16th—20th day of pregnancy are distinctly less marked in the liver, but the placenta tissue demonstrates an increase in radiation damages (MITZNEGG *et al.*, 1970).

b) Irradiation before Partial Hepatectomy

Biochemical and autoradiographic investigations showed that partial hepatectomy after irradiation produced a decrease in and a delayed onset of DNA synthesis (ISHIKAWA, 1973; KALASHNIKOVA, 1963a, b) that could still be demonstrated after 256 days (LADDAGA and ROMAGNOLI, 1961; ALBERT and BUCHER, 1960; VAN LANCKER, 1959, 1960). This temporary blockage of mitosis, however, decreases in intensity with time and is influenced by circadian rhythm. Thus the inhibition of incorporation of metabolic precursors of DNA synthesis is most strongly marked in the morning (MYERS, 1960). On irradiation in rats of only the right lateral lobule with 1,500 R MYERS (1960) observed histologically, a decrease of DNA synthesis and of the content of nuclei in only this lobule, but not in the ones which were covered. This finding suggests a strictly local effect of irradiation.

FABRIKANT's (1964) extensive investigations, on the contrary, proved that irradiation does delay the onset of DNA synthesis and the mitosis of parenchymal cells, but that the regenerative capacity of the liver is not essentially influenced after repeated hepatectomies despite the persistent radiation-induced chromosomal damages.

Morphologically, the marked chromosome aberrations could be regarded as an expression of the manifestation of latent radiation damage after partial hepatectomy (WEINBREN *et al.*, 1960; OEHLERT, 1973; WENIG, 1974). Atypical mitotic configurations as an expression of latent radiation damage could also be made visible in the bile duct epithelia if a ligature of the ductus choledochus was made immediately or 3 months after irradiation of 2 exteriorized lobules with 5,000 R (WEINBREN and GHORPADE, 1960; WEINBREN *et al.*, 1960). At the same time, the rate of proliferation of the bile duct epithelia was markedly reduced.

In contrast to FABRIKANT's findings (1964), the investigations of STEGNER (1974), and of WENIG (1974) demonstrate that after 3 partial hepatectomies, a distinct delay of the regenerative process occurs within 9 months, if the rats were irradiated with a dose of only 800 R 3 months before the first partial hepatectomy. After the 3rd partial hepatectomy, still about 80% of all mitoses showed atypical configuration. This delay in the proliferative process even after repeated partial hepatectomies is the more remarkable because in non-irradiated animals repeated partial hepatectomies produce an increasing acceleration of the regenerative process (INGLE, 1954, 1957; SIMPSON and FINCKH, 1963). In investigations of LEONG *et al.* (1961), the mitotic indices of pre-irradiated, repeatedly partially hepatectomized rats were 50—60% less then those of non-irradiated animals.

WENIG's (1974) histological findings after irradiation and subsequent repeated partial hepatectomies are remarkable. Besides the many atypically configurated mitoses and the delayed regeneration, he found particularly after the 3rd partial hepatectomy, i.e., 9 months after irradiation with 800 R a marked periportal fibrosis of the parenchyma with numerous foci of bile duct proliferation and transition into liver cirrhosis. The Kupffer cells and littoral cells proliferate extensively. These findings must be regarded as late sequelae of irradiation. They were also observed—as already mentioned in Section D.II.—in non-hepatectomized livers (LACASSAGNE and HURST, 1963; BRENDLEIN and OEHLERT, 1974); however, they could not be found after repeated partial hepatectomy without irradiation (STÖCKER *et al.*, 1973; SIMPSON and FINCKH, 1963). The experiments of LACASSAGNE and HURST (1963, 1965) and BRENDLEIN and OEHLERT (1974), however, were carried out with much larger radiation doses so that the multiple proliferative stimuli induced by repeated partial hepatectomy intensify the radiation effect.

c) Irradiation of Non-Hepatectomized Animals

If the adult liver is irradiated without previous or subsequent inducement of proliferation, the morphological changes mentioned in Section D.II. occur. Damage to the DNA, however, cannot be traced with either biochemical or autoradiographic methods (FABRIKANT, 1971; VAN LANCKER, 1969). It occurs only—even after a long period—if the hepatocytes are induced to divide. X-ray irradiation interferes with DNA synthesis, with the synthesis of the quickly labeled nuclear RNA and with the cytoplasmatic RNA. The biosynthesis of those proteins which are important for DNA synthesis is also affected (UCHIYAMA *et al.*, 1965, 1966; VAN LANCKER, 1966).

Chromosomal damages are eliminated only slowly in the resting liver (LESHER *et al.*, 1960; FABRIKANT, 1967a, b, d; CURTIS *et al.*, 1964; CURTIS, 1968; COGGLE, 1968). LESHER *et al.* (1960) demonstrated in mice, after continuous gamma irradiation over 350 days (12 R/10—12 hrs/day), that the onset of DNA synthesis was only moderately delayed and possibly was the result of a mitotic disturbance caused by the accumulation of chromosomes. In investigations in mice which received doses of up to 70 rads/day and in rats which received doses up to 50 rads/day over a long period, these changes proved to be dependent on the dose, on the duration of exposure, and on the dose accumulation (FABRIKANT, 1967a, b, c). The influence on proliferation by accumulated chromosomal damages need not be the result of continuous irradiation with large doses (CURTIS and CROWLEY, 1963; CURTIS *et al.*, 1964). Even extensive genetic damage of liver cells is repaired after some months, if the cells are not exposed to a proliferative stimulus (CURTIS, 1968). On the other hand, severe chromosomal damages which are the result of irradiation with fast-moving neutrons are not repaired (CURTIS and CROWLEY, 1963; CURTIS *et al.*, 1964). We can therefore assume that cellular radiation damages which accumulate during continuous irradiation of cells that have a long intermitotic period do not disturb the process of cell proliferation; nor do they disturb the regenerative capacity, at least to that extent for which irradiation is not accountable. Since liver tissue which is not induced to proliferate represents a G_0 population, the radiation stress released in the non-proliferating phase essentially does not seem to influence the ability to recover from radiation damages (FABRIKANT, 1967a; COGGLE, 1968).

To summarize the results of morphological, proliferation kinetic, and biochemical investigations after irradiation of partially hepatectomized animals, two findings emerge as the results of latent radiation damages:

1. In the proliferation-induced liver, a delay in the onset of regeneration occurs which is repaired within a few weeks (ALBERT and BUCHER, 1960; CATER *et al.*, 1956; HOLMES and MEE, 1955).
2. The repair of chromosomal damages which become manifest after induced mitosis, takes several months (ALBERT and BUCHER, 1960; LEONG *et al.*, 1961; WEBER and STICH, 1965), while damages produced by massive irradiation with fastmoving neutrons obviously are not repaired (CURTIS and CROWLEY, 1963; CURTIS *et al.*, 1964).

IV. Effects on Metabolic Activities Other than DNA Synthesis

The biological changes of the liver produced by irradiation are without exception "early" changes. In the late phase, in which morphological changes are unequivocally traceable within the vascular and connective tissues, primary radiation-induced changes in liver metabolism can no longer be demonstrated or cannot be distinguished from secondary changes. When assessing biochemical changes, the comparison of experimental conditions is particularly important but also particularly difficult. The feeding habits of the animals and the time between irradiation and examination must especially be taken into account. About 3–5 days following irradiation, most of the animals do not feed very much; their stomachs, however, are always heavily filled. Hamsters are the exception; they do not show a reduction in food intake after irradiation. Therefore, meaningful findings are possible only when irradiated and non-irradiated starved animals are compared. Since the animals feed again after some time, it is equally difficult to use non-irradiated control animals. Therefore, experimental and control animals should be starved at least 24 hrs before killing.

1. Fat and Carbohydrate Metabolism

In irradiated animals, the relationship between lipid and carbohydrate metabolism is particularly interesting. Therefore, the following paragraph will deal separately with changes in these metabolic activities, and later on, they will be considered together.

a) Changes in Lipid Metabolism

In the early phase after irradiation, the liver exhibits increased lipogenesis. This increase in the intact irradiated liver is due to a decrease of the respiratory quotient (LANE *et al.*, 1955) which results from a reduction of CO_2 expiration during normal oxygen uptake (HEVESY and FORSSBERG, 1951; LANE *et al.*, 1955; RUST *et al.*, 1963). After irradiation with 300–5,000 R, the incorporation of different metabolic precursors—acetate, L-glucose, or fructose, mevalonate or butyrate, and others—into lipids is increased during the first few days (GOULD *et al.*, 1959; HILL *et al.*, 1956; LERNER *et al.*, 1953; VINOGRADOVA, 1962; TRETYAKOVA and GRODZENSKII, 1960; HANSEN *et al.*, 1965; CONIGLIO *et al.*, 1955, 1956, 1957; TRETYAKOVA, 1964; BARTSCH and GERBER, 1966; MOREHOUSE and SEARCY, 1955; GROSSI *et al.*, 1958, 1964) (Fig. 27). In addition to the kind of food, other factors influence the incorporation of these metabolic precursors: 1. the type of metabolic precursor (α); 2. the animal species investigated (β); 3. the age of the animal (γ), and 4. the irradiation dose and the time of examination after irradiation (δ).

α) The increased incorporation of labeled precursors into cholesterol is best seen in trials with ^{14}C-acetate (GOULD *et al.*, 1959). Smaller increases can be observed using ^{14}C-mevalonate and ^{14}C-squalene (GROSSI *et al.*, 1958, 1964). When mevalonate is used as lactone an increase in the incorporation rate cannot be demonstrated (GOULD and POPJAK, 1957). This effect must be regarded as an expression of the loss of the negative feedback control of cholesterol biosynthesis. The loss of this control mechanism can be considered the cause for the increase in cholesterol synthesis (GERBER and ALTMANN, 1970).

β) The increase in the incorporation of ^{14}C-acetate into cholesterol is greater in rats than in mice or in guinea pigs (GOULD *et al.*, 1959). Changes in cholesterol synthesis, however, cannot be demonstrated in irradiated rabbits. Interestingly,

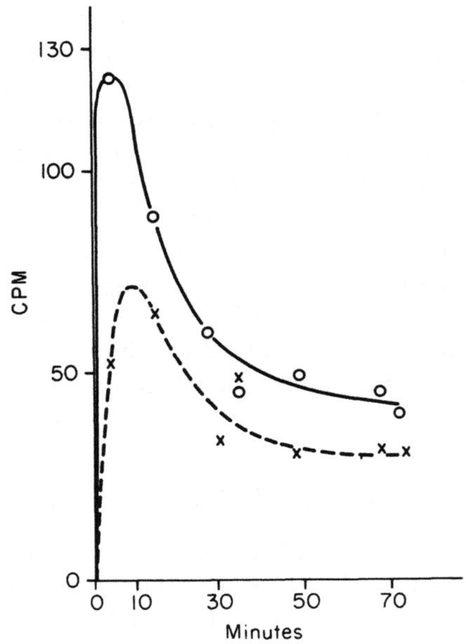

Fig. 27. Lipogenesis from glucose in mouse liver after total body X-irradiation. (o) Specific ^{14}C activity (cpm/100 mg lipid) of hepatic lipids in mice irradiated with 2,000 R X-rays (total body) after subcutaneous injection of glucose-UL-^{14}C. (×) Nonirradiated animals serving as controls for above group. Irradiation began at t_0. All mice were fed until time of exposure to X-rays and were subsequently starved. The ^{14}C activity (ordinate) is expressed in terms of cpm/100 mg lipid. (From LOURAU-PITRES, 1954)

the differing synthesis reactions of the different animals correspond to the degree of inanition.

γ) Increased incorporation of ^{14}C-butyrate (GREENGARD, 1963) or of ^{14}C-L-glucose into the fatty acids of the liver (CONIGLIO *et al.*, 1959; HANSEN *et al.*, 1965) can only be observed in old rats.

δ) The time course of increased lipogenesis is essentially influenced by the degree of irradiation. The labeling intensity of fatty acids and cholesterol following injection of radioactive metabolic precursors is most marked, with a radiation dose of 1,200 R, after 48 hrs and with a radiation dose of 800 R, after 24 hrs (VINOGRADOVA, 1962). On application of 400 R, fatty acids demonstrate the highest labeling intensity after 6 hrs, cholesterol, after 24 hrs (VINOGRADOVA, 1962).

In contrast to these distinct differences in the incorporation of metabolic precursors, the lipid and phospholipid concentrations in the liver are changed only minimally after a single irradiation (SCHWARZ *et al.*, 1961; EBERHAGEN *et al.*, 1965, 1967; SIMONOV, 1965; KAINOVA, 1960; LIM *et al.*, 1967; DEL FAVERO *et al.*, 1965; NOTARIO *et al.*, 1964, 1965; CONIGLIO *et al.*, 1953; BENNETT *et al.*, 1954). When rats are irradiated daily with 50 R for 3 weeks, triglycerides accumulate. Then fatty liver can be demonstrated microscopically. There are no comparable changes when the same dose is applied in a single irradiation (CHEVALLIER and BURG, 1953; AGOSTINI *et al.*, 1964). The concentration of CoA in the liver decreases only when a fatty liver is developing (AGOSTINI *et al.*, 1964), a reaction that can also be observed in fatty livers produced by other toxic influences (BELTZ, 1962). The catabolism of lipids and their transfer to other organs seem to limit the degree of lipid accumulation after irradiation.

b) Changes in Glycogen Synthesis

The glycogen content in the livers of irradiated starved animals is greater than that of non-irradiated starved animals. Compared to fed animals, however, it is small after irradiation (ROSS and ELY, 1951; HANSEN, 1967; MOLE, 1956; ARGAWAL and MEHROTRA, 1964; KAY and ENTENMAN, 1956a, b; WEBER and CANTERO, 1959; CONIGLIO *et al.*, 1955, 1956; Berndt and GAUMERT, 1966; BERNDT and ULBRICH, 1967; STREFFER, 1966a) (Fig. 28). The rate of de novo synthesis of glycogen is increased in those animals that are starved before irradiation, but after irradiation, the small glycogen content increases (MASORO, 1962; BORREBAEK *et al.*, 1964). The increased rate of glycogen synthesis is rendered possible by an increased gluconeogenesis. The degree of glycogen accumulation parallels an increase in blood glucose (STREFFER and LANGENDORFF, 1966).

Little is known about the catabolism of glycogen in the liver following irradiation (BERNDT and GAUMERT, 1966a, b). It is possible that changes in enzymatic activities together with a reduction of the glycolytic activity play a role (BERNDT and GAUMERT, 1966a, b; BERNDT and ULBRICH, 1967; STREFFER, 1966b). These changes, however, cannot be very extensive, as is demonstrated by the increased incorporation of ^{14}C-glucose into the lipids of livers of irradiated rats (LOURAU-PITRES, 1954). A comparison of irradiated and non-irradiated animals fed a carbohydrate-rich diet indicates that, after irradiation, incorporation of fructose into lipids is not disturbed (JARDETZKY *et al.*, 1956). The reduced incorporation of glucose that can, however, be demonstrated is thought to be a consequence of a change in glucokinase activity. The enzymatic phosphorylation of glucose is the most important metabolic step in the glycogen pathway. After irradiation, the decrease in glucokinase activity is less pronounced in starving animals than in non-irradiated starving animals (HILL *et al.*, 1956). Glucokinase is an "adaptive" enzyme (BORREBAEK *et al.*, 1964), the synthesis of which is increased by insulin and is inhibited by glucagon (SOLS *et al.*, 1965). In rats fed a carbohydrate-rich diet, induction of glucokinase is delayed by irradiation. Accordingly, the animals catabolize glucose to CO_2 but are not as able as non-irradiated animals to use it for glycogen or lipid synthesis. In contrast, irradiation has no effect on the utilization of fructose that is phosphorylated by hexokinase and not by glucokinase (HILL *et al.*, 1956).

Extremely large radiation doses (over 5,000 R) *in vivo* as well as *in vitro* cause a degradation of glycogen rather than an accumulation (LELIÈVRE and BELTZ, 1955; LELIÈVRE, 1957; LEVY and RUGH, 1953; MACCARDLE and CONGDON, 1955; MANDEL, 1964; NOYES and SMITH, 1959).

This glycogenolysis may be the result of an increased conversion of phosphorylase A to phosphorylase B. In addition, membrane destruction produces a transfer of Na^+ to K^+ in the cell, whereby K^+ activates phosphorylase B.

On irradiation of rat liver sections *in vitro* with 3,500 R, the incorporation of ^{14}C-glucose into glycogen is reduced by about 30%; however, its oxidation to CO_2 is not influenced (BRESCIANI *et al.*, 1965). Therefore, it is understandable that the rate of incorporation appears sharply decreased because newly formed ^{14}C-glycogen is quickly catabolized.

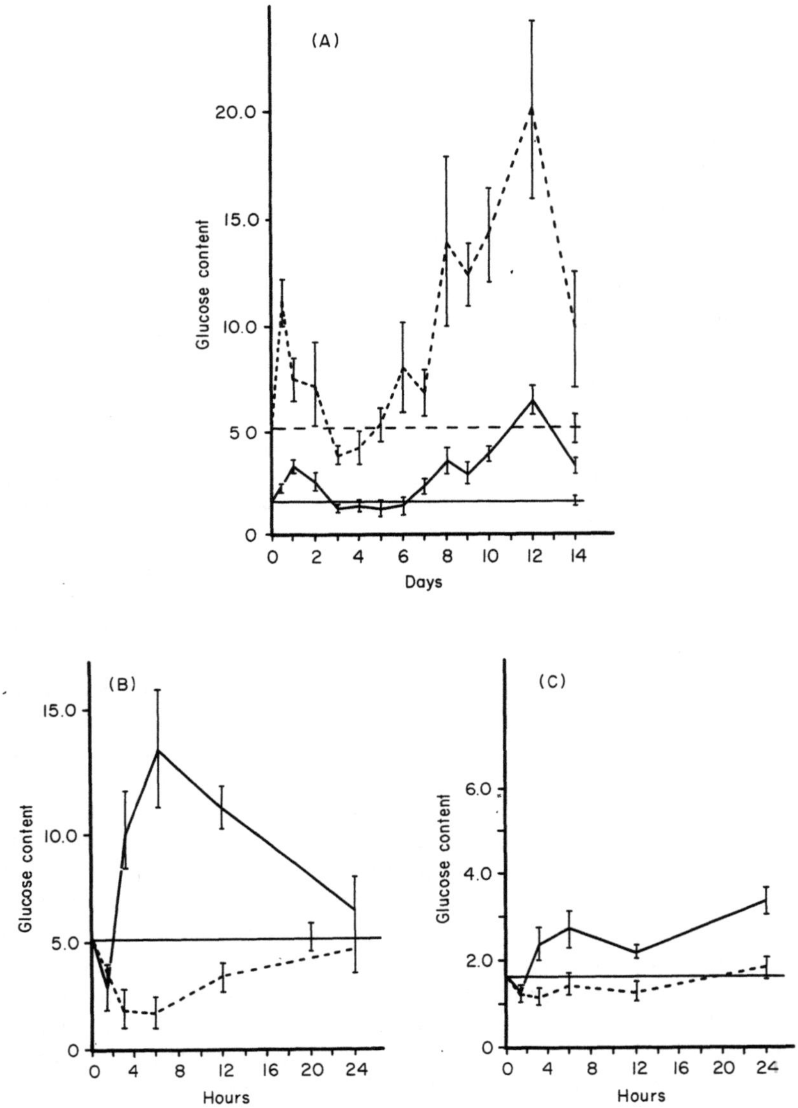

Fig. 28 A—C. Glucose and glycogen contents in X-irradiated mouse liver. Content expressed as μmoles glucose per gram tissue (*A*) Hepatic glycogen and glucose content after total body X-irradiation, examined for 2 weeks following X-irradiation; (————) glucose and (---) glycogen. (*C*) Hepatic glucose content investigated for 24 hrs after exposure. (*B*) Hepatic glycogen content for the first 24 hrs after exposure. The total-body radiation dose was 690 R. All animals were starved 24 hrs before sacrifice. In (*B*) and (*C*) the solid line represents irradiated group, whereas broken line represents the sham-irradiated group. (From STREFFER, 1966a)

c) Relations Between Lipid and Glycogen Metabolism

In the liver of mammalian animals, carbohydrate and lipid metabolic pathways interact through the intermediate, acetyl-CoA. The metabolism of the metabolic precursors in the direction of gluconeogenesis, lipogenesis, or oxidation via the Krebs cycle, can be influenced by changes in acetyl-CoA (Fig. 29). On the first day following irradiation, PEP-carboxykinase activity increases in fed mice, but decreases in starving ones (BERNDT and GAUMER, 1966a, b). Under both dietary conditions, the concentrations of PEP and of acetyl-CoA increase somewhat. The ATP-content of the liver is reduced during the first day, in some cases also during the second day after exposure of the whole body to irradiation with 690—1,400 R (BERNDT and GAUMER, 1966; MAASS, 1960; MAASS and TIMM, 1964; WALDSCHMIDT, 1968; ZICHA *et al.*, 1968). The lactate:pyruvate ratio increases during the first 4—14 hrs after irradiation, but it decreases later on, while the ratio of Beta-hydroxybutyrate and acetacetate decreases "early" after irradiation (STREFFER, 1966a) (Fig. 30). The data on glycogen and lipid metabolism presented so far are not sufficient to explain the mechanisms that are altered by irradiation. Further studies concerning the effect of radiation on glycogenesis, gluconeogenesis, lipogenesis, the Krebs cycle, and protein and citric acid cycles are necessary. It has often been stated that irradiation neutralizes the effects of hunger, i.e., an irradiated animal is not capable of adapting itself to starvation conditions (FITCH *et al.*, 1961). Therefore, substrates are still provided for glycogen and lipid synthesis instead of for oxidation in the citric acid cycle. It is important to note that the activities of glucokinase and other enzymes do not decrease in starving animals

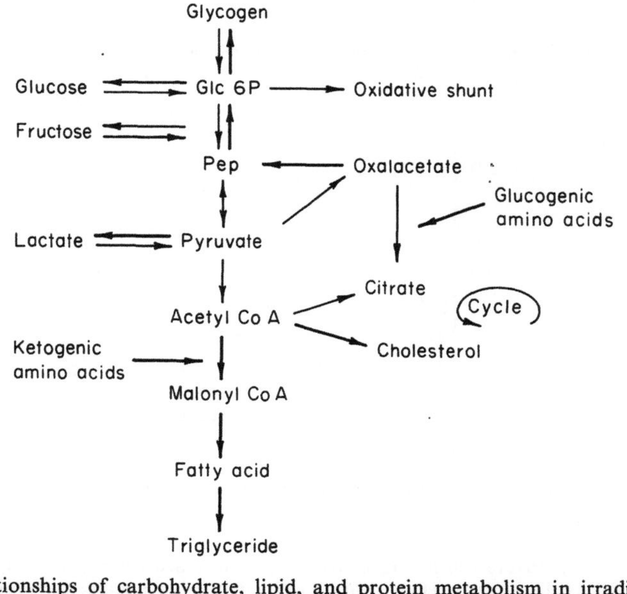

Fig. 29. Interrelationships of carbohydrate, lipid, and protein metabolism in irradiated mammalian liver. Size of arrow indicates approximate extent to which metabolism is thought to proceed in direction of given product, i.e., the heavier the arrow, the greater the metabolic flux in direction of this arrow. (From GERBER and ALTMAN, 1970)

after irradiation (BORREBAEK *et al.*, 1964) and that the incorporation of acetate into lipids does not increase when the irradiated animals are treated with glucose (PANDE *et al.*, 1962). Lipid synthesis and gluconeogenesis can only function if enough substrate is available.

The tissue of radiosensitive organs is destroyed after irradiation. Consequently, a release of glucogenetic and ketogenetic amino acids occurs (RUST *et al.*, 1963; HOLMES, 1956). Thus polypeptide fragments can accumulate in the liver (NIMS

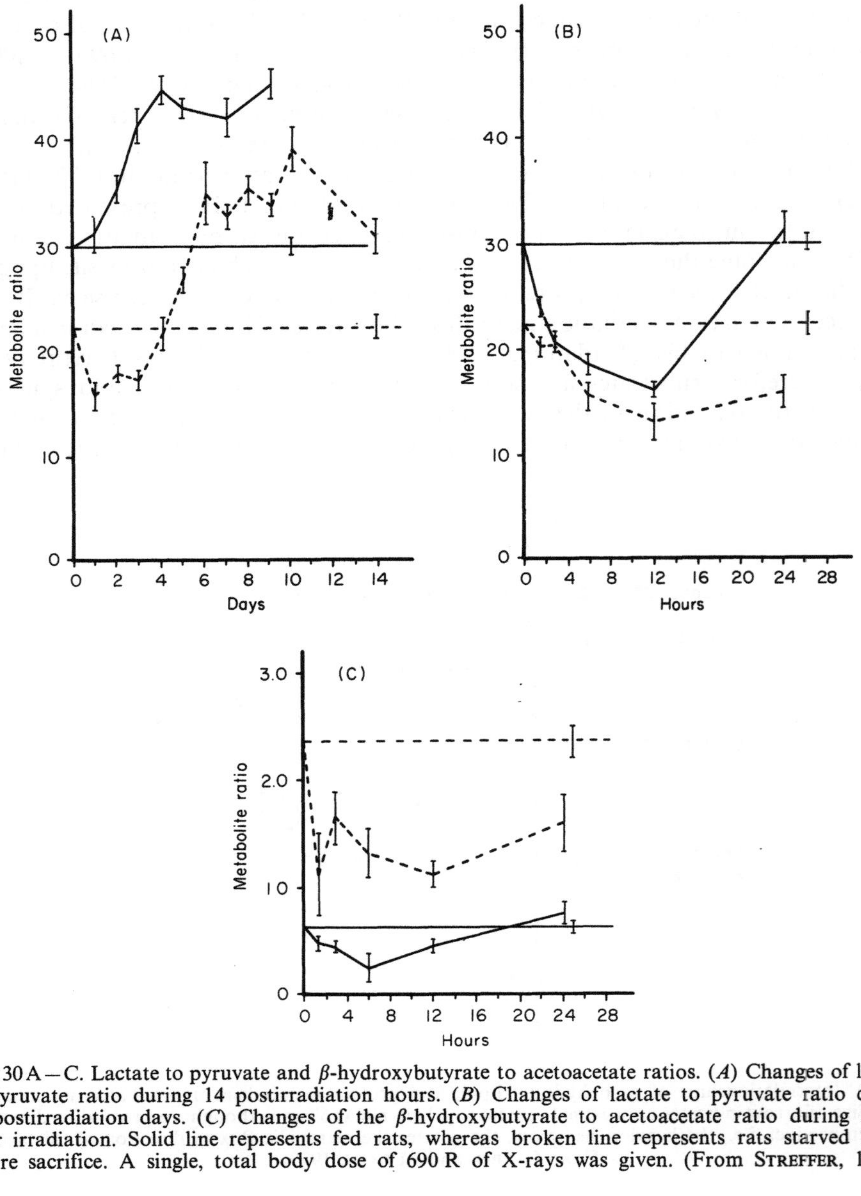

Fig. 30 A—C. Lactate to pyruvate and β-hydroxybutyrate to acetoacetate ratios. (*A*) Changes of lactate to pyruvate ratio during 14 postirradiation hours. (*B*) Changes of lactate to pyruvate ratio during 28 postirradiation days. (*C*) Changes of the β-hydroxybutyrate to acetoacetate ratio during 28 hrs after irradiation. Solid line represents fed rats, whereas broken line represents rats starved 24 hrs before sacrifice. A single, total body dose of 690 R of X-rays was given. (From STREFFER, 1966a)

and SUTTON, 1954). At the same time, the amino acid level in the blood rises (ALTMANN *et al.*, 1949; GERBER *et al.*, 1958; GERBER and REMY-DEFRAIGNE, 1963; LAUENSTEIN *et al.*, 1957; SCHREIER *et al.*, 1954; GRAEVSKAYA and SHCHEDRINA, 1963). An increased conversion of free amino acids into glycogen and lipids may occur (RUST *et al.*, 1963), and ^{14}C-labeled amino acid residues from labeled tissue protein may transfer their radioactivity to liver glycogen (RUSHMER and ALTMANN, 1967). All these observations suggest that during the first phase following irradiation, amino acids are excessively available in the liver.

These observations permit the following interpretation of radiation-induced alterations in lipid and carbohydrate metabolism. After irradiation, an increaed lipogenesis and glycogen accumulation occur because more substrate is available as a consequence of tissue destruction. In this connection, the substrate utilization for lipid and glycogen synthesis prevails over that for oxidation, since irradiated animals are only able to adapt non-oxidative enzymes (GERBER and ALTMANN, 1970).

2. Oxidative Metabolism

Since many enzymes utilized for the respiratory chain, the Krebs cycle, and the oxidation of amino acids are localized in the mitochondria, observations of radiation effects here are particularly interesting. Shortly after X-ray application, the oxidative metabolic activities and the P/O ratio (the ratio of P to O is defined as nmol esterified inorganic phosphate per micron of used oxygen atoms) are still unaltered, though changes such as mitochondrial aggregations and vacuolizations can already be observed under the electron microscope (BRAUN, 1962). Even if very small doses of X-rays are applied (about 50 R), isolated mitochondria from the livers of young rats demonstrate a loss of different enzyme activities of the Krebs cycle (FRITZ-NIGGLI, 1955). On doses of 500–2,000 R soft X-rays (60 KV) render these organelles extremely vulnerable (SCHERER, 1956a); quantitative measurements, predominantly of succinate dehydrogenase, showed a distinct loss of activity. In contrast, RAJEWSKI and co-workers (1957) observed on application of still softer X-rays (45 KV) that in the mitochondrial fractions of mouse liver sections a disturbance of oxidative phosphorylation and an inactivation of different enzymes occurred only after doses of 1,000,000 R. In a later phase, enlargement of the mitochondria and destruction of mitochondrial membranes could be seen (BRAUN, 1963; SCHERER, 1956a, b). Radiosensitivity of liver mitochondria depends partially on the localization of liver cells in the liver lobule. Thus, after irradiation with 500 R changes in central and intermediate parts of the liver lobule could be demonstrated, but not in cells in the peripheral parts of the lobule (MACCARDLE and CONGDON, 1955). After radiation doses of 1,000–9,600 R the number or mitochondria per cell decreases (BRAUN, 1962). The question arises whether these early structural changes are in agreement with biochemical changes. This question cannot be answered yet, because the results so far obtained are contradictory (BARRON, 1954; ORD and STOCKEN, 1953, 1960; SCOTT, 1937). These differences may partially be due to different experimental conditions, e.g., local irradiation or exposure of the whole body, nutritional state, etc. (JAMIESON, 1966; RAJEWSKY *et al.*, 1957; SCAIFE and HILL, 1962). SCAIFE and ALEXANDER (1961) concluded from their tests with mitochondrial suspensions from the livers of different animals (rats, mice, hamsters, rabbits, guinea pigs, and cats) that the permeability of the mitochondria is not altered by X-rays. The permeability of these organelles for molecules of different sizes could neither be altered immediately nor after 15 min of permanent incubation with 9,000 R of unfiltered X-rays (250 KV). The enzyme activities of different dehydrogenases were not disturbed either.

The cellular redox state of the liver and the formation of NADH have shown that even at supralethal radiation doses the NAD+/NADH ratio is not disturbed (JAMIESON, 1966; ZICHA *et al.*, 1968). Some days after irradiation, the NAD+ and the NADH contents of the liver possibly decrease as a consequence of a disturbance in the biosynthesis of pyridine nucleotides (KALASHNIKOVA, 1963; KUSNETS, 1960; MYERS, 1960; SCHNEIDER *et al.*, 1962; STREFFER, 1966b, 1967, 1968; ZICHA *et al.*, 1968).

If we take the P/O ratio as a criterion for the effectiveness of oxidative phosphorylation, then following *in vivo* irradiation, a marked reduction can only be demonstrated in especially radiosensitive organs, particularly in those of the lymphatic tissue (BEKKUM, 1956; SCAIFE and HILL, 1963; THOMSON, 1964). Only small changes in this ratio can be seen in the liver (ALTENBRUNN and KOBERT, 1961; SCAIFE and HILL, 1963; THOMSON and RAHMAN, 1962; THOMSON, 1964; TOPOROVA, 1957; WALDSCHMIDT, 1965). A reduced P/O ratio was, however, also observed in normal liver after exposure of the whole body to irradiation (BENJAMIN and YOST, 1960; BERNDT, 1967; CLARK, 1967; GOLDFEDER, 1956; HALL *et al.*, 1963; KHANSON, 1965; YOST *et al.*, 1964a, b, 1967a, b) or after local irradiation (JACKSON and ENTENMAN, 1961). In the regenerating liver, too, a reduction of this ratio can be shown 24 hrs after operation, if an irradiation was performed 24 or 72 hrs before killing (WEN-MEI, 1963). In these investigations, artifacts due to preparation play an important role. Above all, contamination with lysosomal acid phosphatase may cause a distinct change in the P/O ratio by a change in the concentration of the phosphate acceptors (THOMSON, 1964).

The results of the investigations of oxidative phosphorylation of isolated liver mitochondria after *in vivo* irradiation show that the effectiveness of phosphorylation remains unchanged on lethal or sublethal doses for the first hour following exposure, but that it decreases after 12—24 hrs. It is open to question whether the changes in the later phase are a direct effect of irradiation or whether they are an effect of artifacts (THOMSON, 1964). Irradiation has no effect of oxygen consumption or esterification of inorganic phosphate within 4 hrs after irradiation. On *in vivo* irradiation, the first changes in the mitochondria occur about 30 min after exposure. *In vitro* irradiation with doses under 10^5 R does not alter oxidative phosphorylation (RAJEWSKY *et al.*, 1957).

3. Lipid Peroxides and Lysosomal Damage

Lipidperoxidation due to irradiation can be observed in triglycerides, but not in phospholipids (MCCAY and MACFARLANE, 1963). The formation of lipidperoxides is bound up with the effect of irradiation on the membranes of cellular particles, specifically of lysosomes (WILLS and WILKINSON, 1966). The increase of enzyme activity and the release of lysosomal hydrolases as well as the bursting of lysosomes occur after relatively small radiation doses of 100—700 R (DESAI *et al.*, 1964; GLAVIND *et al.*, 1965; GLAVIND and FARBER, 1966; GOUTIER-PIROTTE and GOUTIER, 1962; RENÉ *et al.*, 1971; OKADA and PEACHEY, 1957). *In vitro*, however, much larger radiation doses are necessary to damage the lysosomes (WILLS and WILKINSON, 1966). In this connection, different factors influence the escape of enzymes of *in vitro* irradiated lysosomes of the rat liver (WILLS and WILKINSON, 1966). Anaerobic conditions essentially reduce the enzymatic release, while it is altered by high oxygen pressure. Ascorbic acid and ferric ions increase the enzymatic release. It is, however, suppressed by vitamin E. The release of enzymes reaches a maximum about 20 hrs after irradiation.

Lipid peroxidation precedes the escape of enzymes from *in vitro* irradiated lysosomes (WILLS and WILKINSON, 1966) and appears to be an obligatory step on the way to membrane destruction. Lysosomal membranes are single-layered membranes and therefore seem to be more radiosensitive than the double membranes of the mitochondria. The mitochondria contain linolen and arachidon acid in the phosphadylcholin fraction, which may explain the membrane protection (JACKSON and ENTENMAN, 1961).

4. Amino Acid and Protein Metabolism

The liver is a central organ for the metabolism of amino acids and proteins. It takes up free amino acids from the portal circulation, transforms them into other metabolites or incorporates them into liver or serum proteins. One of the essential changes in the liver after irradiation is a noticeable protein catabolism. It begins primarily with the destruction of radiosensitive cells by lethal or sublethal radiation doses. Proteolytic enzymes are activated and released following the destruction of cellular structures (HAGEN, 1959). It is specifically kathepsins that are affected by this. Without the influence of preceding radiation, an activity increase of kathepsins in the liver cannot be observed. On the other hand, it was proved that extracts from livers of irradiated rats have a greater digestive effect than those from non-irradiated animals (HAGEN, 1958).

a) Effects on Amino Acid Metabolism

The pool of free amino acids in the liver is not excessively altered by irradiation and reaches values that amount to only 150% of those of the controls (STREFFER and MELCHING, 1964). The determination of the amount of excreted radioactive hippuric acid in the urine of animals injected with ^{14}C-glycine before irradiation shows that the pool of free glycine increases as a result of a degradation of tissue proteins (GERBER *et al.*, 1958; LAUENSTEIN *et al.*, 1957). The findings were confirmed by studies of hippuric acid synthesis in the isolated perfused rat liver (GERBER and REMY-DEFRAIGNE, 1963).

On the first day following irradiation, the amount of urea excreted in the urine increases (FRIEDMAN, 1942; KAY *et al.*, 1957; SYROMATNIKOVA, 1956; WHITE *et al.*, 1955). Correspondingly, the urea (WALDSCHMIDT, 1966) and ornithine (STREFFER and MELCHING, 1965) content goes down for several days after whole body-irradiated of mice with 690 R. In contrast, the ammonia content increases. If, however, 15 min before irradiation, ornithine is injected, then the ammonia content goes down and the urea content remains unchanged (WALDSCHMIDT, 1966). This effect of ornithine, however, cannot be produced in isolated perfused livers of irradiated animals (MILLER, 1960). The changes in the ammonia concentration are very difficult to explain. On the one hand, an increased catabolism of urea by intestinal bacteria may be responsible for it; on the other hand, a disturbance of urea synthesis may be the cause. The degradation of urea is not increased after irradiation, not even with doses that produce lethal damage of the gastrointestinal tract.

b) Changes in Detoxication Activity

The liver is the primary place for the conjugation of metabolites and for the detoxication of drugs and other foreign substances. Conjugation reactions, in many cases, use the same reaction partners, specifically sulphate, glucuronate, and acetyl. Many investigators regarded a disturbance in detoxication as a possible cause of radiation disease. BIRZLE and co-workers (1967) administered N-acetyl-P-amino-phenol to rabbits through a stomach tube. A single dose of 1,000 R led to a reduction in the formation and excretion of sulphoconjugates. This disturbance lasted up to 2 weeks. In contrast, fractionated application of 6,000 R with daily doses of 300 R did not disturb the sulphoconjugation mechanism (BIRZLE *et al.*, 1967). Further investigations, however, showed that the ability of the liver to carry out glucuronization, conjugation, and sulphation is disturbed only minimally by irradiation, in the intact animal as well as *in vitro* (GERBER and REMY-DEFRAIGNE, 1963a, b; CHIRIBOGA, 1963; HARTIALA *et al.*, 1959; WERNZE *et al.*, 1962). In investigations of isolated perfused rat liver, 24 hrs after irradiation of the whole body, GERBER and REMY-DEFRAIGNE (1966) could not see a disturbance of bile salt conjugation. SMYTH and WHIPPLE (1924) observed in dogs with an Eck's fistula that the secretion of bile salts after X-ray treatment remained unchanged and was only slightly reduced after the largest radiation dose. When parts of rat liver were irradiated with soft X-rays of 200 R at that moment (11 o'clock a.m. and 7 o'clock p.m.) when the physiological rhythm of formation and storage of bile and glycogen in the liver cells varies, an inversion of this rhythm takes place (FISHEL, 1941).

Thus production of bile increases at the moment at which it should be reduced to a minimum.

The acetylation capacity of the liver is distinctly diminished by irradiation (HAGEN *et al.*, 1956; HANEL and WILIAN-ULRICH, 1959; ROMANTSEV and ZEMLANOVA, 1956). FENDRICH and GROSSMANN (1966), on the other hand, observed that acetylation of P-aminobenzoic acid was not disturbed by sublethal doses in intact animals.

c) Changes in Enzyme Activities

Amino transferases play a central role in the metabolism of amino acids, because they are necessary for the conversion of N, of alpha-amino acids, to NH_3. They thus prepare for the possible biosynthesis of non-essential amino acids. Amino transferases, particularly those of the liver and muscles, react sensitively on tissue destruction and are emitted into the blood stream. The activities of these enzymes are influenced by the nutritional state and rise distinctly on starvation (Streffer and Melching, 1965). In irradiated animals, however, starvation is not the only factor responsible for changes in amino transferase activities. In starved and fed animals, irradiation with doses between 450 and 9,000 R produces an increase in the total activities as well as an increase in the cytoplasmic activities of aspartate-amino transferase, of alanine-amino transferase, of thyrosine-amino transferase, of aspartate-carbamoyl transferase, and of kynurenin-amino transferase (Braun *et al.*, 1963; Brin and McKee, 1956; Streffer and Melching, 1965; Streffer and Langendorff, 1966). In contrast, the activity of L-glutamate dehydrogenase is not changed (Streffer and Melching, 1965). The enzymatic changes induced by radiation are also influenced by the time of investigation and by the species. In rats fed with a 60% glucose diet, the activity of alanine-amino transferase but not that of aspartate-amino transferase increases after irradiation with 900–1,000 R (Brin and McKee, 1956; Ernst, 1962). After exposure of mice to 450–690 R the activities of both enzymes increase (Braun *et al.*, 1963; Brin and McKee, 1956). In rats, a comparable dose produces a decrease in enzymatic activities 4–6 days later (Braun *et al.*, 1965), while larger doses (1,000 R; Brin and McKee, 1956) cause an increase in activity. It is not clear whether these differences are a result of different radiosensitivities of both species or are dependent on the nutritional state of the animals.

The expulsion of enzymes from subcellular particles into the cytoplasm does not seem to be responsible for the change in activities of liver amino transferases. This allegation is deduced from findings with glutamate-dehydrogenase, which is a mitochondrial enzyme. This enzyme is not discharged into the cytoplasm after irradiation. Enzyme activity/g liver weight after irradiation decreases parallel to the protein content (Streffer and Melching, 1965), which permits the conclusion that these changes are a result of a decrease in the number of organelles and not of a reduction in enzyme activity per organelle. It is doubtful that the change in activities of liver amino transferases by irradiation is important for amino acid metabolism *in vivo*, since the changes are not very extensive, they depend on the species, and do not influence ammonia formation (Waldschmidt, 1966).

d) Changes in Protein Synthesis

Many authors observed an increased incorporation of labeled amino acids into proteins of the normal liver following whole-body irradiation (Altmann *et al.*, 1949; Baeyens and Goutier, 1967; Blokhina and Romantsev, 1966; Butler *et al.*, 1957; Hempelmann *et al.*, 1950; Hevesy, 1949a; Hidvegi *et al.*, 1968; Kay and Entenman, 1956; Maass *et al.*, 1967; Richmond *et al.*, 1957; Ricotti and Notario, 1962; Sarkar *et al.*, 1961). There are, however, contradictory observations (Holmes and Mee, 1955; Notario *et al.*, 1965). In the regenerating liver, a decrease in amino acid incorporation into proteins was observed. Thus, *in vitro* for example, the incorporation of ^{14}C-leucine into nucleoproteins was decreased 24 hrs after partial hepatectomy when the animals were irradiated 2–6 hrs after the operation. This effect could not be observed when irradiation was performed as late as 16 hrs after the operation (Sestan, 1965). Similar observations were made after *in vivo* incorporation of ^{14}C-leucine into cytoplasmic proteins or regenerating livers (SCHUBERT *et al.*, 1958). *In vitro* irradiation of liver homogenates with doses up to 5,000 R did not influence the incorporation of ^{14}C-alanine (SCHUBERT *et al.*, 1958). Since *in vitro* investigations often do not produce data on the specific activities of amino acids, it is difficult to decide whether the change in incorporation of labeled precursors is a result of changes in protein synthesis, in the amino acid pool, or in both.

Further investigations of the change in protein synthesis were carried out at the ribosomal level (BAEYENS and GOUTIER, 1967; HIDVEGI *et al.*, 1968; YATVIN and LATHROP, 1966). In normal rat and guinea pig livers, the ratio of polysomes to monomeric ribosomes increases after irradiation with doses of 600–6,000 R after 12–24 hrs (BAEYENS and GOUTIER, 1967; HIDVEGI *et al.*, 1968). After 24 hrs the heavy polysomal fraction increases about 10% at the expense of the lighter particles (BAEYENS and GOUTIER, 1967). After irradiation with 1,000–3,000 R, the capacity of those fractions that are enriched with polysomes to incorporate labeled amino acids into proteins is increased by about 50% as compared to non-irradiated controls (BAEYENS and GOUTIER, 1967; HIDVEGI *et al.*, 1968).

Protein synthesis in both the regenerating and non-regenerating livers is influenced by whole-body irradiation (BAEYENS and GOUTIER, 1967). On alteration of the radiation dose and the time of investigation, YATVIN and LATHROP (1966) got differing results. Their investigations showed that irradiation of the whole body with 1,500–6,000 R 6, 9, or 12 hrs after partial hepatectomy suppressed the occurrence of heavy polysomes in the regenerating liver up to 24 hrs after the operation. After 36 hrs, they again found newly synthesized heavy polysomes. It is unlikely that hunger is responsible for these changes in non-regenerating livers also. It produces an increase of monomeric ribosomes (HIDVEGI *et al.*, 1968).

In the non-regenerating liver, there seem to be definite indications for an increased incorporation of amino acids into liver proteins as a consequence of radiation. The contradictory findings in the regenerating liver (BAEYENS and GOUTIER, 1967; YATVIN and LATHROP, 1966) seem to be, at least partially, due to different experimental conditions.

The synthesis of plasma proteins, specifically of gamma globulins, constitutes one of the most important metabolic functions of the mammalian liver. The effects of irradiation on concentration and metabolism of plasma proteins were often examined because these macromolecules are easily demonstrated. The net biosynthesis of fibrinogen and alpha-1-acid glycoproteins rises in the isolated rat liver perfused with rabbit blood 4–6 days after irradiation (MILLER *et al.*, 1970). This could be shown by the simultaneous measurement of ^{14}C-lysine incorporation into these proteins and by the determination of the amount of rat proteins by special immunological techniques. The increase in the net synthesis of alpha-1-acid glycoproteins is particularly interesting, because it appears to be a useful indicator for radiation damages. In the isolated perfused rat liver the incorporation of tryptophan (REUTER *et al.*, 1967) or tyrosine (SASSEN *et al.*, 1965) is increased after irradiation. Compared to proteins which decrease to a lower level, there is, however, no change in labeling observed. Catabolism of serum proteins in the liver is not particularly influenced by irradiation (GERBER *et al.*, 1959; REUTER *et al.*, 1967). As neither synthesis nor catabolism appears responsible for the decrease of serum proteins in the liver after irradiation, we must assume the existence of extrahepatic catabolism or of loss into extracellular spaces. In fact, labeled serum proteins disappear more quickly from circulation after irradiation (REUTER *et al.*, 1967; SHABER and MILLER, 1963). ^{14}C-labeled proteins are more quickly degraded to CO_2 in irradiated deviscerated animals than in non-irradiated ones (MILLER *et al.*, 1970).

e) Influence of Irradiation on the Inducibility of Enzymes

The effects of irradiation on substrate- or hormone-induced proteins can be studied particularly well in the liver. This applies to some enzyme proteins and to specific messenger RNA. Moreover, one can compare the effect of radiation to that of inhibitors on different levels of protein synthesis and thus delimit the radiation effect. The general idea is that the induction of enzymes by hormones produces a synthesis of messenger RNA, while induction by substrate influences existing messenger RNA (GREENGARD, 1963). Actinomycin suppresses hormone induction (CATER *et al.*, 1956; GREENGARD, 1963; HOMES and MEE, 1955; KRÖGER and GREUER, 1965), but it has little or no effect on substrate induction. In contrast, puromycin is a general inhibitor of protein synthesis: It inhibits induction by hormones, as well as that by substrates. The induction of L-tryptophan-pyrrolase by tryptophan, is inhibited following irradiation of the whole body in the intact and in the regenerating liver just as it is by actinomycin D (KRÖGER and GREUER, 1965). In contrast to actinomycin or puromycin (KRÖGER and GREUER, 1965; GREENGARD, 1966), irradiation has no effect on stimulation of this enzyme by cortisone or hydrocortisone. Whole-body irradiation blocks the induction of tryptophan-pyrrolase by the substrate in normal as well as in adrenalectomized animals, but it has no influence on hormone induction (HOLMES and MEE, 1955; KRÖGER and GREUER, 1965; THOMSON and MIKUTA, 1954; THOMSON and KLIPFEL, 1957). The opposite effect, however, has also been observed (MISHKIN and SHORE, 1968). Six hours after irradiation, the induction of tryptophan-pyrrolase by substrate is slightly increased (CATER *et al.*, 1956; THOMSON and MIKUTA, 1954) and is then markedly decreased (GREENGARD, 1966; KRÖGER and GREUER, 1965). The lowest values are obtained after 15 days following irradiation with 500 R (GREENGARD, 1966). YATVIN *et al.* (1972) reported that hormone induction of tyrosine-transaminase and tryptophan-pyrrolase by gamma-irradiation (6,000 R Co 60), is possible only in the presence of actinomycin D. These observations make it improbable that the inhibition of induction due to radiation has a direct effect on the messenger RNA. Comparable observations were made with other enzymes, e.g., tyrosine-amino-transferase or L-serine-dehydratase (PITOT *et al.*, 1965).

In starving rats, puromycin and X-rays inhibit the induction of tyrosine-amino transferase, while actinomycin D has no effect (GREENGARD, 1966). Like actinomycin D, ionizing rays inhibit induction of L-serine-hydrolase by casein-hydrolysate in dogs (PITOT and PERAINO, 1964; PITOT *et al.*, 1965, 1968). These findings demonstrate that the mechanisms of actinomycin and irradiation are not the same in enzyme induction by substrates or hormones. Therefore, the way in which irradiation inhibits substrate induction and how it influences the places of synthesis of existing templates remains unclear. It is also unclear why irradiation does not inhibit induction by hormones, when this process is inhibited by actinomycin.

V. Effects on Liver Function by a Combination of Radiation and Drugs

Because of the generally unspecific alterations in liver tissue, it is extremely difficult to decide to what degree the effects of ionizing rays and of other noxae mutually influence each other, i.e., whether one effect or the other is stronger or weaker. The fact that there are not many publications on this problem and that the results are contradictory underline this statement.

In this context, investigations of alterations in radiosensitivity and in the influence of chemical liver carcinogens are particularly important.

1. Changes of Liver Radiosensitivity

Radiosensitizing substances are important for therapy. They must get into the tissue in such high concentrations that at the target spot, for example in tumor tissue, sensitization against ionizing rays develops (STREFFER and SCHWEIGER, 1972). In the partially hepatectomized liver, it could be shown that halogenized pyrimidines, such as the thymidine analogues 5-bromouracil and 5-iodouracil, have an effect only if the rate of proliferation is increased. This produces a greater rate of incorporation of the sensitizer into DNA and thus an increase of the sensitizing effect. At the same time, 5-fluorouracil has a synchronizing effect on the proliferating cells (LOMAKINA *et al.*, 1967; STREFFER and SCHWEIGER, 1972). Inhibitors of protein synthesis such as actinomycin D and puromycin inhibit enzyme induction by cortisol when applied—like ionizing radiation—in doses which have no effect when given alone (ELKIND *et al.*, 1970; STREFFER and SCHWEIGER, 1972; STREFFER and SCHAFFERUS, 1971).

Radioresistance and animal tryptophan metabolism are closely correlated. Thus whole-body irradiation of mice with 600—800 R caused a decrease in activity of the enzymes kynureninase and 5-hydroxytryptophan-decarboxylase (STREFFER, 1968; STREFFER, 1967, 1971).

In this situation, the animals are in such a bad metabolic state that their natural radioresistancy is abolished. This effect can be intensified by previous hypoxy (STREFFER *et al.*, 1970) and by vitamin B_6-deficiency (VENINGA and MORSE, 1965; WISS and WEBER, 1964).

In contrast, an additional intake of ethyl-lineolate combined with liquid nutrition enhances the radioresistance of the liver tissue 24 hrs after irradiation with 1,000 rads ^{60}Co. Mitochondrial swelling does not occur and the mitochondrial oxidative capacity of succinate is not altered (SKIDMORE, 1973). The radio-protecting effect of cysteamine in mouse liver is assumed to be due to a passing arrest of DNA synthesis, which later allows an accelerated repair (MITZNEGG, 1973).

2. Effect of Radiation on Experimental Chemical Carcinogenesis of the Liver and Non-Carcinogenic Alteration

According to the investigations of LACASSAGNE and coworkers (LACASSAGNE *et al.*, 1960; LACASSAGNE and HURST, 1962), the carcinogenic effect of p-dimethylaminoazobenzene(DAB) on the rat liver is delayed with radiation doses ranging from 500—3,000 R even if the carcinogen is still continuously applied one month after irradiation. This same effect occurs if a part of the liver is shielded from the radiation. As a consequence of the toxic effect of DAB in the initial phase, the weight compensation of the radiation-atrophic liver section by the shielded one is delayed. Hypertrophy of the non-irradiated liver portion occurs when damage from DAB becomes irreversible (Fig. 31). Detoxication of DAB solutions *in vitro* is stimulated by the homogenate of irradiated livers treated with DAB, because the carcinogen-induced decrease of flavine-coenzyme content in the liver is checked by irradiation (Emanoil-Revicovitch *et al.*, 1962). In contrast, in combined X-ray and N,N′-2,7-fluorenylen-bis-acetamide application, an accelerated induction of hepatomas was observed by Nagayo *et al.* (1970). Williams and coworkers (1973) demonstrated that the injection of $5-20 \times 10^6$ rat liver epithelia incubated *in vitro* with aflatoxin B_1, dimethylnitrosamine, N-nitroso-methyl-urea, N-hydroxy-N-2-fluorenylacet-amid, and 7,12-dimethylbenz-(a)-anthracene respectively into whole-body irradiated rats leads to a growth of carcinomas within 2—8 months.

Lacassagne *et al.* (1944) drew a connection between the mode of action of physical (radiation) and chemical (hydrocarbons) carcinogens: "In either case, the cancerisation occurs abruptly, after a latency period that is always relatively long, at the moment when the cell has undergone an evolution which leads to what could be termed the threshold of cancerous mutation. By analogy with what happens with radiations, the massive absorption of a great number of toxic molecules causes the cell to die, either immediately or within a short while. But in the case of the action of a weak dose the threshold of mutation could be reached by a summation of punctual lesions of the substratum which controls cell division; whether these lesions are due to radiation or to the fixation of toxic molecules,

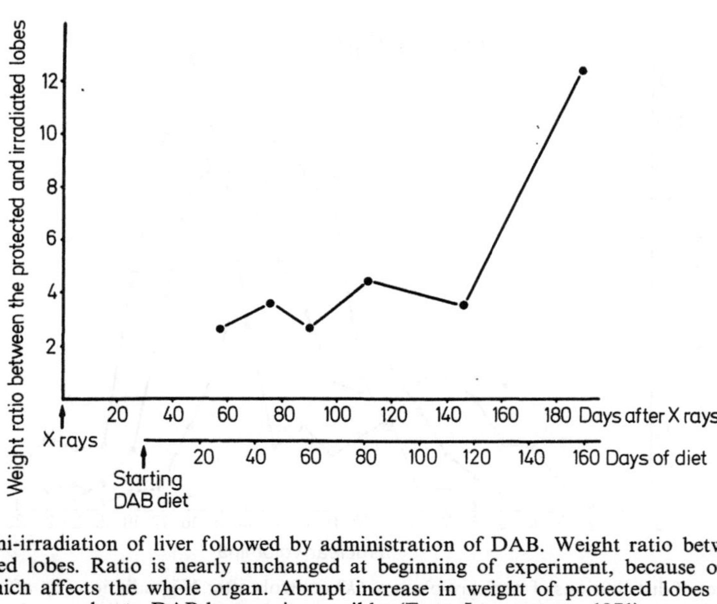

Fig. 31. Hemi-irradiation of liver followed by administration of DAB. Weight ratio between shielded and irradiated lobes. Ratio is nearly unchanged at beginning of experiment, because of toxic effect of DAB, which affects the whole organ. Abrupt increase in weight of protected lobes when lesions due to DAB become irreversible. (From Lacassagne, 1971)

there is always the possibility that the irreversible damage will finally advene which is responsible for the cancerisation."

A change in the reaction of the liver to chemical noxae can also be seen after application of the amino sugar D-galactosamine, which is not carcinogenic when applied once. In the rat liver, galactosamine can induce disseminated parenchymal damage with a mesenchymal reaction, which can be seen in a comparable form in human viral hepatitis (KEPPLER *et al.*, 1968; REUTTER, *et al.*, 1968). Reparative regeneration produces a complete restitution within 48—72 hrs (LESCH *et al.*, 1970). If the animals are irradiated with a single dose of 800 R before the single galactosamine application, and if they are killed up to 3 months after galactosamine application, a histological picture closely related to that of chronic hepatitis develops (LESCH *et al.*, 1972; OEHLERT, 1973). Bile duct proliferation occurs, and atypical mitoses and single-cell necroses can be demonstrated in the parenchyma. Nuclear measurements have shown that the volumina are clearly enlarged after this combined damage, which is partly attributed to massive nuclear edema (SCHNEIKERT, 1973) (Fig. 32). A satisfactory explanation of these phenomena cannot be given yet; one reason may be the lability of the lysosomal membrane which is effective over a long period of time. Similar effects can be seen after combined galactosamine and vitamin A application (LESCH *et al.*, 1972). On the one hand, these investigations show that damage induced by a small radiation dose which cannot be traced by morphologic criteria alone, can be unmasked by a second noxa. On the other hand, it can be assumed that every irradiation of the liver, even if in small doses which do not produce any traceable changes, causes a conditioning of the liver tissue which is able to change decisively the reaction pattern of the pre-irradiated liver following additional damages (OEHLERT, 1973).

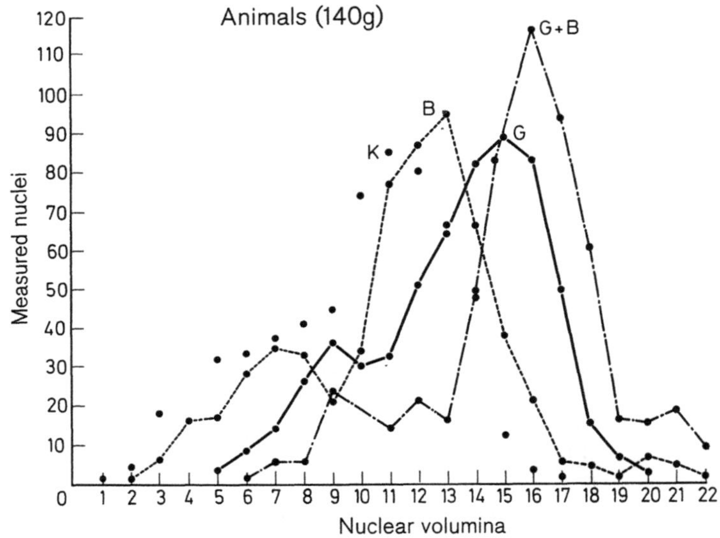

Fig. 32. Curves of distributions of nuclear volumes. (*K*) controls after X-irradiation (*B*), after application of D-galactosamine (*G*); after X-irradiation and glactosamine application (*G*+*B*)

Abbreviations

ATP	Adenosinetriphosphate
CoA	Coenzyme A
DAB	para-dimethylaminoazobenzene
dCR	Deoxy-cytidine
DNA	Deoxyribonucleic Acid
DNase	Deoxyribonuclease
dTR	Thymidine
NAD	Nicotineamide-adenine-dinucleotide
PEP	Phosphoenolpyruvate
RNA	Ribonucleic Acid

References

ADACHI, R.: Experimentelle Untersuchungen über Thorotrast als mikroradioaktive Substanz. Nippon Acta Radiol. **17**, 289 (1940).

AGOSTINI, C., SESSA, A., FENAROLI, A., CICCARONE, P.: Production of "fatty liver" by X-irradiation. Radiat. Res. **23**, 350 (1964).

ALBERT, M.D., BUCHER, N.L.R.: Latent injury and repair in rat liver induced to regenerate at intervals after X-irradiation. Cancer Res. **20**, 1514 (1960).

ALBERTI, W., POLITZER, G.: Über den Einfluß der Röntgenstrahlen auf die Zellteilung. Arch. Entwickl.-Mech. mikr. Anat. **100**, 83 (1923).

ALTENBRUNN, H.J., KOBERT, E.: Der Einfluß von Röntgenstrahlen auf die oxydative Phosphorylierung von isolierten Mitochondrien. Acta biol. med. germ. **7**, 251 (1961).

ALTMAN, K.I., CASARETT, G.W., NOONAN, T.R., SALOMON, K.: Radiation effects on tissues, studies with C^{14}-labeled glycine. Fed. Proc. **8**, 349 (1949).

ARGAWAL, S.K., MEHROTRA, R.M.L.: Changes in liver following total body irradiation in albino rats. Indian J. med. Res. **52**, 1073 (1964).

ARIEL, I.M.: The effect of single massive doses of roentgen radiation upon the liver. An experimental study. Radiology **57**, 561 (1951).

ARNOLD, A., BAILEY, P., LAUGHLIN, J.S.: Effects of betatron radiations on the brain of primates. Neurology (Minneap.) **4**, 165 (1954).

AUSTONI, B.: Epithelioma mammario maschile in sede die mastite cronica da thorotrast. Chirurgia **5**, 145 (1950).

BACQ, Z.M., ALEXANDER, P.: Fundamentals of Radiobiology. Oxford-London-New York-Toronto-Paris: Pergamon 1966.

BAEYENS, W., GOUTIER, R.: Effect of total body X-irradiation on the properties of polyribosomes in normal and regenerating rat liver. Arch. intern. Physiol. Biochim. **75**, 875 (1967).

BANNASCH, P., REISS, W.: Histogenese und Cytogenese cholangio-cellulärer Tumoren bei Nitrosomorpholin-vergifteten Ratten. Zugleich ein Beitrag zur Morphogenese der Cystenleber. Z. Krebsforsch. **76**, 193 (1971).

BARBASON, H.: Influence of X-irradiation of the different stages of the cell cycle in regenerating rat liver. Virschows Arch. Abt. B **16**, 363 (1974).

BARDEEN, C.R.: Abnormal development of toad ova fertilized by spermatozoa exposed to the roentgen rays. J. exp. Zool. **4**, 1 (1907).

BARONCHELLI, A.: Sull' azione dei raggi X suul fegato. Ricerche istochimiche nell ratto. Path. Clin. Med. **33**, 327 (1957).

BARRON, E.S.G.: in: Biological Effects of External and Internal X and Gamma Radiation (R.E. ZIRKLE, ed.). New York: McGraw-Hill 1954.

BARTSCH, G.G., GERBER, G.B.: Incorporation of the acetate-1-^{14}C into lipids by the perfused liver of normal, X-irradiated, or partially hepatectomized rats. J. Lipid Res. **7**, 204 (1966).

BASERGA, R.: Biochemistry of the cell cycle. A review. Cell Tiss. Kinet. **1**, 107 (1968).

BASERGA, R., YOKOO, H., HENEGAR, G.C.: Thorotrast-induced cancer in man. Cancer (Philad.) **13**, 1021 (1960).

BATZENSCHLAGER, A., DORNER, M., WEILL-BOUSSON, M.: La pathologie tumorale du thorotrast chez l'homme. Oncologia **16**, 28 (1963).

BATZENSCHLAGER, A., WILHELM, E.: Cancer primitif de la travée hépatique sur cirrhose thorotrastique. Ann. Anat. path. **2**, 39 (1957).
BAUER, K.H.: Referat über Berufsschäden und Krebs. Dtsch. Ges. Path. **30**, 239 (1937).
BAUER, K.H.: Thorotrast und Krebsgefahr. Chirurg **15**, 204 (1943).
BAUER, K.H.: Über Thorotrastschäden und Thorotrastsarkomgefahr. Chirurg **19**, 387 (1947).
BAUER, K.H.: Das Krebsproblem. Berlin-Göttingen-Heidelberg: Springer 1949.
BEKKUM, D.W. VAN: Oxidative phosphorylation in some radiosensitive tissues after irradiation. Ciba Found. Symp. Ionizing Radiations Cell Metab., p. 77–91 (1956).
BELTZ, R.E.: Comparison of the effect of X-irradiation on the elevation of thymidine kinase and thymidilate synthetase during liver regeneration. Biochem. biophys. Res. Commun. **9**, 78 (1962).
BELTZ, R.E., APPLEGATE, R.L.: X-ray inhibition of enzyme changes associated with DNA synthesis of liver regeneration. Biochem. biophys. Res. Commun. **1**, 298 (1959).
BELTZ, R.E., VAN LANCKER, J.L., POTTER, V.R.: Nucleic acid metabolism in regenerating liver. IV. The effect of X-radiation of the whole body on nucleic acid synthesis in vivo. Cancer Res. **17**, 688 (1957).
BENJAMIN, T.L., YOST, H.T.: The mechanism of uncoupling of oxidative phosphorylation in rat spleen and liver mitochondria after whole-body irradiation. Radiat. Res. **12**, 613 (1960).
BENNETT, E.L., KELLY, L., KREUCKEL, B.: Effects of X-irradiation upon the incorporation of adenine-4, 6-C^{14} in mice. Fed. Proc. **13**, 181 (1954).
BERDJIS, C.C.: The cell. In: Pathology of Irradition, ed. C.C. BERDJIS. Baltimore: Williams and Wilkins 1971.
BERG, T.L., GOUTIER, R.: La synthèse de l'acide ribonucléique dans la foie de rat en régeneration et sa sensibilitée à l'irradiation corporelle totale. Arch. int. Biochim. **74**, 909 (1966).
BERG, T.L., GOUTIER, R.: X-radiation induced disturbances of RNA metabolism in regenerating rat liver. Arch. int. Physiol. Biochim. **75**, 49 (1967).
BERGONIE, J., TRIBONDEAU, L.: Action des rayons-X sur les testicules du rat blanc. C.R. Soc. Biol. (Paris) **57**, 400 (1904).
BERNDT, J., GAUMER, R.: Zur Störung des Kohlenhydratstoffwechsels nach Bestrahlung. Einfluß einer Ganzkörperbestrahlung auf den Gehalt an Intermediärproduktion der Glycolyse in der Mäuseleber. In. J. Radiat. Biol. **11**, 593 (1966).
BERNDT, J., GAUMER, R.: Änderung des Acetyl-Coenzym A-Gehaltes in der Mäuseleber nach Strahleneinwirkung in vivo. Naturwissenschaften **53**, 307 (1966a).
BERNDT, J., GAUMER, R.: Die Aktivität der Phosphofruktokinase und der Fruktose-1-6-diphosphatase im Lebergewebe der Maus nach Ganzkörperbestrahlung. Int. J. Radiat. Bil. **12**, 453 (1966b).
BERNDT, J., ULBRICH, O.: Untersuchungen über den biologischen Strahlenschutz. 78. Mitteilung. Die Aktivität der Phosphoenolpyruvat-Karboxykinase und der Pyruvatkinase in der Mäuseleber nach einer Ganzkörperbestrahlung. Ein Beitrag zur Störung des Kohlehydratstoffwechsels nach Bestrahlung. Strahlentherapie **133**, 288 (1967).
BERNDT, T.J.: The content of alpha-glycerophosphate in mouse liver after whole-body X-irradiation. Int. J. Radiat. Biol. **13**, 187 (1967).
BERNHARD, H.J., GEYER, R.W.: Effects of X-irradiation in growing bone. Prelim. report. Radiology **78**, 207 (1962).
BERTALANFFY, F.D., LAU, C.: Cell renewal. Int. Rev. Cytol. **13**, 359 (1962).
BIBIKOVA, A.F.: Histopathological changes in the central nervous system of dogs at remote periods after repeated X-ray irradiation. Bjul. eksp. Biol. Med. **51**, 106 (1961).
BIRKNER, R., FREY, J., ÜBERSCHÄR, K.H.: Frühveränderungen am Knochen erwachsener Meerschweinchen nach Röntgenbestrahlung. Strahlentherapie **100**, 574 (1956).
BIRZLE, H.: Untersuchungen über die Strahlenempfindlichkeit der Leber. Habil.-Schrift, Freiburg (1965).
BIRZLE, H., BECK, K., DIETERICH, E.: Die Wirkung gezielter Röntgentiefenstrahlung der Leber auf die Bildung gepaarter Schwefelsäure nach Belastung mit N-acetyl-p-amino-phenyl beim Kaninchen. Strahlentherapie **133**, 602 (1967).
BIRZLE, H., FLIEGEL, C.: Reaktion der Leber auf gezielte Bestrahlung. Strahlentherapie **128**, 273 (1965).
BLOKHINA, V.D., ROMANTSEV, E.F.: Effect of ionizing radiation on protein synthesis in nuclei of rat tissue cells. Dokl. Akad. Nauk SSSR **168**, 454 (1966).
BLOOM, W.: Histopathology of Irradiation from External and Internal Sources. New York-Toronto-London: McGraw-Hill 1948.
BLÜHBAUM, T., FRICK, K., KALKBRENNER, H.: Eine neue Anwendungsart der Kolloide in der Röntgendiagnostik. Fortschr. Röntgenstr. **37**, 18 (1928).
BOLLIGER, A., INGLIS, K.: Experimental liver disease produced by X-ray irradiation of exposed organ. J. Path. Bact. **36**, 19 (1933).
BOLLUM, F.J., ANDEREGG, J.W., MCELYA, A.B., POTTER, V.R.: Nucleic acid metabolism in regenerating rat liver. VII. Effect of X-radiation on enzymes of DNA synthesis. Cancer Res. **20**, 138 (1960).
BORREBAEK, B., ABRAHAM, S., CHAIKOFF, I.L.: Glucokinase activities and glycogen content of livers of normal and hypophysectomised, X-irradiated rats subjected to different nutritional treatments. Biochim. biophys. Acta (Amst.) **90**, 451 (1964).

BRAS, G., JELLIFFE, D.B., STUART, K.L.: Veno-occlusive disease of liver with non-portal type of cirrhosis, occurring in Jamaica. Arch. Path. **57**, 285 (1954).

BRAS, G., MCLEAN, E.: Toxic factors in veno-occlusive disease. Ann. N.Y. Acad. Sci. **3**, 392 (1963).

BRAUN, H.: Elektronenoptische Untersuchungen an Zellen des Dünndarmepithels nach Röntgenbestrahlung. Exp. Cell Res. **20**, 267 (1960).

BRAUN, H.: Morphologische Frühveränderungen im Zytoplasma der Leberzellen nach Röntgenbestrahlung. Strahlentherapie **117**, 134 (1962).

BRAUN, H.: In: Strahlenpathologie der Zelle (E. SCHERER and H.S. STENDER, eds.). Stuttgart: Thieme 1963.

BRAUN, H., HORNUNG, G., HEISE, E.R.: Die Wirkung der Röntgen-Ganzkörperbestrahlung auf die Fermentaktivität der Leucin-amino-Peptidase, der Glutamat-Oxalat- und Glutamat-Pyruvat-Transaminase in verschiedenen Organen bei Mäusen. Strahlentherapie **122**, 211 (1963).

BRAUN, H., HORNUNG, G., NEUMEYER, M.: Aktivitätsänderungen der Glutamat-Oxalazetat-Transaminase und Glutamat-Pyruvat-Transminase in Herz, Leber, Niere und im Serum von ganzkörperbestrahlten Ratten. Strahlentherapie **126**, 454 (1965).

BREIT, A.: Strahlenbiologie des Rückenmarkes unter besonderer Berücksichtigung der Spätreaktionen. Ärztl. Forsch. **16**, 268 (1962).

BRENDLEIN, F., OEHLERT, W.: The chronic radiation hepatitis in rat. A morphological and autoradiographic study. Radiat. enfironm. Biophys., in press (1974).

BRESCIANI, F., BLASI, F., PUCA, G.A.: Stimulation of glycogenolysis by X-irradiation in rat liver slices in vitro: An ion-mediated effect. Radiat. Res. **26**, 451 (1965).

BRICK, I.B.: Effects of million volt irradiation on the gastrointestinal tract. Arch. intern. Med. **96**, 26 (1955).

BRIN, M., MCKEE, R.W.: Effects of X-irradiation, cortisone and adrenalectomy on transaminase activity in the rat. Arch. Biochem. Biophys. **61**, 384 (1956).

BRODY, H., CULLEN, M.: Carcinoma of the breast 18 years after mammography with thorotrast. Surgery **42**, 600 (1957).

BROOKS, B., HILLSTROM, H.T.: The effect of roentgen rays on bone growth and bone regeneration. Amer. J. Surg. **20**, 599 (1933).

BUCHER, N.L.R.: Regeneration of mammalian liver. Int. Rev. Cytol. **15**, 245 (1963).

BUCHER, N.L.R., MALT, R.A.: Regeneration of Liver and Kidney. Boston: Little, Brown & Co. 1971.

BUSSE, J., BRONCK, G., STRAUCH, M., OEHLERT, W.: Die Leberregeneration nach Teilhepatektomie bei vorbestrahlten Ratten. Comm. Czech. Soc. histochem.-cytochem. **3**, 11 (1969).

BUTLER, J.A.V., COHN, P., CRATHORN, A.R.: In: Advances in Radiobiology. Edinburgh-London: Oliver and Boyd 1957.

CARLSON, J.G.: Immediate effects of 250 r of X-rays on the different stages of mitosis in neuroblasts of grasshopper: Chortophago viridifasciata. J. Morph. **66**, 11 (1940).

CAROLI, J., ETÉVÉ, J., PLATTEBORSE, R.: Thorotrast et hemangioréticulome malin du foie. Rev. méd. chir. Mal. Foie **31**, 53 (1956).

CASE, J.T., WARTHIN, A.S.: The occurrence of hepatic lesions in patients treated by intensive deep roentgen irradiation. Amer. J. Roentgenol. **12**, 27 (1924).

CATER, D.B., HOLMES, B.E., MEE, L.K.: Cell division and nucleic acid synthesis in the regenerating liver of the rat. Acta radiol. (Stockh.) **46**, 655 (1956).

CHANG, L.O., LOONEY, W.B.: Incorporation of tritiated thymidine into mitochondrial and nuclear DNA in normal and regenerating rat liver before and after irradiation. Int. J. Radiat. Biol. **12**, 187 (1967).

CHEVALLIER, A., BURG, C.: Sur la production de stéatose hépatique par la rayonnement X (Production of fatty liver by X-irradiation) Ann. Nutr. (Paris) **7**, 81 (1953).

CHIRIBOGA, J.: Glucuronide excretion and the detoxication mechanism in whole-body irradiated rats. Nature (Lond.) **198**, 803 (1963).

CHRISTOV, K., RIEDE, U.N., HELIN, H., ROHR, H.P.: Ultrastructural morphometric studies on the effect of irradiation on hepatic parenchymal cells in rats. Pathologia Europea. Int. J. exp. cell. Path. **9**, 11 (1974).

CLARK, J.B.: Effect of irradiation in vitro on mitochondrial metabolism. Oxidation of citric acid cycle substrates. Europ. J. Biochem. **2**, 19 (1967).

CLEAVER, J.E.: Thymidine Metabolism and Cell Kinetics. Amsterdam: North-Holland Publishing Comp. 1967.

COGGLE, J.E.: Effect of cell cycle on recovery from radiation damage in the mouse liver. Nature (Lond.) **217**, 180 (1968).

CONCANNON, J.P., EDELMAN, A., FROCK, J.C., JR., KUNKEL, G.: Localized "radiation hepatitis" as demonstrated by scintillation scanning. Radiology **89**, 136 (1967).

CONIGLIO, J.G., CATE, D.L., BENSON, B., HUDSON, G.W.: Oxidation to C^{14} and conversion to fatty acids of C^{14}-glucose in livers of normal, fasted and X-irradiated rats. Amer. J. Physiol. **197**, 674 (1959).

CONIGLIO, J.G., DARBY, W.J., WILKERSON, M.D., STEWART, W., STOCKELL, A., HUDSON, G.W.: Effect of X-irradiation on fat balance and on lipid and vitamin A content of the liver. Amer. J. Physiol. **172**, 86 (1953).

CONIGLIO, J.G., HUDSON, G.W., MCCARMICK, D.B.: Liver glycogen and fatty acid synthesis in normal and irradiated rats. Fed. Proc. **14**, 30 (1955).

CONIGLIO, J.G., KIRSCHMAN, I.C., HUDSON, G.W.: Hepatic glycogen, lipogenesis and glucose-6-phosphatase in X-irradiated and control rats. Amer. J. Physiol. **191**, 350 (1957).

CONIGLIO, J.G., MCCORMICK, D.B., HUDSON, G.W.: Biosynthesis of fatty acids in liver and intestine of intact normal, fasted and X-irradiated rats. Amer. J. Physiol. **185**, 577 (1956).

Council of Pharmacy and Chemistry: Thorotrast. J. Amer. med. Ass. **99**, 2183 (1932).

CROMPTON, M.R., LAYTON, D.D.: Delayed radionecrosis of the brain following therapeutic X-radiations of the pituitary. Brain **84**, 85 (1961).

CURTIS, H.J.: Recovery of mammalian chromosomes from radiation injury. In: Recovery and repair mechanisms in radiobiology. Brookhaven symp. Biol. **20**, 223 (1968).

CURTIS, H.J., CROWLEY, C.: Chromosome aberrations in liver cells in relation to the somatic mutation theory of aging. Radiat. Res. **19**, 337 (1963).

CURTIS, H.J., TILLEY, J., CROWLEY, C.: Elimination of chromosome aberrations in liver cells by cell division. Radiat. Res. **22**, 730 (1964).

DACQUISTO, M.P., HARTGERING, J.B.: Status of treatment of the acute radiation syndrome. Med. Ann. D.C. **28**, 200 (1959).

DAHLGREN, S.: Thorotrast tumours. Acta path. microbiol. scand. **53**, 147 (1961).

DELCLOS, L., BRAUN, E.J., HERRERA, J.R., JR., SAUPIERE, V.A., ROOSENBEECK, E. VAN: Whole abdominal irradiation by Cobalt-60 mooning strip technique. Radiology **81**, 632 (1963).

DEL FAVERO, A., PASOTTI, C., NICROSINI, F.: Variazione della componente lipidica epatica nel topino dopo panirradiazione con dose letale. Minerva Radiol. Fisiol., Radiobiol. **10**, 380 (1965).

DESAI, I.D., SAWANT, P.L., TAPPEL, A.L.: Peroxidative and radiation damage to isolated lysosomes. Biochim. biophys. Acta (Amst.) **86**, 277 (1964).

DIEM, K., LEUTNER, C. eds.: Wissenschaftliche Tabellen, Basel: J.R. Geigy AG, Pharma 1968.

DIENSTBIER, Z.: New metabolic and hematologic aspects in pathophysiology of the post-irradiation changes. Acta Univ. Carol. Med. **11**, 3 (1965).

DIHLMANN, W.: Die Strahlenspätschäden im Zentralnervensystem und ihre Beziehungen zur Strahlenschädigung in anderen Organen. Med. Welt (Berl.) 1375 (1961).

DOMAGK, G.: Die Röntgenstrahlenwirkung auf das Gewebe, im besonderen betrachtet an den Nieren. Morphologische und funktionelle Veränderungen. Beitr. path. Anat. **77**, 525 (1927).

DUNLAP, C.E.: Effects of radiation. In: Pathology. St. Louis: C.V. Mosby 1961.

DUPLAN, J.F.: Effect de l'irradiation X sur la fonction hémopoiétique du foie foetal. Nouv. Rev. franç. Hémat. **3**, 121 (1963).

DUPLAN, J.F., IZADIAN, H.: Conséquences de l'irradiation localisée du foie foetal de la Souris. C.R. Soc. Biol. (Paris) **153**, 1111 (1959).

EBERHAGEN, D., HARTUNG, R., ZÖLLNER, N.: Die Lipidveränderungen in verschiedenen Rattenorganen nach Ganzkörperbestrahlung mit letalen Röntgendosen. II. Das Verhalten der Leberphosphatide und ihrere Fettsäuren. Strahlentherapie **126**, 601 (1965).

EBERHAGEN, D., HARTUNG, R., ZÖLLNER, N.: Die Lipidveränderungen in verschiedenen Rattenorganen nach Ganzkörperbestrahlung mit letalen Röntgendosen. IV. Das Verhalten der einzelnen Leberphosphatide. Strahlentherapie **132**, 441 (1967).

EDDINGTON, D.N.: The estimation of thorium and uranium at the submicrogram level in bone by neutron activation. Int. J. appl. Radiat. **18**, 11 (1967).

ELKIND, M.M., KANO, E., SAKAMOTO, K.: In: Radiation Protection and Sensitization. London: Taylor and Francis 1970.

ELLINGER, F.: Response of liver to irradiation. Radiology **44**, 241 (1945).

ELLINGER, F.: Medical Radiation Biology. Springfield USA: Thomas 1957.

EMANOIL-REVICOVITCH, R., HERISSON-CAVET, C., ROSENBERG, A.J.: Effect de l'irradiation sur la détoxication du p-diméthyl-aminoazobenzene (DAB) sur le foie du rat au cours de la cancérisation. Bull. Soc. Clin. Biol. **44**, 867 (1962).

ERNST, H.: Strahlenbedingte Frühveränderungen an Zellkern-Proteinen. II. Vergleichende Untersuchungen über die Konzentration nuclearer Globuline und Histone in lymphatischen und parenchymatischen Geweben. Z. Naturforsch. **17**b, 300 (1962).

ERNST, H.: Röntgenbestrahlung isolierter Leberzellkerne. Naturwissenschaften **50**, 227 (1963a).

ERNST, H.: Zur Frage der Dosisabhängigkeit der strahleninduzierten Nukleoprotein-Verminderung im Zellkern von Leber, Milz und Thymus. Naturwissenschaften **50**, 333 (1963b).

EVANS, N.T.S., NAYLOR, P.F.D.: The effect of oxygen breathing and radiotherapy upon the tissue oxygen tension of some human tumours. Brit. J. Radiol. **36**, 418 (1963).

FABRIKANT, J.I.: Studies on Cell Proliferation in the Regenerating Liver and the Effect of Prior Continous Irradiation. Ph. D. Thesis, University of London (1964).

FABRIKANT, J.I.: Cell proliferation in the regenerating liver and the effect of prior continous irradiation. Radiat. Res. **32**, 804 (1967a).
FABRIKANT, J.I.: Cell proliferation in the regenerating liver of continously irradiated mice. Brit. J. Radiol. **40**, 487 (1967b).
FABRIKANT, J.I.: The effect of prior continous irradiation on the G_2, M, and S phases of proliferating parenchymal cells in the regenerating liver. Radiat. Res. **31**, 304 (1967c).
FABRIKANT, J.I.: Accumulation of chromosome damage under continously low dose rate exposure. Radiology **88**, 767 (1967d).
FABRIKANT, J.I.: Rate of cell proliferation in the regenerating liver. Brit. J. Radiol. **41**, 71 (1968a).
FABRIKANT, J.I.: The kinetics of cellular proliferation in regenerating liver. J. Cell Biol. **36**, 551 (1968b).
FABRIKANT, J.I.: Radiation effects on a conditional cell renewal system under continous low dose-rate exposure. Amer. J. Roentgenol. **102**, 811 (1968c).
FABRIKANT, J.I.: The effect of continuous irradiation. In: Pathology of Irradiation. Baltimore: The Williams and Wilkins Comp. 1971.
FASSKE, E., THEMANN, H.: Der Zellkern. In: Strahlenpathologie der Zelle. Stuttgart: Thieme 1963.
FAUSTO, N., VAN LANCKER, J.L.: Molecular mechanisms of liver regeneration. IV. Thymidylic kinase and deoxyribonucleic acid polymerase activities in normal and regenerating liver. J. biol. Chem. **240**, 1247 (1965).
FEDERLIN, K., SCIOR, H.: Spätschäden und Tumorentwicklung nach Thorotrastinjection. Frankfurt. Z. Path. **68**, 225 (1957).
FELLAS, V.M., MESCHAN, I., DAY, P.L., DOUGLAS, C.D.: Effect of total body Xirradiation on desoxyribonuclease activity of rat spleen. Proc. Soc. exp. Biol. (N.Y.) **87**, 231 (1954).
FELLOWS, K.E., VAUTER, G.F., TEFFT, M.: Hepatic effects following abdominal irradiation in children: Detection by Au^{198} scan and confirmation by histologic examination. Amer. J. Roentgenol. **103**, 422 (1968).
FENDRICH, Z., GROSSMANN, V.: Vylucovani Podane p-Aminobenzoove Kyseliny Moci U. Ozarenych Krys. Čs. Fysiol. **15**, 414 (1966).
FISHEL, E.: Recherches expérimentales sur l'influence des rayons X sur la production de la cellule hépatique. Schweiz. med. Wschr. **71**, 764 (1941).
FITCH, M.F., CHAIKOFF, I.L., HILL, R.: Effects of dietary hexoses on changes induced in hepatic enzyme activities of the rat by a lethal dose of X-rays. Arch. Biochem. Biophys. **94**, 387 (1961).
FLACHI, Q., PIEROTTI, P.: Frattu a bilaterale des collo del femore consequente a telecobaltoterapia della pelvi. Radiol. med. (Torino) **49**, 847 (1963).
FLIEDNER, TH.M., STODTMEISTER, R.: Experimentelle und klinische Strahlenhämatologie. München: J.F. Lehmann 1962.
FOULDS, L.: The production of transplantable carcinoma and sarcoma in guinea pigs by injection of thorotrast. Amer. J. Cancer **35**, 363 (1939).
FREEZE, P., KEMNITZ, P.: Beitrag zur Entstehung bösartiger Geschwülste nach Thorotrast. Zbl. allg. Path. path. Anat. **105**, 161 (1964).
FRIEDMAN, M.: Calculated risks of radiation injury of normal tissue in the treatment of cancer of the testis. Proc. IInd Nat. Cancer Conf., New York, Amer. Cancer Soc. **1**, 390 (1954).
FRIEDMAN, N.B.: Effects of radiation on the gastrointestinal tract, including the salivary glands, the liver and the pancreas. Arch. Path. **34**, 749 (1942).
FRITZ, J.: Erscheinungsbild der Radionekrose im Scham- und Sitzbein. Strahlentherapie **109**, 510 (1959).
FRITZ-NIGGLI, H.: Hemmung der Enzymaktivität isolierter Mitochondrien durch kleine Röntgendosen. Naturwissenschaften **42**, 585 (1955).
FRÜHLING, L., GROS, C.M., BATZENSCHLAGER, A.: Sarcome endothelial angioplastique généralisé chez un malade ayant subi 12 ans auparavant une injection intraarteriélle de Thorotrast. Bull. Ass. franç. Cancer **42**, 559 (1955).
FRÜHLING, L., GROS, C.M., BATZENSCHLAGER, A., DORNER, M.: La maladie du thorotrast. Ann. Méd. **57**, 297 (1956).
FRYDL, V.: Zusammenfassendes Referat über morphologische Veränderungen in der Leber durch Bestrahlung. Z. Ges. inn. Med. **17**, 624 (1962).
GERBAULET, K., MAURER, W., BRÜCKNER, J.: Autoradiographische Untersuchung über die Inkorporation von ^3H Aminosäuren im Zellkern während der G_1-Phase und der S-Phase bei normalen und röntgenbestrahlten Mäusen. Biochim. biophys. Acata (Amst.) **68**, 462 (1963).
GERBER, G.B., ALTMAN, K.I.: Tissues and body fluids. In: Radiation Biochemistry. New York-London: Academic Press 1970.
GERBER, G.B., GERBER, G., ALTMAN, K.I.: The catabolism of tissue nucleic acid in the rat. I. The replacement time of deoxyribonucleic acid. J. biol. Chem. **235**, 1433 (1960).
GERBER, G.B., GERBER, G., ALTMAN, K.I., HEMPELMANN, L.H.: Radiation-induced tissue breakdown. Radiat. Res. **9**, 119 (1958).
GERBER, G.B., GERBER, G., ALTMAN, K.I., HEMPELMANN, L.H.: Radiation-induced tissue breakdown. IV. The source of degraded amino-acids in irradiated rats. Int. J. Radiat. Biol. **1**, 277 (1959).

GERBER, G.B., REMY-DEFRAIGNE, J.: Studies on detoxication by the perfused liver. I. Hippuric acid synthesis after irradiation. Int. J. Radiat. Biol. **7**, 53 (1963a).
GERBER, G.B., REMY-DEFRAIGNE, J.: Studies on detoxication by the perfused liver. II. Bilirubin conjugation and excretion after irradiation. Int. J. Radiat. Biol. **7**, 59 (1963b).
GERBER, G.B., REMY-DEFRAIGNE, J.: DNA metabolism in perfused organs. II. Incorporation into DNA and catabolism of thymidine at different levels of substrate by normal and X-irradiated liver and intestine Arch. int. Physiol. Biochim. **74**, 785 (1966).
GILBERT, R.: Die experimentelle Geschwulsterzeugung durch radioaktive Substanzen. Clin. **11**, 59 (1942).
GIUDICE, G., NOVELLI, G.D.: Effect of actinomycin D on the synthesis of DNA polymerase in hepatectomized rats. Biochem. biophys. Res. Commun. **12**, 383 (1963).
GLASSER, O., CLUINSKY, E.H., TAYLOR, L.S., WEATHERWAX, J.L.: Physical Foundations of radiology. New York: P.B. Hoeber Inc. 1949.
GLAUSER, O.: Elektronenmikroskopische Untersuchungen an Rattenlebern nach Röntgenbestrahlung. Schweiz. Z. allg. Path. **19**, 150 (1956).
GLAVIND, J., FARBER, M.: Antioxidants and lipoperoxides in the organs of irradiated rats. II. The influence of ionizing radiation on the amount of the individual antioxidants in rat organs. Int. J. Radiat. Biol. **11**, 445 (1966).
GLAVIND, J., HANSEN, L., FARBER, M.: Antioxidants and lipoperoxides in the organs of irradiated rats. Int. J. Radiat. Biol. **9**, 409 (1965).
GOLDFEDER, A.: In: Progress in Radiobiology. Springfield, Illinois: Thomas 1956.
GOULD, R.G., BELL, V.L., LILLY, E.H.: Stimulation of cholesterol biosynthesis from acetate in rat liver and adrenals by whole body X-irradiation. Amer. J. Physiol. **196**, 1231 (1959).
GOULD, R.G., POPJAK, G.: Biosynthesis of cholesterol in vivo and in vitro from DL-ß-hydroxy-ß-methyl-d-(2-^{14}C)-valerolactone. Biochem. J. **66**, 51P (1957).
GOUTIER, R.: Effects of X-rays on nucleic acid biosynthesis and on the activity of nucleases in mammalian cells. Progr. Biophys. **11**, 53 (1961).
GOUTIER, R.: Irradiation, radioprotection et synthèse de l-acide désoxyribonucléique. Bruxelles: Edition Arscia 1967.
GOUTIER-PIROTTE, M., GOUTIER, R.: Acid deoxyribonuclease and acid phosphatase activities in regenerating rat liver after whole-body X-irradiation. Radiat. Res. **16**, 728 (1962).
GRABIGER, R.: Osteoradionekrose des Schenkelhalses nach Telekobalttherapie. Strahlentherapie **123**, 282 (1964).
GRAEVSKAYA, B.M., SHCHEDRINA, R.N.: Investigation of the nature of the action of X-rays on the tissue protease activity. Radiobiologiya **3**, 168 (1963).
GRAMPA, G., TOMMASINI DEGNA, A.: Hemangioendothelioma of the liver following intravenous injection of thorotrast. Acta genet. (Basel) **8**, 65 (1958).
GRASES, P.J.: Lesiones hepatosplenicas tardas producidas por el Thorotrast. G.E.N. **20**, 755 (1966).
GRASES, P.J., BECKER, S.: Veno-occlusive disease of the liver. A case from Venezuela. Amer. J. Med. **53**, 511 (1972).
GRAUL, E.J., SCHERER, E.: Die Strahlenwirkungen auf den Magendarmkanal, auf Leber und Pankreas. In: Lehrbuch der Strahlenheilkunde. Stuttgart: Ferdinand Enke 1958.
GREENGARD, O.: The role of coenzymes, cortisone and RNA in the control of liver enzyme levels. Advanc. Enzyme Regul. **1**, 61 (1963).
GREENGARD, O.: Effects of irradiation and starvation on the regulation of rat liver enzymes. Proc. nat. Acad. Sci. (Wash.) **56**, 1303 (1966).
GRISHAM, J.W.: A morphologic study of deoxyribonucleic acid synthesis and cell proliferation in regenerating rat liver, autoradiography with thymidine-H^3. Cancer Res. **22**, 842 (1962).
GROS, C.M., FRÜHLING, L., BATZENSCHLAGER, A., KEILING, R.: L'autoradiographie dans le cancer du foie au thorotrast. Acta Un. int. Canc. **16**, 429 (1960).
GROS, C.M., FRÜHLING, L., KEILING, R.: Injection de thorotrast dans le sinus maxillaire; 15 ans après apparition d'un épithélioma malpighien. Bull. Ass. franç. Cancer **42**, 556 (1955).
GROSSI, E., PAOLETTI, P., PAOLETTI, R.: Effetto della irradiazione sulla incorporazione di alcuni precursori nel colesterolo e negli acidi grassi epatici. Minerva nucl. **2**, 343 (1958).
GROSSI, E., POGGI, M., PAOLETTI, R.: In: Response of the Nervous System to Ionizing Radiation. Boston: Little & Brown 1964.
GROSSIORD, A., ROUCRAYROL, J.C., DUPERRAT, B., CECCALDI, P.F., MEEUSBITH, L.: Adenocancer du foie avec cirrhose 21 ans après une arteriographie au thorotrast. Sem. Hôp. Paris **32**, 1728 (1956).
GUARINO, M., PERONI, L.: Le alterazioni morfologiche da radiozioni ionizzanti di alcune strutture nervose nel sottocutaneo, alla luce delle più recenti acquisizioni in tema di fisiopatologia del sistema nervoso periferico. Riv. Anat. pat. **19**, 359 (1961).
GUIMARES, J.P., LAMERTON, L.F., CHRISTENSEN, W.R.: The late effects of thorotrast administration. A review and an experimental study. Brit. J. Cancer **9**, 253 (1955).
HAGEN, U.: Zur Frage der Strahlenaktivierung von Fermenten. Strahlentherapie **106**, 277 (1958).
HAGEN, U.: Labilization of deoxyribonucleic acid in thymus nucleoprotein after whole-body irradiation. Nature (Lond.) **187**, 1123 (1960).

HAGEN, U., KOCH, R., LANGENDORFF, H.: Die Wirkung von Röntgenstrahlen auf die Azetylierungsvorgänge in der Rattenleber. Fortschr. Röntgenstr. **84**, 604 (1956).
HAHN, P.F., JACKSON, M.H., GOLDIE, H.: Liver cirrhosis with ascites, induced in digs by chronic massive hepatic irradiation with radioactive colloidal gold. Science **114**, 303 (1951).
HALL, J.C., GOLDSTEIN, A.L., SONNENBLICK, B.P.: Recovery of oxidative phosphorylation in rat liver mitochondria after whole body irradiation. J. biol. Chem. **23**, 1137 (1963).
HANEL, H.K., WILIAN-ULRICH, J.: The utilization of acetate in rat liver after whole-body roentgen irradiation. I. The incorporation of 2-^{14}C-acetate into fatty acids of liver and the acetylation of sulphanilamide. Int. J. Radiat. Biol. **1**, 366 (1959).
HANSEN, H.J.M., HANSEN, L., FABER, M.: The effect of whole-body X-irradiation on the synthesis of individual fatty acids in liver slices from normal and fasted rats. Int. J. Radiat. Biol. **9**, 25 (1965).
HANSEN, L.: The increase in liver glycogen in nonfasted rats after irradiation. A comparison with pair-fed animals. Int. J. Radiat. Biol. **12**, 367 (1967).
HARTIALA, K., NÄNTÖ, V., RINNE, U.K.: Studies of the effect of X-rays on the glucuronide synthesis by the liver. Acta physiol. scand. **45**, 231 (1959).
HEILMEYER, L.: Die hämatologische Form des Strahlenschadens, ihre Erkennung und Behandlung. In: Strahlenschutz in Forschung und Praxis. Freiburg: Verlag Rombach 1961.
HELD, F.: Die Bedeutung der Strahlenqualität für die schädigende Wirkung ionisierender Strahlung auf die Tibia-Epiphysenfuge der Albinoratte. Radiobiol. Radiother. (Berl.) **2**, 151 (1925).
HELLRIEGEL, W.: zitiert nach BIRZLE, H.: (1965).
HEMPELMANN, L.H., CARR, S., FRANTZ, I.D., MASTERS, R., LAMDIN, E.: Effect of body exposure to X-rays on rate of incorporation of C^{14} carboxyl labeled alanine into mouse protein. Fed. Proc. **9**, 183 (1950).
HERTWIG, G.: Die Radiumkrankheit tierischer Keimzellen. Ein Beitrag zur experimentellen Zeugungs- und Vererbungslehre. Arch. mikr. Anat. **77**, 1 (1911).
HERTWIG, G.: Das Radiumexperiment in der Biologie. Eine literarische Zusammenfassung. Strahlentherapie **11**, 821 (1920).
HEVESY, G. DE: Effect of X-rays on the incorporation of carbon-14 into animal tissue. Nature (Lond.) **164**, 269 (1949).
HEVESY, G. DE, FORSSBERG, A.: Effect of irradiation by X-rays on the exhalation of carbon dioxide by the mouse. Nature (Lond.) **168**, 692 (1951).
HIDVEGI, E.J., HOLLAND, J., BÖLÖNI, E., LONAI, P., VARTERESZ, V.: The effect of whole body X-irradiation of guinea pigs on liver ribosomes. Biochem. J. **109**, 495 (1968).
HIERONYMI, G.: Kritische Untersuchung sogenannter Thorotrasttumoren nebst Mitteilung zweier Fälle. Zbl. allg. Path. path. Anat. **97**, 513 (1958).
HILL, R., KIYASU, J., CHAIKOFF, I.L.: Metabolism of glucose and fructose in liver of the rat subjected to whole-body X-irradiation. Amer. J. Physiol. **187**, 417 (1956).
HOFER, O.: Kieferhöhlenkarzinom durch radiumhaltiges Kontrastmittel hervorgerufen. Dtsch. zahnärztl. Z. **7**, 736 (1952).
HOHENSTATT, H.: Multiple hemangiosarcomas of the liver following cerebral angiography with thorotrast. Hippokrates (Stuttg.) **36**, 227 (1965).
HOLMES, B.E.: Influence of radiation on metabolism of regenerating rat liver. Ciba Foundation Symp. Ionizing Rad., p. 225 (1956).
HOLMES, B.E., MEE, L.K.: In: Radiobiology Symposium. New York: Academic Press 1955.
HOLTHUSEN, H.: Die biologische Dosierung in der Strahlentherapie der einzelnen Gewebe. Strahlenempfindlichkeit der normalen und pathologischen Gewebe. In: Handbuch der gesamten Strahlenheilkunde II. München: J.F. Bergmann 1931.
HOLTHUSEN, H.: In: Einführung in die Röntgenologie. Stuttgart: Thieme 1947.
HORTA DA SILVA, J., COLLECTE, J., RORIZ, M. DA LUZ: Circulation lymphatique du foie. Visualisation du réseau lymphatique du foie chez des individus injectés avec le thorotrast. Arch. Vecchi **35**, 1 (1961).
HORVATH, J., HORVATH, F., JUHASZ, E., URBANYI, L.: Über die Strahlenschädigung wachsender Knochen. Strahlentherapie **118**, 462 (1962).
HÜBNER, G., BERNHARD, W.: Das submikroskopische Bild der Leberzelle nach temporärer Durchblutungssperre. Beitr. path. Anat. **125**, 1 (1961).
HUDELLET, G.: Etude expérimentale de l'action des rayons X sur le foie. C.R. Soc. Biol. (Paris) **61**, 639 (1906).
HUDELLET, G.: Action des rayons X sur le foie. Arch. Élect. méd. **15**, 7 (1907).
HULTH, A., WESTERBORN, O.: Early changes of the growth zone in the rabbit following roentgen irradiation. Acta orthop. scand. **30**, 155 (1960).
HULTH, A., WESTERBORN, O.: Early changes of the growth zone in the rabbit following roentgen irradiation: Autoradiographic investigation after administration of radiosulphate. Brit. J. exp. Path. **43**, 137 (1962).
INGLE, D.J.: Technic of repeated partial hepatectomy in the rat. Proc. Soc. exp. Biol. (N.Y.) **87**, 251 (1954).

INGLE, D.J., BAKER, B.L.: Histology and regenerative capacity of liver following multiple partial hepatectomies. Proc. Soc. exp. Biol. (N.Y.) **95**, 813 (1957).

INGOLD, J.A., REED, G.B., KAPLAN, H.S., BAGSHAW, M.A.: Radiation hepatitis. Amer. J. Roentgenol. **93**, 200 (1965).

IRWIN, D.A.: Experimental intravenous administration of colloidal thorium dioxide. Canad. med. Ass. J. **27**, 130 (1932).

ISHIKAWA, N.: Radiation effect on the liver indicated by the regenerative capacity. Showa-igaku Zasshi **30**, 974 (1973).

JACKSON, K.L., ENTENMAN, C.: USNRDL **TR-504**, 45 (1961), cit. by GERBER, G.B. and ALTMAN, K.I., The liver. In: Radiation Biochemistry (K.I. ALTMAN, G.B. GERBER and S. OKADA, eds.), vol. II. New York and London: Academic Press 1970.

JACOBSON, L.E., ROSENBAUM, D.: Postmortem findings and radioactivity determinations five years after injection of thorotrast. Radiology **31**, 601 (1938).

JAFFE, J.J., LAJTHA, L.G., LASCELLES, J., ORD, M.G., STOCKEN, L.A.: The effect of X-irradiation on the processes leading to DNA synthesis in regenerating rat liver. Intern. J. Radiat. Biol. **1**, 241 (1959).

JAKOB, A., WACHSMUTH, E.: Über die Sekundärstrahlung von Kontrastmitteln. Klin. Wschr. **26**, 20 (1948).

JAMIESON, D.: Ionizing radiation and the intracellular oxidation-reduction state. Nature (Lond.) **209**, 361 (1966).

JARDETZKY, C.D., BARNUM, C.P., VERMUND, H.: Deoxyribonucleic acid and phospholipid metabolism in regenerating liver and the effect of X-irradiation. J. biol. Chem. **222**, 421 (1956).

JOHNSON, P.M., GROSSMAN, F.M., ATKINS, H.L.: Radiation induced hepatic injury. Its detection by scintillation scanning. Amer. J. Roentgenol. **99**, 453 (1967).

JORDAN, S.W., DEAN, PH.N., AHLQUIST, J.: Early ultrastructural effects of ionizing radiation. I. Mitochondrial and nuclear changes. Lab. Invest. **27**, 538 (1972).

JUSTIN-BESANCON, L., PEQUINOT, H., RUBENS-DUVAL, A., DORMONT, J.: Cancer primitif du foie et radiations ionisantes. Arch. Anat. path. **6**, 204 (1958).

KADOWAKY, I.: Studies on the morphological changes produced by X-rays in rat liver. Med. J. Osaka Univ. **7**, 369 (1956).

KADRNKA, S.: Roentgenologic demonstration of the parenchyma of the spleen and liver by means of a new intravenous contrast medium (thorotrast). Radiology **18**, 371 (1932).

KAINOVA, A.S.: Effect of ionizing radiations on phospholipid metabolism in the liver. Biokhimyia **25**, 540 (1960).

KALASHNIKOVA, M.M.: Reparative regeneration of the rat's liver after a local X-irradiation. Dokl. Akad. Nauk. SSSR **151**, 213 (1963b).

KALASHNIKOVA, V.P.: On nicotinic acid metabolism in the irradiated organism. Med. Radiol. **8**, 58 (1963a).

KAMPMANN, H., KRAUSS, O., RÜGER, W., SCHEER, J.E., LORENZ, W.J.: Quantitative Organverteilungsuntersuchungen mit Thorotrast durch Neutronenaktivierungs-Analyse. 6. Jahrestag. d. Ges. I. Nuklearmed., Wiesbaden 1968.

KAMPMANN, H., WESCH, H., WEGENER, K.: Quantitative Thoriumbestimmungen in 30 Organen bei menschlicher Thorotrastose. 7. Jahrestag. d. Ges. f. Nuklearmed., Zürich 1969.

KAPLAN, H.S., BAGSHAW, M.A.: Radiation hepatitis: possible prevention by combined isotopic and external radiation therapy. Radiol. **91**, 1214 (1968).

KAUFMANN, B.P.: Chromosomal aberrations induced in animal cells by ionizing radiations. In: Radiation Biology, vol. 6, p. 627. New York: McGraw-Hill 1954.

KAUL, A., HEYDER, J.: Kinetik der Verteilung und Ausscheidung von Radio-Isotopen nach Thorotrastinjektion. Biophysik **7**, 74 (1971).

KAY, R.C., EARLY, J.C., ENTENMAN, C.: Increased urinary excretion of taurine and urea by rats after X-irradiation. Radiat. Res. **6**, 98 (1957).

KAY, R.E., ENTENMAN, C.: The conversion of glycine-1-C^{14} to protein-C^{14} and $C^{13}O_2$ in liver slices from X-irradiated rats. Arch. Biochim. Biophys. **62**, 419 (1956a).

KAY, R.E., ENTENMAN, C.: Hyperglycemia and increased liver glycogen in rats after X-irradiation. Proc. Soc. exp. Biol. (N.Y.) **91**, 143 (1956b).

KELLY, L.S.: Effect of radiation on DNA synthesis in mammalian cells. Progr. Biophys. **8**, 143 (1957).

KELLY, L.S., PAYLE, A.H.: The effect of irradiation on DNA turnover in regenerating liver normal mouse tissues. Acta radiol. (Suppl.) **116**, 693 (1953).

KEPPLER, D., LESCH, R., REUTTER, W., DECKER, K.: Experimental hepatitis induced by D-Galactosamine. Exp. molec. Path. **9**, 279 (1968).

KHANSON, K.P.: The effect of whole-body irradiation on the processes coupled with oxidative phosphorylation and certain regulatory mechanisms in rat liver mitochondria. Radiobiologyia **5**, 71 (1965).

KLOUWEN, H.M.: Radiosensitivity of nuclear RNA. Biochim. biophys. Acta (Amst.) **42**, 366 (1960).

KNOTT, J.C.A., WILLS, E.D.: The role of testosterone in the regulation on oxidative drug metabolism in normal and irradiated animals. Biochem. Pharmacol. **23**, 793 (1974).

KOHOUTEK, J., NOVAK, D.: Cholangiogenni, karcinom jater po Thorotrastu. Čs. Rentgenol. **14**, 110 (1960).
KOLAR, J., BABICKY, A.: Untersuchungen zum Kalziumstoffwechsel in der Epi- und Metaphyse nach lokaler Röntgenbestrahlung. Strahlentherapie **109**, 483 (1959); **119**, 236, 435 (1962); **120**, 98 (1963).
KONERMANN, G.: Periodische Kompensationsreaktionen im Verlaufe des postnatalen Wachstums von Leber und Gehirn bei der Maus nach fraktionierter Röntgenbestrahlung während der Embryogenese. Habil. Schrift, Freiburg, 1975.
KOSCHITZ-KOSIC, J.: Über Schenkelhalsfrakturen als Folge von Strahlenschäden. Klin. Med. (Wien) **16**, 277 (1961).
KOVACS, L.: Morphologische Leberveränderungen nach experimenteller fraktionierter lokaler Röntgenbestrahlung. Strahlentherapie **142**, 227 (1971).
KRÖGER, H., GREUER, B.: Einfluß von Antagonisten des Nukleinsäure-Stoffwechsels und von Röntgenstrahlen auf die Induktion von Enzymen. Biochem. Z. **341**, 190 (1965).
KURNICK, N.B., MASSEY, B.W., SANDEEN, G.: The effect of radiation on tissue deoxyribonuclease. Radiat. Res. **11**, 101 (1959).
KUROHARA, S.S., SWENSON, N.L., USSELMAN, J.A., GEORGE, F.M.: Response and recovery of liver to radiation as demonstrated by photoscans. Radiology **89**, 129 (1967).
KUSNETS, E.: The effect of X-rays on tissue respiration. Dokl. Akad. Nauk SSSR **130**, 657 (1960).
LACASSAGNE, A.: Les cancer produits par les rayonnements corpusculaires. Paris: Hermann & Cie 1945.
LACASSAGNE, A.: The liver. In: Pathology of Irradiation. Baltimore: The Williams & Wilkins Comp. 1971.
LACASSAGNE, A., BULL-HOI, N.P., CAGNIANT, P.: Association d'hydrocarbures polycycliques et mécanisme de la cancérisation. C.R. Soc. Biol. (Paris) **138**, 16 (1944).
LACASSAGNE, A., HURST, L.: Effects of the combined action of roentgen rays and chemical carcinogen (DAB) on the rat's liver. Amer. J. Roentgenol. **87**, 536 (1962).
LACASSAGNE, A., HURST, L.: Changements produits dans le foie du rat par une irradiation partielle unique. Rev. franç. Étud. clin. biol. **8**, 20 (1963).
LACASSAGNE, A., HURST, L.: Changements produits dans le foie du rat entre les 4e et 19e mois après une irradiation partielle de l'organe. Rev. franç. Étud. clin. biol. **10**, 198 (1965).
LACASSAGNE, A., HURST, L., ROSENBERG, A.J.: Effect de l'irradiation X du foie du rat sur la production de l'hépatome par intoxication on para-diméthyl-aminoazobenzène. C.R. Acad. Sci. (Paris) **251**, 1053 (1960).
LACASSAGNE, A., MONOD, O.: Les caryocinèses atypiques provoquées dans les cellules cancéreuses par les rayons X et Y, et leur rôle dans la regression des tumeurs malignes irradiées. Arch. Franc. Path. Gen. Anat. Path. **1**, (1922).
LADDAGA, M., ROMAGNOLI, U.: Sulla possibilita svelare alcune lesioni latenti nelle cellula epatica. Minerva nucl. **5**, 294 (1961).
LAMARQUE, P.: La restauration après irradiations par les rayons roentgen. Acta radiol. (Stockh.), Suppl. **116**, 448 (1954).
LAMERTON, L.F., FRY, R.M.J.: Cell Proliferation. Oxford: Blackwell Scientific Publ. 1963.
LANE, J.L., WILDING, J.L., RUST, J.R., TRUM, B.F., SCHOOLAR, J.C.: Changes in respiratory gases of burros after prolonged fractionated total-body γ-irradiation. Radiat. Res. **2**, 64 (1955).
LANSING, A.M., DAVIS, W.M., BRIZEL, H.E.: Radiation hepatitis. Arch. Surg. **96**, 878 (1968).
LAUENSTEIN, K., HABERLAND, G.L., HEMPELMANN, L.K., ALTMAN, K.I.: Cellular destruction and protein breakdown induced by exposure to X-rays. III. The use of hippuric acid for the simultaneous assessment of two "free" amino acid pools. Biochim. biophys. Acta (Amst.) **26**, 421 (1957).
LAVEDAN, J., COURTIAL. J.: cit. by K.H. Bauer, 1949.
LEABHART, J.W., BONFIGLIO, M.: The treatment of irradiation fracture of the femoral neck. J. Bone Jt Surg. **43**A, 1056 (1961).
LEBEDINSKIY, A.V., NAKHIL-NITSKAYA, Z.N.: Effects of Ionizing Radiation on the Nervous System. Amsterdam: Elsevier 1963.
LEBLOND, C.P.: In: Control of cell division and the induction of cancer. Nat. Cancer Inst. Monogr. **14**, 119 (1964).
LEBLOND, C.P., WALKER, B.F.: Renewal of cell populations. Physiol. Rev. **36**, 255 (1956).
LEHNERT, S.M., OKADA, S.: DNA-synthesis in nuclei isolated from regenerating rat liver after whole-body irradiation. Intern. J. Radiat. Biol. **5**, 323 (1962).
LEHNERT, S.M., OKADA, S.: Nuclear factors involved in the radiation-induced depression of DNA synthesis of deoxyribonucleic acid. Nature (Lond.) **199**, 1108 (1963).
LEHNERT, S.M., OKADA, S.: Nucleoprotein changes in regenerating liver nuclei after X-irradiation. Int. J. Radiat. Biol. **8**, 75 (1964).
LEHNERT, S.M., OKADA, S.: Effect of irradiation on DNA synthesis in the regenerating livers of rats. Int. J. Radiat. Biol. **10**, 601 (1966).
LELIÈVRE, P.: Modification du glycogène et de la glycémie chez la souris après fortes doses de rayons X. C.R. Soc. Biol. (Paris) **149**, 1296 (1957).

LELIÈVRE, P., BELTZ, E.H.: Les variations de la glycémie au cours de l'irradiation à fortes doses de R.X. C.R. Soc. Biol. (Paris) **149**, 2034 (1955).
LEONG, G.F., PESSOTTI, R.L., KREBS, J.S.: Liver cell proliferation in X-irradiated rats after single and repetitive partial hepatectomy. J. nat. Cancer Inst. **27**, 131 (1961).
LERNER, S.R., WARNER, W.L., ENTENMAN, C.: Lipogenesis from acetate-1-C^{14} by liver slices from X-irradiated rats. Fed. Proc. **12**, 85 (1953).
LESCH, R., BAUER, CH., REUTTER, W.: The development of cholangiofibrosis and hepatomas in galactosamine induced cirrhotic rat livers. Virchows Arch. Abt. B **12**, 285 (1973).
LESCH, R., KEPPLER, D., REUTTER, W., RUDIGIER, J., OEHLERT, W., DECKER, K.: Entwicklung einer experimentellen Leberzirrhose durch D-Galaktosamin. Histologische, biochemische und autoradiographische Untersuchungen an Ratten. Virchows Arch. Abt. B **6**, 57 (1970).
LESCH, R., OEHLERT, W.: Histochemistry in pathological diagnosis, e.g. tumors, autoradiography. Atti del settimo Congresso Internazionale dell' Accademia Internazionale di Patologia, Milano, 1968.
LESCH, R., OEHLERT, W., HEISSMEYER, H.: Die Veränderung des Reaktionsverhaltens der Rattenleber bei der Kombination verschiedener Noxen. Sofia: Kongress der bulg. Ges. f. Pathologie 1972.
LESCH, R., REUTTER, W., KEPPLER, D., DECKER, K.: Liver restitution after acute galactosamine hepatitis: autoradiographic and biochemical studies in rats. Exp. molec. Path. **12**, 58 (1970).
LESHER, S., STROUD, A.N., BRUES, A.M.: The effects of chronic irradiation on DNA synthesis in regenerating mouse liver. Cancer Res. **20**, 1341 (1960).
LEVY, B., RUGH, R.: Hepatic glycogen in acute radiation death. Proc. Soc. exp. Biol. (N.Y.) **82**, 223 (1953).
LEWIN, K., MILLIS, R.R.: Human radiation hepatitis. A morphological study with emphasis on the late changes. Arch. Path. **96**, 21 (1973).
LIKHACHEV, Y.P., NEMIROVSKAYA, N.A.: Injuries of the spinal cord in radiation therapy. Med. Radiol. (Mosk.) **8**, 27 (1963).
LIM, J.K., PIANTADOSI, C., SNYDER, F.: A comparison of phospholipid biosynthesis in irradiated bone marrow and liver. Proc. Soc. exp. Biol. (N.Y.) **124**, 1158 (1967).
LOGAN, R.: The effect of X-irradiation on the uptake of nucleic acids and protein precursors by isolated rabbit-liver, appendix and thymus nuclei. Biochim biophys. Acta (Amst.) **35**, 251 (1959).
LOGAN, R., ERRERA, M., FICQ, A.: The effect of X-rays and ultraviolet light on the uptake in vitro of 8-^{14}C adenine and 2-^{14}C phenylamine by isolated nuclei. Biochim. biophys. Acta (Amst.) **32**, 147 (1959).
LOMAKINA, L.J., ZHILINA, M.V., SAGDEEVA, L.G.: The Action of 5-Fluoro-2'-Deoxyuridine and Aminopterin on the Mitotic Cycle Events in the Culture of Chinese Hamster Cells. Citologiya, Leningrad, **9**, 1155 (1967) (in Russian)
LOONEY, W.B.: An investigation of the late clinical findings following thorotrast (thorium dioxide) administration. Amer. J. Roentgenol. **83**, 163 (1960).
LOONEY, W.B., CAMPBELL, R.C., HOLMES, B.E.: The effect of irradiation on the replication of deoxyribonucleic acid in hepatocytes. Proc. nat. Acad. Sci. (Wash.) **46**, 698 (1960).
LOONEY, W.B., CHANG, L.O.: The effects of X-radiation on thymidine-labeled DNA of regenerating rat liver. Radiat. Res. **37**, 525 (1969).
LOONEY, W.B., CHANG, L.O., WILLIAMS, S.S., FORSTER, J., HAYDOCK, I., BANGHART, F.W.: An autoradiographic and biochemical study of the effects of radiation on deoxyribonucleic acid synthesis in the intact animal. Radiat. Res. **24**, 312 (1965).
LOURAU-PITRES, M.: Incorporation du ^{14}C dans les graisses et le glycogène du foie chez des souris irradiées ayant reçu une injection de glucose manqué par du ^{14}C. Ark. Kemi **7**, 211 (1954).
LÜDIN, M., JR.: Haemangio-Endotheliomatose von Leber und Milz bei Thorotrastspeicherung. Schweiz. Z. allg. Path. **16**, 987 (1953).
MAASS, H.: Adeninnucleotidgehalt in verschiedenen Organen der Ratte nach Ganzkörperbestrahlung. Z. ges. exp. Med. **133**, 97 (1960).
MAASS, H., JENNER, E., HÖLZEL, F.: Der Einfluß einer Röntgen-Ganzkörperbestrahlung auf den Einbau von 2-^{14}C-Glycin in die Proteine der Leber, Milz und des Blutes von Ratten. Z. Naturforsch. **22**b, 634 (1967).
MAASS, H., TIMM, M.: Nukleosidphosphatgehalte in verschiedenen Organen der Ratte nach Ganzkörperbestrahlung. Strahlentherapie **123**, 64 (1964).
MACCARDLE, R.C., CONGDON, C.C.: Mitochondrial changes in hepatic cells of X-irradiated mice. Amer. J. Path. **31**, 725 (1955).
MACH, J.: Beitrag zur Osteoradionekrose. Zbl. Chir. **87**, 1665 (1962).
MACMAHON, H.E., MORPHY, A.S., BATES, M.I.: Endothelial-cell sarcoma of liver following thorotrast injections. Amer. J. Path. **23**, 585 (1947).
MAHLUM, D.D., STKOV, M.R., KASHIMA, M.: Effects of hepatic irradiation by plutonium. Intern. Symposium on Hepatotoxicity, Tel Aviv/Israel, March 25–30, 1973.
MANDEL, P.: Free nucleotides in animal tissues. Progr. Nucleic Acid Res. **3**, 299 (1964).
MASCIOCCHI, A., CAZZOLA, G.: Complicazioni neurologiche in soggetto affetto da tigna tricofitica

trattato con irradiazioni roentgen. Studio clinico, elettro encefalografico, pneumonencefalografico, arteriografico. Cervello **38**, 59 (1962).
MASORO, E.J.: Biochemical mechanism related to the homeostatic regulation of lipogenesis in animals. J. Lipid Res. **3**, 149 (1962).
MATTHES, T.: Thorotrastschäden und Krebsgefahr. Arch. Geschwulstforsch. **6**, 162 (1954).
MATTHES, T.: Zur Frage der Entstehung eines Carcinoms auf dem Boden einer Thorotrast-Narbenleber. Strahlentherapie **99**, 94 (1956).
MCCAY, P., MACFARLANE, M.G.: Lipid peroxide in livers of irradiated rats. Nature (Lond.) **198**, 98 (1963).
MCLEAN, E.K.: The toxic actions of pyrrolizidine (senecio) alkaloids. Pharmacol. Rev. **22**, 428 (1970).
MCLEAN, F.C., BUDY, A.M.: Radiation, Isotopes and Bones. New York: Academic Press 1964.
MELCHING, H.J.: Grundlagen des biologisch-chemischen Strahlenschutzes. III. Intern. Kongr. Hygiene u. Präventivmed. Wien, **27** (1962).
MESSIER, B., LEBLOND, C.P.: Cell proliferation and migration as revealed by radioautography after injection of thymidine-H^3 into male rats and mice. Amer. J. Anat. **106**, 247 (1960).
MILLER, L.L.: Entstehungsorte, Speicherorte und Umsatz der Serumproteine. Verh. dtsch. Ges. inn. Med. **66**, 250 (1960).
MILLER, L.L., JOHN, D.W., CLOUTIER, P.F.: Cit. in GERBER, G.B. and ALTMAN, K.I. The liver. In: Radiation Biochemistry (K.I. ALTMAN, G.B. GERBER and S. OKADA, eds.), vol. II. New York and London: Academic Press 1970.
MIRONESCU, S., DRAGOMIR, C.: Nucleolar behaviour in regenerating liver of normal and whole-body irradiated rats. Cancer Res. **27**, 1819 (1967).
MISHKIN, P.E., SHORE, M.L.: Interference by X-irradiation with the induced synthesis of tryptophan pyrrolase. Radiat. Res. **33**, 437 (1968).
MITZNEGG, P.: Die Wirkung der Strahlenschutzsubstanz auf die Leber weißer Mäuse in Abhängigkeit vom Lebensalter. Acta geront. (Milano) **3**, 753 (1973).
MITZNEGG, P., HEIM, F., SÄBEL, M., PAULY, H.: Über die Hemmung des Wachstums fetaler Rattenlebern und Plazenten durch ionisierende Strahlen. Strahlentherapie **139**, 251 (1970).
MÖBIUS, G., LEMBCKE, K.: Thorotrasttumoren der Leber. Zbl. allg. Path. **105**, 41 (1963).
MÖLBERT, E., GUERRITORE, G.: Elektronenmikroskopische Untersuchungen am Leberparenchym bei akuter Hypoxie. Beitr. path. Anat. **117**, 32 (1957).
MOLE, R.H.: Whole body irradiation and the idea of stress. Brit. J. exp. Path. **37**, 528 (1956).
MOORE, R.: Ionizing radiation and chromosomes. J. Coll. Radiol. Aust. **9**, 272 (1965).
MOORE, T.A., FERRANTE, W.A.: Hepatoma two decades after radiation for hepatic hemangioma. Digestive Disease Week, Amer. Ass. for the Study of the Liver, San Francisco, May 19–25 (1974).
MOREHOUSE, M.G., SEARCY, R.L.: ^{14}C-acetate incorporation into liver lipids and glycogen of irradiated rats. Science **122**, 158 (1955).
MORGAN, A.D., JAYNE, W., MARRACK, D.: Primary liver cell carcinoma 24 years after intravenous injection of thorotrast. J. clin. Path. **11**, 7 (1958).
MORGENROTH, K., JR., THEMANN, H.: Elektronenmikroskopische Untersuchungen der Wirkung ionisierender Strahlen auf die Feinstruktur von Leber und Milz von Mäusen. Strahlentherapie **124**, 4 (1964).
MORI, R., SAKAI, T., NOZUE, Y., OKAMOTO, T., WADA, T., TANAKA, R., TSUYA, A.: Malignancy and other injuries following thorotrast administration: Follow-up study of 147 cases in Japan. Strahlentherapie **134**, 229 (1967).
MORIYAMA, I.M., STEER, A., HAMILTON, H.B., RUSSELL, W.J., SHIMIZU, K., DOCK, D.S.: Radiation effects on atomic bomb survivors. ABCC. Technical Report 6–73 (1973).
MUTH, H.: In: Die Supervolttherapie. Stuttgart: Thieme 1961.
MUTH, H., HEYER, J., VAN KAICK, G., KAUL, A., KEMMER, W., KOEPPE, P., LORENZ, D., OBERHAUSEN, E., ROEDER, D., SCHNEIDLIN, P.: Results of biophysical and clinical examination of thorotrast patients and their importance for better knowledge about radiation late effects. 4. U.N. Conf. peaceful use Atom. Energ. Genf, 1971.
MYERS, D.K.: Synthesis of diphosphopyridine nucleotide in irradiated rats. Nature (Lond.) **187**, 1124 (1960).
MYERS, D.K.: Biochemical effects on liver regeneration. Canad. J. Biochem. **38**, 1059 (1960).
MYERS, D.K., DE WOLFE, D.E.: Effects of X-irradiation on enzyme synthesis during liver regeneration. Canad. J. Biochem. **40**, 619 (1962).
NAGAYO, T., ITO, M., YAMADA, S.: Accelerated induction of hepatoma in rats fed N,N′-2,7-fluorenylene-bis-acetamide by X-irradiation to the target area. Gann **61**, 81 (1970).
NETTLESHIP, A., FING, W.J.: Neoplasms of the liver following injection of thorotrast. Amer. J. clin. Path. **35**, 422 (1961).
NICAUD, P., HAMBURGER, M.: Cancer du poumon à petites cellules à metastases multiples sans semiologie pulmonaire: anaemie pernicieuse aigue après traitment par le thorium. Bull. Soc. méd. Hôp. Paris **53**, 1310 (1937).

NIELSEN, G., KRACHT, J.: Zur Cancerogenese nach diagnostischer Thorotrastanwendung. Frankfurt. Z. Path. **68**, 661 (1958).
NIMS, L.F., SUTTON, E.: Adrenal cholesterol, liver glycogen and water consumption of fastig and X-irradiated rats. Amer. J. Physiol. **177**, 51 (1954).
NOTARIO, A., DI MARCO, N., DONEDA, G., ZANNETTI, A., SLAVIERO, G.: Analisi gascromatografica degli acidi grasse del fegato di ratti normali ed irradiati. Minerva nucl. **9**, 237 (1964).
NOTARIO, A., SLAVIERO, G., DONEDA, G., SANTAGATI, G.: Metabolism of glycine-1-^{14}C in the normal and in the irradiated rat. Experientia (Basel) **21**, 264 (1965).
NOYES, P.P., SMITH, R.E.: Quantitative changes in rat liver mitochondria following whole body irradiation. Exp. Cell Res. **16**, 15 (1959).
NYGAARD, O.F., POTTER, R.L.: Effect of X-irradiation on DNA metabolism in various tissues of the rat. I. Incorporation of C^{14}-thymidine into DNA during the first 24 hours post irradiation. Radiat. Res. **10**, 462 (1959).
OBERLING, CH., GUERIN, M.: Action du thorotrast sur le sarcome de Jensen du rat blanc. Bull. Cancer **22**, 469 (1933).
OEHLERT, W.: Zur Histopathologie des Strahlenschadens. In: Strahlenschutz in Forschung und Praxis. Freiburg: Verlag Rombach 1971.
OEHLERT, W.: Zur Strahlenempfindlichkeit der Leber. In: Strahlenempfindlichkeit von Organen und Organsystemen der Säugetiere und des Menschen; Strahlenschutz in Forschung und Praxis, vol. XIII. Stuttgart: Thieme 1973.
OEHLERT, W., HÄMMERLING, W., BÜCHNER, F.: Der zeitliche Ablauf und das Ausmaß der Desoxyribonukleinsäure-Synthese in der regenerierenden Leber der Ratte nach Teilhepatektomie. Beitr. path. Anat. **126**, 91 (1963).
OEHLERT, W., LESCH, R.: Autoradiographische Untersuchungen an menschlichen Geweben und Zellen. Dtsch. med. Wschr. **91**, 1940 (1966).
OGATA, K., HIZAWA, K., YOSHIDA, M., KITAMURO, T., AKAGI, G., KAGAWA, K.K., FUKUDA, F.: Hepatic injury following irradiation. A morphologic study. Tokushima J. Exp. Med. **9**, 240 (1963).
OKA, M.: Eine neue Methode zur röntgenologischen Darstellung der Milz. Fortschr. Röntgenstr. **40**, 497 (1929).
OKADA, S., PEACHEY, L.D.: Effect of γ-irradiation on the deoxyribonuclease II activity of isolated mitochondria. J. biophys. biochem. Cytol. **3**, 239 (1957).
OKINAKA, S., NAKAO, K., IBAYASHI, K., NAKAIDZIMI, M., KAKEHI, H., SUGIMURA, T.: A case report on the development of biliary tract cancer 11 years after the injection of thorotrast. Amer. J. Roentgenol. **78**, 812 (1957).
O'MALLEY, B., D'ANGIO, G.J., VAWRER, G.F.: Late effects of roentgen therapy given in infancy. Amer. J. Roentgenol. **89**, 1067 (1963).
ORD, M.G., STOCKEN, L.A.: Biochemical aspects of the radiation syndrome. Physiol. Rev. **33**, 356 (1953).
ORD, M.G., STOCKEN, L.A.: In: Mechanisms in Radiobiology, vol. 1, p. 285. Anabolic Processes. Liver and Plasma: Academic Press 1960.
PALLIS, C.A., LOUIS, S., MORGAN, R.L.: Radiation myelopathy. Brain **84**, 460 (1961).
PALMIERI, G.C., MICELLI, R.: Über den Einfluß des natürlichen und künstlichen Winterschlafes auf die Strahlenempfindlichkeit der lebenden Zellen und Gewebe. Proc. Soc. exp. Biol. (N.Y.) **101**, 161 (1959).
PANDE, S.V., RAMAIAH, A., VENKITASUBRAMANIAN, T.A.: Effect of X-irradiation on the hepatic synthesis of fatty acids and cholesterol. Biochim. biophys. Acta (Amst.) **65**, 516 (1962).
PAPPAS, A.M., COHEN, J.: The abscopal effect of X-irradiation on bone growth in rats. J. Bone Jt Surg. A **45**, 765 (1963).
PATT, J.M., QUASTLER, H.: Radiation effects on cell renewal and related systems. Physiol. Rev. **43**, 357 (1963).
PECH, A., CLEMENT, R., BOUDOURESQUES, J., AVIERINOS, R.: A-propos d'une observation de myélite cervicale post-cobaltthérapique (Irradiation pour néo du cavum). Rev. oto-neuro-ophtal. **33**, 78 (1961).
PFEIFFER, I., BUTTENBERG, H.: Osteoradionekrose im Hüftgelenksgebiet. Strahlentherapie **109**, 200 (1959).
PITOT, H.C., PERAINO, C.: Studies on the induction and repression of enzymes in rat liver. I. Induction of threonine dehydrase and ornithin-d-transaminase by oral intubation of casein hydrolysate. J. biol. Chem. **239**, 1783 (1964).
PITOT, H.C.,PERAINO, C., LAMAR, C., JR.: Comparative effects of actinomycin and ionizing radiation on enzyme synthesis in mammalian cells in vitro. Radiat. Res. **33**, 599 (1968).
PITOT, H.C., PERAINO, C., LAMAR, C., JR., LESHER, S.: Effect of gamma radiation on dietary and hormonal induction of enzymes in rat liver. Science **150**, 901 (1965).
PIZZARELLO, D.H., WITCOFSKI, R.L., LYONS, E.A.: Variations in survival time after whole-body irradiation at two times of day. Science **139**, 349 (1963).
POHLE, E.A.,BUNTING, C.H.: Histological changes in the liver of rats following exposure to single graded doses of filtered roentgen rays. Acta radiol. (Stockh.) **13**, 117 (1932).

POHLE, E.A., RITCHIE, G.: Histological studies of liver, spleen and bone marrow in rabbits following intravenous injection of thorium dioxide. Amer. J. Roentgenol. **31**, 512 (1934).
POPPER, L., KLEIN, E.: Über Hepato-Lienographie. Münch. med. Wschr. **78**, 1829 (1931).
PRICE, D.: Dynamics of Proliferating Tissues. Chicago: Univ. of Chicago Press 1958.
RABES, H., TUCZEK, H.V., WIRSCHING, R.: Kinetics of hepatocellular proliferation after partial hepatectomy as a function of structural and biochemical heterogeneity. III workshop on experimental liver injury, Freiburg, Oct. 15—16, 1973.
RADT, P.: Eine Methode zur röntgenologischen Sichtbarmachung von Milz und Leber. Klin. Wschr. **46**, 2128 (1929).
RADT, P.: Eine neue Methode zur röntgenologischen Sichtbarmachung von Leber und Milz durch Injektion eines Kontrastmittels. Med. Klin. **26**, 1888 (1930).
RAJEWSKI, B.: Strahlendosis und Strahlenwirkung. Stuttgart: Thieme 1956.
RAJEWSKY, B., GERBER, B., PAULY, H.: Die Beeinflussung der energieliefernden Prozesse der Zelle durch Röntgenstrahlen. Strahlentherapie **102**, 517 (1957).
REED, G.B., COX, A.J.: The human liver after radiation injury. A form of veno-occlusive disease. Amer. J. Path. **48**, 597 (1966).
REUTER, A.M., GERBER, G.B., KENNES, F., REMY-DEFRAIGNE, J.: Catabolism of serum proteins after X-irradiation. Radiat. Res. **30**, 725 (1967).
RENÉ, A.A., DARDEN, J.H., PARKER, J.L.: Radiation-induced ultrastructural and biochemical changes in lysosomes. Lab. Invest. **25**, 230 (1971).
Report of the United Nations Scientific Committee on the effects of atomic radiation. General Assembly: Official Record Suppl. **16**, (A/5216) U.N. New York 1962.
REUTTER, W., LESCH, R., KEPPLER, D., DECKER, K.: Galaktosamin-Hepatitis. Naturwissenschaften **55**, 497 (1968).
RICHMOND, J.E., ORD, M.G., STOCKEN, L.A.: The effect of X-irradiation in vivo on protein and nucleoprotein metabolism in the rat. Biochem. J. **66**, 123 (1957).
RICOTTI, V, NOTARIO, A.: Metabolic changes in hepatic tissue in mice after panirradiation with lethal doses. Experimental research conducted with the use of labelling substance. Minerva nucl. **7**, 18 (1962).
RIGLER, L.G., KOUCKY, R., ABRAHAM, A.L.: The effects of thorium dioxide sol (thorotrast) on the human liver. Radiology **25**, 521 (1935).
ROBACK, S.A., NESBIT, M.E., JR., SHARP, H.L., D'ANGIO, G.J., LEONHARD, A.S.: Portal hypertension following surgery X-radiation and actinomycin D therapy of nephroblastoma. J. Pediat. **78**, 1031 (1971).
RÖSSLE, R.: Spätschäden nach Thorotrast. Zbl. allg. Path. path. Anat. **85**, 227 (1949).
ROMANTSEV, E.F., ZEMLANOVA, Z.I.: Acetylation of sulfanilamide in animals irradiated with roentgen rays. Biokhimiya **21**, 685 (1956).
ROSENBAUM, F.J.: Lebersarkom nach Thorotrast. Dtsch. med. Wschr. **84**, 428 (1959).
ROSS, J.M.: A case illustrating the effects of prolonged action of radium. J. Path. Bact. **35**, 899 (1932).
ROSS, M.H., ELY, J.O.: Radiation effects on liver glycogen in the rat. J cell. comp. Physiol. **37**, 163 (1951).
ROTBLAT, J., WARD, G.B.: Tissue dosage from thorotrast in the body. Nature (Lond.) **172**, 769 (1953).
ROTBLAT, J., WARD, G.: The radioactivity from thorotrast and its retention in tissues. Phys. in Med. Biol. **1**, 125 (1956).
ROTH, J.S., EICHEL, H.J., WASE, A., ALPER, C., BOYD, M.J.: Effect of total body X-irradiation in some enzymes of rat tissues. Arch. Biochim. Biophys. **44**, 95 (1953).
ROTHE, F.: Thorotrastkarzinom der Bronchien. Zbl. allg. Path. path. Anat. **96**, 417 (1957).
ROUSSY, G., GUERIN, M.: Le cancer expérimental provoqué par le dioxide de thorium. Presse méd. **2**, 761 (1941).
ROUSSY, G., OBERLING, E., GUERIN, M.: Action cancérigène du dioxide de thorium chez le rat blanc. Bull. Acad. Méd. (Paris) **112**, 809 (1934).
RUBIN, P., CASARETT, G.W.: Clinical Radiation Pathology. Philadelphia-London-Toronto: W.B. Saunders 1968.
RUDNICKI, T.: Beitrag zur biologischen Wirkung der 30-MeV-Elektronen. Fortschr. Röntgenstr. **98**, 187 (1963).
RUDOLPHI, H.: Spätentwicklung eines Unterlidkarzinoms nach Thoriumoxydinjektion. Beitr. path. Anat. **111**, 158 (1950).
RÜBER, W.: Das EEG bei fraktionierter Bestrahlung des Gehirns. Strahlentherapie **119**, 442 (1962).
RUGH, R.: X-rays: Are there cyclic variations in radiosensitivity? Science **142**, 53 (1963).
RUGH, R.: Damage to cells by ionizing radiation. Atompraxis **14**, 13 (1968).
RUSHMER, H.N., ALTMAN, K.I.: Unpublished experiments (1967), cit. in: GERBER, G.B. and ALTMAN, K.I., The liver. In: Radiation Biochemistry (K.I. ALTMAN, G.B. GERBER and S. OKADA, eds.,), vol. II. New York and London: Academic Press 1970.
RUST, J.H., LEROY, G.V., SPRATT, J.L., HO, G.B., ROTH, L.J.: Effect of radiation on intermediary metabolism of the rat. Radiat. Res. **20**, 703 (1963).

Sabin, F.R., Doan, C.A., Forkner, C.E.: The production of osteogenic sarcomata and the effect on lymph nodes and bone marrow of intravenous injection of radium chloride and mesothorium in rabbits. J. exp. Med. **56**, 267 (1932).

Samuels, J.D., Grosfield, J.I., Kartha, M.: Radiation hepatitis in children. J. Pediat. **78**, 68 (1971).

Sarkar, N.K., Devi, A, Hempelmann, L.H.: Effects of irradiation on the incorporation of amino-acid into normal and regenerating rat liver. Nature (Lond.) **192**, 179 (1961).

Sarrazin, D., Guy, E., Schweisguth, O.: Séquelles osseuses radiothérapiques des tumeurs de la fosse lombaire chez l'enfant. Ann. Radiol. (Paris) **4**, 767 (1961).

Sassen, A., Gerber, G.B., Kennes, F., Remy-Defraigne, J.: Incorporation of H^3-phenylamine into serum proteins by the perfused liver of normal and X-irradiated rats. Radiat. Res. **25**, 158 (1965).

Scaife, F.J., Alexander, P.: Inability of X-rays to alter the permeability of mitochondria. Radiat. Res. **15**, 658 (1961).

Scaife, F.J., Hill, B.: The uncoupling of oxidative phosphorylation by ionizing radiation. Canad. J. Biochem. **40**, 1025 (1962).

Scaife, F.J., Hill, B.: Uncoupling of oxidative phosphorylation by ionizing radiation. II. The stability of mitochondrial lipids and cytochrome C. Canad. J. Biochem. **41**, 1223 (1963).

Scheer, K.E., Krauss, O., Varga, L.: Neutronen-Aktivierungsanalyse zur Bestimmung von Thorotrast in Gewebsproben. Atompraxis **13**, 451 (1967).

Scheibe, G.: Generalisierte Thorotrastspätschäden. Med. Welt **24**, 1709 (1973).

Scherer, E.: Morphologische und fermenthistochemische Studien zur Strahlenwirkung auf den Organismus. Strahlentherapie **99**, 230 (1956a).

Scherer, E.: Morphologische und fermenthistochemische Studien zur Strahlenwirkung auf den Organismus. II. Fermenthistochemische Untersuchungen an Organen der weißen Maus. Strahlentherapie **99**, 243 (1956b).

Scherer, E.: Cytologische und karyometrische Untersuchungen zur Strahlenwirkung auf Leber und Milz bei Anwendung von Total- und Teilbestrahlung. I. Mitteilung: Untersuchungen an der Leber der weißen Maus. Strahlentherapie **100**, 86 (1956).

Scherer, E.: In: Strahlenpathologie der Zelle. Stuttgart: Thieme 1963.

Scherer, E., Stender, H.S.: Strahlenpathologie der Zelle. Stuttgart: Thieme 1963.

Schinz, H.R.: Strahlenschäden des Rückenmarkes. Dtsch. med. Wschr. **89**, 796 (1964).

Schneider, M., O'Rourke, F., Redetzki, H.M.: X-irradiation and diphosphopyridine nucleotide (DPN) levels in ascitestumor cells and liver tissue of mice. Int. J. Radiat. Biol. **5**, 183 (1962).

Schneider, W.C., Brownell, L.W.: Deoxyribosidic compounds in regenerating liver. J. nat. Cancer Inst. **18**, 579 (1957).

Schneikert, D.: Kerngrößenveränderungen in der Rattenleber nach Röntgenbestrahlung und Galaktosamin-Applikation. Inaug.-Diss. Freiburg, 1973.

Scholtz, W.: Über die physiologische Wirkung der Radiumstrahlen und ihre therapeutische Verwendung. Dtsch. med. Wschr. **1**, 94 (1904).

Schreiber, W.M., Kato, H., Roberston, J.D.: Primary carcinoma of the liver in Hiroshima and Nagasaki, Japan. J. Hiroshima med. Ass. **24**, 794 (1971).

Schreier, K., Diferrante, N., Gaffney, G.W., Hempelmann, L.H., Altman, K.I.: Cellular destruction and protein breakdown induced by exposure to X-rays. Arch. Biochem. Biophys. **50**, 417 (1954).

Schreiner, L.: Über Thorotrastschäden mit Entstehung eines sarkomatösen Hämanioendothelioms der Leber. Z. Krebsforsch. **64**, 169 (1961).

Schubert, G., Bettendorf, G., Künkel, H., Maass, H., Rathgen G.H.: Untersuchungen zum Einfluß von Röntgenstrahlen auf den C^{14}-Alanin-Einbau in die Proteine von Leberhomogenaten und Tumorzellen. Strahlentherapie **106**, 483 (1958).

Schümmelfeder, N.: Die experimentelle Strahlenschädigung des Zentralnervensystems. Ergebn. allg. Path. path. Anat. **42**, 34 (1962).

Schwanzer, A.W., Federlin, K.: Salpingographie mit Thorotrast vor 23 Jahren und Entstehung eines Ovarialkarzinoms. Geburtsh. u. Frauenheilk. **17**, 225 (1957).

Schwarz, H.P., Dreisbach, L., Barrionuevo, M., Kleschick, A., Kosty,, J.: The effect of ionizing irradiation on the lipid composition of the liver mitochondria of rats. Arch. Biochem. Biophys. **92**, 133 (1961).

Scott, C.M.: Some quantitative aspects of the biological action of X and γ rays. Med. Res. Council, Spec. Rep. Ser. **223**, 5, 74 (1937).

Selbie, F.: Tumors in rats and mice following injection of thorotrast. Brit. J. exp. Path. **19**, 100 (1938).

Selding, M.: Über die Wirkung der Röntgen- und Radiumstrahlen auf innere Organe der Tiere. Fortschr. Röntgenstr. **7**, 322 (1904).

Sestan, N.: Effect of whole-body X-irradiation on ^{14}C-leucine incorporation into proteins of cell nuclei of regenerating rat liver. Nature (Lond.) **205**, 615 (1965).

Shaber, G.S., Miller, L.L.: Studies on fibrinogen turnover before and after whole-body X-irradiation in the rat. Proc. Soc. exp. Biol. (N.Y.) **113**, 346 (1963).

SILVA-HORTA, J.: Lebersarkom einer Frau 3 Jahre und 2 Monate nach Thorotrastinjektion. Chirurg **24**, 218 (1953).

SILVA-HORTA, J.: Late lesions in man caused by colloidal thorium dioxide (thorotrast). Arch. Path. **62**, 403 (1956).

SIMONOV, V.V.: Fosfolipidy mitokhondrii kletock pecheni i podvergnutykh obshchemii gamma-obluchemilu. Radiobiologiya **5**, 907 (1965).

SIMPSON, G.E.C., FINCKH, E.S.: The pattern of regeneration of rat liver after repeated partial hepatectomies. J. Path. Bact. **86**, 361 (1963).

SKIDMORE, W.D.: Respiratory control and swelling in rat liver mitochondria: Effect of ^{60}Co Gamma radiation and injected nutrient. J. Nutr. **103**, 836 (1973).

SMITH, K.C., LOW-BEER, B.V.A.:The effect of whole-body X-irradiation on the enzymatic activity of several rat tissues toward uridine, uridylic acid, cytidine, and cytidylic acid. Radiat. Res. **6**, 521 (1957).

SMYTH, F.S., WHIPPLE, G.H.: Bile salt metabolism. II. Proteose and X-rays intoxication. J. biol. Chem. **59**, 636 (1924).

SOLS, A., SILLERO, A., SALAS, J.: Insulin-dependent synthesis of glucokinase. J. cell. comp. Physiol. **66**, 23 (1965).

SOSKA, J., SKALKA, M., BEZDEK, M.: Effect of ionizing radiation on the free deoxyribonucleoside and deoxyribonucleotide content of regenerating rat liver. Folia biol. (Prague) **8**, 239 (1962).

STACEY, K.A.: The inhibition of DNA synthesis by calf thymus polymerase by X-irradiation of the primer DNA. Biochem. biophys. Res. Commun. **5**, 486 (1961).

STEER, A.: Personal communication (1974).

STEGNER, W.: Das Regenerationsverhalten vorbestrahlter Rattenlebern nach wiederholter Teilhepatektomie. Inaug.-Diss. Freiburg, 1974.

STEMMERMANN, G.N.: Adenocarcinoma of the intrahepatic tree following thorotrast. Amer. J. clin. Path. **34**, 446 (1960).

STIRRET, L.A., YUHL, E.T., CASSEN, B.: Clinical applications of hepatic radioactivity surveys. Amer. J. Gastroent. **21**, 310 (1954).

STÖCKER, E.: Altersabhängige Proliferationskinetik im Leberepithel der Ratte. Exp. Gerontologie. Stuttgart: Thieme 1974.

STÖCKER, E., ALTMANN, H.-W.: Die DNS-Synthese in Leberparenchymzellen und Gallengangsepithelien von normalen und Thioazetamidbehandelten Ratten. Naturwissenschaften **51**, 15 (1964).

STÖCKER, E., WULLSTEIN, H.K., BRÄU, G.: Zur Regenerationskapazität des Leberepithels junger, wiederholt teilhepatektomierter Ratten. Autoradiographische Untersuchungen nach kontinuierlicher Dauerinfusion von ^{3}H-Thymidin. Virchows Arch. Abt. B **14**, 93 (1973).

STOLMAN, F., JR.: The Kinetics of Cellular Proliferation. New York: Grune & Stratton 1959.

STRANGEWAYS, T.S.P., OAKLEY, H.E.H.: The immediate changes observed in tissue cells after exposure to soft X-rays while growing in vitro. Proc. Soc. roy. Biol. **95**, 373 (1923).

STREFFER, CH.: Untersuchungen über den Energiestoffwechsel im Lebergewebe der Maus nach Ganzkörperbestrahlung. Int. J. Radiat. Biol. **11**, 179 (1966a).

STREFFER, CH.: Tryptophan und seine Metabolite in der Radiobiologie und im chemischen Strahlenschutz. Radiol. clin. (Basel) **35**, 358 (1966b).

STREFFER, CH.: The formation of nicotinamide-adenine dinucleotide from tryptophan after whole-body irradiation. Germ. med. Mtn. **12**, 35 (1967).

STREFFER, CH.: Beziehungen zwischen biochemischen Veränderungen und Mortalität nach Ganzkörperbestrahlung von Mäusen. Int. J. Radiat. Biol. **12**, 487 (1967).

STREFFER, CH.: The biosynthesis of NAD in the liver of irradiated mice. J. Vitaminol. **14**, 130 (1968).

STREFFER, CH.: Metabolic changes in mice after modification of radiosensitivity. Biophysical Aspects of Radiat. Qual. 1971.

STREFFER, CH., LANGENDORFF, H.-U.: Zum Abbau des Tryptophans und Kynurenins nach Ganzkörperbestrahlung im Lebergewebe der Maus. Int. J. Radiat. Biol. **11**, 455 (1966).

STREFFER, CH., MELCHING, H.J.: Untersuchungen über einen biologischen Strahlenschutz. 58. Mitteilung: Der Gehalt von Aminosäuren in der Leber und Niere weißer Mäuse nach Ganzkörperbestrahlung. Strahlentherapie **125**, 341 (1964).

STREFFER, CH., MELCHING, H.J.: Untersuchungen über einen biologischen Strahlenschutz. 65. Mitteilung: Ein Beitrag zum Glutamatstoffwechsel in der Leber von Mäusen nach Ganzkörperbestrahlung. Strahlentherapie **128**, 406 (1965).

STREFFER, CH., SCHAFFERUS, S.: The induction of liver enzymes by cortisol after combined treatment of mice with X-irradiation and inhibitors of protein biosynthesis. Int. J. Radiat. Biol. **20**, 301 (1971).

STREFFER, CH., SCHWEIGER, K.: Zur biochemischen Wirkung einiger strahlensensibilisierender Substanzen. Strahlentherapie **143**, 244 (1972).

STREFFER, CH., TRIBUKAIT, B., SCHAFFERUS, S.: Über die Änderungen der natürlichen Strahlenresistenz der Maus nach mehrtägigem Aufenthalt in Hypoxie: Enzymaktivitäten des Tryptophan- und Cysteinstoffwechsels. Strahlentherapie **139**, 626 (1970).

SUCKOW, E., HENEGAR, G.D., BASERGA, R.: Tumors of the liver following administration of thorotrast. Amer. J. Path. **38**, 663 (1961).

SUSSMAN, H.: Kerngröße von Leberzellen der Maus nach Röntgenbestrahlung. Oncologia **9**, 373 (1956).

SYROMATNIKOVA, N.V.: Certain aspects of the proteinic function of the liver observed in the course of the development of radiation disease. Dokl. Akad. Nauk SSSR **111**, 730 (1956).

SZCZUREK, Z.: Die Pathomorphologie der Leber in experimentell hervorgerufener Strahlenkrankheit bei Kaninchen. Int. Arch. Gewerbepath. Gewerbehyg. **23**, 19 (1967).

TAFT, R.B.: Demonstration of gamma radiation from living patients following thorotrast injection. Radiology **29**, 530 (1937).

TAPLIN, G.V., MEREDITH, O.M., JR., KADE, H.: The radioactive (J^{131} tagged) rose bengal uptake excretion test for liver function using external gamma-ray scintillation counting techniques. J. Lab. clin. Med. **45**, 665 (1955).

TEFFT, M.: Irradiation of the liver in children: Review of experience in the acute and chronic phases and in the intact normal and partially resected. Amer. J. Roentgenol. **108**, 365 (1970).

TESLUK, H., NORDIN, W.A.: Hemangioendothelioma of liver following thorium dioxide administration. Arch. Path. **60**, 493 (1955).

THOMAS, S.F., HENRY, G.W., KAPLAN, H.S.: Hepatolienography: Past, present and future. Radiology **57**, 669 (1951).

THOMSON, J.F.: Effects of total-body X-irradiation on phosphate esterification and hydrolysis in mitochondrial preparations of rat spleens. Radiat. Res. **21**, 46 (1964).

THOMSON, J.F., KLIPFEL, F.J.: Effect of X-irradiation on increase in rat liver tryptophan peroxidase produced by adrenal steroids. Proc. Soc. exp. Biol. (N.Y.) **95**, 108 (1957).

THOMSON, J.F., MIKUTA, E.T.: The effect of cortisone and hydrocortisone on the tryptophan peroxidase-oxidase activity of rat liver. Endocrinology **55**, 232 (1954).

THOMSON, J.F., RAHMAN, Y.E.: Effect of X-irradiation on distribution and properties of cytoplasmic particulates of rat liver. Radiat. Res. **17**, 573 (1962).

TOPOROVA, G.P.: The actions of X-rays on nucleic acid metabolism in the liver. Dokl. Akad. Nauk SSSR **114**, 454 (1957).

TRASINO, M., MACARINI, N., GANDOLFO, E.: Ricerche istologiche ed istochimiche sul tessuto epatico e pancreatico di animali trattati con raggi roentgen. Minerva fisioter. **4**, 144 (1959).

TRETYAKOVA, K.A.: Vkliuchemie C^{14}-atsetata kholesterin i zhirneye kisloty pecheni adrenalektomirovangykh krys usloviiakh obluchemiia. Byull. éksp. Biol. Med. **57**, 47 (1964).

TRETYAKOVA, K.A., GRODZENSKII, D.E.: The rate of synthesis of cholesterol and fatty acids in the adrenals, testes and liver of young and old rats in normal conditions and after the irradiations. Biokhimiya **25**, 399 (1960).

TRIBONDEAU, L., HUDELLET, G.: Action des rayons X sur le foie du chat nouveau-né. C.R. Soc. Biol. (Paris) **62**, 102 (1907).

TRIPOLI, C.J., HAAM, E.V.: Effects of toxic and non-toxic doses of thorium dioxide in various animals. Proc. Soc. exp. Biol. (N.Y.) **29**, 1053 (1932).

TRÜBESTEIN, G.K., CITOLER, P.: Drei Fälle von Thorotrast-Spätschäden. Med. Klin. **68**, 1442 (1973).

TSCHASSOWRIKOW, N.: Über die Wirkung der Röntgenstrahlen auf den feinen Bau der Leberzellen beim Frosch. Virchows Arch. path. Anat. **269**, 166 (1928).

TSUCHIYA, T., HAYAKAWA, J.-I., MURAMATSU, S., ETO, H., SUGAHARA, T.: Radiosensitivity and thyroid function in mice. Radiat. Res. **19**, 316 (1963).

TSUKADA, K., LIEBERMAN, I.: Metabolism of nucleolar ribonucleic acid after partial hepatectomy. J. biol. Chem. **239**, 1564 (1964).

TSUZUKI, M.: Erfahrungen über radioaktive Schädigung der japanischen Fischer durch Bikini Asche. Münch. med. Wschr. **97**, 988 (1955).

TUDWAY, R.C.: The age factor in the susceptibility of man and animals to radiation. III. The age of the patient and tolerance to radiation. Brit. J. Radiol. **35**, 36 (1962).

UCHIYAMA, R., FAUSTO, N., VAN LANCKER, J.L.: Metabolic alterations after total body doses of X-irradiation. The effects of X-irradiation on rapidly labeled RNA. Arch. Biochem. Biophys. **110**, 191 (1965).

UCHIYAMA, T., FAUSTO, N., VAN LANCKER, J.L.: Molecular mechanisms of liver regeneration. V. The effect of X-irradiation on the incorporation of ^{14}C orotic acid into rapidly labeled nuclear RNA. J. biol. Chem. **241**, 991 (1966).

UMEGAKI, Y., MATSUZAWA, T.: Deoxygenation radiotherapy. Nippon Acta radiol. (Stockh.) **22**, 1327 (1963).

UNGER, E.: Histologische und histochemische Beobachtungen an der Rattenleber nach lokaler und nach Ganzkörperbestrahlung. Rad. biol. ther. **9**, 723 (1968).

UNNEWEHR, F., KAUL, A., STAHLHOFEN, W.: Messung von ^{232}Th, ^{228}Th und deren Folgeprodukten in Gewebeproben von Thorotrastpatienten. Atomenergie **9**, 181 (1964).

USSELMAN, J.A.: Liver scanning in the assessment of liver damage from therapeutic external irradiation. J. nucl. Med. **7**, 761 (1966).

VANDERGOTEN, R., GOUTIER, R.: Effect of total-body X-irradiation and of chemical protector AET administration on the activity of nuclear RNA polymerase in regenerating rat liver. Int. J. Radiat. Biol. **11**, 449 (1966).

VAN LANCKER, J.L.: Inhibition of incorporation of ^{3}H thymidine in tissue homogenate after total body doses of X-radiation. Biochim. biophys. Acta (Amst.) **33**, 587 (1959).

VAN LANCKER, J.L.: Metabolic alterations after total body doses of X-irradiation. II. Incorporation of deoxycytidylic and thymidylic acid into purified DNA and nuclei in presence of regenerating-liver supernatant. Biochim. biophys. Acta (Amst.) **45**, 63 (1960).

VAN LANCKER, J.L.: Molecular pathology of irradiation. Lab. Invest. **15**, 192 (1966).

VAN LANCKER, J.L.: In: Biochemistry of Cell Division. Springfield, Illinois: Thomas 1969.

VELLENGA, L.R.: A case of hemangiosarcoma of the liver occurring 25 years after injection of thorotrast for cerebral aniography. Acta leidensia **33**, 226 (1965).

VENINGA, T.S., MORSE, H.: Contributions to the study of immediate and early X-ray reactions with regard to chemoprotection. X. The effect of pyridoxine-deficiency in mice on their radiosensitivity. Int. J. Radiat. Biol. **9**, 399 (1965).

VERGA, V., CALL, A.: Veränderungen des Lebergewebes der Ratte und insbesondere des argentophilen Gerüstes nach direkter fraktionierter Röntgenbestrahlung der Leber. Strahlentherapie **112**, 608 (1960).

VINOGRADOVA, M.F.: Influence of X-ray irradiation on the rate of the renewal of lipids and cholesterol in the liver of white rats. Vestn. Leningr. Univ., Ser. Biol. **17**, 102 (1962).

VÖGTLIN, J., MINDER, W.: Über Thorotrastschäden nach Bronchographie, retrograder Pyelographie, Salpingographie und Arteriographie. Radiol. clin. (Basel) **21**, 96 (1952).

WACHSMUTH, W.: Untersuchungen über die gewebeschädigende Wirkung von Thorotrast. Chirurg **19**, 390 (1948).

WACHTLER, F.: Über strahlenbedingte Schäden im knöchernen Skelett. Radiol. austriaca **12**, 253 (1961).

WALDSCHMIDT, M.: Das Verhalten von Bernsteinsäure-Dehydrogenase und NADH-Cytochrom-C-Reduktase in Leber-, Milz- und Thymusmitochondrien von Ratten nach Bestrahlung *in vivo*. Strahlentherapie **128**, 586 (1965).

WALDSCHMIDT, M.: Harnstoff- und Ammoniakgehalt der Leber nach Bestrahlung *in vivo*. Int. J. Radiat. Biol. **11**, 429 (1966).

WALDSCHMIDT, M.: Änderungen des Gehalts einiger energiereicher Phosphatverbindungen in der Mäuseleber in vivo. Strahlentherapie **135**, 695 (1968).

WARREN, S.L.: The physiological effects of radiation upon organ and body systems. In: Biological Effects of Radiation. New York: McGraw-Hill 1936.

WARREN, S., FRIEDMAN, N.: Effects of radiation on normal tissues. IV. Effects of radiation on the gastro-intestinal tract, including the salivary glands, the liver and the pancreas. Arch. Path. **31**, 749 (1942).

WARREN, SH., GATES, O.: Spontaneous and induced tumors of the guinea pig. Cancer Res. **1**, 65 (1941).

WARTHIN, A.S.: Changes produced in kidneys by roentgen irradiation. Amer. J. med. Sci. **133**, 736 (1907).

WEBER, G., CANTERO, A.: Effect of X-irradiation on hepatic carbohydrate enzymes in control and hypophysectomized rats. Amer. J. Physiol. **197**, 1284 (1959).

WEBER, M.M., STICH, H.F.: Formation of cell colonies in X-irradiated regenerating livers of rats. Canad. J. Biochem. **43**, 817 (1965).

WEGENER, K., KAMPMANN, H., WESCH, H.: Lymphknotenveränderungen bei menschlichen Thorotrastosen (pathologisch-anatomische, autoradiographische und quantitative Untersuchungen mittels der Neutronenaktivierungsanalyse). In: Strahlenempfindlichkeit von Organen und Organsystemen der Säugetiere und des Menschen vol. 18. Stuttgart: Thieme 1973.

WEGENER, K., WESCH, H., KAMPMANN, H.: Retikuloendotheliales System und Thorotrastose nach diagnostischer Angiographie. Dtsch. med. Wschr. **96**, 1977 (1971).

WEGENER, K., ZAHNERT, R.: Bericht über pathologisch-anatomische und autoradiographische Untersuchungen an 9 Fällen menschlicher Thorotrastose. Virchows Arch. Abt. A **351**, 316 (1970).

WEINBREN, K., FITCHEN, W., COHEN, M.: The unmasking by regeneration of latent irradiation effects in the rat liver. Brit. J. Radiol. **33**, 419 (1960).

WEINBREN, K., GHORPADE, K.V.: The effect of bile duct ligation on latent irradiation effects in the rat liver. Brit. J. Radiol. **33**, 426 (1960).

WELLING, W., COHEN, J.A.: Disturbance of RNA turnover in the cell nucleus by X-irradiation in the early phase of rat liver regeneration. Biochim. biophys. Acta (Amst.) **42**, 181 (1960).

WENIG, W.: Der latente Strahlenschaden der Leber. Inaug.-Diss. Freiburg (1974).

WEN-MEI, S.: Oxidative phosphorylation and optical density of mitochondria of normal and regenerating livers of rats subjected to general irradiation by X-rays. Radiobiologiya **3**, 159 (1963).

WERNZE, H., BRAUN, H., GABAR, M.: Über die hepatische Farbstoffexkretion bei verändertem Bromsulphthalein-Metabolismus nach Röntgenbestrahlung. Klin. Wschr. **40**, 1220 (1962).

WERTHEMANN, A.: Über Spätschäden verschiedener Organe durch Thorotrast und autoradiographischer Nachweis desselben. Schweiz. Z. Path. **22**, 350 (1959).

WESELOH, G., NIKFETRAT, A., GREGL, A., EGER, W.: Beiträge zu Spätveränderungen der Rattenleber nach Ganzkörper- und Lokalbestrahlung. Strahlentherapie **133**, 86 (1967).

Wetterer, J.: Handbuch der Röntgen- und Radium-Therapie. Leipzig-München: Keim und Nemnich 1922.
Wharton, J.T., Delclos, L., Gallager, S., Smith, J.P.: Radiation hepatitis induced by abdominal irradiation with the Cobalt 60 moving strip technique. Amer. J. Roentgenol. **117**, 73 (1973).
White, J., Burr, B.E., Cool, H.T., David, P.W., Ally, M.S.: Level of protein intake and nitrogen excretion in rats following total-body X-irradiation. J. nat. Cancer Inst. **15**, 1145 (1955).
Wiley, A.L., Jr., Vogel, H.H., Jr., Clifton, K.H.: The effect of variations in LET and cell cycle on radiation hepatocarcinogenesis. Radiat. Res. **54**, 284 (1973).
Williams, G.M., Elliott, J.M., Weisburger, J.H.: Carcinoma after malignant conversion in vitro of epithelial-like cells from rat liver following exposure to chemical carcinogens. Cancer Res. **33**, 606 (1973).
Willis, D.A., Bachem, A.: The effects of roentgen rays upon the kidney. Amer. J. Roentgenol. **18**, 334 (1927).
Wills, E.D., Wilkinson, A.E.: Release of enzymes from lysosomes by irradiation and the relation of lipid peroxide formation to enzyme release. Biochem. J. **99**, 657 (1966).
Wilson, M.E., Stowell, R.E.: Cytological changes following roentgen irradiation of the liver in mice. J. nat. Cancer Inst. **13**, 1123 (1953).
Wiss, O., Weber, R.: In: Vitamines and Hormones. New York-London: Academic Press 1964.
Wolff, S.: Chromosome aberrations and the cell cycle. Radiat. Res. **33**, 609 (1968).
Yatvin, M.B., Lamar, C., Jr., Pitot, H.C.: The effect of gamma-radiation and actinomycin on cortisone induction of liver enzymes. Proc. Soc. exp. Biol. (N.Y.) **139**, 1220 (1972).
Yatvin, M.B., Lathrop, T.P.: Polyribosome response in regenerating liver following ionizing radiation. Biochem. biophys. Res. Commun. **25**, 535 (1966).
Yost, H.T., Jr., Glickman, R.M., Beck, L.H.: Studies on the effects of irradiation of cellular particulates. IV. The time sequence of phosphorylation changes in vivo. Biol. Bull. **127**, 173 (1964a).
Yost, H.T., Jr., Richmond, S.S., Beck, L.H.: Studies on the effects of irradiation of cellular particulates. V. Acceleration of recovery of phosphorylation by polyanions. Biol. Bull. **127**, 526 (1964b).
Yost, H.T., Jr., Yost, M.T., Robson, H.H.: Studies on the effects of irradiation of cellular particulates. VI. Comparison of uncoupling at the three phosphorylating sites. Biol. Bull. **133**, 697 (1967a).
Yost, M.T., Robson, H.H., Yost, H.T., Jr.: Uncoupling of oxidative phosphorylation in rat liver and spleen mitochondria by exposure to total-body irradiation. Radiat. Res. **32**, 187 (1967b).
Zeman, W.: Die Wirkung ionisierender Strahlen auf das Nervensystem. Dtsch. med. Wschr. **86**, 1196 (1961).
Zicha, B., Benes, J., Dienstbier, Z.: The effect of ionizing radiation on stationary concentration of the metabolites of anaerobic glycolysis in the liver of rats whole-body irradiated by the dose of 1400 R. Strahlentherapie **135**, 467 (1968).
Zollinger, H.U.: Ein Spindelzellsarkom der Niere, 16 Jahre nach Thorotrast-Pyelographie. Schweiz. med. Wschr. **79**, 1266 (1949).
Zollinger, H.U.: Radio-Histologie und Radio-Histopathologie. In: Handbuch der allgemeinen Pathologie, vol. X/1. Berlin-Heidelberg-Göttingen: Springer 1960.
Zuppinger, A.: Die Aufgabe der Strahlenbiologie im Rahmen der Strahlentherapie. Schweiz. med. Wschr. **93**, 845 (1962).

Experimental Production of Gallstones

JOB HARENBERG

In Western communities the major component of gallstones is cholesterol, which is held in solution in the bile by formation of micelles in which phospholipid and bile salts are involved. The ratio of cholesterol to bile salts and phospholipids determines cholesterol solubility. The most effective method for the experimental formation of gallstones is brought about by supersaturation with cholesterol. On the basis of the above-mentioned ratio, supersaturation results either by an overproduction of cholesterol or by diminishing the excretion of bile salts or phospholipids of liver cells. DENBESTEN et al. (1974) found that the formation of gallstones in prairie dogs induced by a high cholesterol diet was preceded by a shift of cholic acid to chenodeoxycholic acid concentration in bile salts. This seems to be of great importance, because it could lead to development of a method to predict gallstone formation in man.

A. A Fat- and Cholesterol-Free Diet in Hamsters

DAM and CHRISTENSEN (1952) fed hamsters a cholesterol-free and nearly fat-free "284" dietary regimen (Table 1) or the same diet slightly modified by omission of vitamin E or by its replacement with tetraethyl-thiuram-disulfide (Antabuse). After 87 days the animals were killed; 16 of 18 had gallstones while of those killed earlier, only 1 of 14 had such stones.

Further studies of "284" diet were made by ROBINS and FASULO (1973). By direct analysis of this diet they found that it contained only 0.08% total lipid and 0.04% total essential fatty acids, present entirely as linoleic acid. This "essential

Table 1. Diet "284": To each 100 g of the diet were added 20 mg of 1 tocopherol-acetate. Vitamins A and D were given as an aqueous solution, 1 ml of which contained 7000 IU vitamine A "natural ester and 103 IU of vitamin D_2 in 0.114 mg peanut oil in a 0.1 g. Tween 80 solution protected against autoxidation by 1.0 mg ethyl gellate. Each animal received 5 drops a week. (From DAM and CHRISTENSEN, 1952)

Casein "low vitamin"	20.0 g
Sucrose	74.3 g
Salt mixtures	5.0 g
Choline chloride	0.2 g
Vitamin mixture	0.5 g
	100.0 g

fatty acid-deficient" EFAD diet was fed to male Syrian hamsters. They formed lithogenic hepatic bile and gallstones of high cholesterol content. At 30 days of age animals were caged in pairs and fed ad lib. either the gallstone-inducing EFAD diet or one of the two lipid-containing diets which do not result in gallstone production: Purina lab chow or a synthetic diet of the same composition as the EFAD diet but with 5% safflower oil added. Because synthetic diets apparently modify bile acid turnover, kinetic studies were performed in animals after at least 2 weeks of dietary equilibration. Through a small laparotomy incision a tracer amount of sodium cholate-carboxyl ^{14}C (0.9–1.1 μc) was injected directly into the duodenal lumen. Upon recovery hamsters were individually housed in cages with attached tunnels through which combined feces and urine were collected at daily intervals of 4–6 days. After this period of isotope excretion, each animal was reoperated to determine the cholate pool and the bile salt secretion rate. Cholate specific activity and cholate and total bile salt output were determined from the first 30-min bile collection. The cumulative excretion of radioactivity in stool and urine was substracted from the amount of radioactivity administered. The calculated amount of radioactivity remaining in the animal at the time that bile cholate specific activity was determined was used to represent radioactivity at "zero-time." Thus, the pool size could be measured by dividing "zero-time" radioactivity by bile salt specific activity. In some experiments after the 30-min period of bile collection, total cholesterol was determined in plasma and in liver. Plasma volume was assumed to average 4.9% of hamster body weight and total plasma cholesterol was expressed in milligrams per gram of body weight ×100. In these studies 11% of hamsters (1 of 9) had stones after 10 days on the EFAD diet, 48% (5 of 11) had stones at 18 days, and 75% (9 of 12) had stones after 24 days. Furthermore, gallstones were larger and more numerous after a longer period on the EFAD diet. After 24 days up to 2 months the incidence of stone production did not increase and remained about 75–80%. Gallstones were at no time observed in hamsters fed the Purine lab chow or the safflower oil-enriched diet. The fractional excretion and daily amount of cholate excretion was significantly different in the two dietary groups. The most pronounced effect of EFAD feeding was on bilary cholesterol secretion, which in the two control groups was almost identical as shown (Table 2). In contrast, in EFAD-fed hamsters bilary cholesterol secretion was two- to three-fold greater than in the control group,

Table 2. Effect of control and EFAD diets on bile volume and secretion rate of bile salts, phospholipids, and cholesterol. Measruements obtained from first 30-min bile collection after common diet shown as mean ± SD, EFAS-essential fatty acid supplemented. (From ROBINS and FASULO, 1974)

Diet group	No. of animals	Days on diet	Gallstones in animals (%)	Bile volume (μl/½ h)	Secretion rate		
					Bile salts (μg/½ h)	Phospholipids (μg/½ h)	Cholesterol (μg/½ h)
Control (CF)	12	17–60	0	102±28	1219±392	239± 97	25±11
Control (EFAS)	8	10–45	0	102±35	847±380	196±106	23± 9
EFAD	5	10	11	151±37	1611±650	205± 67	47±14
	15	17–24	48	129±43	1320±663	210± 85	45±25
	13	38–60	75	138±39	1420±545	435±197	77±49

and was significantly increased even after 10 days of feeding. In 10 of the 33 EFAD hamsters, shown in Table 2, gallstones were not observed, but cholesterol secretion was also significantly increased compared with the control group. (41 ± 12 vs. 24 ± 10 μg/30-min). The EFAD hamsters secreted excessive amounts of cholesterol in the bile in the prestone period and after gallstone production. The lithogenic potential of hepatic bile in these animals can be related directly to the hepatic cholesterol output.

B. A Lithogenic Diet Supplemented with Chenodeoxycholic Acid

Hamsters fed a lithogenic diet showed a significantly stronger tendency to gallstone formation if the diet was supplemented with 0.5% chenodeoxycholic acid (BERGMAN and VAN DER LINDEN, 1973). Sixten hamsters of both sexes were randomly divided into two equal groups. One group was fed the gallstone-inducing diet "284". The other group was given the same diet supplemented with 0.5% chenodeoxycholic acid. At the end of the dietary period, the common bile duct was ligated at its terminal and enough time (about 30 min) was allowed to complete filling of the gallbladder, which was rhen removed and its contents collected. Free bile acids were separated by thin-layer chromatography together with cholic acid, chenodeoxycholic acid, and cholic acid standards with DC Fertigplatten Kieselgel F_{254} (Merck, Darmstadt, West Germany). After spraying with 15% phosphomolybdic acid in ethanol, the plates were heated to 110° C for 10 min. The spots were quantified by means of a Vitatron densitometer U.F.D. (Vitatron, Dioren, Holland) equipped with a 578 mμ filter. After 1 week they were killed and analyzed in the prescribed way. In a second experiment 24 hamsters received the same diet as the first group and were sacrificed after 28 days. In the third and fourth experiments, hamsters were killed after either 1 week or 4 weeks on the following diet: vitaminized commercial chow (Harald Fors, Holmsund, Sweden) supplemented by either 0.5% cholic acid plus 1% cholesterol, 0.5% chenodeoxycholic acid plus 1% cholesterol, or 1% cholesterol.

After 4 weeks on the chenodeoxycholic acid-supplemented gallstone-inducing diet "284", gallstone formation in hamsters was significantly higher than in the control groups and they contained only cholesterol stones (Table 3).

Analysis of gallbladder bile after 1 week on the "284" diet without supplement and with 0.5% chenodeoxycholic acid in hamsters in the first experiment reveals a shift in gallbladder bile acids from cholic acid to chenodeoxycholic acid. The same shift in bile salts was observed in the third experiment in which the hamsters

Table 3. Concretions in hamsters fed gallstone-inducing diet "284" with and without chenodeoxycholic acid. (From BERGMAN and VAN DER LINDEN, 1973)

Diet	No.	Cholesterol stones	Mixed stones	Pigmented stones	No stones
With chenodeoxycholic acid	9	8	0	0	1
Without chenodeoxycholic acid	11	2	0	1	8

were fed the lab chow supplemented with 1% cholesterol and 0.5% chenodeoxycholic acid.

However, in the third group no gallstones occurred, whereas in the group fed 1% cholesterol and 0.5% cholic acid gallstones were present. Hamsters in the last group were found to have cholic acid as the main bile salt. For these results two factors may be responsible: (1) chenodeoxycholic acid is known to be able to dissolve a greater quantity of cholesterol, and (2) this acid was found to have a higher turnover rate and to eliminate cholesterol more rapidly than cholic acid. The results of the first and second experiments lead to the hypothesis that gallstone formation is preceded by a rapid shift from cholic acid to chenodeoxycholic acid in bile salts in hamsters fed a gallstone inducing diet supplemented with 0.5% chenodeoxycholic acid.

C. A High Cholesterol Diet in Prairie Dogs

BRENNEMAN et al. (1972) studied the formation of abnormal bile and cholesterol gallstones in praire dogs. They fed 24 adult male dogs a high cholesterol, egg yolk diet; 13 control animals received a cholesterol-free diet. After a period on a low cholesterol diet, the animals were divided into two groups, each was fed a different synthetic diet as shown in Table 4. The control diet (diet 1) was free of cholesterol and contained 4% fat of the total calories. The lithogenic diet (diet 2) had a cholesterol content of 1.2% contained in the egg yolk and 41% fat of the total calories. Both diets contained ample essential fatty acids. The duration of the experiments was either 2–3 months or 6 months. Cholesterol $4^{14}C$ was added to the egg yolk diet for the last 4 months of the experiment in six dogs to establish an isotopic steady state: 150 g of chow with 1 μCi of purified cholesterol $4^{14}C$

Table 4. Composition of diets. (From BRENNEMAN et al. 1972)

	Diet 1—control diet (g/100 g)	Diet 2—lithogenic diet (g/100 g)
Ingredients		
Soya assay protein	20.23	7.48
Egg yolk powder	—	36.60
Crystalline cholesterol	—	0.40
Corn starch	—	14.00
Cane sugar	70.57	33.94
Corn oil	1.62	—
Salt mix (Phillips Hart)	4.00	4.00
Vitamin supplement GBI	1.00	1.00
Nonnutritive fiber	2.58	2.58
Cholesterol source		
Egg yolk	0	0.8
Crystalline	0	0.4
Total	0	1.2
Calories	Percent total	Percent total
Fat	4	41
Carbohydrate	76	44
Protein	20	15

Table 5. Cholesterol content of gallbladder bile and serum in prairie dogs fed a cholesterol-free and egg yolk diet. (From BRENNEMAN et al. 1972)

Diet and duration	Number of animals	Gallstone incidence	Gallbladder bile	Serum
2–3 months				
Control	8	0	165± 74	179± 84
Egg yolk	14	14	408±264	1165±430
P values			<0.05±	<0.001
6 months				
Control	5	0	180± 82	156± 53
Egg yolk	10	10	644±338	1572±684
P values			<0.02	<0.001

dissolved in ether. Ether was evaporated and the dogs were fed the chow ad lib. Animals consumed an average of 0.1 μCi of cholesterol 4^{14} C/day. Total bile acids were measured by the steroid dehydrogenase method and the individual bile acids were determined by gas liquid chromatography. To determine cholesterol radioactivity, the sample was saponified with alcoholic KOH. The nonsaponifiable residue was extracted with hexane, dried, and then dissolved in 10 ml of scintillation mixture (4 g 2.5 diphenyl-oxazole and 100 mg 1.4 bis (2-5 phenyloxazole) benzene in 1 l of toluene). Samples were counted in a Packard Tri-Carb/scintillation spectrometer at an efficiency of 89% and the cholesterol activity was expressed in disintegrations/min/mg of cholesterol.

Gallstones developed in all prairie dogs fed a high cholesterol egg yolk diet (Table 5). No gallstones were found in animals of the control group. Gallstones were found only in the gallbladder. The cholesterol content in animals fed 6 months was 74±17% of dry weight and in dogs fed 2–3 months, 80±12%. As shown in Table 5, the cholesterol concentration of gallbladder bile from animals fed the lithogenic diet significantly increased after egg yolk diet from 165 to 408 mg/100 ml in dogs fed 2–3 months and from 180 to 664 mg/100 ml in animals fed 6 months. Complete analysis of the bile components, cholesterol, phospholipid, and bile acids, was determined in five animals in group 1 and in seven animals in group 2. There was a significant ($P<0.001$) shift in group 2 from cholic acid to chenodeoxycholic acid as shown (Table 6). The bile acid/cholesterol molar ratios decreased significantly in gallbladder bile and hepatic bile. The specific activities of cholesterol in serum was 923, in gallbladder bile 838, and in gallstones 893 disintigrations/min/mg of cholesterol. The isotopic data indicated that about 70% of cholesterol in serum, bile, and gallstones was from the diet.

Table 6. Cholic acid and chenodeoxycholic acid content of gallbladder bilde. (From BRENNEMAN et al. 1972)

Bile	No. of animals	Diet	Cholic acid	Chenodeoxycholic acid
Gallbladder	5	Control	77.7± 5.3	18.0± 3.5
	7	Egg yolk	30.3±11.6	67.7±11.3
P values			<0.001	<0.001

DENBESTEN et al. (1974) found early changes in gallbladder bile after 36 h with the same method as described by BRENNEMAN et al. (1972). The serum cholesterol level increased in the high cholesterol diet group from 143 mg/100 ml to 427 mg/100 ml. The bile cholesterol concentration was greater in the cholesterol-fed animals (5.2 vs. 2.2% of total bile composition). After 36 h a significant decrease of cholic acid (87.5 vs. 76.3%) and an increase of chenodeoxycholic acid (10.9 vs. 17.6) was noted. Total bile acids decreased significantly from 90.8 to 85.0 and phospholipids increased from 7.0 to 9.7 ($P<0.05$). After 5 days on the cholesterol and fat-rich diet, the first small crystals in gallbladder were observed in all animals. From the results of these experiments it seems to be possible to predict gallstone formation by analyzing gallbladder bile for a shift from cholic acid to chenodeoxycholic acid.

D. A Diet Supplemented with D-Thyroxine in Hamsters

D-thyroxine, the optical isomer of naturally occurring L-thyroxine, is known as a cholesterol depressant agent in serum. BERGMAN and VAN DER LINDEN found (1964) that sodium D-thyroxine favors the formation of gallstones in Syrian hamsters when given over a relatively short period. They divided 24 young hamsters of both sexes, 5–7 weeks old, into groups of 12 and fed them a sucrose-rich diet as shown in Table 7. The first group received in addition sodium D-thyroxine (A-B Pharmacia, Uppsala, Sweden) in a dose of 5 mg/100 g food. These animals were housed in cages containing two to five hamsters of the same sex. In a second experiment with the same conditions as in the first one, hamsters were caged individually. All animals were sacrificed and investigated for gallstones after 1 month. Of 10 animals in the first group, 8 were fed the sucrose-rich diet with 5 mg % sodium D-thyroxine and none of the control group developed gallstones. The second experiment showed that 7 of 9 developed gallstones on the same diet. There was no difference noted in serum cholesterol levels between the two dietary groups. All animals that produced gallstones showed a fatty degeneration of the liver. The results show that sodium D-thyroxine, when added to a sucrose-rich diet, favors the formation of gallstones and gives rise to fatty degeneration of the liver. It should be pointed out that the dose of D-thyroxine used in this experiment is about 7 times higher than the usual therapeutic dose in man.

Table 7. Basal sucrose-rich diet fed to hamsters in addition to D-thyroxine resulting in formation of gallstones. (From BERGMAN and VAN DER LINDEN, 1964)

Sucrose	48.2 g
Rice starch	24.1 g
Caseine (crude)	20.0 g
Salt mixture	5.0 g
Vitamin mixture	0.5 g
Choline chloride	0.2 g
Lard	2.0 g
	100.0 g

E. A Fat- and Cholesterol-Rich Diet in Squirrel Monkeys

OSUGA and PORTMAN (1971) fed 33 male and female squirrel monkeys, weighing from 540–885 g, a basal semipurified diet (840 calories), not associated with atherosclerosis, in which 15% of the calories were supplied as corn oil. A second group of 33 monkeys was maintained on the same semipurified diet plus high butter plus cholesterol, which was consistently associated with hypercholesterolemia and atherosclerosis, containing 0.1 g additional cholesterol/100 calories. Monkeys were killed from 2 weeks to 13 months after the start of the semipurified diets. A control group of 19 monkeys was given a "natural" diet (Purina monkey chow—25) for 4 months, immediately sacrificed, and the gallbladders were removed. The gallstones were washed 4 times in distilled water, dried at 80° C, and weighed. They were then dissolved in chloroform and the solution was applied to silica H plates with or without 5% $AgNO_3$ and subjected to thin-layer chromatography. The extracts were chromatographed alone or with various combinations of cholesterol and cholestan-3β-ol. Each spot was detected and cholesterol was quantified using a Farrand UIS-US thin-layer analyzer. No stones were found in the control group of the 19 squirrel monkeys fed the Purina monkey chow diet. Of the 33 monkeys fed the basal semipurified diet, which supplied 15% of the calories as corn oil, 3 developed gallstones after 3–6 months. The mean weight of these gallstones was 5.5 and 5.0 mg. As shown in Table 8, 10 of the 33 monkeys fed the atherogenic diet high in butter and cholesterol developed gallstones after 3 months. The gallstones in this group were much greater than in those of the other diet group and increased in size, number, and weight with the duration of the diet. The gallstones, which were completely soluble in chloroform, showed only one spot on thin-layer chromatography, had the same Rf of cholesterol when chromatographed with purified cholesterol, and were clearly separable from cholestan-3β-ol. In gallbladder bile the ratio of cholesterol to phospholipids was highest in monkeys fed the atherogenic high-butter and cholesterol diet. The animals with

Table 8. Incidence of gallstones in squirrel monkeys fed different diets (m = male; f = female). (From OSUGA and PORTMAN, 1971)

Duration of diet (months)	Basal diet 840 calories (15% of calories as corn oil)			Basal diet 840 calories +high butter +0.1 g cholesterol/100 cal		
	No. of monkeys	No. of stones	Mean weight of stones (mg)	No. of monkeys	No. of stones	Mean weight of stones (mg)
0– 2	8 m 2 f	0		9 m 2 f	0	
3	7 f	2	5.5	3 f	1	23.0
4	2 m 2 f	0		2 m 2 f	1 m 1 f	16.5
6	4 f	1	5.0	6 f	2	85.0
8	3 f	0		3 f	0	
9	2 f	0		2 f	2	96.5
10	1 f	0		2 f	1	73.0
13	2 f	0		2 f	2	162.0
	33	3		33	10	

gallstones had the highest ratios of all. There was no sex difference in incidence of gallstones.

Experimental study in suitable animal models of the physiologic and pathologic mechanisms leading to gallstone formation suggests that an understanding of cholesterol and bile salt excretion, precipitation and growth of gallstones, will lead to methods to predict, prevent, and dissolve gallstones in man.

Abbreviations

diet "284"	nearly fat- and cholesterin-free diet
EFAD	essential fatty acid deficient diet
C	carbon
f	female
g	gram
m	male
μCi	mikro-Curie
mg	milligram
μg	mikrogram
R_f	Ratio front
S_D	Standard deviation

References

BERGMAN, F., VAN DER LINDEN, W.: Influence of D-thyroxine on gallstone formation in hamsters. Acta chir. scand **129**, 547—552 (1964).

BERGMAN, F., VAN DER LINDEN, W.: Liver morphology and gallstone-formation in hamsters and mice treated with chenodeoxycholic acid. Acta path. microbiol. scand. A **81**, 213—221 (1973).

BOUCHIER, J.A.D.: Gallstone formation. Lancet **1971 I**, 711—715.

BRENNEMAN, D.E., CONNOR, W.E., FORKER, E.L., DENBESTEN, L.: The formation of abnormal bile and cholesterol gallstones from dietary cholesterol in prairie dog. J. clin. Invest. **51**, 1495—1503 (1972).

DAM, H., CHRISTENSEN, F.: Alimentary Production of gallstones in hamsters. Acta path. microbiol. scand. **30**, 236—242 (1952).

DENBESTEN, L., SAFAIE-SHIRAZI, S., CONNOR, W.E., BELL, S.: Early changes in bile composition and gallstone formation induced by a high cholesterol diet in prairie dogs. Gastroenterology **66**, 1036—1045 (1974)

FRESTON, J.W., BOUCHIER, J.A.D.: Experimental cholelithiasis. Gut **9**, 2—4 (1968).

OSUGA, T., PORTMAN, D.W.: Experimental formation of gallstones in the squirrel monkey. Proc. Soc. exp. Biol. Med. (N.Y.) **135**, 722—727 (1971).

ROBINS, S.J., FASULO, J.: Mechanism of lithogenic bile production: Studies in the hamsters fed an essential fatty acid-deficient diet. Gastroenterology **65**, 104—114 (1973).

SMALL, D.M.: Gallstones. New Engl. J Med. **279**, 588—593 (1968).

Author Index

Page numbers in *italics* refer to bibliography
Numbers shown in square brackets are the numbers in the bibliography

Subject Index

Handbuch der experimentellen Pharmakologie
Handbook of Experimental Pharmacology

Heffter-Heubner, New Series

Vol. 4:	A. J. CLARK: **General Pharmacology**	
Vol. 10:	O. EICHLER: **Die Pharmakologie anorganischer Anionen**	
Vol. 11:	W. GRAUBNER, G. PETERS: **Lobelin und Lobeliaalkaloide**	
Vol. 12:	O. SCHAUMANN: **Morphin und morphinähnlich wirkende Verbindungen**	
Vol. 14:	Part 1:	**The Adrenocortical Hormones I.** Editor: H. W. DEANE
	Part 2:	**The Adrenocortical Hormones II.** Editors: H. W. DEANE, B. L. RUBIN
	Part 3:	**The Adrenocortical Hormones III.** Editors: H. W. DEANE, B. L. RUBIN
Vol. 15:	**Cholinesterases and Anticholinesterase Agents.** Editor: G. B. KOELLE. Out of print	
Vol. 17:	Part 1:	**Ions alcalino-terreux I.** Systèmes isolés. Editeur: Z. M. BACQ
	Part 2:	**Ions alcalino-terreux II.** Organismes entiers. Editeur: Z. M. BACQ
Vol. 18:	Part 1:	**Histamine.** Editor: M. ROCHA E SILVA
	Part 2:	**Anti-Histanimics.** In preparation
Vol. 19:	**5-Hydroxytryptamine and Related Indolealkylamines.** Editor: V. ERSPAMER	
Vol. 20:	Part 1:	**Pharmacology of Fluorides I.** Editor: F. A. SMITH
	Part 2:	**Pharmacology of Fluorides II.** Editor: F. A. SMITH
Vol. 21:	G. KIMMERLE: **Beryllium**	
Vol. 22:	Part 1:	**Die Gestagene I.** Herausgeber: K. JUNKMANN
	Part 2:	**Die Gestagene II.** Herausgeber: K. JUNKMANN
Vol. 23:	**Neurohypophysial Hormones and Similar Polypeptides.** Editor: B. BERDE	
Vol. 24:	**Diuretica.** Herausgeber: H. HERKEN	
Vol. 25:	**Bradykinin, Kallidin and Kallikrein.** Editor: E. G. ERDÖS. Technical Editor: A. F. WILDE	

Vol. 26: H. FISCHER: **Vergleichende Pharmakologie von Überträgersubstanzen in tiersystematischer Darstellung**

Vol. 27: **Anticoagulantien.** Herausgeber: F. MARKWARDT

Vol. 28: Part 1: **Concepts in Biochemical Pharmacology I.** Editors: B. B. BRODIE, J. R. GILLETTE

Part 2: **Concepts in Biochemical Pharmacology II.** Out of print

Part 3: **Concepts in Biochemical Pharmacology III.** Editors: J. R. GILLETTE, J. R. MITCHELL

Vol. 29: **Oral wirksame Antidiabetika.** Herausgeber: H. MASKE

Vol. 30: **Modern Inhalation Anesthetics.** Editor: M. B. CHENOWETH

Vol. 31: R. CHARLIER: **Antianginal Drugs.** Out of print

Vol. 32: Part 1: **Insulin I.** Herausgeber: E. DÖRZBACH

Part 2: **Insulin II.** Editors: A. HASSELBLATT, F. v. BRUCHHAUSEN

Vol. 33: **Catecholamines.** Out of print

Vol. 34: **Secretin, Cholecystokinin, Pancreozymin and Gastrin.** Editors: J. E. JORPES, V. MUTT

Vol. 35: Part 1: H. E. VOSS, G. OERTEL: **Androgene I**

Part 2: **Androgens II and Antiandrogens/Androgene II und Antiandrogene**

Vol. 36: **Uranium – Plutonium – Transplutonic Elements.** Editors: H. C. HODGE, J. N. STANNARD, J. B. HURSH

Vol. 37: **Angiotensin.** Editors: I. H. PAGE, F. M. BUMPUS

Vol. 38: Part 1: **Antineoplastic and Immunosuppressive Agents I.** Editors: A. C. SARTORELLI, D. G. JOHNS

Part 2: **Antineoplastic and Immunosuppressive Agents II.** Editors: A. C. SARTORELLI, D. G. JOHNS

Vol. 39: **Antihypertensive Agents.** In preparation

Vol. 40: **Organic Nitrates.** Editor: P. NEEDLEMAN

Vol. 41: **Hypolipidemic Agents.** Editor: D. KRITCHEVSKY

Vol. 42: **Neuromuscular Junction.** Editor: E. ZAIMIS

Springer-Verlag Berlin Heidelberg New York

MIX
Papier aus verantwortungsvollen Quellen
Paper from responsible sources
FSC® C105338

If you have any concerns about our products,
you can contact us on
ProductSafety@springernature.com

In case Publisher is established outside the EU,
the EU authorized representative is:
Springer Nature Customer Service Center GmbH
Europaplatz 3, 69115 Heidelberg, Germany

Printed by Libri Plureos GmbH
in Hamburg, Germany